Small Animal Clinical Nutrition
Quick Consult

Small Animal Clinical Nutrition
Quick Consult

EDITED BY

Michael S. Hand, DVM, PhD
Diplomate, American College of Veterinary Nutrition
Chair, Board of Directors, Mark Morris Institute
Arroyo Hondo, New Mexico

Steven C. Zicker, DVM, PhD, MS
Diplomate, American College of Veterinary Internal Medicine (Internal Medicine)
Diplomate, American College of Veterinary Nutrition
Associate, Mark Morris Institute
Veterinary Clinical Nutritionist, Science and Technology
Hill's Pet Nutrition, Inc.
Topeka, Kansas

Bruce J. Novotny, DVM
Board of Directors, Mark Morris Institute
Owner, Managing Partner
Helios Communications, LLC
Bandon, Oregon

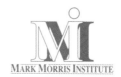

MARK MORRIS INSTITUTE

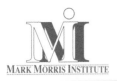
MARK MORRIS INSTITUTE

Small Animal Clinical Nutrition QUICK CONSULT
ISBN-13: 978-0-945837-03-9

NOTICE

Companion animal practice, clinical nutrition and commercial pet foods are ever changing. The authors and editors of Small Animal Clinical Nutrition, 5th edition, from which this textbook was derived, carefully checked trade names, nutrient levels and recommended uses of listed commercial pet foods, to ensure that the information provided was precise and in accordance with standards accepted at the time of publication. Readers are advised, however, to check the most current product information provided by the manufacturer of each food to ensure that a product's nutrient profile, feeding guide and contraindications for feeding are accurate.

These same precautions have been taken to ensure that recommendations for drug therapy, when provided, are also accurate. And, as with foods, readers are advised to check the manufacturer's information for each drug to be used to verify that the recommended dose and the method and duration of administration are accurate and to be aware of potential contraindications.

These precautions are particularly important in regards to new or infrequently used foods or drugs. It is the responsibility of those recommending a food or administering a drug, relying on their professional skill and experience, to determine the best treatment for the patient. This includes the appropriate food and/or drug and its proper administration. Neither the publisher nor the editors assume any liability for any injury and/or damage to animals or property arising from the use of this publication.

Although this textbook is intended to be a global reference for companion animal nutrition, only North American products are listed in the food tables. Also, the regulatory guidelines used herein are those of the Association of American Feed Control Officials and the United States Food and Drug Administration. Regulatory agencies, regulation of foods, nutrients, supplements, drugs and claims may be different in geographies outside North America.

THE PUBLISHER

For more information about this book contact:
Mark Morris Institute
P.O. Box 2097
Topeka, Kansas 66601-2097
Phone 785-286-8101
Facsimile 785-286-8173

Last digit is the print number 9 8 7 6 5 4 3 2

Preface

About Nutrition in Veterinary Practice

Dogs and cats have enjoyed unique relationships with people that date back thousands of years. Today, they are appreciated as special companions in our society and deserve our best efforts to maximize both the quality and length of their lives. Proper dietary management is one of the most important, cost-effective tools in our arsenal for improving pet health and performance, managing disease and increasing longevity. Many pet owners are aware of the importance of nutrition to their own health and expect state-of-the-art nutritional services for their pets.

Advancing the practice of veterinary nutrition has been the chief objective of the American College of Veterinary Nutrition (ACVN) for more than two decades. ACVN diplomates occupy positions in veterinary schools, private practice and industry. Many of these specialists authored chapters in *Small Animal Clinical Nutrition, 5th Edition* (*SACN5*), which is intended to enhance the nutritional knowledge of small animal veterinarians. ACVN diplomates contributed to the development of the American Animal Hospital Association's (AAHA) "Nutritional Assessment Guidelines for Dogs and Cats" (www.aahanet.org/resources/NutritionalGuidelines.aspx), which was published in 2010. These groundbreaking AAHA guidelines underscore the importance of nutrition to pet health. The guidelines are available to assist veterinary hospitals in developing protocols for integrating nutrition into daily practice and emphasize a two-part process for every patient at every visit: 1) nutritional assessment and 2) specific dietary recommendations. The guidelines state that feeding plans should consider foods, treats, feeding methods, feeding frequency and where the pet is fed. Efforts are underway to establish nutritional status as the "fifth vital assessment" along with temperature, heart rate, respiratory rate and pain.

About this Book

The Mark Morris Institute (MMI) was incorporated to support the betterment of companion animals through a global veterinary nutrition education program. In addition to offering the University Teaching Program (www.markmorrisinstitute.org), MMI publishes the *Small Animal Clinical Nutrition* (*SACN*) textbook series. The first edition of *SACN* was published in 1983. Since then, *SACN* has been printed in five languages. *The Small Animal Clinical Nutrition Quick Consult* (*Quick Consult*) augments the 5th edition of *SACN*. The purpose of the *Quick Consult* is to provide practical, informative, readily accessible, succinct feeding plans for healthy and diseased dogs and cats. It is intended for use by busy veterinary health care team members as a clinical tool in treatment/exam rooms.

The *Quick Consult* is not intended as a reference for diagnostics, medicine or surgery. Readers should consult other texts (including *SACN5*) for that information. In most cases, it is assumed that the reader already has a diagnosis and is seeking specific information on how and what to feed the patient. The *Quick Consult* is intended to be a source of feeding plans, which are the "how-tos" of veterinary nutrition.

Each chapter is arranged into five sections including clinical points, key nutritional factors, feeding plans, followup and miscellaneous. Specific icons are included in the headers for each of these sections to facilitate finding specific categories of information. (**Figure 1**.)

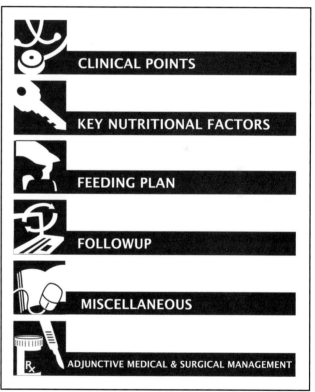

Figure 1. Icons used in the *Quick Consult* to facilitate location of information.

Clinical points sections briefly summarize demographics, prevalences, causes, diagnostics and prognostics. Also, where applicable, chapters covering specific diseases summarize adjunctive medical and/or surgical management.

Key nutritional factors encompass nutrients of concern and other food characteristics. The concept of nutrients of concern greatly simplifies the approach to clinical nutrition because most commercial pet foods sold in the United States provide at least the Association of American Feed Control Officials' (AAFCO) allowances of all nutrients. Thus, if a commercial food is fed, veterinary health care teams need only to understand and focus on delivering the target levels

Preface, continued

of a few nutrients (nutrients of concern) rather than the 40 plus nutrients currently recognized for dogs and cats. Other food characteristics may include desirable non-nutritional effects (e.g., the urinary pH produced by a food).

The feeding plans that make up the core of each chapter include food selection, management of treats/snacks, how much to feed, how to offer the food, switching foods and food/water receptacle hygiene. Food selection is based on AAFCO nutritional assurance statements (see product labels) and key nutritional factors. The key nutritional factor content of selected foods is presented in comparative food tables included in each chapter. Because some foods are modified/ improved over time and other foods enter/leave the market place, updates of the food tables will be published regularly at www.markmorrisinstitute.org.

The information provided in the *Quick Consult* was adapted and summarized from *SACN5*. The contributing authors of the original chapters in *SACN5* are acknowledged at the end of each *Quick Consult* chapter. During the writ-

ing of the *Quick Consult*, *SACN5* authors often provided additional information and suggestions for the *Quick Consult* editors; thus, some new information is included. Throughout the chapters, readers are encouraged to refer to the *SACN5* textbook for more detailed information about prevalences, demographics, causes, patient assessment specifics, etio-pathogeneses, derivation of the KNFs and case reports. Also, readers should refer to *SACN5* for information about feeding small pet mammals, reptiles and birds.

The *Quick Consult* is our attempt to summarize and outline the practical aspects of canine and feline veterinary clinical nutrition to encourage fulfillment of ACVN and AAHA goals. We would appreciate your feedback so we can improve future editions. Send comments to Mark Morris Institute, P.O. Box 2097, Topeka, Kansas 66601-2097 or contact us through the MMI website at: www.markmorrisinstitute.org.

THE EDITORS

Acknowledgement

Writing book chapters can be a relatively thankless task and though the rewards of textbook chapter writing are largely intangible, the importance of textbooks to veterinary education/continuing education is difficult to overstate. The editors and the Mark Morris Institute would like to recognize the numerous contributors to the *Small Animal Clinical Nutrition* series.

Contents

Contents

Feeding Young Adult Dogs: Before Middle-Age

CLINICAL POINTS

- Depending on breed, dogs 1 through 5-7 years of age are considered young adults.
- Feeding goals for young adult dogs: maximize health, longevity and quality of life (disease prevention).
- Overweight/obesity conditions are more prevalent in female dogs and have a higher prevalence in neutered dogs of either sex.
- Provide nutritional counseling to prevent obesity when dogs are neutered.
- Record body weight and BCS in the patient's file.

KEY NUTRITIONAL FACTORS

- Foods should provide recommended allowances of all required nutrients (nutritional adequacy), but should also contain specific levels of KNFs.
- **Table 1** lists important diseases with nutritional associations for adult dogs.
- **Table 2** lists KNF recommendations for foods for young adult dogs that are of normal body condition or are inactive/obese prone. A detailed description of these recommendations can be found in Chapter 13, Small Animal Clinical Nutrition, 5th edition. Water is always a key nutritional factor.

FEEDING PLAN

Assess and Select the Food

Ensure the Food's Nutritional Adequacy. AAFCO nutritional adequacy statements are usually found on a product's label. AAFCO approval does not ensure the food will be effective in preventing long-term health problems.

Compare the Food's KNF Content with the Recommended Levels. Tables 3 and 4 compare KNF profiles for selected commercial foods. Contact the manufacturer for this information if the food in question cannot be found in these tables. Manufacturers' contact information is listed on product labels. A new food should be selected if discrepancies are noted; the new food should best approximate the recommended KNF levels.

Manage Treats and Snacks. If treats/snacks are fed, commercial treats that match the nutritional profile recommended for young adult dogs (see product label) are best. Otherwise, treats/snacks should not be fed excessively (<10% of the total diet on a volume, weight or calorie basis). See Appendix B for more information about treats/snacks.

Abbreviations

AAFCO = Association of American Feed Control Officials
BCS = body condition score (Appendix A)
KNF = key nutritional factor

Table 1. Important diseases for mature adult dogs that have nutritional associations.

Disease/ health concern	Incidence/prevalence/ mortality/pet owner concern
Dental disease	Most prevalent disease; numerous associated health risks (e.g., kidney disease)
Obesity	Approximate 30% prevalence; associated health risks (e.g., diabetes mellitus, musculoskeletal disease); major concern
Cognitive dysfunction	32% of dogs ≥8 years had >2 categories of DISHA; concern
Kidney disease	Second leading cause of nonaccidental death; major concern
Arthritis	6% prevalence; primary concern
Cancer	Primary cause of death; primary concern
Skin/coat problems	Second most common cause of disease (26% prevalence); second most common health concern

Key: DISHA = disorientation, alterations in interactions with people and other pets, alterations in sleep-awake cycles, house soiling, alterations in activity levels (see Chapter 35 in Small Animal Clinical Nutrition, 5th edition).

Table 2. Key nutritional factors for foods for young adult dogs.

Factors	Recommended food levels* Normal weight and body condition	Inactive/ obese prone
Water	Free access	Free access
Energy density (kcal ME/g)	3.5-4.5	3.0-3.5
Energy density (kJ ME/g)	14.6-18.8	12.5-14.6
Fat and essential fatty acids (%)	10-20	7-10
Crude fiber (%)**	≤5	≥10
Protein (%)	15-30	15-30
Phosphorus (%)	0.4-0.8	0.4-0.8
Sodium (%)	0.2-0.4	0.2-0.4
Chloride (%)	1.5 x Na	1.5 x Na
Antioxidants (amount/kg food)		
Vitamin E (IU)	≥400	≥400
Vitamin C (mg)	≥100	≥100
Selenium (mg)	0.5-1.3	0.5-1.3
Food texture (VOHC Seal of Acceptance)	Plaque	Plaque

Key: DM = dry matter, kcal = kilocalories, kJ = kilojoules, ME = metabolizable energy, VOHC = Veterinary Oral Health Council Seal of Acceptance.
*Dry matter basis. Concentrations presume an energy density of 4.0 kcal/g. Levels should be corrected for foods with higher energy densities.
**Crude fiber measurements underestimate total dietary fiber levels in food.

Assess and Determine the Feeding Method

Determine How Much to Feed. Appropriate intake levels of basic nutrients and KNFs are determined by the amounts in food, and by how much food is consumed. If the dog has an ideal BCS (2.5/5 to 3.5/5), the amount being fed is likely appropriate. In the case of a new food, the amount fed can be estimated either from feeding guides on product labels or by calculation (Appendix C). Feeding guidelines and calculations are based on population averages and may need to be adjusted for individual dogs (See Followup below.)

Consider How to Offer the Food. Both free-choice and restricted-feeding methods have advantages and disadvantages (Appendix D). Although free-choice feeding is most popular, it is most likely to result in overeating in young adult dogs. Food-restricted feeding is less likely to result in overweight/obesity. Pet owners often overestimate food needs and feed too much; most people do not recognize overweight/obesity in their own dog.

Manage Food Changes. Most healthy dogs adapt well to new foods, but a transition period to avoid GI upsets is good practice. Example: to change to a new food, replace 25% of the old food with the new food on Day 1 and continue this incremental change daily until the change is complete on Day 4. Appendix E provides additional information.

Food and Water Receptacle Husbandry. Food and water bowls should be washed regularly with warm soapy water and rinsed well. Dishes used for moist food need daily cleaning. Discard moist or moistened dry foods after 2-4 hours of room temperature exposure to avoid foodborne illnesses (Appendix F).

FOLLOWUP

Owner Followup

Owners should weigh their dog (if possible) and/or grade its BCS monthly. If a trend of increasing or decreasing body weight or BCS is noticed, the amount fed should be changed by 10% increments and the dog's weight rechecked every 2 weeks for 1 month. At that point, if necessary, the amount fed should be changed again and the cycle repeated.

Veterinary Health Care Team Followup

Healthy young adult dogs should be examined every 6-12 months. More frequent assessment is recommended if homemade food is a significant part of a dog's total food intake.

MISCELLANEOUS

See Chapter 13, Small Animal Clinical Nutrition, 5th edition, for more information. See Appendix G for information about abnormal (alternative) eating behaviors.

Authors

Condensed from Chapter 13, Small Animal Clinical Nutrition, 5th edition, authored by Jacques Debraekeleer, Kathy L. Gross and Steven C. Zicker.

References

See Chapter 13, Small Animal Clinical Nutrition, 5th edition, on the website www.markmorrisinstitute.org for references.

Table 3. Selected nutrient levels in commercial foods for young adult dogs (normal body condition) compared to recommended levels of KNFs.*
(Numbers in red match optimal KNFs.)

Dry foods	Energy density (kcal/cup)**	Energy density (kcal ME/g)	Fat (%)	Fiber (%)	Protein (%)	P (%)	Na (%)	Vit E (IU/kg)	Vit C (mg/kg)	Se (mg/kg)	VOHC plaque (Yes/No)
Recommended levels (normal body condition)	-	3.5-4.5	10-20	≤5	15-30	0.4-0.8	0.2-0.4	≥400	≥100	0.5-1.3	-
Hill's Science Diet Lamb Meal & Rice Recipe	364	4.0	16.0	2.5	23.0	0.67	0.29	582	174	0.54	No
Hill's Science Diet Oral Care Adult	273	3.8	15.5	10.1	25.1	0.65	0.24	564	175	0.62	Yes
Iams Adult Lamb Meal & Rice Formula	330	4.0	14.2	4.2	25.1	1.6	0.65	123	52	0.37	No
Iams Chunks	381	4.4	17.8	2.9	29.8	1.1	0.6	103	43	0.27	No
Iams Eukanuba Medium Breed Adult	404	4.7	17.9	2.1	27.8	1.16	0.55	na	na	na	No
Iams ProActive Health Chunks	374	4.0	17.0	1.9	28.9	1.21	0.58	na	na	na	No
Medi-Cal Dental Formula	290	na	12.7	5.3	19.7	0.9	0.4	na	na	na	No
Medi-Cal Preventive Formula	340	na	16.3	2.7	23.9	0.8	0.4	na	na	na	No
Nutro Natural Choice Dental Care Lamb Meal and Rice	287	3.7	15.4	4.4	23.6	1.54	0.22	275	71	1.65	No
Nutro Natural Choice Lamb Meal and Rice	342	3.8	14.3	2.2	24.2	1.54	0.33	220	66	0.77	No
Purina Dog Chow	430	4.2	11.4	5.1	23.9	0.91	0.42	144	na	0.64	No
Purina ONE Total Nutrition Lamb & Rice Formula	451	4.7	20.1	1.8	30.5	1.09	0.52	na	na	na	No
Purina Pro Plan Chicken & Rice Formula	489	4.8	16.9	3.4	33.8	1.22	0.46	na	na	na	No
Royal Canin MINI Adult 27	352	4.3	17.4	1.6	29.3	0.87	0.43	717	326	0.22	No
Royal Canin MINI Dental Hygiene 24	320	4.2	15.4	1.8	26.4	0.77	0.33	659	330	0.21	No
Waltham Pedigree Small Crunchy Bites	290	3.8	13.7	2.0	26.0	1.55	0.65	256	80	na	No

Moist foods	Energy density (kcal/can)**	Energy density (kcal ME/g)	Fat (%)	Fiber (%)	Protein (%)	P (%)	Na (%)	Vit E (IU/kg)	Vit C (mg/kg)	Se (mg/kg)	VOHC plaque (Yes/No)
Recommended levels (normal body condition)	-	3.5-4.5	10-20	≤5	15-30	0.4-0.8	0.2-0.4	≥400	≥100	0.5-1.3	-
Hill's Science Diet Adult Advanced Savory Chicken Entrée	345/13 oz.	3.9	17.1	1.3	26.7	0.67	0.25	200	na	1.00	No
Medi-Cal Preventive Formula	435/396 g	na	20.1	3.3	23.8	0.7	0.3	na	na	na	No
Purina Pro Plan Adult Chicken & Rice Entrée Classic	426/13 oz.	4.9	36.6	0.9	40.4	1.36	0.47	na	na	na	No

Key: KNF = key nutritional factor, ME = metabolizable energy, Fiber = crude fiber, P = phosphorus, Na = sodium, Se = selenium, VOHC = Veterinary Oral Health Council, na = information not available from manufacturer, g = grams.
*From manufacturers' published information or calculated from manufacturers' published as-fed values; all values are on a dry matter basis unless otherwise stated.
**Energy density values are listed on an as fed basis and are useful for determining the amount to feed; cup = 8-oz. measuring cup. To convert to kJ, multiply kcal by 4.184.

Table 4. Selected nutrient levels in commercial foods for young adult dogs (inactive/obese prone) compared to recommended levels of KNFs.* (Numbers in red match optimal KNFs.)

Dry foods	Energy density (kcal/cup)**	Energy density (kcal ME/g)	Fat (%)	Fiber (%)	Protein (%)	P (%)	Na (%)	Vit E (IU/kg)	Vit C (mg/kg)	Se (mg/kg)	VOHC plaque (Yes/No)
Recommended levels (inactive/obese prone)	-	3.0-3.5	7-10	≥10	15-30	0.4-0.8	0.2-0.4	≥400	≥100	0.5-1.3	-
Hill's Science Diet Light Adult	295	3.3	8.8	14.6	24.5	0.58	0.23	586	276	0.45	No
Iams Eukanuba Medium Breed Weight Control	275	4.2	10.5	1.9	21.3	0.76	0.50	206	42	0.34	No
Iams Weight Control	328	4.2	12.5	2.8	22.2	0.85	0.37	103	44	0.35	No
Medi-Cal Weight Control/Mature	320	na	8.5	4.0	19.5	0.8	0.2	na	na	na	No
Nutro Natural Choice Lite	244	3.4	7.2	4.4	16.7	1.22	0.33	161	67	0.44	No
Purina Pro Plan Chicken & Rice Weight Management	337	3.7	10.2	2.7	30.5	1.06	0.27	503	na	0.33	No
Royal Canin MINI Weight Care 30	326	3.8	12.0	6.2	32.6	0.82	0.33	652	326	0.16	No

Moist foods	Energy density (kcal/can)**	Energy density (kcal ME/g)	Fat (%)	Fiber (%)	Protein (%)	P (%)	Na (%)	Vit E (IU/kg)	Vit C (mg/kg)	Se (mg/kg)	VOHC plaque (Yes/No)
Recommended levels (inactive/obese prone)	-	3.0-3.5	7-10	≥10	15-30	0.4-0.8	0.2-0.4	≥400	≥100	0.5-1.3	-
Hill's Science Diet Light Adult	322 kcal/13 oz.	3.4	8.6	9.7	19.5	0.51	0.31	385	na	0.78	No
Medi-Cal Weight Control/Mature	370 kcal/396 g	na	10	5.5	21.5	0.6	0.3	na	na	na	No

Key: KNF = key nutritional factor, ME = metabolizable energy, Fiber = crude fiber, P = phosphorus, Na = sodium, Se = selenium, VOHC = Veterinary Oral Health Council, na = information not available from manufacturer, g = grams.
*From manufacturers' published information or calculated from manufacturers' published as-fed values; all values are on a dry matter basis unless otherwise stated.
**Energy density values are listed on an as fed basis and are useful for determining the amount to feed; cup = 8-oz. measuring cup. To convert to kJ, multiply kcal by 4.184.

CLINICAL POINTS

- Depending on breed, dogs 6-8 years of age and older are considered mature adults; this term includes dogs considered to be "middle-aged," "senior" and "geriatric."
- Feeding goals: optimize quality and longevity of life (disease prevention).

KEY NUTRITIONAL FACTORS

- Foods should provide recommended allowances of all required nutrients (nutritional adequacy), but should also contain specific levels of KNFs (certain nutrients and nonnutritional food ingredients or food features that can influence important diseases).
- Table 1, Chapter 1, lists disease prevalences, which are increased in mature adult dogs; adherence to respective KNF recommendations in this age group is even more important than in young adult dogs.
- **Table 1** lists KNF recommendations for foods for mature adult dogs that are either of normal body condition or inactive/obese prone. A detailed discussion of these recommendations can be found in Chapters 13 and 14, Small Animal Clinical Nutrition, 5th edition. Water is always a KNF; mature adult dogs are more prone to dehydration perhaps due to medications (e.g., diuretics) and subclinical CKD.

FEEDING PLAN

Assess and Select the Food

Ensure the Food's Nutritional Adequacy. AAFCO nutritional adequacy statements are usually found on a product's label. AAFCO approval does not ensure a food will be effective in preventing long-term health problems.

Compare the Food's KNF Content with the Recommended Levels. Table 2 compares KNF profiles for selected commercial foods. A new food should be selected if discrepancies are noted; the new food should best approximate the recommended KNF levels.

Manage Treats and Snacks. If treats/snacks are fed, commercial treats that match the nutritional profile recommended for mature adult dogs (see product label) are best. Otherwise, treats/snacks should not be fed excessively (<10% of the total diet on a volume, weight or calorie basis). See Appendix B for more information about treats/snacks.

Abbreviations

AAFCO = Association of American Feed Control Officials
BCS = body condition score (Appendix A)
CKD = chronic kidney disease
KNF = key nutritional factor

Table 1. Key nutritional factors for foods for mature dogs.

Factors	Recommended food levels*	
	Normal weight and body condition	**Inactive/ obese prone**
Water	Free access	Free access
Energy density (kcal ME/g)	3.0-4.0	3.0-3.5
Energy density (kJ ME/g)	12.5-16.7	12.5-14.6
Crude fat (%)	10-15	7-10
Crude fiber (%)**	≥2	≥10
Protein (%)	15-23	15-23
Phosphorus (%)	0.3-0.7	0.3-0.7
Sodium (%)	0.15-0.4	0.15-0.4
Chloride (%)	1.5 x Na	1.5 x Na
Antioxidants (amount/kg food)		
Vitamin E (IU)	≥400	≥400
Vitamin C (mg)	≥100	≥100
Selenium (mg)	0.5-1.3	0.5-1.3
Food texture (VOHC Seal of Acceptance)	Reduced plaque accumulation	Reduced plaque accumulation

Key: kcal = kilocalories, kJ = kilojoules, ME = metabolizable energy, VOHC = Veterinary Oral Health Council Seal of Acceptance (Chapter 36).
*All foods expressed on a dry matter basis unless otherwise noted. If the caloric density of the food is different, the nutrient content in the dry matter must be adapted accordingly.
**Crude fiber measurements underestimate total dietary fiber levels in food.

Assess and Determine the Feeding Method

Determine How Much to Feed. Appropriate intake levels of basic nutrients and KNFs are determined by the amounts in food and by how much food is consumed. If the patient has an ideal BCS (2.5/5 to 3.5/5), the amount being fed is likely appropriate. In the case of a new food, the amount fed can be estimated either from feeding guides on product labels or by calculation (Appendix C). Feeding guidelines and calculations are based on population averages and may need to be adjusted for individual dogs (see Followup below).

Consider How to Offer the Food. Free-choice and restricted-feeding methods have advantages and disadvantages (Appendix D). Although free-choice feeding is most popular, it can facilitate overeating. Meal feeding is usually best because it is less likely to result in overweight/obesity conditions, which can exacerbate existing problems; however, free-choice feeding may be preferred for underweight, very old dogs to facilitate increased food intake. Pet owners often overestimate food needs and feed too much; most people do not recognize overweight/obesity in their own dog.

Manage Food Changes. Most healthy dogs adapt well to new foods but a transition period to avoid GI upsets is good practice. Example: to change to a new food, replace 25% of the old food with the new food on Day 1 and continue this incremental change daily until the change is complete on Day 4. Appendix E provides additional information.

Food and Water Receptacle Husbandry. Food and water bowls should be washed regularly with warm soapy water and rinsed well. Dishes used for moist foods need daily cleaning. Discard moist or moistened dry foods after 2-4 hours of room temperature exposure to avoid foodborne illnesses (Appendix F).

FOLLOWUP

Owner Followup
Owners should weigh their dog (if possible) and/or determine its BCS monthly. If a trend of increasing or decreasing body weight or BCS is noticed, the amount fed should be changed by 10% increments and the dog rechecked every 2 weeks for 1 month. At that point, if necessary, the amount fed is changed again and the cycle is repeated.

Veterinary Health Care Team Followup
Assessments by a veterinarian or other members of the health care team should take place regularly. Healthy mature adult dogs should be examined every 6-12 months, usually more frequently than young adults. More frequent assessment is recommended if homemade food is a significant part of a dog's total food intake.

MISCELLANEOUS

See Chapters 13 and 14, Small Animal Clinical Nutrition, 5th edition, for more information. See Appendix G for information about apparently abnormal (alternative) eating behaviors.

Authors
Condensed from Chapter 14, Small Animal Clinical Nutrition, 5th edition, authored by Jacques Debraekeleer, Kathy L. Gross and Steven C. Zicker.

References
See Chapter 14, Small Animal Clinical Nutrition, 5th edition, on the website www.markmorrisinstitute.org for references.

Table 2. Comparison of recommended levels of key nutritional factors for foods for mature adult dogs with levels in selected commercial foods.* (Numbers in red match optimal KNFs.)

Dry foods	Energy density (kcal/cup)**	Energy density (kcal ME/g)	Fat (%)	Fiber (%)	Protein (%)	P (%)	Na (%)	Vit E (IU/kg)	Vit C (mg/kg)	Se (mg/kg)	VOHC plaque*** (Yes/No)
Recommended levels (normal body condition)	-	3.0-4.0	10-15	≥2	15-23	0.3-0.7	0.15-0.4	≥400	≥100	0.5-1.3	-
Hill's Science Diet Mature Adult 7+ Original	363	4.0	15.8	4.2	19.3	0.58	0.18	700	271	0.41	No
Hill's Science Diet Oral Care Adult	273	3.8	15.5	10.1	25.1	0.65	0.24	564	175	0.62	Yes
Iams Eukanuba Medium Breed Senior	350	4.6	12.8	2.2	29.3	0.95	0.40	236	83	na	No
Medi-Cal Dental Formula	280	na	12.7	5.3	19.7	0.9	0.40	na	na	na	No
Nutro Natural Choice Senior	267	3.8	12.1	2.2	23.1	1.21	0.27	275	99	0.49	No
Purina ONE Senior Protection Formula	375	4.1	14.0	3.4	32.3	1.12	0.30	1,012	na	0.99	No
Purina Pro Plan Chicken & Rice Senior	408	4.2	15.6	2.3	30.4	1.14	0.44	na	na	na	No
Royal Canin MINI Aging Care 27	378	4.3	17.4	1.7	29.3	0.71	0.33	717	326	0.22	No

Moist foods	Energy density (kcal/can)**	Energy density (kcal ME/g)	Fat (%)	Fiber (%)	Protein (%)	P (%)	Na (%)	Vit E (IU/kg)	Vit C (mg/kg)	Se (mg/kg)	VOHC plaque*** (Yes/No)
Recommended levels (normal body condition)	-	3.0-4.0	10-15	≥2	15-23	0.3-0.7	0.15-0.4	≥400	≥100	0.5-1.3	-
Hill's Science Diet Gourmet Beef Entrée Mature Adult 7+	164/5.8 oz. 368/13 oz.	4.0	14.4	1.6	18.8	0.52	0.16	316	na	0.70	No
Hill's Science Diet Gourmet Turkey Entrée Mature Adult 7+	369/13 oz.	4.1	12.8	2.1	19.4	0.62	0.17	426	na	0.83	No
Hill's Science Diet Savory Chicken Entrée Mature Adult 7+	155/5.8 oz. 347/13 oz.	3.8	13.1	1.6	18.4	0.57	0.16	520	na	0.82	No

Dry foods†	Energy density (kcal/cup)**	Energy density (kcal ME/g)	Fat (%)	Fiber (%)	Protein (%)	P (%)	Na (%)	Vit E (IU/kg)	Vit C (mg/kg)	Se (mg/kg)	VOHC plaque*** (Yes/No)
Recommended levels (inactive/obese prone)	-	3.0-3.5	7-10	≥10	15-23	0.3-0.7	0.15-0.4	≥400	≥100	0.5-1.3	-
Hill's Science Diet Light Adult	295	3.3	8.8	14.6	24.5	0.58	0.23	586	276	0.45	No
Iams Eukanuba Medium Breed Weight Control	275	4.2	10.5	1.9	21.3	0.76	0.50	206	42	0.34	No
Iams Weight Control	328	4.2	12.5	2.8	22.2	0.85	0.37	103	44	0.35	No
Medi-Cal Weight Control/Mature	320	na	8.5	4.0	19.5	0.8	0.2	na	na	na	No
Nutro Natural Choice Lite	244	3.4	7.2	4.4	16.7	1.22	0.33	161	67	0.44	No
Purina Pro Plan Chicken & Rice Weight Management	337	3.7	10.2	2.7	30.5	1.06	0.27	503	na	0.33	No
Royal Canin MINI Weight Care 30	326	3.8	12.0	6.2	32.6	0.82	0.33	652	326	0.16	No

Moist foods†	Energy density (kcal/can)**	Energy density (kcal ME/g)	Fat (%)	Fiber (%)	Protein (%)	P (%)	Na (%)	Vit E (IU/kg)	Vit C (mg/kg)	Se (mg/kg)	VOHC plaque*** (Yes/No)
Recommended levels (inactive/obese prone)	-	3.0-3.5	7-10	≥10	15-23	0.3-0.7	0.15-0.4	≥400	≥100	0.5-1.3	-
Hill's Science Diet Light Adult	322/13 oz.	3.4	8.6	9.7	19.5	0.51	0.31	385	na	0.78	No
Medi-Cal Weight Control/Mature	370/396 g	na	10.0	5.5	21.5	0.6	0.3	na	na	na	No

Key: ME = metabolizable energy, Fiber = crude fiber, Se = selenium, P = phosphorus, Na = sodium, VOHC = Veterinary Oral Health Council, na = information not available from manufacturer, g = grams.
*From manufacturers' published information or calculated from manufacturers' published as-fed values; all values are on a dry matter basis unless otherwise stated.
**Energy density values are listed on an as fed basis and are useful for determining the amount to feed; cup = 8-oz. measuring cup. To convert to kJ, multiply kcal by 4.184.
***An adequate periodontal management program should be in place (veterinarian/client/patient) to ensure that there is sufficient periodontal health to enable the patient to chew these products.
†The manufacturers of most of the foods listed for inactive/obese-prone dogs recommend these foods for young adults.

CLINICAL POINTS

- Reproducing dogs: bitches involved in breeding, gestation or lactation and breeding studs.
- Feeding goals: optimize conception, number of puppies per litter, parturition and puppy viability.
- Mating: no special nutritional needs; feed studs and bitches with a normal BCS the same as sexually intact young adults (Chapter 1). Breed only dogs with a normal BCS.
- Mating: obese bitches are at risk for lower ovulation rates, smaller litter size, insufficient lactation, silent heat, prolonged interestrous intervals and anestrus. Overweight bitches should lose weight before breeding.
- Flushing: unnecessary for a bitch with a normal BCS.
- Gestation: properly fed bitches gain 15-25%, mostly in the last trimester. Postpartum bitches should weigh 5-10% more than their pre-breeding weight (**Figure 1**). Excessive weight gain may increase dystocia risk, predisposing puppies to hypoxia and hypoglycemia. Inadequate food intake may lead to smaller litter size, lower birth weights and compromised lactation.
- Lactation: success depends on body condition before breeding and adequate nutrition throughout gestation and lactation; food needs are related to milk production, which depends on the number of nursing pups.
- Typically, pups begin to eat solid food during Weeks 3-4; as a result, the bitch's milk production declines and so does its nutrient needs.

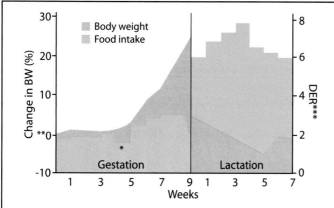

- * Transient decrease in food intake around the fourth week after conception is indicative of pregnancy.
- ** Prebreeding body weight
- *** Daily energy requirement. Numbers are multiples of resting energy requirement.

Figure 1. Typical changes in body weight and food intake of a bitch during gestation and lactation. A bitch only weighs 5 to 10% above pre-breeding weight after parturition, and should not lose more than 5% of its body weight during the first month of lactation. Food intake may drop precipitously during the last days of gestation.

Abbreviations
AAFCO = Association of American Feed Control Officials
BCS = body condition score (Appendix A)
KNF = key nutritional factor

Table 1. Key nutritional factors for reproducing dogs.

Factors	Recommended levels in food (DM)	
	Mating*	Gestation/lactation
Water	Fresh water should always be available	Fresh water should always be available
Energy density (kcal ME/g)**	3.5-4.5	≥4.0
Energy density (kJ ME/g)**	14.6-18.8	≥16.7
Crude protein (%)	15-30	25-35
Crude fat (%)	10-20	≥20
DHA (%)	-	≥0.02
Digestible carbohydrate (%)	≥23	≥23
Calcium (%)	0.5-1.0	1.0-1.7
Phosphorus (%)	0.4-0.7	0.7-1.3
Ca:P ratio	1:1-1.5:1	1:1-2:1
Digestibility	Foods with higher energy density are more likely to have higher digestiblity	Foods with higher energy density are more likely to have higher digestibility

Key: DM = dry matter, ME = metabolizable energy, kcal = kilo-calories, kJ = kilojoules, DHA = docosahaexaenoic acid.
*Foods for most breeding males and females are usually similar to those for young and middle-aged adults (Tables 3 and 4, Chapter 1).
**If the caloric density of the food is different, the nutrient content in the DM must be adapted accordingly.

KEY NUTRITIONAL FACTORS

During lactation a bitch's nutrient demands are greater than at any other adult lifestage; only extreme exercise is more energy demanding. **Table 1** summarizes KNFs for breeding males and females and pregnant and lactating bitches. Note that digestible carbohydrate is important for gestation/lactation. A detailed description of these recommendations can be found in Chapter 15, Small Animal Clinical Nutrition, 5th edition. Water is an often overlooked KNF and is needed in large quantities for lactation.

FEEDING PLAN

Assess and Select the Food
Ensure the Food's Basic Nutritional Adequacy. AAFCO

Table 2. Comparison of key nutritional factors in selected commercial foods for reproducing (gestation and lactation) bitches to recommended levels.* (Numbers in red match optimal KNFs.)

Dry foods	Energy density (kcal/cup)**	Energy density (kcal ME/g)	Protein (%)	Fat (%)	DHA (%)	Carbohydrate (%)	Ca (%)	P (%)	Ca:P
Recommended levels	-	≥4.0	25-35	≥20	≥0.02	≥23	1.0-1.7	0.7-1.3	1:1-2:1
Hill's Science Diet Nature's Best Chicken & Brown Rice Dinner Puppy	445	4.3	30.2	22.1	0.20	37.7	1.43	1.05	1.4:1
Hill's Science Diet Nature's Best Lamb & Brown Rice Dinner Puppy	442	4.2	30.1	22.1	0.17	36.5	1.5	1.1	1.4:1
Hill's Science Diet Puppy Healthy Development Original	384	4.2	31.8	22.9	0.22	33.2	1.59	1.21	1.3:1
Hill's Science Diet Puppy Lamb Meal & Rice Recipe	377	4.2	31.7	21.7	0.22	35.3	1.58	1.1	1.4:1
Iams Smart Puppy	428	4.7	32.1	19.9	na	38.7	1.37	1.04	1.3:1
Medi-Cal Development Formula	425	na	28.4	17.5	0.09	na	1.2	1.1	1.1:1
Purina ONE Healthy Puppy Formula	465	4.6	31.7	20.6	na	38.4	1.61	1.11	1.5:1
Purina Pro Plan Chicken & Rice Formula Puppy Food	473	4.6	31.6	20.7	na	36.6	1.23	1.04	1.2:1
Purina Puppy Chow	416	4.2	30.7	13.6	na	41.7	1.25	1.02	1.2:1
Royal Canin Veterinary Diet Development Formula	322	4.3	28.4	17.0	na	45.0	1.32	0.99	1.3:1

Moist foods	Energy density (kcal/can)**	Energy density (kcal ME/g)	Protein (%)	Fat (%)	DHA (%)	Carbohydrate (%)	Ca (%)	P (%)	Ca:P
Recommended levels	-	≥4.0	25-35	≥20	≥0.02	≥23	1.0-1.7	0.7-1.3	1:1-2:1
Hill's Science Diet Puppy Healthy Development Savory Chicken Entrée	205/5.8 oz. 459/13 oz.	4.1	28.2	23.6	na	39.2	1.33	0.96	1.4:1
Medi-Cal Development Formula	445/396 g	na	32.2	14.1	0.02	na	1.3	0.9	1.4:1
Royal Canin Veterinary Diet Development Formula	430/396 g	4.6	31.8	19.6	na	40.4	1.45	1.2	1.2:1

Key: ME = metabolizable energy, Ca = calcium, P = phosphorus, Ca:P = calcium-phosphorus ratio, na = information not available from manufacturer, g = grams, DHA = docosahexaenoic acid.
*From manufacturers' published information or calculated from manufacturers' published as-fed values; all values are on a dry matter basis unless otherwise stated. Digestibility: Foods with higher energy density are more likely to have higher digestibility. Foods for most breeding males and females are usually similar to those for young and middle-aged adults (Tables 3 and 4, Chapter 1).
**Energy density values are listed on an as fed basis and are useful for determining the amount to feed; cup = 8-oz. measuring cup. To convert to kJ, multiply kcal by 4.184.

nutritional adequacy statements are usually found on a product's label and should ensure that the product is intended for gestation/lactation. Many of these foods are also marketed for puppy growth and are sometimes referred to as growth/reproduction-type foods. Feed this type of food throughout gestation and lactation, particularly for giant-breed bitches. Transition to this type of food should occur at least one week before breeding (see Managing Food Changes below).

Compare the Food's KNF Content with the Recommended Levels. Table 2 compares KNF profiles for selected commercial foods. Contact manufacturers for this information for foods not in the table (manufacturer contact information is listed on product labels). A new food should be selected if discrepancies are noted; the new food should best approximate the recommended KNF levels.

Dry Foods vs. Moist Foods. Dry foods are more nutrient dense, as fed, and have higher levels of carbohydrates. Dry foods may benefit bitches experiencing weight loss and those spending little time eating. Moist foods are often higher in fat and provide additional water to support lactation. They may be more palatable to some dogs. Feeding both forms during gestation and lactation is an accepted practice.

Manage Treats and Snacks. If treats/snacks are fed, commercial treats that match the nutritional profile recommended for gestation/lactation or growth (see product label) are best. Otherwise, treats/snacks should not be fed excessively (<10% of the total diet on a volume, weight or calorie basis). Appendix B contains more information about treats/snacks.

Assess and Determine the Feeding Method
Determine How Much Food to Feed.

BREEDING MALES. Feed the same amount as intact adult dogs (Chapter 1). Some studs in heavy service may have inadequate food intake and lose weight; in these cases, increase the amount fed and/or switch to a more energy-dense food (also rule out other possible causes of weight loss).

Table 3. Periparturient hypoglycemia.

1. Occurs infrequently.
2. If it does occur, typically it will be in the last 2-3 weeks of gestation.
3. Neurologic signs of hypoglycemia predominate; differentiation from eclampsia is not always easy.
4. Clinical hypoglycemia (glucose values <45 mg/dl or 2.5 mmol/l).
5. Elevated serum ketones (mainly β-hydroxybutyrate); ketonemia may be missed with strips or tablets containing nitroprusside for ketone detection. Nitroprusside primarily detects acetone and acetoacetate.
6. Risk factors: poor body condition during pregnancy and malnutrition, which may include a high-fat, digestible carbohydrate-free food.
7. Emergency/acute treatment: 50% glucose, 1 ml/kg IV slow bolus (1-3 min.); this can be followed by IV 5% glucose at 2 ml/kg/hour to effect.
8. Soon after, or even during, the glucose infusion, feed small amounts of a good quality commercial gestation/lactation food (**Table 2**); continue feeding this food, at the exclusion of the previous food, for the duration of the pregnancy and lactation.

Table 4. Eclampsia (puerperal tetany) in the bitch.

1. Acute, life-threatening condition due to a sudden decrease in extracellular calcium.
2. Timing: highest risk is during Weeks 2-3 of lactation; less common during Weeks 1 and 4 of lactation and rarely during the last 2 weeks of gestation. Occasionally occurs at or just before whelping.
3. Usually primiparous small bitches with relatively large litters (low body weight-to-litter size ratio); typically less than 4 years of age.
4. Clinical signs vary based on severity and time course and include: anxiety, panting, whining, hypersalivation, vomiting, ataxia, stiff gait, muscle tremors, tetany, seizures, hyperthermia and tachycardia.
5. Low serum ionized calcium (<0.8 mmol/l).
6. Some bitches may not exhibit clinical signs and some may be normocalcemic.
7. Suggested causes: excessive dietary calcium supplementation during pregnancy (may down-regulate parathyroid gland secretion, impairing calcium mobilization from skeletal stores; as calcium demand increases during late gestation/lactation, serum calcium homeostasis cannot be maintained) or inadequate dietary calcium intake during late gestation and lactation combined with increased calcium demand (fetal development and lactation).
8. Initial treatment: slow IV infusion (5-10 minutes) of 10% calcium gluconate (0.5-1.5 ml/kg) usually results in rapid improvement; administer to effect. Monitor heart rate and stop infusion temporarily if bradycardia occurs. If an ECG is available, QT interval shortening is also an indication to stop infusion temporarily. Monitor body temperature because hypothermia may also occur.
9. When the IV route is unavailable, subcutaneous calcium gluconate, diluted with an equal volume of saline, can be used at the IV dose, above (undiluted may cause necrosis).
10. Following correction of acute signs provide oral vitamin D (calcitriol) at a loading dose of: 0.02-0.03 µg/kg/day divided q12h for 4 days followed by a maintenance dose of 0.005-0.015 µg/kg/day divided q12h (adjust as necessary to maintain normocalcemia). Discontinue at the end of lactation.
11. Also provide oral calcium supplementation (e.g., calcium carbonate, 100 mg/kg/day, divided with meals) throughout lactation.
12. If possible, separate puppies from the bitch for the first 24 hours of treatment and feed them canine milk replacer by bottle or orogastric tube (Chapter 4).
13. If tetany recurs during the same lactation, wean the puppies.
14. Prevention: for subsequent pregnancies feed a high quality commercial growth/reproduction-type food (**Table 2**) and avoid calcium supplements.
15. Prognosis: good to excellent if properly managed.

BITCHES DURING ESTRUS. Feed the same amount as intact adult dogs (Chapter 1). Bitches tend to have a depressed appetite during estrus; a decrease in food intake can be expected.

BITCHES DURING GESTATION. First 2 trimesters: feed the same amount as intact adult dogs (Chapter 1). Expect a normal decrease in appetite during Weeks 3-4 of gestation, which may result in a 30% reduction in food intake (**Figure 1**). Last 3 weeks: increase the amount fed by about two-thirds (or more in large breeds) to maintain a normal BCS. Postpone mating in bitches with inadequate body condition (BCS <2/5) and feed to improve BCS for the next breeding. If breeding cannot be postponed, such bitches should be fed increased amounts throughout gestation.

BITCHES DURING LACTATION. At peak lactation, a bitch's energy needs may be 3-4 times greater than requirements for adult maintenance. Do not underfeed. If bitches maintain a normal BCS (2.5/5 to 3.5/5) and puppy growth rate is normal, the amount being fed is appropriate. The amount to feed can be estimated by calculation (Appendix C) or by referring to feeding guides on product labels. A rough estimate: bitches should ingest their maintenance amount of food + 25% more for each nursing puppy.

BITCHES DURING WEANING. Reducing the amount of food fed to the bitch will help decrease lactation, which helps prevent excessive mammary gland distention/discomfort (Table 6, Chapter 4).

Consider How to Offer the Food.

BITCHES DURING ESTRUS. Occasional vomiting may occur in bitches due to a variety of stressors. If so, feed small meals or do not feed immediately before or after mating.

BITCHES DURING GESTATION. Overfeeding has similar negative effects as underfeeding; small- and medium-sized bitches should be food-restricted fed and be offered 1-2 meals/day during the first half of pregnancy. Two or more meals per day should be provided in the last half of pregnancy. Giant breeds and bitches pregnant with large litters may be fed free choice.

BITCHES DURING LACTATION. Feed free choice, except when a bitch has only 1 puppy and a tendency to gain weight. Free-choice feeding will allow nervous bitches to eat on their own schedule. If food-restricted fed, they should receive at least 3 meals/day. At about 3 weeks, puppies will begin to eat the bitch's food; make sure owners allow them access.

Manage Food Changes. Most healthy dogs adapt well to new foods but a transition period to avoid GI upsets is good practice. Example: to change to a new food, replace 25% of the old food with the new food on Day 1 and continue this incremental change daily until the change is complete on Day 4. Appendix E provides additional information.

Food and Water Receptacle Husbandry. Food and water bowls should be washed regularly with warm soapy water and rinsed well. Dishes used for moist foods need daily cleaning. Discard moist or moistened dry foods after 2-4 hours of room temperature exposure to avoid foodborne illnesses (Appendix F).

FOLLOWUP

Owner Followup
Owners should be instructed to contact their veterinarian if the bitch's food intake decreases before or during lactation or it exhibits hypersalivation, muscle contractions, seizures and/or weakness (**Tables 3** and **4**). Puppy weight gain is an indication of milk production; therefore, the owner should note puppy weights daily. Failure to gain weight for more than 1 day and/or continuous vocalization can be due to inadequate nutrition or health issues.

Breeders can be taught to assess body condition. During gestation, the BCS process should exclude the abdominal component, focusing on muscle mass and fat covering the ribs and bony prominences (Appendix A). Stools normally vary from soft to firm during reproduction. Constipation and diarrhea are always considered abnormal. The bitch's BCS should be about 3/5 throughout lactation.

If body condition is abnormal, adjustments should be made in the amount of food fed, assuming other potential causes of weight loss are ruled out. The amount fed should be changed by 10% increments and rechecked in 2 weeks. At that point, if necessary, the amount fed should be changed again and the cycle repeated. A bitch should not lose more than 5% of body weight during the first month of lactation and optimal body weight should be reached within 1 month after lactation ceases.

Veterinary Health Care Team Followup
Breeding bitches should be examined at least one month before the upcoming estrus. Problems detected by the assessment still may be corrected before breeding. Ideally, the bitch should be examined again at the time of pregnancy diagnosis, 1 week before parturition and at Week 3 or 4 of lactation. See Chapters 13 and 15, Small Animal Clinical Nutrition, 5th edition, for more information.

MISCELLANEOUS

Authors
Condensed from Chapter 15, Small Animal Clinical Nutrition, 5th edition, authored by Jacques Debraekeleer, Kathy L. Gross and Steven C. Zicker.

References
See Chapter 15, Small Animal Clinical Nutrition, 5th edition, on the website www.markmorrisinstitute.org for references.

Chapter 4

Feeding Nursing and Orphaned Puppies from Birth to Weaning

CLINICAL POINTS

- Feeding goal: through proper feeding and husbandry produce healthy, viable weaned puppies.
- Pre-weaning puppy mortality is 10-30%: two-thirds of deaths occur during Week 1. Mortality is highly correlated to low birth weight.
- Proper medical, husbandry and nutritional practices are closely intertwined: see Chapter 16, Small Animal Clinical Nutrition, 5th edition, for nonnutritional puppy health management recommendations.
- Orphans can be raised successfully with proper nutrition and husbandry practices.
- Pups that are orphaned, rejected or cannot be raised by the bitch can be fed by fostering, partial orphan rearing or handfeeding.
- Fostering: least labor intensive, best nutrition, lower mortality and better immune status, physical environment and social development.

Abbreviations
AAFCO = Association of American Feed Control Officials
BCS = body condition score (Appendix A)
DER = daily energy requirement (Appendix C)
Ig = immunoglobulin
KNF = key nutritional factor

- Partial orphan rearing: allows pups to stay with the dam in a normal environment and facilitates natural socialization.
- Handfeeding: most common method of feeding orphaned pups; typically, eyedroppers, syringes, bottles or stomach tubes are used.
- Weaning: important, stressful time for puppies and the bitch.

KEY NUTRITIONAL FACTORS

- Mature milk: complete (including water) food for neonates. The nutrient composition of milk (**Table 1**) is designed to support the normal growth of neonates and represents the KNFs for foods for nursing pups. Bitch's milk is more nutrient dense than cow's milk.

Table 1. Key nutritional factors for foods for nursing puppies (the nutritional content of bitch's milk).

Nutrient	Per 100 g milk, as fed	DM basis*
Moisture (g)	77.3	0
Dry matter (g)	22.7	100
Crude protein (g)	7.5	33
Arginine (mg)	420	1.85
Fat (g)	9.5	41.8
Linoleic acid (g)	1.11	4.9
Lactose (g)	3.3	14.5
Calcium (mg)	240	1.06
Phosphorus (mg)	180	0.79
Sodium (mg)	80	0.35
Potassium (mg)	120	0.53
Magnesium (mg)	11	0.05
Copper (mg)	0.33	0.0015
Iron (mg)	0.7	0.003
ME (kcal)	146 (610 kJ)	6.43 kcal/g (26.9 kJ/g)
Osmolarity (mOsm/kg)	569	Not applicable
DM digestibility	>95%	>95%

Key: DM = dry matter, ME = metabolizable energy.
*Units are expressed in percentages unless otherwise indicated.

- Colostrum: mammary secretion during the 1-7 days postpartum after which it changes to mature milk. Colostrum is higher in IgG, energy and other selected nutrients than milk and has a mild laxative effect. Its high viscosity can make nursing more difficult, especially for weaker puppies. Ensure colostrum intake by pups within 12-24 hours of age for adequate Ig uptake. If bitch colostrum is unavailable, use colostrum from other species.

FEEDING PLAN

Assess and Select the Food

Nursing Pups. Milk from a healthy bitch is the food of choice. Insufficient milk production and/or deficient milk quality may result in puppy growth failure (see Followup below), weakness, abdominal enlargement and abnormal behavior (e.g., restlessness, continuous vocalization). If these signs are present, the bitch's BCS, food and feeding method should be assessed (see Chapter 3).

Orphaned Pups. Milk from a healthy bitch is the food of choice but is rarely available. **Table 2** lists selected commercial milk replacers and their nutrient profiles compared to bitch's milk. **Table 3** lists 3 homemade recipes and **Table 4** compares their nutrient profiles to bitch's milk. Commercial (preferred) and homemade milk replacers should closely mimic the profile of bitch's milk. Ruminant milk may be used as a base for homemade formulas but doesn't meet the nutritional needs of puppies; goat's milk provides no benefit over cow's milk.

Weaning. Food for weaning should be a good quality growth/reproduction-type food such as the lactating bitch's food (Table 2, Chapter 3 and Table 3, Chapter 5).

Food Form. Foods should be liquid until nursing puppies and orphans are 3-4 weeks old after which semisolid to solid foods should be introduced.

Assess and Determine the Feeding Method

Nursing Pups. Day 1, if necessary, to ensure colostrum ingestion, position puppies on the bitch's nipples at feeding time and encourage a nervous bitch to lie quietly while pups nurse. Week 1, pups should nurse 8-12 times/day; after Week 1, at least 3-4 times/day. Competition may prevent smaller/weaker pups from nursing, predisposing to dehydration and hypoglycemia.

Orphaned Pups.

FOSTERING. Best method for feeding orphaned or rejected puppies. Bitches readily accept additional puppies during lactation. Fostering works best when there are fewer than 14 days age difference between the bitch's own pups and the orphans, otherwise large pups may crowd out smaller ones. Owners should supervise feeding until orphans can fend for themselves. Initially, owners should observe for signs of rejection or impending cannibalism by the dam. Pups should be accepted immediately and allowed to nurse. Foster mothers should be well fed.

PARTIAL ORPHAN REARING. Pups that cannot be raised by the bitch may be left with the mother but given supplemental feeding, including handfeeding (see below) or timed feedings using a surrogate bitch. Pups may also be reared "communally" by dividing a litter into 2 equal groups. One group remains with the bitch while the other is removed and fed milk replacer. The groups are exchanged 3-4 times/day. Owners should always feed the separated group just before it is returned to the bitch so the puppies will be less inclined to immediately nurse. Partial orphan rearing may be necessary to assist a foster mother.

HANDFEEDING.

Bottle Feeding. Bottle feeding is more successful in vigorous puppies with good nursing reflexes (**Figures 1** and **2**). Bottle-fed neonates will nurse until satiated and reject the formula when full. Bottle feeding can be time consuming, especially with large litters. Most puppies will readily suckle small pet nursing bottles, which are available in pet stores (**Figure 3**). Nursing bottles for dolls or bottles for premature human infants are alternatives.

Only 1 drop at a time should fall from the nipple of an inverted bottle. Fluid should be sucked never squeezed from the bottle. Too rapid flow may cause aspiration, choking and pneumonia.

Pups should be held horizontally with the head in a natural position (**Figure 1**), which reduces the risk of aspiration. Pups that prefer a different position (**Figure 2**) should be observed closely because the risk of aspiration is increased.

Tube Feeding. Pups that are weak or suckle poorly may be tube fed. Tube feeding is faster than bottle feeding and is often used when 1 person must care for several orphans. Bottle feeding allows puppies to control the amount of food intake, whereas tube feeding bypasses this control mechanism. Infant feeding tubes (5-8 Fr.) or soft urethral or intravenous catheters are used (**Figure 3**).

Measure and mark the tube before insertion so that its tip will be in the lower esophagus (~75% of the distance from the nose to the last rib). Recheck the mark every few days to allow for growth.

During feeding, position orphans as in **Figure 1**. Lubricate the tube and open the mouth with the same hand that steadies the head. Gently advance the tube to the mark. The tube may be in the trachea if resistance is encountered or the pup struggles. After proper tube placement, attach the syringe and administer the warmed formula over 1-2 minutes.

Table 2. Nutrient content of milk replacers compared with that of bitch's milk/100 grams of milk, as fed*

Nutrients**	Bitch's milk	Esbilac Liquid	Esbilac Reconstituted Powder	Nurturall C Puppy Liquid[†]	Nurturall-C Reconstituted Powder[†]	Just Born Puppy Liquid[†]	Just Born Reconstituted Powder[†]	Goat's Milk Esbilac Liquid	Goat's Milk Esbilac Reconstituted Powder
Manufacturer	-	PetAg	PetAg	VPL	VPL	Farnam	Farnam	PetAg	PetAg
Dilution***	na	na	1+2	na	1+2	na	1+2	na	1+2
Moisture (g)	77.3	84.9	na	80.1	85.7	80.1	85.7	84.2	-
Dry matter (g)	22.7	15.1	na	19.9	14.3	19.9	14.3	15.9	-
Crude protein (g)	7.5	5.1	6.2	7.6	4.5	7.6	4.5	4.7	6.12
Arginine (mg)	420	290	390	200	102	200	102	210	390
Lysine (mg)	380	370	470	na	na	na	na	360	470
Fat (g)	9.5	6.4	7.5	4.3	4.4	4.3	4.4	6.2	7.5
Linoleic acid (g)	1.1	na	0.4	na	na	na	na	-	0.86
Carbohydrate									
NFE (g)	3.8	2.9	2.7	6.4	4.3	6.4	4.3	2.9	2.7
Lactose (g)	3.3	na	-	na	na	na	na	-	-
Crude fiber (g)	na	0	0	<0.1	<0.1	<0.1	<0.1	0	0
Minerals									
Total ash (g)	1.2	0.8	1.3	1.5	1.1	1.5	1.1	1.2	1.3
Calcium (mg)	240	145	220	254	215	254	215	150	207
Phosphorus (mg)	180	110	178	221	186	221	186	-	149
Sodium (mg)	80	65	53	na	na	na	na	110	94
Potassium (mg)	120	130	194	113	186	113	186	250	142
Magnesium (mg)	11	12	12.6	6.5	7.0	6.5	7.0	18	14.2
Copper (mg)	0.33	0.18	0.23	0.2	0.16	0.2	0.16	0.22	0.46
Iron (mg)	0.70	0.60	0.82	2.70	2.17	2.7	2.17	1.90	0.83
Energy									
ME (kcal)	146	82	95	86	68	86	68	82	94.7
ME (kJ)	610	343	396	358	285	358	285	343	396
Osmolarity (mOsm/kg, $H_2O\pm SD$)	568.7±41.2	na	-	na	na	na	na	na	-

Nutrient content of milk replacers compared with that of bitch's milk/100 kcal metabolizable energy[††]

Protein (g)	5.20	6.21	6.56	8.89	6.63	8.89	6.63	5.70	6.46
Arginine (mg)	288	354	411	234	149	234	149	256	412
Lysine (mg)	260	451	495	na	na	na	na	439	496
Fat (g)	6.40	7.78	7.92	5.03	6.41	5.03	6.41	7.55	7.94
Linoleic acid (g)	0.76	na	0.43	na	na	na	na	na	0.91
Carbohydrate									
NFE (g)	2.60	3.51	2.80	7.49	6.29	7.49	6.29	3.51	2.81
Lactose (g)	2.3	na	na	na	na	na	na	na	na
Crude fiber (g)	na	0	0	<0.1	<0.1	<0.1	<0.1	0	0
Minerals									
Total ash (g)	0.82	0.98	1.32	1.75	1.62	1.75	1.62	1.46	1.38
Calcium (mg)	164	177	232	297	314	297	314	183	219
Phosphorus (mg)	123	134	187	258	272	258	272	0	157
Sodium (mg)	55	79	56	na	na	na	na	134	99
Potassium (mg)	82	159	204	132	272	132	272	305	150
Magnesium (mg)	7.5	14.6	13.3	7.6	10.2	7.6	10.2	22.0	15.0
Copper (mg)	0.23	0.22	0.24	0.23	0.24	0.23	0.24	0.27	0.49
Iron (mg)	0.48	0.73	0.86	3.16	3.18	3.16	3.18	2.32	0.88

Key: na = not applicable/available, NFE = nitrogen-free extract, ME = metabolizable energy, mOsm = milliosmoles.
*Manufacturers' data; nutrient content for reconstituted powdered products are manufacturers' calculations based on the recommended dilution. Nutrient data per 100 ml would be reduced slightly (between 1 to 2%) because the specific gravity of milk is greater than that of water.
**g/100 g = %.
***The first number is the milk powder, the second the water (e.g., 1+2 = one part of powder plus two parts of water).
[†]Nutrients in liquid and powder forms are averages from the yearly laboratory analyses of composite samples from 2004 to date.
[††]The nutrient levels per 100 kcal ME were calculated from the nutrient and energy levels in the top portion of the table.

Table 3. Homemade milk replacers for puppies.

Recipe 1		Recipe 2		Recipe 1 (modified)	
Skim milk	43.8 g	Cow's milk**	800 ml	Skim milk	64 g
Low-fat curd*	40 g	Half cream***	200 ml	Low-fat curd*	15 g
Egg yolk (2/3)	10 g	Bone meal	6 g	One egg yolk	15 g
Vegetable oil	6 g	Citric acid	4 g	Vegetable oil	3 g
Vitamin-mineral mix	0.2 g	One egg yolk	15 g	Vitamin-mineral mix	2.5 g
-	-	Vitamin A	2,000 IU	$CaCO_3$	0.5

*Do not use cottage cheese because it may increase the risk of clotting in the neonate's stomach.
**3% fat.
***12% fat (i.e., half cream in the UK).

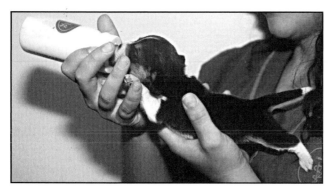

Figure 1. This is the preferred position for bottle feeding puppies. This position mimics the normal nursing position and decreases the likelihood of aspiration.

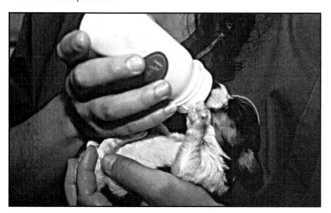

Figure 2. Some neonates prefer different positions for bottle feeding. This puppy prefers nursing in dorsal recumbency. Close observation is required because this position may predispose to aspiration.

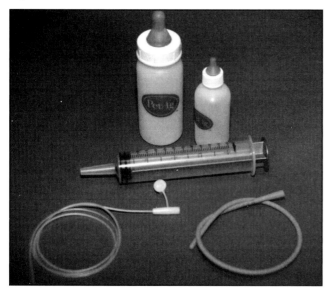

Figure 3. Various bottles and feeding tubes can be used for hand-feeding orphaned puppies.

Palpate the stomach to determine the degree of distention. Stop delivery if the stomach becomes taut or there is resistance to formula flow. If regurgitation occurs, withdraw the tube and discontinue feeding until the next scheduled meal.

Table 4. Comparisons between bitch's milk and homemade milk replacers for puppies (See **Table 3**).

Nutrients*	Bitch's milk	Homemade milk replacers		
		Recipe 1**	Recipe 2**	Recipe 1 (modified)***
	-			
Moisture (g)	77.3	76.6	85.3	79.9
Dry matter (g)	22.7	23.4	14.7	20.1
Crude protein (g)	7.5	9.9	3.5	7.5
Fat (g)	9.5	9.5	5.5	8.1
NFE (g)	3.8	3.3	4.6	3.5
Ash (g)	1.2	0.8	0.7	1.3
Calcium (mg)	240	92.6	290	287
Phosphorus (mg)	180	177	200	186
Sodium (mg)	80	32	50	34
Potassium (mg)	127	96	150	110
Copper (mg)	0.33	0.03	na	0.05
Iron (mg)	0.7	0.68	na	0.95
Zinc (mg)	0.95	0.79	na	1.01
Energy				
ME (kcal)†	146	130	80	110
ME (kJ)†	610	544	335	460

Key: NFE = nitrogen-free extract, ME = metabolizable energy.
*g/100 ml or g/100 g = %.
**Calculated before addition of the vitamin-mineral mix.
***Calculated based on the addition of 2.5 g Pecutrin (Bayer).
†Calculated except for bitch's milk, for which the actual energy density was known from the literature.

Table 5. Recommendations for energy intake of orphaned puppies as a basis for determining orphan formula dose.*

Feeding period	kcal ME/100 g BW	kJ ME/100 g BW
Days 1-3	15	60
Days 4-6	20	85
>6 days	20-25	85-105

Key: ME = metabolizable energy, BW = body weight.
*Do not over feed orphan formulas initially. The feeding amount for the first six days intentionally provides less energy than would normally be provided, which is gradually increased so that the orphaned puppies' energy requirements are being met after about one week.

Feeding Schedule: Amount, Rate and Formula Temperature

Daily amount to feed: estimate the pup's DER (**Table 5**) and divide the DER by the energy density of the milk replacer = amount/day. It is usually best to follow label instructions when using commercial milk replacers. Properly diluted, most milk replacers will provide ~1 kcal/ml. To meet fluid needs, orphans should be fed ~180 ml of milk replacer/kg/day. Add water to the milk replacer if necessary to provide the total recommended amount.

During Week 1 of life, the gastric capacity of small breeds may be 10-15 ml/feeding. Young neonates and weak pups should be fed every 2-4 hours. Older pups should be fed every 4-6 hours.

Warm the milk replacer to 38°C (100°F) and deliver slowly (1-2 ml/min.). Cold foods, rapid feeding and overfeeding may result in regurgitation, aspiration, bloating and diarrhea. If diarrhea occurs, reduce the amount fed or dilute the milk replacer with water. Gradually return to the previous dilution to meet energy needs. It is better to underfeed than overfeed.

Hygiene

Use stringent hygienic measures for orphans because they may

Table 6. Weaning.

1. Weaning actually begins when puppies voluntarily start eating the bitch's food between 3-4 weeks of age.
2. Weaning food: if fed correctly, the bitch should already be eating the type of food recommended for the weaning process (high quality growth/reproduction-type food (Table 2, Chapter 3 and Table 3, Chapter 5); using it as the weaning/postweaning food will facilitate transition of the pups to their growth/reproduction-type food.
3. 3-week-old pups can also be offered gruel to stimulate food intake. To make a gruel, blend a moist growth/reproduction-type food with an equal volume of warm water or use 1 part crushed dry food mixed with 3 parts of warm water (volume basis). Encourage pups to eat gruel by dipping a fingertip in the gruel and then into the pup's mouth.
4. Progressively reduce the gruel's water content.
5. By Week 5, the bitch's milk production is usually declining. By then, the pups should be eating sufficient quantities of solid food.
6. After 3 weeks of age, separate puppies from the bitch for short periods, progressively increasing separation time to ~4 hours/day by 6 weeks of age.
7. Weaning should be done at 6-7 weeks of age.
8. Day 1 of the weaning process: separate the bitch and puppies; withhold the bitch's food but allow the puppies to eat their weaning food. Reunite the bitch and puppies that night and remove all food for the night. Reducing the amount of food fed to the bitch will decrease lactation, which helps prevent excessive mammary gland distention/discomfort.
9. Day 2: separate the bitch and puppies again and allow the puppies to eat their weaning food but feed the bitch 25% of the amount fed before breeding and do not reunite them.
10. At this point, the puppies are considered weaned and are only fed their weaning food. Gradually increase the amount fed to the bitch so that by Day 5 or 6, the prebreeding amount is fed.
11. As pups transition to solid foods, they are prone to GI upsets. If a GI disturbance occurs, gruel can be made from a highly digestible moist food intended for treatment of diarrhea (Table 3, Chapter 42).

Table 7. Average daily weight gain of puppies.

Week	% of current body weight
1	8 (5-10)
2	6
3	4
4	3.5

Table 8. Treatment of hypoglycemia, hypothermia and dehydration in neonates.

(See Chapter 16, Small Animal Clinical Nutrition, 5th edition, for diagnosis and etiopathogenesis information).
1. Treatment goals: optimize core body temperature, normalize glucose levels, provide adequate hydration and restore to normal feeding.
2. Chilled pups (<35°C [<95°F]) should receive a mixture of equal amounts of PSS (or LRS) and DFW SQ before rewarming (1 ml/30 g body weight).
Slow (1-3 hrs) warming of hypothermic pups increases digestive enzyme activity to prevent diarrhea.
    Body heat: place pup in the inside pocket of a loose garment, which provides slow warming and gentle massage. Warm water (36.5°C [98°F]) or a warm water heating blanket is a good alternative. Incubator humidity should be ~60%.
3. Infection risk: administration of antibiotics may be lifesaving.
4. Oral fluids and/or nursing care should begin when normal body temperature is restored.
5. Prevent hypothermia and dehydration with early treatment: implement tube feeding, administer SQ fluids and manage temperature immediately.
Key: PSS = physiologic saline solution, LRS = lactated Ringer's solution, DFW = sterile 5% dextrose in water.

have received less colostrum and be more susceptible to infections. Clean feeding equipment and boil in water between uses.

Ingredients for homemade milk replacers should be fresh and refrigerated until used. Prepare only 24 hours worth of milk replacer at a time. Discard milk replacer after 1 hour at room temperature.

Orphans should be washed gently with a soft moistened cloth at least twice a week to simulate cleaning by the dam's tongue.

Weaning
Wean at 6-7 weeks as described in **Table 6**. After weaning, feed according to recommendations in Chapter 5 (growing puppies).

FOLLOWUP

Owner Followup
Record body weights of pups using a gram scale every 1-2 days for the 1st month, then weekly. Puppy growth is a good indicator of the quality/quantity of milk produced by the bitch and milk consumption and health status of the puppies (**Table 7**). Puppy weight loss/failure to gain for more than 1 day suggests disease in the pups or bitch, inadequate milk production or inability to nurse. Evaluate growth rate in relation to changes in behavior (e.g., restlessness and continuous vocalization).

Orphans may gain less because they are fed at a lower energy intake and milk replacers are not the same quality as bitch's milk.

Veterinary Health Care Team Followup
Consider weekly veterinary checkups for inexperienced owners during the first month. Assess pups for alertness, muscle tone, temperature and response to handling. Healthy puppies may cry but will soon stop and return to sleep. Ask the owner if the pups are nursing. Small/weak pups may appear to nurse and have an enlarged abdomen but fail to thrive. They are often restless and vocalize excessively. If orphans do not thrive when fed a milk replacer, consider a different product or formula. **Table 8** summarizes treatment for pups that develop clinical hypoglycemia, hypothermia and dehydration.

MISCELLANEOUS

See Chapters 15 and 16, Small Animal Clinical Nutrition, 5th edition, for more information.

Authors
Condensed from Chapter 16, Small Animal Clinical Nutrition, 5th edition, authored by Jacques Debraekeleer, Kathy L. Gross and Steven C. Zicker.

References
See Chapter 16, Small Animal Clinical Nutrition, 5th edition, on the website www.markmorrisinstitute.org for references.

Chapter 5

Feeding Growing Puppies: Postweaning to Adulthood

CLINICAL POINTS

- Puppies should be weaned at 6-7 weeks. Most breeds are considered adults at 10-12 months.
- Feeding goals: achieve healthy growth and create a healthy adult (optimize trainability and immune function; minimize obesity and DOD).
- Feed pups to grow at optimal rates for body condition and bone development; don't feed for maximal growth rates.
- Certain breeds are at risk for obesity (**Table 1**), as are neutered puppies.
- BCS: most practical indicator of whether or not a puppy's growth rate is healthy.
- All puppies should have a body condition evaluation (BCS) every 2 weeks so that, if necessary, timely adjustments can be made in the amount fed to achieve optimal growth.
- BCS: should be in the range of 2/5 to 3/5; the lower end of the range is better for breeds/genders at risk for obesity or for large-/giant-breed puppies at risk for DOD.
- Underfeeding during the postweaning growth phase is healthier than overfeeding and results in the same mature size.
- Chapter 27, Small Animal Clinical Nutrition, 5th edition, discusses diseases associated with obesity in adults.
- Limiting energy (food) intake early in life has the greatest positive nutritional influence on the incidence of phenotypic hip dysplasia.
- Chapter 33, Small Animal Clinical Nutrition, 5th edition, provides in-depth recommendations for feeding large- and giant-breed puppies (>25 kg adult weight) to prevent DOD.
- Thin pups should be fed carefully; owners are often tempted to overfeed so their puppies can "catch up."

Table 1. Breeds at increased risk for obesity.

Basset hounds
Beagles
Cairn terriers
Cavalier King Charles spaniels
Cocker spaniels
Dalmatian dogs
Golden retrievers
Labrador retrievers
Longhaired dachshunds
Pugs
Shetland sheepdogs

Abbreviations

AAFCO = Association of American Feed Control Officials
BCS = body condition score (Appendix A)
DHA = docosahexaenoic acid
DOD = developmental orthopedic disease
KNF = key nutritional factor
RER = resting energy requirement (Appendix C)

KEY NUTRITIONAL FACTORS

- Foods should provide recommended allowances of all required nutrients (nutritional adequacy), but should also contain specific levels of KNFs (certain nutrients and nonnutritional food ingredients or food features that can influence important diseases).
- **Table 2** lists KNF recommendations for growth foods. A detailed discussion of these recommendations can be found in Chapter 17, Small Animal Clinical Nutrition, 5th edition. Most nutrients supplied in excess of the amounts needed for growth cause little/no harm. However, excess energy and calcium are of special concern; energy for small-/medium-sized breeds (obesity prevention) and energy, calcium and the calcium:phosphorus ratio for large-/giant-breed puppies (skeletal health). Adequate DHA is important for normal neural development and improved trainability of all puppies. Water is always a KNF.

Table 2. Key nutritional factors for foods for growing puppies.*

Factors	Recommended levels in food (DM) Puppies with an adult BW <25 kg	Recommended levels in food (DM) Puppies with an adult BW >25 kg
Energy density (kcal ME/g)	3.5-4.5	3.5-4.5
Energy density (kJ ME/g)	14.6-18.8	14.6-18.8
Crude protein (%)	22-32	22-32
Crude fat (%)	10-25	10-25
DHA (%)	≥0.02	≥0.02
Calcium (%)	0.7-1.7	0.7-1.2
Phosphorus (%)	0.6-1.3	0.6-1.1
Ca:P ratio	1:1-1.8:1	1:1-1.5:1
Digestibility	See energy density recommendations, above; foods with higher energy density values tend to be more digestible	See energy density recommendations, above; foods with higher energy density values tend to be more digestible

Key: DM = dry matter, BW = body weight, kcal = kilocalories, kJ = kilojoules, ME = metabolizable energy, DHA = docosahexaenoic acid.
*For large- and giant-breed dogs (adult BW >25 kg), also see Table 33-5 in Chapter 33, Small Animal Clinical Nutrition, 5th edition.

FEEDING PLAN

Assess and Select the Food

Ensure the Food's Nutritional Adequacy. AAFCO nutritional adequacy statements are usually found on a product's label. AAFCO approval does not ensure a food will be effective in preventing important health problems associated with puppy growth such as obesity and DOD. Adult dog foods may not be balanced for healthy puppy growth.

Compare the Food's KNF Content with the Recommended Levels. Table 3 compares the KNF profiles for selected commercial foods for puppy growth. Many of these foods are also formulated/marketed for gestation and lactation and are sometimes referred to as growth/reproduction-type foods or foods for all lifestages. Contact the manufacturer for this information for foods not in the table (manufacturer contact information is listed on product labels). A new food should be selected if discrepancies are noted; the new food should best approximate the recommended KNF levels.

Table 3. Comparison of recommended levels of key nutritional factors for small- to medium-breed puppies (adult BW <25 kg) to the key nutritional factor content of selected commercial foods marketed for healthy puppy growth.* For large- to giant-breed puppies (adult BW >25 kg), see foods and recommended levels in Table 3, Chapter 22. (Numbers in red match optimal KNFs.)

Dry foods	Energy density (kcal/cup)**	Energy density (kcal ME/g)***	Protein (%)	Fat (%)	DHA (%)	Ca (%)	P (%)	Ca:P
Recommended levels	-	3.5-4.5	22-32	10-25	≥0.02	0.7-1.7	0.6-1.3	1:1-1.8:1
Hill's Science Diet Puppy Healthy Development Original	384	4.2	31.8	22.9	0.22	1.59	1.21	1.3:1
Hill's Science Diet Puppy Lamb Meal & Rice Recipe	377	4.2	31.7	21.7	0.22	1.58	1.10	1.4:1
Hill's Science Diet Nature's Best Chicken & Brown Rice Dinner Puppy	445	4.3	30.2	22.1	0.20	1.43	1.05	1.4:1
Hill's Science Diet Nature's Best Lamb & Brown Rice Dinner Puppy	442	4.2	30.1	22.1	0.17	1.50	1.10	1.4:1
Iams Eukanuba Medium Breed Puppy	463	4.1	31.7	19.2	na	1.50	1.07	1.4:1
Iams ProActive Health Smart Puppy	432	4.2	30.8	18.9	na	1.30	1.10	1.2:1
Medi-Cal Veterinary Diet Development Formula	425	na	28.4	17.5	na	1.20	1.10	1.1:1
Nutro Natural Choice Puppy Lamb Meal and Rice	333	3.8	29.7	14.3	na	1.98	1.54	1.3:1
Purina ONE Healthy Puppy Formula	465	4.6	31.7	20.6	na	1.61	1.11	1.5:1
Purina Puppy Chow	416	4.2	29.8	15.6	na	1.31	1.01	1.3:1
Purina Pro Plan Chicken & Rice Formula Puppy	473	4.6	31.6	20.7	na	1.23	1.04	1.2:1
Royal Canin Medium Puppy 32	402	4.6	35.6	20.0	na	1.12	0.88	1.3:1

Moist foods	Energy density (kcal/can)**	Energy density (kcal ME/g)***	Protein (%)	Fat (%)	DHA (%)	Ca (%)	P (%)	Ca:P
Recommended levels	-	3.5-4.5	22-32	10-25	≥0.02	0.7-1.7	0.6-1.3	1:1-1.8:1
Hill's Science Diet Puppy Healthy Development Savory Chicken Entrée	205/5.8 oz. 459/13 oz.	4.1	28.2	23.6	na	1.33	0.96	1.4:1
Purina Pro Plan Puppy Chicken & Rice Entrée Classic	459/13 oz.	4.9	42.4	38.4	na	1.92	1.48	1.3:1

Key: BW = body weight, ME = metabolizable energy, DHA = docosahexaenoic acid, Ca = calcium, P = phosphorus, na = not available from manufacturer.
*From manufacturers' published information or calculated from manufacturers' published as-fed values; all values are on a dry matter basis unless otherwise stated.
**Energy density values are listed on an as fed basis and are useful for determining the amount to feed; cup = 8-oz. measuring cup.
***Energy density also reflects digestibility; foods with higher energy density are likely to have better digestion than foods with lower energy density; for kJ/g, multiply kcal/g by 4.184.

Table 4. Recommendations for initial estimate of energy intake of growing dogs.

Time frame	x RER	kcal/BW$_{kg}^{0.75}$	kJ/BW$_{kg}^{0.75}$
Weaning to 50% of adult BW*	3	210	880
50 to 80% of adult BW	2.5	175	735
≥80% of adult BW	1.8-2.0	125-140	525-585

Key: RER = resting energy requirement, kcal = kilocalories, kJ = kilojoules, BW = body weight. RER can be obtained from Table 5-2, Small Animal Clinical Nutrition, 5th edition, or calculated. If calculating RER, use one of these two formulas: for puppies of all body weights, $RER_{kcal} = 70(BW_{kg}^{0.75})$; or for puppies weighing more than 2 kg, $RER_{kcal} = 30(BW_{kg}) + 70$. To convert kcal to kJ, multiply by 4.184. *Great Dane puppies may need 25% more energy during the first two months after weaning = 250 kcal or 1,050 kJ/BW$_{kg}^{0.75}$. See text.

Manage Treats and Snacks. If treats/snacks are fed, commercial treats that match the nutritional profile recommended for postweaning puppies (see product label) are best. Otherwise, treats/snacks should not be fed excessively (<10% of the total diet on a volume, weight or calorie basis). See Appendix B for more information about treats/snacks.

Assess and Determine the Feeding Method

Determine How Much Food to Feed. The amount to feed can be obtained from the product label or it can be calculated (**Table 4** and Appendix C). The amount to feed is related to a puppy's energy requirement, which depends on its growth phase (**Table 4**). Great Dane puppies may have energy requirements 20-25% higher than those of other breeds; young Great Dane puppies may not grow optimally when the daily energy intake is less than 2.5 x RER. However, do not extrapolate this information to puppies of other giant breeds. Feeding guides and calculated amounts are starting points; BCS should be used to adjust these estimates to individual puppies (see Followup below). Do not overfeed.

Consider How to Offer the Food. Use food-restricted feeding and avoid free-choice feeding. When proper amounts are used, food-restricted feeding is less likely to cause obesity and DOD. Divide the daily amount fed into 2-4 feedings.

Manage Food Changes. If a food change is necessary, a transition period is good practice to avoid GI upsets. Example: to change to a new food, replace 25% of the old food with the new food on Day 1 and continue this incremental change daily until the change is complete on Day 4. Appendix E provides additional information.

Food and Water Receptacle Husbandry. Food and water bowls should be washed regularly with warm soapy water and rinsed well. Dishes used for moist foods require daily cleaning. Discard moist or moistened dry foods after 2-4 hours of room temperature exposure to avoid foodborne illnesses (Appendix F).

FOLLOWUP

Owner Followup
Teach puppy owners to perform body condition scoring; they should monitor BCS at least every 2 weeks and adjust the amount fed by 10% increments to maintain a BCS of 2/5 to 3/5. Owners should record body weights and food intake (including snacks and treats) weekly.

Veterinary Health Care Team Followup
During office calls for routine vaccinations, review the growth rate and food consumption records and compare the owner's BCS evaluation to a BCS done by a member of the health care team. This level of attention to BCS helps owners manage a healthy BCS throughout the life of their dog.

MISCELLANEOUS

See Chapters 15-17, Small Animal Clinical Nutrition, 5th edition, for more information.

Authors
Condensed from Chapter 17, Small Animal Clinical Nutrition, 5th edition, authored by Jacques Debraekeleer, Kathy L. Gross and Steven C. Zicker.

References
See Chapter 17, Small Animal Clinical Nutrition, 5th edition, on the website www.markmorrisinstitute.org for references.

CLINICAL POINTS

- Working and sporting dogs are defined by the wide range of activities they undertake (**Tables 1** and **2**); depending on the activity, there is a need for athletic performance, scent detection or both.
- Feeding goals: optimize exercise and olfactory performance and long-term health.
- **Table 1** also lists the 3 basic types of physical activity performed by working/sporting dogs.
- Matching the food and feeding method to the type of activity allows sporting/working dogs to perform to their genetic potential and level of training.
- Exercise type is linked to genetics, which dictates working/sporting dogs' predominant muscle fiber type.
- Exercise and muscle fiber types determine the preferred metabolic substrates and thus the optimal nutrient profile of foods for working/sporting dogs.
- Sprinting uses Type II muscle fibers and depends on anaerobic metabolism of carbohydrate (glucose and glycogen), which is supported by high-carbohydrate foods.
- Endurance running uses Type I fibers, is completely aerobic and relies mostly on oxidation of fatty acids.
- Intermediate exercise uses both fiber types but mostly Type I fibers, is usually of low-to-moderate intensity, but may also include short periods of high-intensity work; both fats and carbohydrates are important fuels.
- Most working/sporting dogs do intermediate-type work.
- Exercise amount can be quantified as hours/day or week.
- Exercise frequency: how often the exercise occurs: daily, weekly, weekends only or seasonally. Hunting dogs often only work on weekends during hunting season ("part time"); livestock dogs may work several hours every day ("full time").
- Scent detection is important to what many working/sporting dogs are expected to do.
- Proper nutrition can optimize olfaction directly.
- Nutrition and training that optimize physical activity can improve olfaction indirectly: a dog cannot pant and sniff at the same time.
- Disorders (**Table 3**) and drugs (**Table 4**) can also negatively affect olfaction (e.g., dexamethasone can reduce olfactory acuity after only 1 week); many hunting dogs receive corticosteroid therapy for skin or musculoskeletal disorders.
- Most dogs that perform intermediate exercise are fed commercial foods; racing sprint and endurance dogs are often fed homemade foods or more commonly a mixture of commercial food and other ingredients. Supplement use is prevalent with all types of working/sporting dogs.

Abbreviations
AAFCO = Association of American Feed Control Officials
BCS = body condition score (Appendix A)
DER = daily energy requirement
KNF = key nutritional factor
RER = resting energy requirement

Table 1. Working and sporting dog activities listed by exercise type.

Exercise type	Activity
Sprint (high-intensity physical activity that can be sustained less than two minutes)	Coursing (sight hounds) Racing (greyhounds, whippets) Weight pulling
Intermediate (physical activity lasting a few minutes to a few hours)	Agility Border patrol, customs Drug detection Exercise with people (running, bicycling) Field trials Frisbee trials Guarding Hunting (game birds, rabbits) Livestock management (cattle, sheep,) Military Police work Pursuit (raccoon, coyote, fox, deer, wild boar) Search and rescue Service work (guide dogs, assistance dogs) Tracking
Endurance (physical activity that lasts many hours)	Sled pulling (racing, expedition)

Table 2. Various scent-detection activities conducted by working and sporting dogs.

Brown tree snake detection
Cadaver detection
Conservation work
Drug detection
Explosives detection
Fire accelerant detection
Game hunting
Identification of individuals
Pipeline leak detection
Search and rescue
Termite detection
Tracking for work or sport
War dogs

- Homemade foods can be complicated mixtures of many ingredients. Chapter 10, Small Animal Clinical Nutrition, 5th edition, discusses assessment of homemade foods in detail.

Table 3. Disorders affecting olfaction in people.*

Disorder	Effect on olfaction
Adrenal cortical insufficiency	Increased detection
Allergic rhinitis	Absent or diminished
Bronchial asthma	Absent or diminished
Chronic kidney failure	Absent or diminished
Cobalamin deficiency	Absent or diminished
Cushing's syndrome	Absent or diminished
Diabetes mellitus	Absent or diminished
Head trauma	Absent or diminished
Hepatic cirrhosis	Absent or diminished
Hypothyroidism	Absent, diminished or distorted
Nasal polyposis	Absent or diminished
Upper respiratory infections	Absent, diminished or distorted
Viral hepatitis (acute)	Absent, diminished or distorted

*Many of these diseases would also be expected to cause similar problems in dogs. Adapted from: Schiffman SS. Taste and smell in disease. New England Journal of Medicine 1983; 308: 1275-1279.

Table 4. Drugs that can cause changes in the sense of smell in dogs and people.*

Drug	Effect on olfaction
Amiodarone	Abnormal sense of smell reported in 1 to 3% of human patients
Amlodipine	Disturbance of smell reported rarely in human patients; resolves after drug withdrawal
Bromocriptine	Olfactory hallucination in 9% of human patients receiving 0.5 to 5 mg/day
Cimetidine	Decrease in olfactory acuity in human patients; reported rarely
Dexamethasone	Reduced olfactory acuity in dogs after only one week
Doxycycline	Loss or distortion of sense of smell in a small number of human patients
Nifedipine	Disturbance of sense of smell in human patients; rare and symptoms resolve after drug withdrawal
Phenylephrine	Decreased ability to smell in 1% of human patients

*Adapted from: Bleasel AF, McLeod JG, Brown ML. Anosmia after doxycycline use. Medical Journal of Australia 1990; 152: 440. Ezeh PI, Myers LJ, Hanrahan LA, et al. Effects of steroids on olfactory function of the dog. Physiology and Behavior 1992; 51: 1183-1187. Henkin RL. Drug induced taste and smell disorders: Incidence, mechanisms and management related primarily to treatment of sensory receptor dysfunction. Drug Safety 1994; 11: 318-377. Levenson JL, Kennedy K. Dysosmia, dysgeusia and nifedipine. Annals of Internal Medicine 1985; 1102: 135-136. Product Information: Amiodarone, 2004.

- Homemade food recipes for working/sporting dogs often use commercial dry dog food as a base; if dry dog food constitutes 50-75% of the mixture on a weight basis, and most additions are wet ingredients or fat, vitamin and mineral deficiencies are unlikely.
- Raw meat and by-products used in some homemade foods contain bacteria and bacterial toxins that are health risks for people handling the foods and the dogs that eat them. Chapter 11, Small Animal Clinical Nutrition, 5th edition, discusses food safety.
- The primary focus of this chapter is the use of commercial foods for most working/sporting dogs (i.e., dogs involved in intermediate level activity).

KEY NUTRITIONAL FACTORS

- Foods should provide recommended allowances of all required nutrients (nutritional adequacy), but should also contain specific levels of KNFs (certain nutrients and nonnutritional food ingredients or food features that can influence physical and olfactory performance and important diseases [Table 1, Chapter 1]).
- **Table 5** lists KNF recommendations for foods for working/sporting dogs. A detailed description of these recommendations can be found in Chapter 18, Small Animal Clinical Nutrition, 5th edition. Note that antioxidants are KNFs. Exercise-induced free radical production can overwhelm innate antioxidant systems. Prolonged oxidative stress may lead to chronic muscle fatigue ("overtraining syndrome"). Proper dietary antioxidant levels augment innate systems and improve performance; however, excessive levels may impair performance. Water is always a KNF. Even mild dehydration can limit exercise performance and probably limits olfaction and appetite. Hydration status is the most important determinant of endurance capacity. Water requirements may double when ambient temperatures reach 45°C (113°F).

FEEDING PLAN

Assess and Select the Food

Ensure the Food's Nutritional Adequacy. AAFCO nutritional adequacy statements are usually found on a product's label. AAFCO approval does not ensure a food will support optimal physical and olfactory performance when fed to working/sporting dogs or that it will help prevent certain diseases (Table 1, Chapter 1).

Compare the Food's KNF Content with the Recommended Levels. **Table 6** lists the KNFs for the categories of working/sporting dogs and compares them to the KNF content of selected commercial foods. Contact manufacturers for this information for foods not in the table (manufacturer contact information is listed on product labels). A new food should be selected if discrepancies are noted; the new food should best approximate the recommended KNF levels. The energy density of most commercial foods is not high enough for dogs engaged in true endurance activity. **Table 6** also provides energy density information for commercial foods supplemented with vegetable oil to meet the increased energy needs of endurance athletes.

Manage Treats, Snacks and Supplements.

SPRINT AND INTERMEDIATE ACTIVITY. Products are available to support energy levels during exercise. Timing of their use is important (see Feeding Methods below). Included are hydratable powders used in drinking water or dry snacks. Check online or at pet/sporting goods stores. Small amounts of a high-carbohydrate, low-fat commercial dog food or treats are also effective. For some foods, increasing the unsaturated fatty

Table 5. Key nutritional factors for foods for working and sporting dogs.

Factors	Sprint activity	Intermediate activity (low/moderate duration and frequency)	Intermediate activity (high duration and frequency)	Endurance activity
Water	Unlimited access except just before a race	Unlimited access	Unlimited access	Unlimited access
Energy density	Use food with 3.5 to 4.0 kcal ME/g DM	Use food with 4.0 to 5.0 kcal ME/g DM	Use food with 4.5 to 5.5 kcal ME/g DM	Use food with >6.0 kcal ME/g DM
Fat	Use food with 8 to 10% DM fat or 20 to 24% of calories from fat	Use food with 15 to 30% DM fat or 30 to 55% of calories from fat	Use food with 25 to 40% DM fat or 45 to 65% of calories from fat	Use food with >50% DM fat or >75% of calories from fat
Unsaturated fatty acids	-	>60% unsaturated fatty acids to optimize olfaction	>60% unsaturated fatty acids to optimize olfaction	-
Digestible carbohydrate	Use food with 55 to 65% DM NFE or 50 to 60% of calories from NFE	Use food with 30 to 55% DM NFE or 20 to 50% of calories from NFE	Use food with 30 to 35% DM NFE or 15 to 30% of calories from NFE	Use food with <15% DM NFE or <10% of calories from NFE
Protein	Use food with 22 to 28% DM protein or 20 to 25% of kcal (ME) from protein	Use food with 22 to 32% DM protein or 20 to 25% of kcal (ME) from protein	Use food with 22 to 32% DM protein or 18 to 25% of kcal (ME) from protein	Use food with 28 to 34% DM protein or 18 to 22% of kcal (ME) from protein
Digestibility	DM digestibility >80%	DM digestibility >80%	DM digestibility >80%	DM digestibility >80%
Antioxidants				
Vitamin E	≥500 IU vitamin E/kg food (DM)	≥500 IU vitamin E/kg food (DM)	≥500 IU vitamin E/kg food (DM)	≥500 IU vitamin E/kg food (DM)
Vitamin C	150 to 250 mg vitamin C/kg food (DM)	150 to 250 mg vitamin C/kg food (DM)	150 to 250 mg vitamin C/kg food (DM)	150 to 250 mg vitamin C/kg food (DM)
Selenium	0.5 to 1.3 mg/kg food (DM)	0.5 to 1.3 mg/kg food (DM)	0.5 to 1.3 mg/kg food (DM)	0.5 to 1.3 mg/kg food (DM)

Key: ME = metabolizable energy, DM = dry matter, NFE = nitrogen-free extract (represents digestible [soluble] carbohydrate fraction).

acid content by adding vegetable oil (see below) may improve olfaction.

ENDURANCE ACTIVITY. Vegetable oil can be added to commercial food to increase energy density for support of endurance activity (**Table 6**). One tablespoon of corn oil/lb of dry food will increase total fat content by 3-4 percentage points (e.g., 2 tablespoons of corn oil added to 1 lb of dry food containing 20% fat will result in a food/corn oil mixture containing 27% fat). Addition of oil should be done gradually. Steatorrhea and reduced palatability indicate that fat tolerance has been exceeded. When modifying foods, adequate time (~6 weeks) should be allowed to take full advantage of the new nutrient profile.

Assess and Determine the Feeding Method

Determine How Much Food to Feed. Feeding guidelines on pet food labels are seldom correct for active working/sporting dogs; thus, the initial food dosage is often calculated. The nutrients in commercial foods are balanced to the food's energy density, which allows for the food dose calculation to be based on the dog's DER (Appendix C). A dog's DER is the product of its RER and a factor that accounts for activity. To ensure energy balance, determine the BCS regularly and adjust the food dose accordingly (see Followup below). Dogs working in environmental temperature extremes typically do not require more energy intake for thermoregulation.

SPRINT ACTIVITY. Feeding guidelines on product labels of foods properly formulated for active dogs will often be a good starting point for food dosages for sprint dogs. If the amount to feed is calculated, the DER range is 1.6 to 2 x RER.

INTERMEDIATE ACTIVITY (TRAINING/WORKING/HUNTING). Food dosage is highly variable, depending on duration and frequency of activity. The DER range for food dosage calculation is 2-5 x RER. Compared to product label feeding guidelines this is 1-2.5 x as much food as recommended for sprint dogs. Initially, assess body condition frequently and adjust food intake accordingly. **Table 7** provides energy expenditure information that can help estimate DER. Idle dogs in this category should be fed as a typical adult dog (Chapter 1).

ENDURANCE ACTIVITY. Food dosage is highly variable, depending on duration and frequency of activity. The DER range for food dosage calculations is 5-11 x RER. Compared to product label feeding guidelines this is 2.5-5.5 x as much food as recommended for sprint dogs. Initially, assess body condition frequently and adjust food intake accordingly. **Table 7** provides energy expenditure information that can help estimate DER. Idle dogs in this category should be fed as typical adult dogs (Chapter 1). Sled dogs are often fed so they begin a long-distance race with 1-2 kg of extra body fat, which is used to support energy needs.

Consider How to Offer the Food. Food-restricted feeding is best because the amount consumed is known. Feed at the right time in relation to exercise. Elevated insulin levels decrease fatty acid mobilization and deplete glycogen stores, impairing endurance. Feed at least 4 hours before exercise to help decrease insulin and improve glucose homeostasis at the onset of exercise. However, small amounts of high-carbohydrate food/treats or supplements offered during exercise may aid glucose homeostasis. Proper timing of high-carbohydrate meals postexercise (0.5-2 hours) improves glycogen resynthesis and is a form of "carbo-

Table 6. Levels of key nutritional factors (DM) in selected dry commercial foods used for working and sporting dogs compared to recommended key nutritional factor values.* (Numbers in red match optimal KNFs.)

Recommended levels for sprint activity

Foods	Energy density (kcal/cup)** -	Energy density (kcal ME/g)*** 3.5-4.0	Fat (%) 8-10	Carbohydrate (%) 55-65	Protein (%) 22-28	Vitamin E (IU/kg) ≥500	Vitamin C (mg/kg) 150-250	Selenium (mg/kg) 0.5-1.3
Hill's Science Diet								
Adult Lamb Meal & Rice Recipe	364	_4.0_	16.0	52.9	_23.0_	_582_	_174_	_0.54_
Hill's Science Diet Adult Active	560	5.0	27.2	35.4	29.8	_556_	_152_	_0.54_
Iams Eukanuba Premium								
Performance Sporting Dog Food	431	4.8	22.2	33.8	33.3	na	na	na
Iams Proactive Health								
Lamb Meal & Rice Formula	330	_4.0_	14.2	46.3	_25.1_	123	52	0.37
Nutro Natural Choice High Energy	396	4.3	23.1	32.4	34.1	na	66	0.33
Nutro Natural Choice								
Lamb Meal & Rice Formula	342	_3.8_	14.3	50.0	_24.2_	220	66	_0.77_
Pedigree Small Crunchy Bites								
Dog Food	290	_3.8_	13.7	48.1	_26.0_	256	80	na
Purina Dog Chow	430	4.2	11.4	51.9	_23.9_	144	na	_0.64_
Purina Pro Plan								
Performance Formula	493	4.8	23.2	31.3	35.0	na	na	na
Royal Canin Energy 4800	591	5.2	33.3	15.8	35.6	_856_	389	0.28
Royal Canin Maxi								
German Shepherd 24	314	4.5	21.2	37.0	_26.8_	_670_	na	0.22
Royal Canin Maxi								
Golden Retriever 25	412	4.1	14.7	38.7	_27.5_	_769_	na	0.20
Royal Canin Maxi								
Labrador Retriever 30	321	4.1	14.3	35.3	33.0	_659_	na	0.18
Royal Canin Medium								
Active Special 25	349	4.6	18.9	na	_27.8_	_667_	333	0.16

Recommended levels for intermediate activity (low/moderate duration and frequency)

Foods	Energy density (kcal/cup)** -	Energy density (kcal ME/g)*** 4.0-5.0	Fat (%) 15-30 (>60% unsaturated)†	Carbohydrate (%) 30-55	Protein (%) 22-32	Vitamin E (IU/kg) ≥500	Vitamin C (mg/kg) 150-250	Selenium (mg/kg) 0.5-1.3
Hill's Science Diet								
Adult Lamb Meal & Rice Recipe	364	_4.0_	_16.0_ (na)	_52.9_	_23.0_	_582_	_174_	_0.54_
Hill's Science Diet Adult Active	560	5.0	_27.2 (64% unsaturated)_	_35.4_	_29.8_	_556_	_152_	_0.54_
Iams Eukanuba Premium								
Performance Sporting Dog Food	431	_4.8_	_22.2_ (na)	_33.8_	33.3	na	na	na
Iams Proactive Health								
Lamb Meal & Rice Formula	330	_4.0_	14.2 (na)	_46.3_	_25.1_	123	52	0.37
Nutro Natural Choice High Energy	396	_4.3_	_23.1_ (na)	_32.4_	34.1	na	66	0.33
Nutro Natural Choice								
Lamb Meal & Rice Formula	342	3.8	14.3 (na)	_50.0_	_24.2_	220	66	_0.77_
Pedigree Small Crunchy Bites								
Dog Food	290	3.8	13.7 (na)	_48.1_	_26.0_	256	80	na
Purina Dog Chow	430	_4.2_	11.4 (na)	_51.9_	_23.9_	144	na	_0.64_
Purina Pro Plan								
Performance Formula	493	_4.8_	_23.2_ (na)	_31.3_	35.0	na	na	na
Royal Canin Energy 4800	591	5.2	33.3 (na)	15.8	35.6	_856_	389	0.28
Royal Canin Maxi								
German Shepherd 24	314	_4.5_	_21.2_ (na)	_37.0_	_26.8_	_670_	na	0.22
Royal Canin Maxi								
Golden Retriever 25	412	_4.1_	14.7 (na)	_38.7_	_27.5_	_769_	na	0.20
Royal Canin Maxi								
Labrador Retriever 30	321	_4.1_	14.3 (na)	_35.3_	33.0	_659_	na	0.18
Royal Canin Medium								
Active Special 25	349	_4.6_	_18.9_ (na)	na	_27.8_	_667_	333	0.16

hydrate loading." This is more important for dogs that perform strenuous exercise on consecutive days. Feeding more than 4 hours before exercise may also aid endurance by stimulating bowel evacuation before work begins. Working/sporting dogs should not be fed high-fat meals immediately before or during intense exercise.

SPRINT ACTIVITY. Provide food or a snack at least 4 hours before activity. Offer a high-carbohydrate food/snack within 0.5-2 hours after activity. Water is typically not provided to greyhounds within 2 hours of a race to reduce urine weight and

Recommended levels for intermediate activity (high duration and frequency)

Foods	Energy density (kcal/cup)**	Energy density (kcal ME/g)***	Fat (%)	Carbohydrate (%)	Protein (%)	Vitamin E (IU/kg)	Vitamin C (mg/kg)	Selenium (mg/kg)
	-	4.5-5.5	25-40 (>60% unsaturated)†	30-35	22-32	≥500	150-250	0.5-1.3
Hill's Science Diet Adult Active	560	**5.0**	**27.2 (64% unsaturated)**	35.4	**29.8**	**556**	**152**	**0.54**
Iams Eukanuba Premium Performance Sporting Dog Food	431	**4.8**	22.2 (na)	**33.8**	33.3	na	na	na
Iams Proactive Health Lamb Meal & Rice Formula	330	4.0	14.2 (na)	46.3	**25.1**	123	52	0.37
Nutro Natural Choice High Energy	396	4.3	23.1 (na)	**32.4**	34.1	na	66	0.33
Nutro Natural Choice Lamb Meal & Rice Formula	342	3.8	14.3 (na)	50.0	**24.2**	220	66	**0.77**
Pedigree Small Crunchy Bites Dog Food	290	3.8	13.7 (na)	48.1	**26.0**	256	80	na
Purina Dog Chow	430	4.2	11.4 (na)	51.9	**23.9**	144	na	**0.64**
Purina Pro Plan Performance Formula	493	**4.8**	23.2 (na)	**31.3**	35.0	na	na	na
Royal Canin Energy 4800	591	**5.2**	**33.3** (na)	15.8	35.6	**856**	389	0.28
Royal Canin Maxi German Shepherd 24	314	**4.5**	21.2 (na)	37.0	**26.8**	**670**	na	0.22
Royal Canin Maxi Golden Retriever 25	412	4.1	14.7 (na)	38.7	**27.5**	**769**	na	0.20
Royal Canin Maxi Labrador Retriever 30	321	4.1	14.3 (na)	35.3	33.0	**659**	na	0.18
Royal Canin Medium Active Special 25	349	**4.6**	18.9 (na)	na	**27.8**	**667**	333	0.16

Recommended levels for endurance activity

Foods	Energy density (kcal/cup)**	Energy density (kcal ME/g)***	Fat (%)	Carbohydrate (%)	Protein (%)	Vitamin E (IU/kg)	Vitamin C (mg/kg)	Selenium (mg/kg)
	-	>6	>50††	<15	28-34	≥500	150-250	0.5-1.3
Hill's Science Diet Adult Active	560	5.0	27.2	35.4	**29.8**	**556**	**152**	**0.54**
Iams Eukanuba Premium Performance Sporting Dog Food	431	4.8	22.2	33.8	**33.3**	na	na	na
Nutro Natural Choice High Energy	396	4.3	23.1	32.4	34.1	na	66	0.33
Purina Pro Plan Performance Formula	493	4.8	23.2	31.3	35	na	na	na
Royal Canin Energy 4800	591	5.2	33.3	15.8	35.6	**856**	389	0.28

Key: DM = dry matter, ME = metabolizable energy, na = not available from manufacturer.
*This table lists selected products for which manufacturers' published information is available. **Table 1** provides examples of types of activities conducted by working and sporting dogs.
**Energy density values are listed on an as-fed basis and are useful for determining the amount to feed; cup = 8-oz. measuring cup. To convert to kJ, multiply kcal x 4.184.
***Foods higher in energy density are generally more digestible.
†For improved olfaction, fat sources should provide >60% total unsaturated fatty acids (**Table 7**).
††To increase fat content and energy density, adding two tablespoons of vegetable oil per pound (454 g) of food would increase fat content by approximately 6 percentage points; one tablespoonful of vegetable oil = 125 kcal ME; adding vegetable oil to dry commercial foods intended to support endurance activity is recommended.

the associated time handicap. Water should be offered as soon as possible after exercise; cool water is absorbed more rapidly.

INTERMEDIATE ACTIVITY (TRAINING/WORKING/HUNTING). Provide a high-carbohydrate food/snack at least 4 hours before activity. Offer the same food/snacks during the activity or at the end of breaks within 15 minutes of resuming activity. After exercise, offer the food/treat/snack within 0.5-2 hours. This feeding regimen will also help prevent exercised-induced ("hunting dog") hypoglycemia. Affected dogs initially work normally but develop signs of weakness and tremors that

Table 7. Saturated and unsaturated fatty acid content of selected fat sources used in commercial pet foods.*

Ingredient	Saturated fatty acids (%)	Unsaturated fatty acids (%)**
Beef tallow	47.4	52.6
Choice white grease	38.7	61.3
Lard (swine fat)	28.6	71.4
Poultry fat	28.6	71.4
Fish oil (menhaden)	20.2	79.8
Corn oil	12.7	87.3
Flax oil (linseed)	9.4	90.6
Safflower oil	8.6	91.4
Soybean oil	14.2	85.8
Sunflower oil	8.9	91.1

*National Research Council. Nutrient Requirements of Dogs and Cats. Washington, DC: National Academies Press, 2006; 328-329.
**Includes both polyunsaturated and monounsaturated fatty acids; derived by subtracting % saturated fatty acid values from 100.

may progress to seizures and even death. The condition is more common in hyperactive, under-conditioned dogs. Feeding at the beginning of a 45-minute lunch break may also contribute. Regularly offer cool water to all dogs, particularly those in warm, humid environments. Allow at least 6 weeks for dogs in training to adapt to a new food. Intermediate activity dogs that are idle should be fed as typical adult dogs (Chapter 1).

ENDURANCE ACTIVITY. Feed as for intermediate activity, above. Monitor hydration status frequently.

Manage Food Changes. GI adaptation to changes in fat and carbohydrate intake usually occurs quickly but a transition period is good practice. Example: to change to a new food, replace 25% of the old food with the new food on Day 1 and continue this incremental change daily until the change is complete on Day 4. Appendix E provides additional information. Associated advantageous metabolic changes take longer. Training should be initiated and food changes completed at least 6 weeks before the exercise season.

Food and Water Receptacle Husbandry. Food and water bowls should be washed regularly with warm soapy water and rinsed well. Dishes used for moist foods need daily cleaning. Discard moist or moistened dry foods after 2-4 hours of room temperature exposure to avoid foodborne illnesses (Appendix F).

FOLLOWUP

Owner Followup

Owners should be taught to assess their dog's body condition (Appendix A). During active periods, weekly BCS assessment is the best measure of energy balance. If a trend of increasing or decreasing BCS is noticed, the amount fed should be changed by 10% increments and the dog rechecked weekly. At that point, if necessary, the amount fed should be changed again and the cycle repeated. The target BCS of most working/sporting dogs is 2/5 to 3/5 with a bias towards the low side of this range. Hunting dogs' BCS should be between 2.5/5 to 3.5/5. Unfortunately, some of these dogs' BCS will be greater than 3.5/5 (family pets are more overweight prone). Sight hounds are kept lean (BCS 1/5 to 2/5). Normal racing greyhounds' BCS is 1/5. Racing sled dogs' BCS should be 2.5/5. Owners should avoid use of supplements not approved by a veterinarian. Decreased food consumption is an early indicator of problems; monitor food intake daily.

Veterinary Health Care Team Followup

A thorough physical exam is important in underperforming dogs because the problem may not be nutritional. Obtain a thorough history including all medications, foods/supplements and feeding and training methods being used. Except for certain drugs, generally, what is good for exercise performance is good for olfaction. Besides certain disorders (**Table 3**), specific medications (**Table 4**) can impair olfaction. Make sure adequate water is provided during activity.

MISCELLANEOUS

See Chapters 13 and 18, Small Animal Clinical Nutrition, 5th edition, for more information about feeding working and sporting dogs.

Authors

Condensed from Chapter 18, Small Animal Clinical Nutrition, 5th edition, authored by Philip W. Toll, Robert L. Gillette and Michael S. Hand.

References

See Chapter 18, Small Animal Clinical Nutrition, 5th edition, on the website www.markmorrisinstitute.org for references.

CLINICAL POINTS

- Young adult cats are in the age range of 10-12 months through 6-7 years.
- Feeding goals: maximize health, longevity and quality of life (disease prevention).
- Periodontal disease is the most prevalent disease in cats, is preventable and has important associated health risks; food can play an important role in prevention, if VOHC accepted.
- The mortality risk of obese young adult cats is 2.7 times that of lean cats.
- Neutering increases the risk of overweight/obesity conditions.
- Nutritional counseling to prevent obesity should be provided at the time cats are neutered.

KEY NUTRITIONAL FACTORS

- Foods should provide recommended allowances of all required nutrients but should also contain specific levels of KNFs (certain nutrients and nonnutritional food ingredients or food features that can influence important diseases).
- **Table 1** lists important diseases with nutritional associations for adult cats.
- **Table 2** lists KNF recommendations for foods for young adult cats that are of normal body condition or inactive/obese prone. A detailed description of these recommendations can be found in Chapter 20, Small Animal Clinical Nutrition, 5th edition. Water is always a KNF.

Abbreviations
AAFCO = Association of American Feed Control Officials
BCS = body condition score (Appendix A)
KNF = key nutritional factor
VOHC = Veterinary Oral Health Council

FEEDING PLAN

Assess and Select the Food
Ensure the Food's Nutritional Adequacy. AAFCO nutritional adequacy statements are usually found on a product's label. AAFCO approval does not ensure the food will be effective in preventing long-term health problems.
Compare the Food's KNF Content with the Recommended Levels. **Table 3** compares KNF profiles for selected commercial foods. Contact the manufacturer for this information for foods not in this table (manufacturer contact information is listed on product labels). A new food should be selected if discrepancies are noted; the new food should best approximate recommended KNF levels.
Manage Treats and Snacks. If treats/snacks are fed, commercial treats that match the nutritional profile recommended for adult cats (see product label) are best. Otherwise, treats/snacks should not be fed excessively (<10% of the total diet on a volume, weight or calorie basis). See Appendix B for more information about treats/snacks.

Assess and Determine the Feeding Method
Determine How Much to Feed. Appropriate intake levels of basic nutrients and KNFs are determined by the amounts in food and by how much food is consumed. If the patient has an ideal BCS (2.5/5 to 3.5/5), the amount being fed is likely appropriate. If a new food is needed, the amount fed can be estimated either

Table 1. Important diseases for adult cats that have nutritional associations.

Disease/health concern	Incidence/prevalence/mortality/pet owner concern	References*
Dental disease	Most prevalent disease; numerous associated health issues	Lund et al, 1999
Obesity	Approximate 30% prevalence; numerous associated health issues; neutered and indoor cats are at increased risk	Lund et al, 1999
FLUTD	0.85 to 1.5% per year incidence; 3% prevalence; most common reason cat owners seek veterinary care; kidney/urinary diseases are the most common cat owner concerns	Lawler et al, 1985; Lund et al, 1999; Willeberg, 1984; Westropp et al, 2005; Hostutler et al, 2005; Anon, Vet Economics, 2005; MAF, 2005
Kidney disease	Second leading cause of non-accidental death; kidney/urinary diseases are the most common cat owner concerns	Polzin et al, 2005; Ross et al, 2006; MAF, 1998, 2005
Cancer	Leading cause of non-accidental death	MAF, 1998
Arthritis	Incidence in general population unknown, but 22% in cats over one year of age in one study; overweight cats are three times likelier to have arthritis	Godfrey, 2005; Scarlett and Donoghue, 1998

Key: FLUTD = feline lower urinary tract disease.
*The references for **Table 1** can be found at www.markmorrisinstitute.org.

Table 2. Key nutritional factors for foods for young adult cats.

Factors	Recommended food levels*	
	Normal weight	Inactive/ obese prone
Energy density (kcal ME/g)	4.0-5.0	3.3-3.8
Energy density (kJ ME/g)	16.7-20.9	13.8-15.9
Fat (%)	10-30	9-17
Fiber (%)	<5	5-15
Protein (%)	30-45	30-45
Phosphorus (%)	0.5-0.8	0.5-0.8
Sodium (%)	0.2-0.6	0.2-0.6
Chloride (%)	1.5 x Na	1.5 x Na
Magnesium (%)	0.04-0.1	0.04-0.1
Average urinary pH	6.2-6.4	6.2-6.4
Antioxidants		
Vitamin E (IU/kg)	≥500	≥500
Vitamin C (mg/kg)	100-200	100-200
Selenium (mg/kg)	0.5-1.3	0.5-1.3
VOHC Seal of Acceptance	Plaque control	Plaque control

Key: ME = metabolizable energy, VOHC = Veterinary Oral Health Council (Chapter 36).
*Dry matter basis. Concentrations presume an energy density of 4.0 kcal/g. Levels should be corrected for foods with higher energy densities. Adjustment is unnecessary for foods with lower energy densities.

from feeding guides on the product label or by calculation (Appendix C). Feeding guidelines and calculations are estimates and may need to be adjusted for individual cats (see Followup below). Inform cat owners that a normal decline in food intake can occur from time to time and should not be confused with inappetence due to disease.

Consider How to Offer the Food. Both free-choice and food-restricted feeding methods have advantages and disadvantages (Appendix D). Although free-choice feeding is more popular, it is most likely to result in overeating in young adult cats. Owners often overestimate food needs and feed too much; most people do not recognize overweight/obesity in their own cat. Food-restricted feeding is better because it is less likely to cause overweight/obesity conditions; feeding at least twice daily is preferred. Cats will often return to the feeding bowl for several small feedings. A combination of dry and moist food is often used.

Manage Food Changes. Most healthy cats adapt well to new foods, but a transition period to avoid GI upsets and food refusal is good practice. Example: to change to a new food, replace 25% of the old food with the new food on Day 1 and continue this incremental change daily until the change is complete on Day 4. Appendix E provides additional information.

Food and Water Receptacle Husbandry. Food and water bowls should be washed regularly with warm soapy water and rinsed well. Dishes used for moist foods need daily cleaning. Discard moist or moistened dry foods after 2-4 hours of room temperature exposure to avoid foodborne illnesses (Appendix F). Consider shallow dishes for breeds with less prominent faces (e.g., Persians). For multi-cat households, individual feeding dishes placed at different levels provides a degree of privacy for low-status cats.

Table 3. Selected commercial foods for young adult cats (normal and

Dry foods	Energy density (kcal/cup)**
Recommended levels (normal body condition)	–
Hill's Science Diet Adult Hairball Control Feline	339
Hill's Science Diet Adult Optimal Care Ocean Fish & Rice Recipe	488
Hill's Science Diet Adult Oral Care Feline	337
Hill's Science Diet Nature's Best Ocean Fish & Brown Rice Dinner Adult	470
Iams Eukanuba Adult Chicken Formula	436
Iams Original with Chicken Cat Food	368
Nutro Max Cat Adult Roasted Chicken Flavor	421
Nutro Natural Choice Complete Care Adult	452
Purina ONE Natural Blends Chicken & Oat Meal Formula	450
Purina ONE Total Nutrition Salmon & Tuna Flavor	430
Purina Pro Plan Indoor Care Turkey & Rice Formula	433
Royal Canin Adult Fit 32	351

Moist foods	Energy density (kcal/can)**
Recommended levels (normal body condition)	–
Hill's Science Diet Adult Hairball Control Savory Chicken Entrée Minced	91/3 oz. 168/5.5 oz.
Hill's Science Diet Adult Indoor Cat Savory Chicken Entrée Minced	91/3 oz. 168/5.5 oz.
Hill's Science Diet Adult Optimal Care Gourmet Beef Entrée Minced	93/3 oz. 171/5.5 oz.
Nutro MAX Cat Gourmet Classics Adult Chicken & Liver Formula	169/5.5 oz.
Nutro Natural Choice Complete Care Adult Chicken & Liver Entrée	167/5.5 oz.
Purina Pro Plan Adult Cat Chicken & Rice Entrée in Gravy	78/3 oz.

Dry foods	Energy density (kcal/cup)**
Recommended levels (inactive/obese prone)	–
Hill's Science Diet Adult Hairball Control Light Feline	283
Hill's Science Diet Adult Indoor Cat	281
Hill's Science Diet Adult Light Feline	316
Hill's Science Diet Oral Care Adult Feline	337
Iams Eukanuba Adult Weight Control	315
Nutro Natural Choice Complete Care Indoor Weight Management	359
Nutro Natural Choice Complete Care Weight Management	308
Purina ONE Indoor Advantage Hairball & Healthy Weight Formula	416
Purina ONE Special Care Healthy Weight Formula	362
Purina Pro Plan Weight Management Formula	413
Royal Canin Indoor 27	324
Royal Canin Indoor Light 37	285

Moist foods	Energy density (kcal/can)**
Recommended levels (inactive/obese prone)	–
Hill's Science Diet Adult Indoor Cat Savory Seafood Entrée Minced	90/3 oz. 165/5.5 oz.
Hill's Science Diet Adult Light Liver & Chicken Entrée Minced	75/3 oz. 138/5.5 oz.
Nutro MAX Cat Gourmet Classics Lite with Chicken & Lamb	140/5.5 oz.

Key: ME = metabolizable energy, P = phosphorus, Na = sodium, Mg = magnesium, Se = selenium, VOHC = Veterinary Oral Health Council Seal of Acceptance (Chapter 36), na = information not available from manufacturer, g = grams.

inactive/obese prone) compared to recommended levels of key nutritional factors.* (Numbers in red match optimal KNFs.)

Energy density (kcal ME/g)	Fat (%)	Fiber (%)	Protein (%)	P (%)	Na (%)	Mg (%)	Urinary pH	Vit. E (IU/kg)	Vit. C (mg/kg)	VOHC Se (mg/kg)	plaque (Yes/No)
4.0-5.0	10-30	<5	30-45	0.5-0.8	0.2-0.6	0.04-0.1	6.2-6.4	≥500	100-200	0.5-1.3	Yes
4.1	22.1	8.1	34	0.69	0.31	0.053	6.3	705	119	0.79	No
4.3	22.7	1.2	34	0.72	0.27	0.065	6.3	1,042	197	0.86	No
4.2	22.0	7.5	34.1	0.75	0.37	0.058	6.3	670	171	0.55	Yes
4.3	20.6	1.2	33.9	0.74	0.33	0.088	6.2	739	270	0.83	No
4.4	23.6	1.4	38.5	0.99	0.55	na	na	na	na	na	No
4.1	17.3	1.8	37.3	1.06	0.50	0.109	na	na	na	na	No
4.2	20.9	2.2	36.3	1.1	0.44	0.082	na	132	38	0.49	No
4.3	22.0	2.7	37.4	1.1	0.44	0.088	na	330	88	0.77	No
4.4	17.9	1.9	37.9	1.44	0.60	na	na	na	na	na	No
4.4	15.7	1.8	37.9	1.29	0.52	na	na	na	na	na	No
4.2	15.2	5.3	46.0	1.28	0.48	0.110	na	na	na	na	No
4.2	16.5	8.1	35.2	1.12	0.66	0.121	na	604	220	0.49	No

Energy density (kcal ME/g)	Fat (%)	Fiber (%)	Protein (%)	P (%)	Na (%)	Mg (%)	Urinary pH	Vit. E (IU/kg)	Vit. C (mg/kg)	Se (mg/kg)	VOHC plaque (Yes/No)
4.0-5.0	10-30	<5	30-45	0.5-0.8	0.2-0.6	0.04-0.1	6.2-6.4	≥500	100-200	0.5-1.3	Yes
4.4	23.3	9.8	35.9	0.65	0.49	0.069	6.4	694	241	1.1	No
4.4	23.3	9.8	35.5	0.65	0.49	0.082	6.4	816	257	1.06	No
4.4	22	4.8	37.6	0.72	0.32	0.072	6.4	396	80	1.2	No
4.6	29.8	2.1	42.6	1.28	0.64	0.106	na	170	106	0.43	No
4.7	30.4	1.7	47.8	1.30	0.65	0.10	na	174	261	0.43	No
3.9	15.1	0.4	59.1	0.95	1.38	0.04	na	na	na	na	No

Energy density (kcal ME/g)	Fat (%)	Fiber (%)	Protein (%)	P (%)	Na (%)	Mg (%)	Urinary pH	Vit. E (IU/kg)	Vit. C (mg/kg)	Se (mg/kg)	VOHC plaque (Yes/No)
3.3-3.8	9-17	5-15	30-45	0.5-0.8	0.2-0.6	0.04-0.1	6.2-6.4	≥500	100-200	0.5-1.3	Yes
3.5	9.1	8.3	36	0.72	0.33	0.071	6.2-6.4	689	176	0.68	No
3.5	9.1	8.3	36	0.72	0.33	0.071	6.2	689	176	0.68	No
3.5	9.5	6.9	35.1	0.73	0.4	0.068	6.2	693	189	0.67	No
4.2	22	7.5	34.1	0.75	0.37	0.058	6.3	670	171	0.55	Yes
3.9	14.4	1.8	34.7	0.99	0.54	na	na	na	na	na	No
3.8	13.2	2.7	36.3	0.82	0.22	0.088	na	330	110	0.71	No
3.8	13.2	3.3	37.4	1.10	0.44	0.093	na	330	88	0.60	No
4.1	11.7	3.8	42.9	1.42	0.45	na	na	na	na	na	No
3.7	12.2	3.7	46.1	1.41	0.40	na	na	na	na	na	No
4.2	12.0	3.4	50.5	1.08	0.54	0.84	na	na	na	na	No
4.0	14.3	7.5	29.7	1.08	0.70	0.11	na	604	220	0.49	No
3.5	9.9	10.2	40.7	1.07	0.80	0.11	na	604	220	0.49	No

Energy density (kcal ME/g)	Fat (%)	Fiber (%)	Protein (%)	P (%)	Na (%)	Mg (%)	Urinary pH	Vit. E (IU/kg)	Vit. C (mg/kg)	Se (mg/kg)	VOHC plaque (Yes/No)
3.3-3.8	9-17	5-15	30-45	0.5-0.8	0.2-0.6	0.04-0.1	6.2-6.4	≥500	100-200	0.5-1.3	Yes
4.1	23	9.4	37.9	0.7	0.43	0.094	6.4	961	195	1.72	No
3.6	14.2	10.1	35.6	0.69	0.32	0.077	6.2	401	na	1.46	No
3.9	15.2	1.7	41.3	1.3	1.09	0.104	na	174	87	0.43	No

*From manufacturers' published information or calculated from manufacturers' published as fed values; all values are on a dry matter basis unless otherwise stated.

**Energy density values are listed on an as-fed basis and are useful for determining the amount to feed; cup = 8-oz. measuring cup. To convert to kJ, multiply kcal by 4.184.

FOLLOWUP

Owner Followup

Owners should weigh their cat (if possible) and/or determine its BCS monthly. If a trend of increasing or decreasing body weight or BCS is noticed, the amount fed should be changed by 10% increments and the cat rechecked every 2 weeks for 1 month. At that point, if necessary, the amount fed should be changed again and the cycle repeated.

Veterinary Health Care Team Followup

Healthy young adult cats should be examined every 6-12 months. More frequent assessment is recommended if homemade food is a significant part of a cat's total food intake.

MISCELLANEOUS

See Chapter 19, Small Animal Clinical Nutrition, 5th edition, for information about cats as carnivores; Appendix G provides information about apparently abnormal (alternative) eating behaviors. See Chapter 20, Small Animal Clinical Nutrition, 5th edition, for more information about feeding young adult cats.

Authors

Condensed from Chapter 20, Small Animal Clinical Nutrition, 5th edition, authored by Kathy L. Gross, Iveta Becvarova, P. Jane Armstrong and Jacques Debraekeleer.

References

See Chapter 20, Small Animal Clinical Nutrition, 5th edition, on the website www.markmorrisinstitute.org for references.

Chapter 8

Feeding Mature Adult Cats: Middle-Aged and Older

CLINICAL POINTS

- Cats 7-8 years of age and older are mature adults; this term includes cats considered to be "middle-aged," "senior" and "geriatric."
- Feeding goals: optimize quality and longevity of life (disease prevention).

KEY NUTRITIONAL FACTORS

- Foods should provide recommended allowances of all required nutrients (nutritional adequacy), but should also contain specific levels of KNFs (certain nutrients and nonnutritional food ingredients or food features that can influence important diseases).
- Table 1, Chapter 7, lists disease prevalences, which are increased in mature adult cats; adherence to respective KNF recommendations in this age group is even more important than in young adult cats.
- Table 1 lists KNF recommendations for foods for mature adult cats that are of normal body condition or inactive/obese prone. Relative to urinary pH produced by young adults, urinary pH produced by foods for mature adults should be increased because of the shift in FLUTD risk from struvite to calcium

Abbreviations

AAFCO = Association of American Feed Control Officials
BCS = body condition score (Appendix A)
CKD = chronic kidney disease
FLUTD = feline lower urinary tract disease
KNF = key nutritional factor

oxalate (**Figure 1**) and the decreased ability of older cats to buffer dietary acid due to subclinical CKD. Reduced renal concentrating ability may also predispose to dehydration. Thus, water is an important KNF. A detailed summary of KNF recommendations can be found in Chapters 20 and 21, Small Animal Clinical Nutrition, 5th edition.

FEEDING PLAN

Assess and Select the Food

Ensure the Food's Nutritional Adequacy. AAFCO nutritional adequacy statements are usually found on a product's label. AAFCO approval does not ensure the food will be effective in preventing long-term health problems.

Compare the Food's KNF Content with the Recommended Levels. Table 2 compares the KNF profiles for selected commercial foods. Contact the manufacturer for this information for foods not in this table (manufacturer contact information is listed on product labels). A new food should be selected if

Table 1. Key nutritional factors for foods for older cats.		
Factors	**Recommended food levels***	
	Normal and underweight	**Inactive/ obese prone**
Energy density (kcal ME/g)	4.0-4.5	3.5-4.0
Energy density (kJ ME/g)	16.7-18.8	14.6-16.7
Fat (%)	18-25	10-18
Fiber (%)	≤5	5-15
Protein (%)	30-45	30-45
Calcium (%)	0.6-1.0	0.6-1.0
Phosphorus (%)	0.5-0.7	0.5-0.7
Sodium (%)	0.2-0.4	0.2-0.4
Potassium (%)	≥0.6	≥0.6
Magnesium (%)	0.05-0.1	0.05-0.1
Average urinary pH	6.4-6.6	6.4-6.6
Antioxidants		
Vitamin E (IU/kg)	≥500	≥500
Vitamin C (mg/kg)	100-200	100-200
Selenium (mg/kg)	0.5-1.3	0.5-1.3
VOHC Seal of Acceptance	Plaque control	Plaque control

Key: ME = metabolizable energy, VOHC = Veterinary Oral Health Council (Chapter 36).
*Dry matter basis. Concentrations presume an energy density of 4.0 kcal/g. Levels should be corrected for foods with higher energy densities. Adjustment is unnecessary for foods with lower energy densities.

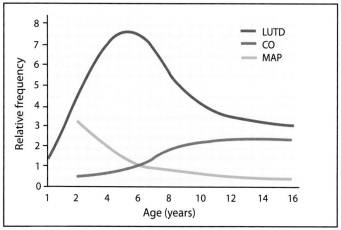

Figure 1. Relative frequency of feline lower urinary tract disease (LUTD), struvite (magnesium ammonium phosphate, MAP) urolithiasis and calcium oxalate (CO) urolithiasis in cats of varying age. Note that LUTD is most common in adult cats, struvite urolithiasis is most common in adult cats less than six years old and calcium oxalate urolithiasis is most common in cats over six years old. (Adapted from Bartges JW. Lower urinary tract disease in older cats: What's common, what's not. Veterinary Clinical Nutrition 1996; 3: 57-62. Thumchai R, Lulich JP, Osborne CA, et al. Epizootiologic evaluation of urolithiasis in cats: 3498 cases (1982-1992). Journal of the American Veterinary Medical Association 1996; 208: 547-551.)

Table 2. Comparison of recommended levels of key nutritional factors for foods for mature adult cats (normal/underweight and inactive/obese prone) with levels in selected commercial foods.* (Numbers in red match optimal KNFs.)

Dry foods	Energy density (kcal/cup)**	Energy density (kcal ME/g)	Fat (%)	Fiber (%)	Protein (%)	Ca (%)	P (%)	Na (%)	K (%)
Recommended levels (normal/underweight)	–	4.0-4.5	18-25	≤5	30-45	0.6-1.0	0.5-0.7	0.2-0.4	≥0.6
Hill's Science Diet Adult Oral Care	337	4.2	22	7.5	34.1	0.82	0.75	0.37	0.69
Hill's Science Diet Mature Adult Hairball Control	326	4.0	20	8	34	0.86	0.70	0.39	0.80
Hill's Science Diet Mature Adult Indoor	326	4.0	20.1	8	34	0.86	0.71	0.39	0.81
Iams Eukanuba Senior Mature Care	414	4.1	19.0	2.0	39.5	1.39	1.12	0.43	0.85
Nutro MAX Cat Senior Roasted Chicken Flavor	359	3.9	14.3	2.2	31.9	1.10	0.99	0.38	0.66
Nutro Natural Choice Complete Care Senior Cat Food	329	4.0	16.5	2.7	34.1	1.10	1.04	0.44	0.66
Purina Cat Chow Vitality 7+ Formula	397	4.1	13.7	5.4	37.6	1.49	1.32	0.40	0.71
Purina ONE Vibrant Maturity 7+ Senior Formula	437	4.4	16.0	1.7	42.0	1.65	1.39	0.48	0.90
Purina Pro Plan Senior 11+ Indoor Care Turkey & Rice Formula Cat Food	513	4.8	19.8	3.1	50.2	1.45	1.25	0.47	0.78
Royal Canin Mature 27	282	4.2	16.5	7.1	29.7	0.86	0.69	0.34	0.92

Moist foods	Energy density (kcal/can)**	Energy density (kcal ME/g)	Fat (%)	Fiber (%)	Protein (%)	Ca (%)	P (%)	Na (%)	K (%)
Recommended levels (normal/underweight)	–	4.0-4.5	18-25	≤5	30-45	0.6-1.0	0.5-0.7	0.2-0.4	≥0.6
Hill's Science Diet Mature Adult Active Longevity Gourmet Turkey Entrée Minced	87/3 oz. 160/5.5 oz.	4.1	20.1	4.8	34.5	0.96	0.64	0.28	0.84
Hill's Science Diet Mature Adult Active Longevity Savory Chicken Entrée Minced	91/3 oz. 168/5.5 oz.	4.4	23.3	3.7	39.2	1.02	0.69	0.49	0.82
Nutro Natural Choice Complete Care Indoor Senior Chicken & Lamb Formula	169/5.5 oz.	4.5	27.1	1.3	39.6	1.25	1.04	0.29	na

Dry foods	Energy density (kcal/cup)**	Energy density (kcal ME/g)	Fat (%)	Fiber (%)	Protein (%)	Ca (%)	P (%)	Na (%)	K (%)
Recommended levels (inactive/obese prone)	–	3.5-4.0	10-18	5-15	30-45	0.6-1.0	0.5-0.7	0.2-0.4	≥0.6
Hill's Science Diet Mature Adult Hairball Control	326	4.0	20	8	34	0.86	0.70	0.39	0.80
Hill's Science Diet Mature Adult Indoor Cat	326	4.0	20.1	8	34	0.86	0.71	0.39	0.81
Hill's Science Diet Adult Light	316	3.5	9.5	6.9	35.1	1.00	0.73	0.4	0.67
Iams Eukanuba Senior Mature Care	414	4.1	19.0	2.0	39.5	1.39	1.12	0.43	0.85
Nutro Natural Choice Complete Care Indoor Senior	364	4.0	16.5	2.7	34.1	1.32	0.88	0.38	0.71
Purina ONE Special Care Healthy Weight Formula	362	3.7	12.2	3.7	46.1	1.42	1.41	0.40	1.15
Purina Pro Plan Senior 11+ Indoor Care Turkey & Rice Formula	513	4.8	19.8	3.1	50.2	1.45	1.25	0.47	0.78
Purina Pro Plan Weight Management Formula	413	4.2	12.0	3.4	50.5	1.19	1.08	0.54	0.82
Royal Canin Indoor Light 37	285	3.5	9.9	10.2	40.7	1.16	1.07	0.80	0.68

Moist foods	Energy density (kcal/can)**	Energy density (kcal ME/g)	Fat (%)	Fiber (%)	Protein (%)	Ca (%)	P (%)	Na (%)	K (%)
Recommended levels (inactive/obese prone)	–	3.5-4.0	10-18	5-15	30-45	0.6-1.0	0.5-0.7	0.2-0.4	≥0.6
Hill's Science Diet Adult Light Liver & Chicken Entrée Minced	75/3 oz. 138/5.5 oz.	3.6	14.2	10.1	35.6	0.85	0.69	0.32	0.77
Nutro MAX Cat Gourmet Classics Lite with Chicken & Lamb	140/5.5 oz.	3.9	15.2	1.7	41.3	1.74	1.30	1.09	1.09
Nutro Natural Choice Complete Care Indoor Senior Chicken & Lamb Formula	169/5.5 oz.	4.5	27.1	1.3	39.6	1.25	1.04	0.29	na

Key: ME = metabolizable energy, g = grams, Ca = calcium, P = phosphorus, Na = sodium, K = potassium, Mg = magnesium, VOHC = Veterinary Oral Health Council Seal of Acceptance (plaque control, Chapter 36), na = information not available from the manufacturer.
*From manufacturers' published information or calculated from manufacturers' published as fed values; all values are on a dry matter basis unless otherwise stated.
**Energy density values are listed on an as-fed basis and are useful for determining the amount to feed; cup = 8-oz. measuring cup. To convert to kJ, multiply kcal by 4.184.

discrepancies are noted; the new food should best approximate recommended KNF levels.

Manage Treats and Snacks. If treats/snacks are fed, commercial treats that match the nutritional profile recommended for mature adult cats (see product label) are best. Otherwise, treats/snacks should not be fed excessively (<10% of the total diet on a volume, weight or calorie basis). See Appendix B for more information about treats/snacks.

Assess and Determine the Feeding Method
Determine How Much Food to Feed. Intake levels of basic nutrients and KNFs are determined by the amounts in food and by how much food is consumed. If the patient has an ideal BCS (2.5/5 to 3.5/5), the amount being fed is probably appropriate. The amount of a new food can be estimated from feeding guides on product labels or by calculation (Appendix C). Feeding guidelines and calculations are estimates and may need to be

Mg (%) 0.05-0.1	Urinary pH 6.4-6.6	Vit. E (IU/kg) ≥500	Vit. C (mg/kg) 100-200	Se (mg/kg) 0.5-1.3	VOHC plaque (Yes/No) Yes
0.06	6.3	670	171	0.7	Yes
0.06	6.6	940	133	0.8	No
0.07	6.6	940	193	0.6	No
na	na	na	na	na	No
0.088	na	330	88	0.9	No
0.088	na	330	99	0.6	No
0.12	na	na	na	na	No
na	na	na	na	na	No
0.09	na	na	na	na	No
0.12	na	725	330	0.4	No
Mg (%) 0.05-0.1	**Urinary pH 6.4-6.6**	**Vit. E (IU/kg) ≥500**	**Vit. C (mg/kg) 100-200**	**Se (mg/kg) 0.5-1.3**	**VOHC plaque (Yes/No) Yes**
0.07	6.5	217	na	1.0	No
0.07	6.5	241	na	1.2	No
na	na	na	na	na	No
Mg (%) 0.05-0.1	**Urinary pH 6.4-6.6**	**Vit. E (IU/kg) ≥500**	**Vit. C (mg/kg) 100-200**	**Se (mg/kg) 0.5-1.3**	**VOHC plaque (Yes/No) Yes**
0.06	6.6	940	133	0.8	No
0.07	6.6	940	193	0.6	No
0.07	6.2	693	189	0.7	No
na	na	na	na	na	No
0.09	na	330	104	0.9	No
na	na	na	na	na	No
0.09	na	na	na	na	No
0.84	na	na	na	na	No
0.11	na	604	220	0.5	No
Mg (%) 0.05-0.1	**Urinary pH 6.4-6.6**	**Vit. E (IU/kg) ≥500**	**Vit. C (mg/kg) 100-200**	**Se (mg/kg) 0.5-1.3**	**VOHC plaque (Yes/No) Yes**
0.08	6.2	401	na	1.5	No
0.10	na	174	87	0.5	No
na	na	na	na	na	No

adjusted (see Followup below). Although a normal decline in food intake can occur, continued inappetence in mature adult cats is more likely due to disease than in younger cats.

Consider How to Offer the Food. Both free-choice and food-restricted feeding methods have advantages (Appendix D). Free-choice feeding is more popular, but may result in overeating. Owners often overestimate food needs and feed too much; most people do not recognize overweight/obesity in their own cat.

Free-choice feeding may be preferred for underweight, very old cats to facilitate increased food intake. For food-restricted feeding, feeding at least twice/day is preferred. Cats will often return for several small feedings. A combination of dry and moist food is often used. Warming moist foods or adding low-salt broth to dry foods may enhance food and water intake.

Manage Food Changes. Most healthy cats adapt well to new foods but a transition period to avoid GI upsets and food refusal is good practice. Example: to change to a new food, replace 25% of the old food with the new food on Day 1 and continue this incremental change daily until the change is complete on Day 4. Appendix E provides additional information.

Food and Water Receptacle Husbandry. Wash food and water bowls regularly and rinse well. Dishes used for moist foods need daily cleaning. Discard moist or moistened dry foods after 2-4 hours of room temperature exposure to avoid foodborne illnesses (Appendix F). Consider shallow dishes for breeds with less prominent faces (e.g., Persians). Individual feeding dishes placed at different levels provide a degree of privacy for low-status cats.

FOLLOWUP

Owner Followup

Owners should weigh their cat (if possible) and/or determine its BCS monthly. If a trend of increasing or decreasing body weight or BCS is noticed, the amount fed should be changed by 10% increments and the cat should be rechecked every 2 weeks for 1 month. At that point, if necessary, the amount fed should be changed again and the cycle repeated. Lean body mass tends to decline as cats reach ~16 years of age; rapid loss of body condition/weight warrant evaluation by a veterinarian.

Veterinary Health Care Team Followup

Healthy mature adult cats should be examined every 6-12 months, usually more frequently than young adults. Even more frequent assessments are recommended if homemade food is a significant part of a cat's total food intake.

MISCELLANEOUS

See Chapters 19 and 21, Small Animal Clinical Nutrition, 5th edition, for information about cats as carnivores and feeding mature cats. Appendix G has information about apparently abnormal (alternative) eating behaviors.

Authors

Condensed from Chapter 21, Small Animal Clinical Nutrition, 5th edition, authored by Kathy L. Gross, Iveta Becvarova and Jacques Debraekeleer.

References

See Chapter 21, Small Animal Clinical Nutrition, 5th edition, on the website www.markmorrisinstitute.org for references.

CLINICAL POINTS

- Reproducing cats: breeding studs and queens that are involved in mating, gestation or lactation.
- Feeding goals: optimize conception, litter size, parturition and kitten viability.
- Mating: no special nutritional needs; tomcats and queens with a normal BCS should be fed as sexually intact young adults (Chapter 7). It is best to breed only queens and tomcats with a normal healthy BCS (3/5). Queens with BCS <2/5 or >4/5 should not be bred.
- Mating: undernourished queens may fail to conceive, abort or may bear small, underweight kittens and have markedly reduced lactation. Obesity is detrimental to reproductive performance (e.g., stillbirths, dystocia). Small variations in BCS can be corrected during pregnancy.
- Gestation: queens fed marginally adequate foods during early gestation experience impaired conception rates and in utero fetal viability.
- Gestation: a steady, linear gain in body weight is an early indicator of conception (**Figure 1**). Normal weight gain during gestation is 700-900 g. At parturition, much of weight gained will not be lost and is used to help sustain lactation.
- Lactation: success depends on the BCS before breeding and adequate nutrition throughout gestation and lactation.
- Lactation: kittens should nurse within the first 6-8 hours to

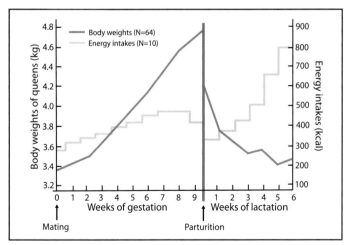

Figure 1. Body weight and energy intake during gestation and lactation in queens. Unlike bitches, which have a dramatic increase in energy intake and body weight during the last trimester, queens have a regular linear increase in both body weight and energy intake throughout gestation. Mobilized stores of body fat provide needed energy during lactation, which accounts for weight loss during this period. Food intake parallels lactation and peaks during the sixth to seventh week. (Adapted from Loveridge GG. Body weight changes and energy intake of cats during gestation and lactation. Animal Technology 1985; 37: 7-15.)

Abbreviations
AAFCO = Association of American Feed Control Officials
BCS = body condition score (Appendix A)
Ig = immunoglobulin
KNF = key nutritional factor

ensure transfer of colostral antibodies; unlike puppies, after 16 hours postpartum Ig absorption is greatly curtailed.
- Encouraging kittens to eat solid food by 3 weeks of age will reduce the queen's nutritional needs.

KEY NUTRITIONAL FACTORS

During lactation a queen's nutrient demands are greater than at any other adult lifestage. **Table 1** summarizes KNFs for breeding males and females and for pregnant and lactating queens. A detailed description of these recommendations can be found in Chapter 22, Small Animal Clinical Nutrition, 5th edition. Water is an often overlooked KNF and is needed in large quantities for lactation.

FEEDING PLAN

Assess and Select the Food

Ensure the Food's Nutritional Adequacy. AAFCO nutritional adequacy statements are usually found on a product's label and should ensure that the product is intended for gestation/lactation. Many of these foods are also marketed for kitten growth and are sometimes referred to as growth/reproduction-type foods or foods for all lifestages. It is best to feed this type of food throughout gestation and lactation. If possible, transition to this type of food at least 1 week before breeding (see Manage Food Changes below).

Compare the Food's KNF Content with the Recommended Levels. **Table 2** compares the KNF profiles for selected commercial foods. Contact manufacturers for this information for foods not in the table (manufacturer contact information is listed on product labels). A new food should be selected if discrepancies are noted; the new food should best approximate the recommended KNF levels.

Dry Foods vs. Moist Foods. Semi-moist foods may produce urinary pH values below desired levels for reproducing queens. Dry foods are more nutrient dense, as fed, and have higher levels of carbohydrates. Dry foods may benefit queens experiencing weight loss and those spending little time eating. Moist foods are often higher in fat and provide additional water to support lactation. They may be more palatable to some cats. Feeding both forms during gestation and lactation is an accepted practice. If both dry and moist foods are fed, it may be desirable to feed dry foods free choice and provide multiple moist food meals daily. Feeding moist foods or adding water to food can improve water intake.

Manage Treats and Snacks. If treats or snacks from human foods are fed, commercial treats that match the nutritional profile recommended for gestation/lactation or growth (see product label) are best. Otherwise, treats/snacks should not be fed excessively (<10% of the total diet on a volume, weight or calorie basis). See Appendix B for more information about treats/snacks.

Assess and Determine the Feeding Method
Determine How Much Food to Feed.

BREEDING TOMCATS. Feed the same amount as is fed to intact adult cats (Chapter 7). Some tomcats in heavy service may have inadequate food intake and lose weight; in these cases, increase the amount fed and/or switch to a more energy-dense food (also rule out other possible causes of weight loss).

QUEENS DURING ESTRUS. Feed the same amount as intact adult cats (Chapter 7). Queens tend to have a depressed appetite during estrus and a decrease in food intake can be expected.

QUEENS DURING GESTATION. Unless obese prone, gestating queens should be allowed to eat as much as they want. Near the end of gestation, food intake is typically increased by 40%. Expect a normal decrease in appetite at about Day 15 of gestation and a more pronounced decline during the last week (**Figure 1**).

QUEENS DURING LACTATION. At peak lactation, a queen's energy needs may be 2.5-3 times greater than requirements for adult maintenance, depending in part on litter size. Do not underfeed. If they maintain a normal BCS (2.5/5 to 3.5/5) and kitten growth rate is normal, the amount being fed is appropriate. The amount to feed can be estimated by calculation (Appendix C) or by referring to feeding guides on product labels. Lactating queens should eat as much as they want.

QUEENS DURING WEANING. Reducing the amount of food fed will help decrease lactation, which helps prevent excessive mammary gland distention/discomfort (Table 6, Chapter 10).
Consider How to Offer the Food.
QUEENS DURING ESTRUS. Free choice is best; food intake often declines due to a variety of stressors.

QUEENS DURING GESTATION. Free choice is best. Obese-prone queens should be fed 3-4 meals per day in controlled portions. Obese queens (BCS ≥4/5) should be fed similarly; they should not be fed to lose weight.

QUEENS DURING LACTATION. Free choice is best. Kittens may begin eating the queen's food at 3-4 weeks of age. Even with this help, queens typically lose weight throughout lactation (**Figure 1**) to near prebreeding weight. Queens with large litters that experience excessive weight loss during lactation should be given additional food to restore body condition before the next breeding. Matted abdominal hair can interfere with nursing in longhaired queens; remove hair accordingly.

Manage Food Changes. Most healthy cats adapt well to new foods but a transition period to avoid GI upsets or food refusal

Table 1. Key nutritional factors for foods for reproducing cats.

Factors (units)*	Mating**	Gestation/lactation
Energy density (kcal ME/g)	4.0-5.0	4.0-5.0
Energy density (kJ ME/g)	16.7-20.9	16.7-20.9
Protein (%)	30-45	35-50
Fat (%)	10-30	18-35
DHA (%)	-	≥0.004
Digestible carbohydrate (%)***	-	≥10
Calcium (%)	-	1.1-1.6
Phosphorus (%)	0.5-0.7	0.8-1.4
Ca:P ratio	-	1:1-1.5:1
Sodium (%)	0.2-0.5	0.3-0.6
Average urinary pH	6.2-6.4	6.2-6.5

Key: ME = metabolizable energy, DHA = docosahexaenoic acid.
*Units expressed on a dry matter basis. Concentrations presume an energy density of 4.0 kcal/g. Levels should be corrected for foods with higher energy densities. Adjustment is unnecessary for foods with lower energy densities.
**Foods for most breeding males and females are usually similar to those for young adult cats (Chapter 7).
***Important for lactation.

is good practice. Example: to change to a new food, replace 25% of the old food with the new food on Day 1 and continue this incremental change daily until the change is complete on Day 4. Appendix E provides additional information.

Food and Water Receptacle Husbandry. Food and water bowls should be washed regularly with warm soapy water and rinsed well. Dishes used for moist foods need daily cleaning. Discard moist or moistened dry foods after 2-4 hours of room temperature exposure to avoid foodborne illnesses (Appendix F). Use care when placing water bowls near neonates to avoid accidental drowning.

FOLLOWUP

Owner Followup
Counseling owners is important because assessment is often performed without direct veterinary supervision. Breeders can be taught to assess body condition. During gestation, body condition assessment should ignore the abdominal component and focus on muscle mass and fat covering ribs and bony prominences (Appendix A). Stools may normally vary from soft to firm during reproduction. Constipation and diarrhea are always considered abnormal.

Queens During Gestation. Owners should note food intake, body weight and the BCS weekly. Inadequate nutrition may be overlooked if body weight is the only monitoring criterion used. Underfed queens may gain weight as the fetuses develop but fail to develop the energy reserves needed for lactation.

Queens/Kittens During Lactation. Kitten growth rate and rate of weight loss in queens indicate food/feeding method adequacy. Weigh queens and kittens within 24 hours after parturition. Queens should weigh 700-900 g above pre-breeding weight and kittens should weigh 85-120 g each. The queen's appetite, which

Table 2. Comparison of recommended key nutritional factor levels in selected commercial foods for reproducing (gestation and lactation) queens to recommended levels.* (Numbers in red match optimal KNFs.)

Dry foods	Energy density (kcal/cup)**	Energy density (kcal ME/g)	Protein (%)	Fat (%)	DHA (%)	Carbohydrate (%)***	Ca (%)	P (%)	Ca:P ratio	Na (%)	Urinary pH
Recommended levels	–	4.0-5.0	35-50	18-35	≥0.004	≥10	1.1-1.6	0.8-1.4	1:1-1.5:1	0.3-0.6	6.2-6.5
Hill's Science Diet Kitten Healthy Development Original	510	4.5	42.3	26.1	0.24	22.2	1.3	1.1	1.1:1	0.39	6.4
Hill's Science Diet Kitten Indoor	510	4.5	42.2	26.1	0.24	22.3	1.3	1.1	1.1:1	0.39	6.4
Hill's Science Diet Nature's Best Chicken & Brown Rice Dinner Kitten	487	4.4	37.6	26.0	0.26	27.6	1.45	1.2	1.2:1	0.46	6.4
Hill's Science Diet Nature's Best Ocean Fish & Brown Rice Dinner Kitten	487	4.4	38.0	26.3	0.23	26.6	1.4	1.1	1.2:1	0.59	6.4
Iams Eukanuba Chicken Formula Kitten	469	4.5	40.0	25.7	na	25.4	1.3	1.1	1.2:1	0.43	na
Iams Kitten	470	5.0	37.8	24.6	na	28.4	1.15	0.9	1.2:1	0.54	na
Nutro Natural Choice Complete Care Kitten	463	4.4	40.7	24.2	0.077	25.3	1.3	1.2	1.1:1	0.44	na
Purina Kitten Chow	457	4.5	44.8	15.6	na	30.8	1.4	1.42	1:1	0.56	na
Purina ONE Healthy Kitten Formula	512	4.8	45.5	21.1	na	24.8	1.3	1.2	1.1:1	0.40	na
Purina Pro Plan Kitten Chicken & Rice Formula	472	4.3	46.0	20.1	na	26.6	1.3	1.2	1.1:1	0.42	na
Royal Canin Babycat 34 Formula	531	4.8	37.4	27.5	na	21.6	1.3	1.1	1.1:1	0.64	na
Royal Canin Kitten 34 Formula	393	4.6	37.4	22.0	na	26.5	1.25	1.1	1.1:1	0.67	na

Moist foods	Energy density (kcal/can)**	Energy density (kcal ME/g)	Protein (%)	Fat (%)	DHA (%)	Carbohydrate (%)***	Ca (%)	P (%)	Ca:P ratio	Na (%)	Urinary pH
Recommended levels	–	4.0-5.0	35-50	18-35	≥0.004	≥10	1.1-1.6	0.8-1.4	1:1-1.5:1	0.3-0.6	6.2-6.5
Hill's Science Diet Kitten Healthy Development Liver & Chicken Entrée Minced	114/3 oz. 210/5.5 oz.	4.7	49.3	23.9	0.243	16.2	1.3	1.0	1.4:1	0.32	6.4
Hill's Science Diet Tender Chunks in Gravy Real Chicken Dinner Kitten	84/3 oz. (pouch)	4.3	47.8	22.6	0.087	19.5	1.2	1.1	1.1:1	0.43	6.3

Key: ME = metabolizable energy, DHA = docosahexaenoic acid, Ca = calcium, P = phosphorus, Na = sodium, na = not available from manufacturer.
*From manufacturers' published information or calculated from manufacturers' published as fed values; all values are on a dry matter basis unless otherwise stated. Digestibility: Foods with higher energy density are more likely to have higher digestibility. Foods for most breeding males and females are usually similar to those for young and middle-aged adults (Chapter 7).
**Energy density values are listed on an as-fed basis and are useful for determining the amount to feed; cup = 8-oz. measuring cup. To convert to kJ, multiply kcal by 4.184.
***Important for lactation.

is reduced 24-48 hours before parturition, should return to normal or to an increased level within 24 hours after parturition. Healthy nursing kittens gain about 100 g/week or 10-15 g/day. Weight gains less than 7 g/day require immediate evaluation of the food, the queen and the kittens. If milk production is inadequate, kittens will be restless and cry excessively. Aerophagia can give the appearance of gastric fullness in kittens, despite inadequate milk intake.

Breeding Tomcats and Queens. Optimal body weight and condition should be achieved before the next breeding.

Table 3. Eclampsia (puerperal tetany) in the queen.

1. Acute, uncommon, life-threatening condition due to a sudden decrease in extracellular calcium.
2. Timing: unlike dogs, highest risk is during the last 3 weeks of pregnancy; should be considered as a diagnostic rule out in queens with vague signs of illness in late gestation.
3. Usually queens with relatively large litters.
4. Often nonspecific clinical signs of lethargy, depression, weakness, tachypnea, mild muscle tremors, vomiting, anorexia, hypothermia, flaccid paralysis, hyperexcitability and other signs of malaise.
5. Low serum ionized calcium (<0.8 mmol/l); blood glucose should also be measured because hypoglycemia may be present concurrently.
6. Suggested cause: excessive dietary calcium supplementation during pregnancy (may down-regulate parathyroid gland secretion, impairing calcium mobilization from skeletal stores; as calcium demand increases during late gestation, serum calcium homeostasis cannot be maintained).
7. Initial treatment: slow IV infusion (10-30 minutes) of 10% calcium gluconate (0.5-1.5 ml/kg) is given to effect. Monitor heart rate and stop infusion temporarily or discontinue if bradycardia or dysrhythmias develop. Glucose may be administered by intravenous bolus (50% solution; 1 ml/kg over 1-3 minutes) or intravenous infusion (5% glucose in saline; 2 ml/kg/hour) to correct hypoglycemia, if present.
8. After correction of acute signs, oral supplementation of calcium carbonate (10-30 mg/kg every 8 hours) is begun and continued throughout gestation and lactation.
9. If eclampsia is diagnosed following parturition, separate kittens from the queen for 24 hours and feed them feline milk replacer by bottle or orogastric tube (Chapter 10).
10. Unlike puppies, it is rarely necessary to wean kittens early.
11. Recurrence has not been reported in cats.

Veterinary Health Care Team Followup

If owners are reluctant to perform certain parts of the above recommendations, the veterinarian should be involved as much as is practical; minimal involvement should include pregnancy diagnosis, another exam 1 week before parturition and again at Weeks 3-4 of lactation. For the next breeding, a prebreeding or interestrous exam might allow problems to be corrected before breeding. Eclampsia in queens is uncommon (**Table 3**).

MISCELLANEOUS

See Chapters 20 and 22, Small Animal Clinical Nutrition, 5th edition, for more information.

Authors

Condensed from Chapter 22, Small Animal Clinical Nutrition, 5th edition, authored by Kathy L. Gross, Iveta Becvarova and Jacques Debraekeleer.

References

See Chapter 22, Small Animal Clinical Nutrition, 5th edition, on the website www.markmorrisinstitute.org for references.

CLINICAL POINTS

- Feeding goal: through proper feeding and husbandry, produce healthy, viable weaned kittens.
- Mortality is 9-63%; low birth weights (<75 g) correlate with very high mortality rates.
- Proper medical, husbandry and nutritional practices are closely intertwined; see Chapter 23, Small Animal Clinical Nutrition, 5th edition, for nonnutritional kitten health management recommendations.
- Orphans can be raised successfully with proper nutrition and husbandry practices.
- Kittens that are orphaned, rejected or cannot be raised by the queen can be fed by fostering, partial orphan rearing or handfeeding.
- Fostering: least labor intensive, best nutrition, lower mortality and better immune status, physical environment and social development.
- Partial orphan rearing: allows kittens to stay with the dam in a normal environment and facilitates natural socialization.
- Handfeeding: most common method of feeding orphaned kittens; typically, eyedroppers, syringes, bottles or stomach tubes are used.
- Weaning: important, stressful time for kittens and the queen; use a good process.

Abbreviations
AAFCO = Association of American Feed Control Officials
BCS = body condition score (Appendix A)
DER = daily energy requirement (Appendix C)
Ig = immunoglobulin
KNF = key nutritional factor

KEY NUTRITIONAL FACTORS

- Mature milk: complete (including water) food for neonates. The nutrient composition of milk (**Table 1**) is designed to support the normal growth of neonates and its nutrient content represents the KNFs for foods for nursing/orphaned kittens.
- Colostrum: mammary secretion during the 1-3 days postpartum after which time it changes to mature milk. Along with nutrients (**Table 1**), colostrum provides growth factors, digestive enzymes and Ig. However, the Ig levels in cat colostrum and mature milk may not be as different as those from other species. Ensure colostrum or milk intake by kittens within the first 6-8 hours for adequate Ig uptake; after 16 hours, passive Ig transfer is greatly diminished in kittens. Sterile serum may be given SQ to kittens if queen's colostrum/milk is unavailable (see Chapter 23, Small Animal Clinical Nutrition, 5th edition).

Table 1. Nutrient comparison among queen's colostrum, queen's milk and milk of selected species.

Nutrients	Queen's colostrum*	Queen's milk*	Bitch's milk**	Cow's milk***	Goat's milk***
Moisture (g/100 g)	–	79	77.3	87.7	87.0
Dry matter (g/100 g)	–	21	22.7	12.3	13
Crude protein (g/100 g)	8.3	7.5	7.5	3.3	3.6
Arginine (mg/100 g)	357	347	420	119	119
Taurine (mg/100 g)	26	27	–	0.13	–
Methionine (mg/100 g)	202	188	–	82	80
Crude fat (g/100 g)	9.3	8.5	9.5	3.6	4.1
Lactose (g/100 g)	3.0	4.0	3.3	4.7	4.0
Minerals					
Calcium (mg/100 g)	46	180	240	119	133
Phosphorus (mg/100 g)	114	162	180	93	111
Potassium (mg/100 g)	–	103	120	150	204
Magnesium (mg/100 g)	11	9	11	14	14
Copper (mg/100 g)	0.04	0.11	0.33	–	–
Iron (mg/100 g)	0.19	0.35	0.70	0.05	0.05
ME (kcal/100 g)	130	121	146	64	69
ME (kJ/100 g)	544	506	610	268	288

Key: ME = metabolizable energy.
*Adapted from Adkins Y, Zicker SC, Lepine A, et al. Changes in nutrient and protein composition of cat milk during lactation. American Journal of Veterinary Research 1997; 58: 370-375. Zottman B, Dobenecker B, Kienzle E, et al. Investigations on milk composition and milk yield in queens (abstract). In: Proceedings. The Waltham International Symposium, Orlando, FL, 1997.
**Adapted from Meyer H, Kienzle E, Dammers C. Milchmenge und Milchzusammensetzung bei und Hündin sowie Futteraufnahme und Gewichtsenwicklung ante und post partum.Fortschritte in der Tierphysiologie und tierernährung (Advances in Animal Physiology and Animal Nutrition) 1985; Suppl. No. 16: 51-72.
***Adapted from Pennington JA. Food Values of Portions Commonly Used. New York, NY: Harper Collins, 1989.

FEEDING PLAN

Assess and Select the Food

Nursing Kittens. Milk from a healthy queen is the food of choice. Insufficient milk production and/or deficient milk quality may result in failure of kittens to grow (see Followup below), weakness, abdominal enlargement and abnormal behavior (e.g., restlessness, continuous vocalization). If these signs are present, the queen's body condition and feeding plan should be assessed (Chapter 9).

Orphaned Kittens. Milk from a healthy queen is the food of choice but is rarely available. **Table 2** lists selected commercial milk replacers and compares their nutrient profiles to queen's milk. **Table 3** lists 2 homemade recipes and **Table 4** compares their nutrient profiles to queen's milk. Commercial (preferred) and homemade milk replacers should closely mimic the profile of queen's milk. Unsupplemented ruminant milk may be used as a base for homemade formulas but by itself doesn't meet the needs of kittens; goat's milk provides no more benefits than cow's milk.

Weaning. Food for weaning should be a good quality growth/reproduction-type food such as the lactating queen's food (Table 2, Chapter 9 and Table 2, Chapter 11).

Food Form. Foods should be liquid until nursing kittens and orphans are 3-4 weeks old after which semisolid to solid foods may be introduced; nursing kittens voluntarily start eating the queen's food at this age.

Assess and Determine the Feeding Method

Nursing Kittens. If necessary, to ensure colostrum ingestion during the first 12 hours, position kittens on the queen's nipples. Week 1, kittens should nurse 6-12 times/day; after Week 1, at least 4-6 times/day. Hypothermic (<35°C [95°F]) kittens will not suckle and may also be hypoglycemic. If kittens fail to respond to warming, provide 2.5% glucose (1 ml/30 g) SQ; repeat as necessary until the suckling reflex returns.

Orphaned Kittens.

FOSTERING. Best method for feeding orphaned or rejected kittens; queens readily accept additional kittens during lactation. The orphans and the queen's own kittens should have no more than 14 days age difference, otherwise large kittens may crowd out smaller ones. Feeding may need to be supervised until orphans can fend for themselves. Initially, owners should observe for signs of rejection or impending cannibalism by the dam. Kittens should be accepted immediately and allowed to nurse. Foster mothers should be well fed.

PARTIAL ORPHAN REARING. Kittens that cannot be raised by the queen may be left with the mother but given supplemental feeding, including handfeeding (see below) or timed feedings using a surrogate queen. Kittens may also be reared communally by dividing a litter into 2 equal groups. One group remains with the queen while the other is removed and fed milk replacer. The groups are exchanged 3-4 times/day. Always feed the separated group just before it is returned to the queen so the kittens will be less inclined to immediately nurse. Partial orphan rearing may be necessary to assist a foster mother.

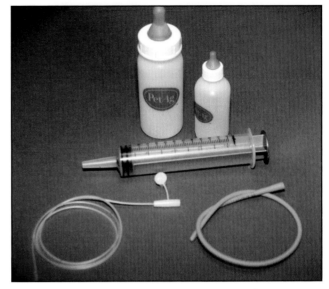

Figure 1. Various bottles and feeding tubes can be used for hand-feeding orphaned kittens.

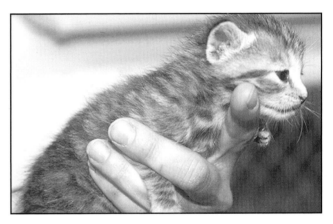

Figure 2. Kittens should be held horizontally in the palm of the hand for tube feeding.

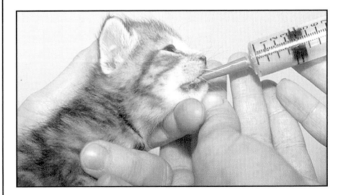

Figure 3. A lubricated tube is gently advanced to the premeasured mark and warm formula is administered over several minutes. The tube should be withdrawn and repositioned if resistance or struggling is encountered.

Table 2. Nutrient content of milk replacers compared with that of queen's milk/100 grams of milk, as fed.*

Nutrients** Manufacturer	Queen's milk -	KMR Liquid PetAg	KMR Reconstituted Powder PetAg	Nurturall C Kitten Liquid[†] VPL	Nurturall-C Reconstituted Powder[†] VPL	Just Born Kitten --Liquid[†] Farnam	Just Born Reconstituted Powder[†] Farnam
Dilution***	na	na	1+2	na	1+1	na	1+1.33
Moisture (g)	79.0	81.7	na	80.1	74.0	80.1	79.1
Dry matter (g)	21.0	18.3	na	19.9	26.0	19.9	21.0
Crude protein (g)	7.5	7.7	7.7	7.7	9.8	7.7	7.9
Arginine (mg)	430	250	310	200	240	200	195
Taurine (mg)	10	10	10	na	na	na	na
Fat (g)	8.5	4.7	4.7	4.4	5.4	4.4	4.5
Linoleic acid (C18:2) (g)	na	na	0.31	na	na	na	na
Arachidonic acid (C20:4) (mg)	na	na	20	na	na	na	na
Carbohydrate							
NFE (g)	na	4.7	3.6	6.2	8.7	6.2	7.0
Lactose (g)	4.0	na	3.1	na	na	na	na
Crude fiber (g)	na	0	0	<0.1	<0.1	<0.1	<0.1
Minerals							
Total ash (g)	0.6	1.2	1.4	1.5	2.1	1.5	1.7
Calcium (mg)	180	190	200	252	373	252	300
Phosphorus (mg)	162	160	200	220	287	220	231
Sodium (mg)	90	80	70	na	na	na	na
Potassium (mg)	103	210	190	102	308	102	248
Magnesium (mg)	9.0	16.0	14.2	18.4	31.5	18.4	25.3
Copper (mg)	0.11	0.26	0.27	0.40	0.73	0.40	0.58
Iron (mg)	0.4	1.2	1.4	0.4	5.5	0.4	4.4
Energy							
ME (kcal)	121	83	79	86	111	86	91
ME (kJ)	505	347	332	360	464	360	379
Osmolarity (mOsm/kg, H_2O±SD)	329±18.7	na	na	na	na	na	na
Nutrient content of milk replacers compared with that of queen's milk/100 kcal metabolizable energy[††]							
Crude protein (g)	6.3	9.3	9.7	9.0	8.9	9.0	8.7
Fat (g)	7.1	5.6	5.9	5.1	4.9	5.1	5.0
Linoleic acid (C18:2)	>1.1	na	390	na	na	na	na
Carbohydrate							
NFE (g)	na	5.71	4.54	7.21	7.85	7.21	7.71
Lactose (g)	3.3	na	3.9	na	na	na	na
Minerals							
Total ash (g)	0.5	1.4	1.8	1.7	1.9	1.7	1.8
Calcium (mg)	150.0	230	250	293	336	293	331
Phosphorus (mg)	135	190	250	256	259	256	255
Sodium (mg)	75	100	90	na	na	na	na
Potassium (mg)	86	250	240	119	278	119	273
Magnesium (mg)	7.5	19.3	17.9	21.4	28.4	21.4	27.9
Copper (mg)	0.10	0.31	0.34	0.50	0.66	0.47	0.64
Iron (mg)	0.3	1.4	1.7	0.5	5.0	0.5	4.9

Key: na = not applicable/available, NFE = nitrogen-free extract, ME = metabolizable energy, mOsm = milliosmoles.
*Manufacturers' data; nutrient content for reconstituted powdered products are manufacturers' calculations based on the recommended dilution. Nutrient data per 100 ml would be reduced slightly (between 1 to 2%), because the specific gravity of milk is greater than that of water.
**g/100 g = %.
***The first number is the milk powder, the second the water (e.g., 1+2 = one part of powder plus two parts of water).
[†]Nutrients in liquid and powder forms are averages from the yearly laboratory analyses of composite samples from 2004 to date.
[††]The nutrient levels per 100 kcal ME were calculated from the nutrient and energy levels in the top portion of the table.

HANDFEEDING.

Bottle Feeding. Bottle feeding is more successful in vigorous kittens with good nursing reflexes. Bottle-fed neonates will nurse until satiated and reject the formula when full. Bottle feeding can be time consuming, especially with large litters. Most kittens will readily suckle small pet nursing bottles available in pet stores (**Figure 1**). Nursing bottles for dolls or bottles for premature human infants are alternatives.

Only 1 drop at a time should fall from the nipple of an inverted bottle. Fluid should be sucked, never squeezed from the bottle. Too rapid flow may cause aspiration, choking and pneumonia.

Kittens should be held horizontally with the head in a natural position (Figure 1, Chapter 4), which reduces aspiration risk. Kittens that prefer a different position (Figure 2, Chapter 4) should be observed closely because the risk of aspiration is increased.

Tube Feeding. Kittens that are weak/suckle poorly may be tube fed. Tube feeding is faster than bottle feeding and is often used when 1 person must care for several orphans. Bottle feeding allows kittens to control the amount of food intake, whereas tube feeding bypasses this control mechanism. Infant feeding tubes (5-8 Fr.) or soft urethral or intravenous catheters are used (**Figure 1**).

Measure and mark the tube before insertion so that its tip will be in the lower esophagus (~75% of the distance from the nose to the last rib). Recheck the mark every few days to allow for growth.

During feeding, position orphans as in **Figure 2**. Lubricate the tube and open the mouth with the same hand that steadies the head. Gently advance the tube to the mark. The tube may be in the trachea if resistance is encountered or the kitten struggles. After proper tube placement, attach the syringe and gently administer the warmed formula over 1-2 minutes (**Figure 3**).

Palpate the stomach to determine the degree of distention. Stop delivery if the stomach becomes taut or there is resistance to formula flow. If regurgitation occurs, withdraw the tube and discontinue feeding until the next scheduled meal.

Feeding Schedule: Amount, Rate and Formula Temperature

Daily amount to feed: estimate the kitten's DER (**Table 5**); divide DER by the energy density of the milk replacer to be fed that day. It is usually best to follow label instructions when using commercial milk replacers. Properly diluted, most milk replacers will provide ~1 kcal/ml. To meet fluid needs, orphans should be fed ~18 ml of milk replacer/100 g/day. Add water to the milk replacer if necessary to provide the total recommended amount.

During Week 1 of life, the capacity of milk intake may be 10-15 ml/feeding. Young neonates and weak kittens should be fed every 2-4 hours. Older kittens should be fed every 4-6 hours.

Warm the milk replacer to 38°C (100°F) and deliver slowly (1-2 min.). Cold foods, rapid feeding and overfeeding may result in regurgitation, aspiration, bloating and diarrhea. If diarrhea occurs, reduce the amount fed or dilute the milk replacer with water. Gradually return to the previous dilution to meet energy needs. It is better to underfeed than overfeed.

Hygiene

Hygienic measures should be more stringent for orphans because they may have received less colostrum and be immunocompromised. Owners should thoroughly clean feeding equipment and boil in water between uses.

Ingredients for homemade milk replacers should be fresh and refrigerated until used. Prepare only 24 hours worth of milk replacer at a time. Discard milk replacer after 1 hour at room temperature.

At least 2 times/week, orphans should be washed gently with a soft moistened cloth to simulate cleaning by the dam's tongue.

Weaning

Wean at 6-9 weeks as described in **Table 6**. After weaning, feed according to recommendations in Chapter 24, Small Animal Clinical Nutrition, 5th edition.

Table 3. Recipes for homemade kitten orphan formulas.

Recipe 1*		Recipe 2**	
Skim milk	70 g	One whole egg, fresh	15 g
Low-fat curd***	15 g	Protein supplement	25 g
Lean beef hash	8 g	Milk, sweetened,	
Egg yolk (1/5)	3 g	condensed	17 ml
Vegetable oil	3 g	Corn oil	7 ml
Lactose	0.8 g	Water	250 ml
Vitamin-mineral mix	0.2 g	-	-
Total	100 g	Total	310 g

*Adapted from Kienzle E. Raising of motherless puppies and kittens. In: Proceedings. World Small Animal Veterinary Association Congress, Vienna, Austria, 1991: 240-242.
**Remillard RL, Pickett JP, Thatcher CD, et al. Comparison of kittens fed queen's milk with those fed milk replacers. American Journal of Veterinary Research 1993; 54: 901-907.
***Do not use cottage cheese because it may increase the risk of clotting in the neonate's stomach.

Table 4. Key nutritional factor content of homemade orphan formulas (**Table 3**) compared to key nutritional factor content of queen's milk.

Nutrients*	Queen's milk	Recipe 1**	Recipe 2**
Moisture (g)	79.3	83.1	86.4
Dry matter (g)	20.7	16.9	13.6
Crude protein (g)	7.5	7.1	6.4
Fat (g)	8.6	4.4	3.4
NFE (g)	4	4.7	2.9
Ash (g)	0.6	0.8	0.7
Calcium (mg)	180	96.2	109
Phosphorus (mg)	162	126	109
Sodium (mg)	90	33.5	90
Potassium (mg)	103	117	113
Copper (mg)	0.11	0.03	0.2
Iron (mg)	0.35	0.6	3.5
Zinc (mg)	na	0.7	1.9
Energy			
ME (kcal)***	121	80	62
ME (kJ)***	506	335	260

Key: NFE = nitrogen-free extract, ME = metabolizable energy.
*Calculated before addition of the vitamin-mineral mix.
**Calculated based on the addition of 2.5 g Pecutrin (Bayer).
***Calculated.

Table 5. Daily energy intake recommendations for orphaned kittens as a basis for determining food dose.*

Age (days)	kcal ME/100 g BW	kJ ME/100 g BW
1-3	15	60
4-6	20	85
>6	20-25	85-105

Key: ME = metabolizable energy, BW = body weight.
*Clients should not overfeed orphan formulas initially; the energy amounts listed for the first six days of the feeding period intentionally underfeed but then gradually increase so that the orphans' energy requirements are being met after about one week. Adapted from Mundt H-C, Thomée A, Meyer H. Zur Energie- und Eiweißversorgung von Saugwelpen über die Muttermilch. Kleintierpraxis 1981; 26: 353-360. Schaefers-Okkens AC. Pediatrie Post University Course, Ghent, Belgium, January 14, 1993. Sheffy BE. Nutrition and nutritional disorders. Veterinary Clinics of North America: Small Animal Practice 1978; 8: 7-29. Monson WJ. Orphan rearing of puppies and kittens. Veterinary Clinics of North America: Small Animal Practice 1987; 17: 567-576. Hoskins JD. Clinical evaluation of the kitten from birth to eight weeks of age. Compendium on Continuing Education for the Practicing Veterinarian 1990; 12: 1215-1225.

Table 6. Weaning

1. Weaning actually begins when kittens voluntarily start eating the queen's food between 3-4 weeks of age (eruption of deciduous teeth).
2. Weaning food: if fed correctly, the queen should already be eating the type of food recommended for the weaning process (high quality growth/reproduction-type food [Table 2, Chapter 9 and Table 2, Chapter 11]); using it as the weaning/postweaning food will facilitate the transition of the kittens to their growth food.
3. 3-4 week-old kittens can also be offered gruel to initially stimulate food intake: blend a moist growth/reproduction-type food with an equal volume of warm water or use 1 part crushed dry food mixed with 3 parts of warm water (volume basis). Encourage kittens to eat gruel by dipping a fingertip in the gruel and then into their mouths.
4. As solid food intake increases, progressively reduce the gruel's water content.
5. By 5-6 weeks, kittens eat ~30% of their energy requirement as solid food; kittens will increase their intake of solid food over time until they are independent of the queen.
6. After 3 weeks of age, some breeders separate kittens from the queen for short periods, progressively increasing separation time to ~4 hours/day by 6 weeks of age.
7. Domestic shorthair kittens are often weaned at 6 weeks and purebred kittens at 8-9 weeks; later weaning allows more time for growth and immune system maturation.
8. Day 1 of the weaning process: separate the queen and kittens; withhold the queen's food but allow the kittens to eat their weaning food. Reunite the queen and kittens that night and remove all food for the night. Reducing the amount of food fed to the queen will decrease lactation, which helps prevent excessive mammary gland distention/discomfort. For queens that are heavy milk producers, restrict the queen's food intake 1-2 days before the weaning process is begun.
9. Day 2: separate the queen and kittens again and allow the kittens to eat their weaning food but feed the queen 25% of the amount fed before breeding and do not reunite them at the end of the day.
10. At this point the kittens are considered weaned and are only fed their weaning food. Gradually increase the amount fed to the queen so that the prebreeding amount is being fed by Day 5 or 6.
11. Kittens are prone to GI upsets as they transition to solid foods. If a GI disturbance occurs, gruel can be made from a highly digestible moist food intended for treatment of diarrhea (Table 4, Chapter 42).

FOLLOWUP

Owner Followup

Kittens should be assessed daily. Body weights of nursing kittens should be recorded at birth (normal is 85-120 g) and then weekly. Nursing/orphaned kittens should gain about 100 g/week (7 g/day minimum) through weaning. Kitten growth is a good indicator of the quality/quantity of milk produced by the queen and milk consumption and health status of the kittens. Poor weight gain/failure to thrive should prompt the owner to seek immediate veterinary attention.

Veterinary Health Care Team Followup

Consider weekly veterinary checkups during the first month for inexperienced owners. Check kittens' body weights and assess for alertness, muscle tone, temperature and response to handling. Ask the owner if the kittens are nursing. Small/weak kittens may appear to nurse and have an enlarged abdomen but fail to thrive. They are often restless and vocalize excessively. If orphans do not thrive when fed a milk replacer, consider a different product or formula.

MISCELLANEOUS

See Chapters 22 and 23, Small Animal Clinical Nutrition, 5th edition, for more information.

Authors

Condensed from Chapter 23, Small Animal Clinical Nutrition, 5th edition, authored by Kathy L. Gross, Iveta Becvarova and Jacques Debraekeleer.

References

See Chapter 23, Small Animal Clinical Nutrition, 5th edition, on the website www.markmorrisinstitute.org for references.

CLINICAL POINTS

- Kittens should be weaned at 6-9 weeks and are considered adults at 10-12 months.
- Feeding goals: achieve healthy growth and create a healthy adult (optimize immune function; minimize obesity).
- Feed kittens to grow at optimal rates for body condition; don't feed for maximal growth rates.
- BCS: the most practical indicator of whether or not a kitten's growth rate is healthy.
- All kittens should have their body condition assessed every 2 weeks so that, if necessary, timely adjustments can be made in amounts fed to achieve optimal growth.
- BCS: should be in the range of 2/5 to 3/5; the lower end of the range is better for kittens at risk for obesity.
- Obesity risks for kittens include living indoors, free-choice feeding, high-fat foods and neutering.
- Chapter 14 discusses diseases associated with obesity in adults.

KEY NUTRITIONAL FACTORS

- Foods should provide recommended allowances of all required nutrients (nutritional adequacy), but should also contain specific levels of KNFs (certain nutrients and nonnutritional food ingredients or food features that can influence important diseases).
- **Table 1** lists KNF recommendations for foods for healthy kitten growth. A detailed description of these recommendations can be found in Chapter 24, Small Animal Clinical Nutrition, 5th edition. Most nutrients supplied in excess of the amounts needed for growth cause little/no harm. However, excess energy is of special concern (obesity prevention). Adequate DHA is important for normal neural development. Foods for young adults may be over acidified for kittens, resulting in reduced bone mineralization. Water is always a KNF.

FEEDING PLAN

Assess and Select the Food
Ensure the Food's Nutritional Adequacy. AAFCO nutritional adequacy statements are usually found on a product's label. AAFCO approval does not ensure a food will be effective in preventing important health problems associated with kitten growth such as obesity. Adult cat foods may not be balanced for healthy kitten growth.

Abbreviations
AAFCO = Association of American Feed Control Officials
BCS = body condition score (Appendix A)
DHA = docosahexaenoic acid
KNF = key nutritional factor
RER = resting energy requirement (Appendix C)

Table 1. Key nutritional factors for foods for growing kittens (postweaning to adult).*

Factors	Recommended food levels**
Energy density (kcal ME/g)	4.0-5.0
Energy density (kJ ME/g)	16.7-20.9
Protein (%)	35-50
Fat (%)	18-35
DHA (%)	≥0.004
Calcium (%)	0.8-1.6
Phosphorus (%)	0.6-1.4
Ca:P ratio	1:1-1.5:1
Potassium (%)	0.6-1.2
Average urinary pH***	6.2-6.5

Key: ME = metabolizable energy, DHA = docosahexaenoic acid.
*Concentrations presume an energy density of 4.0 kcal/g. Levels should be corrected for foods with higher energy densities. Adjustment is unnecessary for foods with lower energy densities.
**Dry matter basis.
***As determined in growing kittens.

Compare the Food's KNF Content with the Recommended Levels. **Table 2** compares KNF profiles for selected commercial foods for kitten growth. Many of these foods are also formulated/marketed for gestation and lactation and are sometimes referred to as growth/reproduction-type foods or foods for all lifestages. Contact the manufacturer for this information for foods not in the table (manufacturer contact information is listed on product labels). A new food should be selected if discrepancies are noted; the new food should best approximate the recommended KNF levels.

Manage Treats and Snacks. If treats/snacks are fed, commercial treats that match the nutritional profile recommended for postweaning kittens (see product label) are best. Otherwise, treats/snacks should not be fed excessively (<10% of the total diet on a volume, weight or calorie basis). Limit milk feeding; intestinal lactase declines shortly after weaning. See Appendix B for more information about treats/snacks.

Assess and Determine the Feeding Method
Determine How Much Food to Feed. The amount to feed can be obtained from the product label or it can be calculated (**Table 3** and Appendix C). The amount to feed is related to a kitten's energy requirement, which depends on its rate of growth (**Table 3**). Feeding guides and calculated amounts are starting points;

Table 2. Comparison of the key nutritional factors recommended for foods for healthy kitten growth to the key nutritional content of selected commercial foods.* (Numbers in red match optimal KNFs.)

Dry foods	Energy density (kcal/cup)**	Energy density (kcal ME/g)	Protein (%)	Fat (%)	DHA (%)	Ca (%)	P (%)	Ca:P ratio	K (%)	Urinary pH
Recommended levels	–	4.0-5.0	35-50	18-35	≥0.004	0.8-1.6	0.6-1.4	1:1-1.5:1	0.6-1.2	6.2-6.5
Hill's Science Diet Kitten Healthy Development Original	510	4.5	42.3	26.1	0.24	1.28	1.13	1.1:1	0.9	6.4
Hill's Science Diet Kitten Indoor	510	4.5	42.2	26.1	0.24	1.28	1.14	1.1:1	0.9	6.4
Hill's Science Diet Nature's Best Chicken & Brown Rice Dinner Kitten	487	4.4	37.6	26.0	0.26	1.45	1.2	1.2:1	0.8	6.4
Iams Eukanuba Chicken Formula Kitten	469	4.5	40.0	25.7	na	1.29	1.07	1.2:1	0.97	na
Iams Kitten	470	5.0	37.8	24.6	na	1.15	0.94	1.2:1	0.86	na
Nutro Natural Choice Complete Care Kitten	463	4.4	40.7	24.2	0.077	1.32	1.21	1.1:1	0.71	na
Purina Kitten Chow	457	4.5	44.8	15.6	na	1.43	1.43	1:1	0.77	na
Purina ONE Healthy Kitten	512	4.8	45.5	21.1	na	1.33	1.20	1.1:1	0.98	na
Purina Pro Plan Kitten Chicken & Rice Formula	472	4.3	46.0	20.1	na	1.33	1.16	1.1:1	0.68	na
Royal Canin Babycat 34 Formula	531	4.8	37.4	27.5	na	1.29	1.12	1.1:1	0.67	na
Royal Canin Kitten 34 Formula	393	4.6	37.4	22.0	na	1.25	1.14	1.1:1	0.71	na

Moist foods	Energy density (kcal/can)**	Energy density (kcal ME/g)	Protein (%)	Fat (%)	DHA (%)	Ca (%)	P (%)	Ca:P ratio	K (%)	Urinary pH
Recommended levels	–	4.0-5.0	35-50	18-35	≥0.004	0.8-1.6	0.6-1.4	1:1-1.5:1	0.6-1.2	6.2-6.5
Hill's Science Diet Kitten Healthy Development Liver & Chicken Entrée Minced	114/3 oz. 210/5.5 oz.	4.7	49.3	23.9	0.243	1.3	0.95	1.4:1	0.88	6.4
Hill's Science Diet Tender Chunks in Gravy Real Chicken Dinner Kitten	84/3 oz. (pouch)	4.3	47.8	22.6	0.087	1.17	1.09	1.1:1	1.04	6.3
Purina Pro Plan Kitten Chicken & Liver Entrée Classic	98/3 oz.	4.6	56.0	31.2	na	2.0	1.96	1:1	1.36	na

Key: ME = metabolizable energy, DHA = docosahexaenoic acid, Ca = calcium, P = phosphorus, K = potassium, na = not available from manufacturer.
*From manufacturers' published information or calculated from manufacturers' published as fed values; all values are on a dry matter basis unless otherwise stated.
**Energy density values are listed on an as fed basis and are useful for determining the amount to feed; cup = 8-oz. measuring cup. Energy density also reflects digestibility; foods with higher energy density are likely to have better digestibility than foods with lower energy density. To convert kcal to kJ, multiply kcal by 4.184.

BCS should be used to adjust these estimates to individual kittens (see Followup below). Do not overfeed.

Consider How to Offer the Food. Free-choice feeding is popular for kittens less than 5 months old (unless they are becoming overweight); after 5 months, food-restricted feeding is preferred. When proper amounts are used, food-restricted feeding is less likely to cause obesity. Divide the daily amount fed into 3-4 feedings until the kittens are 6 months old, then twice/day feedings are adequate. Food-restricted feeding should be used in neutered kittens.

Manage Food Changes. If a food change is necessary, a transition period to avoid GI upsets is good practice. Example: to change to a new food, replace 25% of the old food with the new food on Day 1 and continue this incremental change daily until the change is complete on Day 4. Appendix E provides additional information.

Food and Water Receptacle Husbandry. Food and water bowls should be washed regularly with warm soapy water and rinsed well. Dishes used for moist foods need daily cleaning. Discard moist or moistened dry foods after 2-4 hours of room temperature exposure to avoid foodborne illnesses (Appendix F). Shallow pans facilitate access to food for young kittens.

FOLLOWUP

Owner Followup

Teach kitten owners to assess body condition; they should monitor the patient's BCS and body weight at least every 2 weeks and adjust the amount fed by 10% increments to maintain a BCS of 2/5 to 3/5 and normal growth. Kittens grow at ~100 g/

week until 20 weeks old. Then males typically gain 20 g/day and females gain 11 g/day. Growth rates slow as kittens approach 80% of adult weight (30 weeks old). They should reach adult body weight at 40-52 weeks of age.

Veterinary Health Care Team Followup

During office calls for routine vaccinations, review growth rate and food consumption records and compare the owner's assessment of his/her cat's BCS to a BCS assessment done by a member of the health care team. This level of attention to BCS helps owners manage a healthy BCS throughout the life of their cat.

MISCELLANEOUS

See Chapters 22-24, Small Animal Clinical Nutrition, 5th edition, for more information.

Authors

Condensed from Chapter 24, Small Animal Clinical Nutrition, 5th edition, authored by Kathy L. Gross, Iveta Becvarova and Jacques Debraekeleer.

References

See Chapter 24, Small Animal Clinical Nutrition, 5th edition, on the website www.markmorrisinstitute.org for references.

Table 3. Daily energy requirements of growing kittens.

Age (months)	kcal/kg BW/day	kJ/kg BW/day
Birth	250	1,045
1	240	1,005
2	210	880
3	200	840
4*	175	730
5	145	610
6**	135	565
7	120	500
8	110	460
9***	100	420
10	95	400
11	90	375
12	85	355

Key: RER = resting energy requirement = $70(BW_{kg})^{0.75}$, BW = body weight.
*Up to 50% of adult BW (at about four months of age) or 3.0 x RER.
**Between 50 and 70% of adult BW (around six months of age) or 2.5 x RER.
***Between 70 and 100% of adult BW (around nine to 12 months of age) or 2 x RER.

Chapter 12

Critical Care Nutrition and Enteral-Assisted Feeding

CLINICAL POINTS

- Many hospitalized dogs and cats do not consume enough food to meet their nutrient needs.
- The consequences of undernutrition in sick/injured patients are decreased immunocompetence, decreased tissue repair, altered drug metabolism and increased morbidity/mortality.
- Hospitalized patients not eating for more than 2 days or those eating less than 50% of normal food intake for more than 3 days are candidates for assisted feeding; routine use of hospital feeding notes helps track food intake (**Table 1**).
- Patients scheduled for surgical procedures that preclude normal eating for >2 days are also candidates for assisted feeding; consider placement of an indwelling feeding tube (below) during surgery.
- Initial assessment: special attention should be given to the BCS

Abbreviations

AAFCO = Association of American Feed Control Officials
BCS = body condition score (Appendix A)
CRI = continuous rate infusion
DM = dry matter
EN = enteral nutrition
IBD = inflammatory bowel disease
KNF = key nutritional factor
NPO = nothing by mouth
PN = parenteral nutrition
RER = resting energy requirement

and body weight; specific, practical lab tests that correlate with nutritional status have not been identified.
- A practical goal is to begin nutritional support within 24 hours of hospitalization for the injury or illness.
- Correct a patient's fluid/electrolyte, acid/base balance and

Table 1. Examples of hospital feeding orders.

1. Offer 2 cans of product XX every 6 hr PO.
2. Give 100 ml of product YY gruel every 6 hr via PEG (percutaneous gastrostomy) tube.
3. Administer 300 ml of parenteral solution IV every 8 hr.
   Sometimes the feeding orders should contain special conditions:
4. Begin feeding liquid product ZZ at 10 ml/hr via NG (nasogastric) tube. D/C (discontinue) all feeding if vomiting begins.
5. Administer 300 ml of parenteral solution IV every 8 hr. Check urine glucose and decrease rate to 150 ml every 8 hr if urine is positive. Recheck serum potassium daily and increase to 40 mEq/l if below normal.
6. Give 30 ml of product YY gruel every 6 hr by PEG tube. Increase meal volume fed by 10 ml every 24 hr, decrease volume by 50% if vomiting begins.

Table 2. Key nutritional factors for commercial liquid or blended foods for canine and feline patients requiring enteral nutrition (EN) support.

Factors	Recommended food levels
Water	Correct dehydration with parenteral fluid therapy before starting assisted feeding. Supply at 1 ml/kcal DER unless patient requires fluid restriction or diuresis. Typical daily maintenance fluid requirement is 60 ml/kg body weight.
Electrolytes	Major electrolyte disorders, acid-base abnormalities and blood glucose levels should be corrected before instituting EN support.
Osmolarity	250 (optimal) to 400 mOsm/liter.
Energy density	Supply 1 kcal/ml (as standard minimum). If the patient is not eating at least RER per os, provide nutritional support by assisted-feeding techniques to meet this requirement. By the fifth day of food deprivation or longer, patients should receive the majority (60 to 90%) of their calculated RER as lipid. If using a liquid or blended food, select a product that provides 1.0 to 2.0 kcal/ml (1.0 to 2.0 kcal/g), as fed.
Digestible carbohydrate	Dogs and cats: 2 to 4 g/100 kcal is a safe starting point for refeeding. Increase to 6 to 10 g/100 kcal 3 to 4 days into the refeeding process.
Protein	Dogs: Use a food that provides 5.0 to 12.0 g protein/100 kcal. Cats: Use a food that provides 7.5 to 12.0 g protein/100 kcal.
Arginine	≥146 mg arginine/100 kcal for dogs. ≥250 mg arginine/100 kcal for cats.
Glutamine	≥500 mg/100 kcal.
Fat	Provide a calorically dense food (5 to 7.5 g fat/100 kcal), except in cases in which high fat content is not tolerated. Provide a low-fat content food (2.0 to 3.5 g fat/100 kcal) if fat restriction is required.*

Key: DER = daily energy requirement, RER = resting energy requirement, to convert kcal to kJ, multiply kcal by 4.184.
*For example, patients with pancreatitis.

blood glucose before assisted feeding is begun; nutritional support should not be initiated in unstable patients.
- Progression to the recovery phase and subjective improvement of the patient indicate a positive clinical response and may occur as soon as 36 hours after initiation of feeding.

- Recovery phase is patient dependent; this underscores the need for continued/consistent reassessment/followup so that, if necessary, the feeding plan can be modified in a timely manner.
- Appetite stimulants may be used to induce food consumption but voluntary food intake rarely continues and patients' nutrient needs are often unmet.
- **Figure 1** is a decision-making algorithm for choosing between EN and PN (Chapter 13).
- EN and PN can be done together; sometimes a dual approach is necessary to meet RER.
- Feeding goal: reduce morbidity/mortality in patients that cannot/will not eat by providing appropriate nutritional support for enhanced immunocompetence and tissue repair.

KEY NUTRITIONAL FACTORS

- Foods should provide recommended allowances of all required nutrients (nutritional adequacy), but should also contain specific levels of KNFs (certain nutrients and nonnutritional food ingredients or food features that can influence important diseases).
- Unlike KNF recommendations in the rest of this book, KNFs for EN and PN are expressed on energy rather than a DM basis. **Table 2** summarizes KNFs for dogs and cats requiring EN support. To optimize recovery, these foods have increased fat/protein and decreased carbohydrate. Excess carbohydrate can result in glucose dyshomeostasis and diarrhea.
- Other KNFs to note: osmolarity of liquid foods; arginine and glutamine content. A detailed description of these recommendations can be found in Chapter 25, Small Animal Clinical Nutrition, 5th edition.
- Water is always a KNF and should be available to critically ill patients at all times (unless NPO order). A patient's water requirement in ml is approximately the same as its energy requirement in kcal (or about 60 ml/kg).

FEEDING PLAN

Assess and Determine the Feeding Method
Consider How to Provide the Food. Patient assessment is the first step in developing a feeding plan because it dictates how the food is provided, which dictates the food form (e.g., solid/liquid) for providing assisted feeding.
Oral Feeding.
FOOD BOLUS. This method can be tried first in patients that are physically able to eat but will not do so voluntarily. Placing a bolus of food in the proximal oral cavity stimulates the swallowing reflex and is a good method if tolerated and food intake is sufficient. Discontinue if the patient does not swallow food voluntarily.
SYRINGE FEEDING. Also a good method, if tolerated. See Appendix H for the procedure.
OROGASTRIC TUBE. Useful for 1-2 days of feeding but

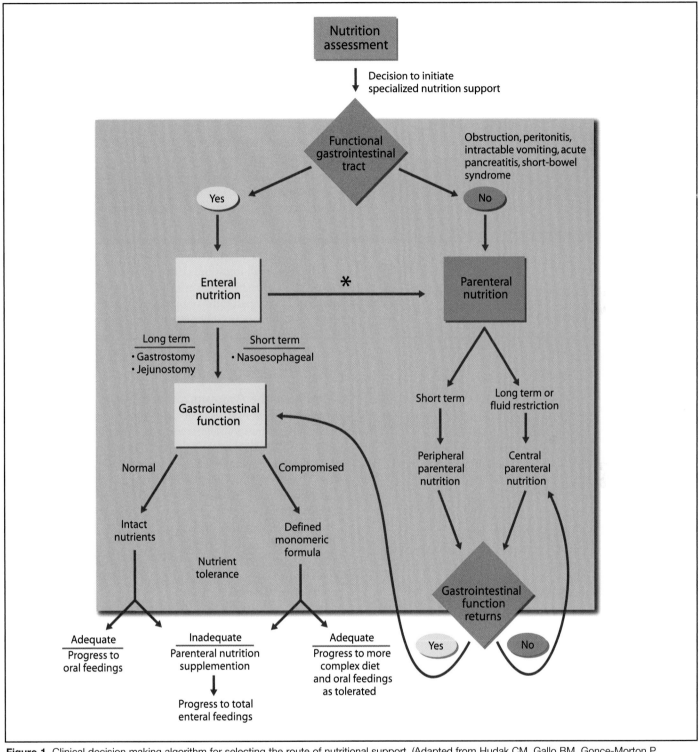

Figure 1. Clinical decision making algorithm for selecting the route of nutritional support. (Adapted from Hudak CM, Gallo BM, Gonce-Morton P, eds. Patient management: Gastrointestinal system. Critical Care Nursing, 7th ed. Philadelphia, PA: Lippincott, 1998; 771.)
*Nasoesophageal tube not tolerated or anesthesia not possible.

requires tube placement at each feeding. Red rubber or polyvinyl chloride tubes (8-24 Fr.)[a] may be used. Tip placement should be in the caudal esophagus or stomach (Appendix H). Anesthesia is not required.

Indwelling Tubes. Easier and less stressful on patients than forced feeding or repeated placement of an orogastric tube and thus better for longer term feeding. Use the most proximal functioning portion of the GI tract possible by the least invasive method. The tubes can also be used to deliver oral medications.

NASOESOPHAGEAL TUBE. Anesthesia or tranquilization is unnecessary, thus this route can provide EN feeding to patients considered anesthetic risks. Polyurethane tubes with or without weighted tips[b] and silicone tubes[c] are used. This route is most often used in the hospital, although capable owners can use them

Table 3. Example using enteral-assisted feeding guidelines.

Patient data needed	Canine patient example
1. Current body weight	12 kg
2. Calculate resting energy requirement (RER) as kcal/day	451 kcal/day
3. Expected daily fluid volume in ml/kg/day	60 ml/kg
4. Size (Fr.) and volume capacity of feeding tube	18-Fr., E-tube (10-ml volume)

Food information needed:
Determine the caloric density of the food or food blend. Liquid foods have a set caloric density (kcal/ml) provided on the product information sheet. Moist foods need to be blended with a liquid (water or liquid food) to make a gruel (food blend) that can be delivered through a feeding tube or syringe.

1. Determine gruel caloric density:

Identify kcal per can of food	569 kcal/12.7 oz. can
Calculate ml/can (XX oz. in can x 30 ml/oz.); assumes 30 ml/weight/oz.	12.7 oz. x 30 = 383 ml
Determine ml of fluid needed to blend with canned food	100 ml warm water
Determine caloric density of fluid if not water*	–
Calculate caloric density of food blend. kcal/ml = (total kcal ÷ total ml)	569 ÷ (383 + 100) = 1.2 kcal/ml

2. Determine water provided in food or food blend:

Calculate water in canned food (ml x % moisture); 75% moisture in canned food obtained from product information sheet	383 x 75% = 287 ml
Calculate water in liquid if not water**	–
Calculate % water in blend (ml total water ÷ total ml)	(287 + 100) ÷ 483 = 79%

3. Provide a feeding protocol:

Method of food delivery (bolus feeding or constant rate infusion)	bolus
Beginning feeding rate (x % of RER)	25% RER
Daily caloric intake goal (kcal/day)***	113 kcal/day
Daily feeding rate	–
Calculate amount (kcal/day ÷ kcal/ml of food blend)	113 kcal ÷ 1.2 kcal/ml = 94 ml food blend/day
Determine meals/day (per 24 hr)	4
Determine feeding dosage (ml/meal/day)	94 ml ÷ 4 meals = 24 ml/ meal; therefore, 24 ml q6hr
Water provided by food or food blend/day (ml)	94 ml x 79% = 74 ml water
Flush required after food delivery (ml)	4 x 10 ml flush = 40 ml water
Additional water needed to meet daily fluid volume (daily requirement = 60 ml/kg)	720 ml/day – (74 + 40) = 606 ml
Provide guidelines for residuals	(see text)
Provide monitoring guidelines	(see text)
Tube maintenance and removal guidelines	(see text)

*If blending the canned food with a commercial liquid food, these foods provide a caloric density greater than 0. Determine the liquid food's caloric density and plug it into the top half of the equation. The caloric density can range between 0.8 and 1.9 kcal/ml depending on the commercial product.
**Every liquid food is part solids and part water, find this information about the product and calculate the absolute water contribution to the food blend, or assume the liquid food to be 100% water, if moisture content is 90% or greater.
***Increase this rate as tolerated by the patient or with a feeding goal to meet the patient's RER by Day 2 or 3.

at home. Appendix H describes placement.

PHARYNGOSTOMY TUBE. The tip of the tube is placed in the caudal esophagus and the tube can be used for long-term (weeks/months) in-hospital or home feedings. Appendix H describes placement.

ESOPHAGOSTOMY TUBE. The tube tip is placed in the caudal esophagus. It can be used for long-term (weeks/months) in-hospital or home feedings. Appendix H describes placement.

GASTROSTOMY TUBE. Gastrostomy tubes (mushroom-tipped, 16 to 28 Fr.)[d] can be placed either surgically (Appendix H) or percutaneously using an endoscope or a gastrostomy tube introduction device[e] (Appendix H). Percutaneous placement is easier, faster, less expensive and less invasive than surgical placement. Gastrostomy tubes are convenient and safe for long-term (weeks to months) in-hospital or home feedings.

JEJUNOSTOMY TUBE. Also called J-tube (5-8 Fr.); placement is within the small intestine, ideally at the time of exploratory celiotomy to bypass the proximal GI tract. J-tubes may also be placed by mini-laparotomy or by threading a small tube through a larger esophagostomy, pharyngostomy or gastrostomy tube and placing the tip of the J-tube in the jejunum. However, even a weighted-tip tube may be pushed back into the stomach by reverse peristalsis.

Determine the Amount to Feed/Feeding Schedule

Amount to Feed. Applies to all feeding routes. **Table 3** provides example guidelines for determining the amount to feed. Generally, feed to meet the patient's RER. Appendix C provides methods for estimating RER. To avoid refeeding complications, do not overfeed. Use Table 9, Chapter 14, to avoid overestimating RER in overweight/obese patients (BCS = 4/5 to 5/5). A patient's energy requirement in kcal is approximately the same as its water requirement in ml, and the energy density of most liquid foods is 1 kcal/ml; thus, when the patient's energy requirement is being met, so are its water needs. If more water is needed to meet the water requirement, it can be provided via the tube (**Table 3** provides an example).

TRANSITION FEEDING. Patients may tolerate feeding an amount of food to meet their estimated RER within the first 24-hour period. Otherwise, use a graduated approach: feed 25-33% of RER on Day 1, with a goal to meet the patient's RER by the end of Day 2 or 3 (**Table 3**).

FOOD BOLUS FEEDING REGIMEN. Tubes that deliver food into the esophagus/stomach allow for bolus or food-restricted feeding schedules because the stomach acts as a food reservoir. The stomach doesn't shrink as a result of a prolonged fast but stretch receptors become more sensitive. Delivery rate is 5 ml/1 min. to allow for uncomplicated gastric expansion. Stop feeding if signs of gastric intolerance occur (salivating, gulping, retching, vomiting), reduce meal size by 50% for 24 hours then increase gradually by 25%/day back to the feeding dose. Also see the residual volume discussion in Followup below.

FOOD BOLUS VOLUME ESTIMATE. Determined by estimating gastric capacity; initially 5-10 ml/kg but may be as high as 45-90 ml/kg when a patient is fully realimented; however, RER can usually be met readily at less than these maximal capacities.

Table 4. Key nutritional factor content of selected commercial veterinary liquid foods, human liquid foods and moist veterinary foods used for enteral-assisted feeding of critically ill dogs compared to key nutritional factor recommended levels.* (Numbers in red match optimal KNFs.)

Factors	Osmolarity (mOsm/l)	Energy density (kcal/ml)	CHO (g)	Protein (g)	Arginine (mg)	Glutamine (mg)	Fat (g)
Recommended levels	250-400**	1-2***	2-4	5-12	≥146	≥500	5-7.5
Liquid veterinary products							
Abbott CliniCare Canine/Feline Liquid Diet	315	1.0	6.8	8.2	350	815	5.1
Abbott CliniCare RF Liquid Diet	235	1.0	5.9	6.3	350	615	6.8
PetAg Formula V Enteral Care HLP	312	1.2	4.2	8.5	413	na	4.8
PetAg Formula V Enteral Care MLP	256	1.1	5.8	7.5	392.6	na	5.7
Liquid human products							
Glucerna Shakes	355	1.0	9.6	4.2	na	na	5.4
Nestlé Impact Advanced Recovery	375	1.0	13.2	5.6	1,250	na	2.7
Nestlé Peptamen AF	390	1.2	8.9	6.3	na	na	4.6
Novartis Resource Diabetic	300	1.1	10.0	6.3	na	na	4.7
Moist veterinary foods†							
Hill's Prescription Diet a/d Canine/Feline	-	1.2	3.2	9.2	495	1,077	6.3
Hill's Prescription Diet n/d Canine	-	1.6	3.7	7.0	544	na	6.1
Iams Veterinary Formula Maximum-Calorie Canine & Feline	-	2.1	2.2	7.2	534	940	6.4
Purina Veterinary Diets Cardiovascular (CV) Feline Formula	-	1.4	4.7	8.8	469	1,169	5.5
Purina Veterinary Diets Dietetic Management (DM) Feline Formula	-	1.2	1.7	11.9	568	1,825	5.0
Royal Canin Veterinary Diet Feline and Canine Recovery RS	-	1.0	1.9	12.3	683	na	7.7

Key: CHO = digestible carbohydrate, na = information not available from the manufacturer.
*Liquid and moist veterinary foods in this table are formulated to meet minimum requirements of the Association of American Feed Control Officials; all nutrient values = units/100 kcal, unless otherwise stated; to convert kcal to kJ, multiply kcal by 4.184.
**250 is optimal.
***Energy density on an as-fed basis.
†**Table 6** contains recipes for blending these foods for tube feeding.

CRI VOLUME ESTIMATE. For patients that cannot tolerate bolus feeding, administer by CRI using a pump or gravity flow. It is best to feed by continuous delivery for patients with J-tubes. The rate should be RER/24 hours.

FEEDING TUBE MAINTENANCE. Flush the tube with water after bolus feeding to clear food residue. Before tube placement, determine the water volume necessary to clean the tube, particularly for volume sensitive patients (**Table 3** provides an example). Fill plugged tubes with water or a nonalcoholic carbonated beverage, cap and allow time for the plug to dissolve. End port tubes are easier to maintain. All tubes except orogastric and nasoesophageal require standard every other day bandage care.

Manage Food Changes. Patients that have recovered and are eating on their own can be fed their regular food. A transition period to avoid GI upsets is good practice. Example: replace 25% of the old food with the new food on Day 1 and continue this incremental change daily until the change is complete on Day 4. If problems occur, return to feeding the previous food fed for several more days before repeating the food change. Appendix E provides additional information.

Assess and Select the Food

Food selection depends on tube size and location within the GI tract. Smaller tubes (<8 Fr., e.g., nasoesophageal and jejunostomy tubes) require use of liquid foods; blended pet foods can be used in larger tubes. High protein intake is handled well by most canine and feline patients; because of the overlap of protein recom-mendations for EN foods for dogs and cats, single EN products are often indicated for use in both species.

Liquid Foods and Modules.

MONOMERIC (ELEMENTAL) FOODS. These are commercial products with hydrolyzed nutrients for easy assimilation in patients with compromised GI function (**Figure 1** [e.g., IBD, lymphangiectasia, parvoviral enteritis and pancreatitis]). These foods can be fed through any size feeding tube. Most human monomeric foods provide adequate protein for adult dogs (except those with excessive protein losses) but not for puppies or cats. Also, they usually do not contain adequate arginine and taurine for cats.

POLYMERIC FOODS. Larger molecular weight nutrient components require normal GI function. Delivery is typically good via small feeding tubes (<8 Fr.). **Tables 4** and **5** list selected foods for dogs and cats, respectively, and compare them to KNF recommendations. Liquid veterinary foods are generally better tolerated than liquid human products and should be AAFCO approved (check label) to help avoid refeeding complications.

BLENDED PET FOODS. Tables 4 and **5** list selected foods for dogs and cats. These are readily available, better tolerated and less expensive than monomeric or polymeric foods. These products are useful for syringe feeding; may require larger bore tubes for tube feeding (product dependent) and more attention to tube maintenance (see above). To enhance delivery by tube, these foods can be blended with liquid foods or additional water. **Table 6** lists moist recovery-type foods with dilution information for delivery through various size tubes. **Table 3** provides an

Table 5. Key nutritional factor content of selected commercial veterinary liquid foods, human liquid foods and moist veterinary foods used for enteral-assisted feeding of critically ill cats compared to key nutritional factor recommended levels.* (Numbers in red match optimal KNFs.)

Factors	Osmolarity (mOsm/l)	Energy density (kcal/ml)***	CHO (g)	Protein (g)	Arginine (mg)	Glutamine (mg)	Fat (g)
Recommended levels	250-400**	1-2	2-4	7.5-12	≥250	≥500	5-7.5
Liquid veterinary foods							
Abbott CliniCare Canine/Feline Liquid Diet	315	1.0	6.8	8.2	350	815	5.1
Abbott CliniCare RF Liquid Diet	235	1.0	5.9	6.3	350	615	6.8
PetAg Formula V Enteral Care HLP	312	1.2	4.2	8.5	413	na	4.8
PetAg Formula V Enteral Care MLP	256	1.1	5.8	7.5	392.6	na	5.7
Liquid human foods							
Glucerna Shakes	355	1.0	9.6	4.2	na	na	5.4
Nestlé Impact Advanced Recovery	375	1.0	13.2	5.6	1,250	na	2.7
Nestlé Peptamen AF	390	1.2	8.9	6.3	na	na	4.6
Novartis Resource Diabetic	300	1.1	10.0	6.3	na	na	4.7
Moist veterinary foods†							
Hill's Prescription Diet a/d Canine/Feline	-	1.2	3.2	9.2	495	1,077	6.3
Iams Veterinary Formula Maximum-Calorie Canine & Feline	-	2.1	2.2	7.2	534	940	6.4
Purina Veterinary Diets Cardiovascular (CV) Feline Formula	-	1.4	4.7	8.8	469	1,169	5.5
Purina Veterinary Diets Dietetic Management (DM) Feline Formula	-	1.2	1.7	11.9	568	1,825	5.0
Royal Canin Veterinary Diet Feline and Canine Recovery RS	-	1.0	1.9	12.3	683	na	7.7

Key: CHO = digestible carbohydrate, na = information not available from the manufacturer.
*Liquid and moist veterinary foods in this table are formulated to meet minimum requirements of the Association of American Feed Control Officials; all nutrient values = units/100 kcal, unless otherwise stated; to convert kcal to kJ, multiply kcal by 4.184.
**250 is optimal.
***Energy density on an as-fed basis.
†Table 6 contains recipes for blending these foods for tube feeding.

Table 6. Recipes for blending selected commercial moist veterinary therapeutic foods in **Tables 4** and **5** for use with feeding tubes.

Feeding tube size			20 Fr.		18 Fr.		16 Fr.		14 Fr.	
Moist veterinary foods	Can size (oz.)	No. of cans	Water added (ml)	Energy density (kcal/ml)*	Water added (ml)	Energy density (kcal/ml)*	Water added (ml)	Energy density (kcal/ml)*	Water added (ml)	Energy density (kcal/ml)*
Hill's Prescription Diet a/d Canine/Feline	5.5	2	30	1.00	40	0.97	45	0.96	50	0.95
Hill's Prescription Diet n/d Canine	12.7	1	95	1.20	100	1.18	110	1.16	120	1.14
Iams Veterinary Formula Maximum-Calorie Canine & Feline	6	2	30	1.74	35	1.72	40	1.70	45	1.68
Purina Veterinary Diets Feline CV	5.5	2	100	1.04	105	1.03	110	1.01	120	0.99
Purina Veterinary Diets Feline DM	5.5	2	55	1.01	60	1.00	70	0.97	75	0.96
Royal Canin Veterinary Diet Feline and Canine Recovery RS	6	2	30	0.88	32.5	0.88	35	0.87	37.5	0.87

*Predicted as fed energy density of blended mixture.

example calculation. Recovering patients can continue to be fed these foods unblended when they start eating on their own, obviating the need for a food change. For specific diseases, moist veterinary therapeutic foods can be blended with water, strained and fed through large-bore feeding tubes (≥14 Fr.). To help avoid refeeding complications, use foods that are AAFCO approved (see product labels).

NUTRIENT MODULES. Concentrated (powdered or liquid) protein, amino acids, fats, carbohydrates or fiber modules are available for supplemental use (**Table 7**). Usually these are used to supplement human liquid products (**Tables 4** and **5**).

HUMAN BABY FOODS. Some canine/feline critical care patients will voluntarily eat moist baby foods. However, these products are not balanced, and some contain onion powder, which can cause Heinz bodies in cats. Use AAFCO approved veterinary foods.

FOLLOWUP

Veterinary Health Care Team Followup

Hospitalized patients: food intake, hydration status and body weight should be monitored daily; monitor TPR as necessary. Evaluate serum potassium, phosphorus, magnesium, glucose and lipids if concerns arise about metabolic complications of refeeding. Other lab values are unlikely to change over a 2-week period. Most patients will subjectively improve within 36 hours of feeding. BCS and body weight should improve over a period of weeks. Diarrhea can occur during refeeding; causes include overfeeding, use of hyperosmolar and/or high carbohydrate formulas; treatment includes reducing the feeding amount and/or changing the food.

Residual Volume. Many patients become intolerant of food administration, which is attributable to GI motility dysfunction. Residual gastric contents may pose risks for underfeeding (due to volume limitation): aspiration, prolonged recovery and increased mortality. Management includes prokinetic medications, feeding plan alterations (e.g., reduced volume/increased frequency, J-tube feeding or supplemental/total PN support).

MONITORING RESIDUAL VOLUME. Before a scheduled food delivery, aspirate gastric contents; if excessive (>20 ml/kg), discard or replace a portion back into the stomach and skip the feeding; if no excess, proceed with the feeding. If a scheduled feeding was skipped, recheck volume at the next feeding. If no excess, proceed with feeding at the usual amount or less. However, if excess volume was again noted and a subsequent recheck still indicates excess, consider additional diagnostics, initiation of prokinetic therapy or an alternate feeding route. Routinely check the residual volume every 12-24 hours when using CRI.

MISCELLANEOUS

See Chapters 25 and 26, Small Animal Clinical Nutrition, 5th edition, for more information.

Authors

Condensed from Chapter 25, Small Animal Clinical Nutrition, 5th edition, authored by Korinn E. Saker and Rebecca L. Remillard.

Table 7. Modules for augmenting foods.

Products	Key features
Arginine (various)	Available OTC as 500-mg capsules in most pharmacies and health food stores
Corn syrup (various)	Mostly maltose, 2.9 kcal/ml
Glutamine (various)	Available as powder from chemical catalogs and most pharmacies and health food stores; check label for concentration
Medium-chain triglyceride oil (Mead Johnson)	Fractionated coconut oil, 8.3 kcal/ml
Pectin (various)	Available OTC as a powder containing <1% crude protein and ~90% soluble fiber
ProMod (Ross Laboratories)	23.6 g protein/100 kcal, 18.2 g glutamine/100 g powder, 1.48 kcal/ml reconstituted
Psyllium fiber (FiberAll Regular, Rydelle Labs)	Available OTC as a powder containing 8% crude protein, 85% total dietary fiber, 72% soluble fiber
Psyllium fiber (Metamucil Regular, Searle)	Available OTC as a powder containing 17% crude protein, 53% total dietary fiber, 44% soluble fiber
Taurine (various)	Available OTC as 250-mg and 500-mg tablets in most pharmacies and health food stores

Key: OTC = over the counter; to convert kcal to kJ, multiply kcal by 4.184.

References

See Chapter 25, Small Animal Clinical Nutrition, 5th edition, on the website www.markmorrisinstitute.org for references.

Endnotes

a. Sovereign Feeding Tube. Sherwood Medical, St Louis, MO, USA.

b. Kangaroo Enteral Feed Tube. Sherwood Medical, St Louis, MO, USA. KeoFeed II Feeding Tube. IVAC Corp., San Diego, CA, USA.

c. Feeding Tube. Cook Veterinary Products, Bloomington, IN, USA.

d. Pezzar Model Catheter. C.R. Bard, Inc., Covington, GA, USA.

e. Gastrostomy Tube Introduction Set. Cook Veterinary Products, Bloomington, IN, USA.

CLINICAL POINTS

- See Chapter 12 for EN Clinical Points that also apply to PN.
- PN in veterinary clinical use is usually partial support because it is typically of short duration (2-7 days). True PN is intended for long-term (months) administration.
- PN candidates: patients that are not eating and cannot tolerate EN or feeding tube installation for several days (Figure 1, Chapter 12).
- This chapter assumes TNA solutions are used for PN.
- TNA solution: PN solution with individual lipid, dextrose and amino acid solutions combined in a single fluid bag with a sufficient mixture to meet a patient's fluid, energy, amino acid, electrolyte and B-vitamin needs for 24 hours.
- Purchasing premixed TNA solutions (see Miscellaneous below), rather than compounding, greatly simplifies PN delivery.
- Before initiation of PN, ensure the patient's cardiovascular hemodynamics and glucose and electrolyte/acid-base status are corrected, if necessary.
- Technical requirements for PN: 1) good catheter technique, 2) ability to provide 24-hour patient care and 3) IV fluid delivery experience and equipment.
- PN is sometimes used with EN, example: simple provision of an IV lipid solution to an EN patient when there is difficulty in providing enough food to meet RER.
- PN goal: provide short-term nutritional support to enhance immunocompetence and tissue repair until the patient can be fed via EN and/or can eat on its own.

KEY NUTRITIONAL FACTORS

- Water is always a KNF; a patient's water requirement in ml is the same as its energy requirement in kcal (or about 60 ml/kg).
- Energy: the preferred sources are admixtures of lipids and glucose. After 3-5 days of food deprivation, at least 60% of calories should be from lipids. PN solutions with high lipid/dextrose ratios result in a better response in septic patients and fewer problems than high-glucose solutions. High-fat solutions fed at RER are even safe for patients with hypertriglyceridemia, hepatic lipidosis or pancreatitis.
- Protein: provide within a ratio of 1-6 g protein (amino acids)/100 kcal of nonprotein energy. Adult dogs should receive 2-3 g/100 kcal and adult cats 3-4 g/100 kcal. Lower protein/calorie ratios are better for renal or hepatic insufficiency patients. Patients with excessive protein losses should receive admixtures with higher protein/calorie ratios.

- Electrolytes: potassium and less often phosphorus are of increased importance because they move out of blood into tissues during refeeding, reducing serum levels.
- Osmolarity: depends on the administration route (e.g., peripheral or central vein infusion.)
- Vitamins: supply water-soluble vitamins daily (provided in TNA).
- A detailed discussion of these KNFs can be found in Chapters 25 and 26, Small Animal Clinical Nutrition, 5th edition.

FEEDING PLAN

Amount to Administer
The patient's RER in combination with the daily water requirement are the bases for determining daily volume to administer. Typically, TNA solutions have non-energy nutrients balanced to their energy density so when administered in amounts that meet the patient's RER, the non-energy nutrients, including water, are in proper proportions. Appendix C provides methods for estimating RER. To avoid refeeding complications (refeeding syndrome), do not feed in excess of RER. Use Table 9, Chapter 14, to avoid overestimating RER in overweight/obese patients (BCS = 4/5 to 5/5).

Administration Routes
Peripheral Veins. High osmolarity solutions can cause phlebitis due to fluid shifts in the vein lumen, attributable to peripheral veins' smaller diameter and slower blood flow. For feeding durations ≥3 days, use TNA solutions with osmolarities between 400-550 mOsm/l. If the feeding duration is <3 days, patients tolerate up to 650 mOsm/l. Peripheral vein catheters are the preferred route for short-term (<7 days) feeding or when CVC access is unavailable. Commonly used veins are the lateral saphenous (dog) and medial saphenous (cat); overlying skin is thinner, making catheter insertion easier. Less commonly used veins are the cephalic and accessory cephalic, femoral and ear veins (dogs with pendulous ears). Less intensive patient monitoring is required compared to CVCs but there is increased risk of patient damage to bandage covers; use Elizabethan collars.

Table 1. Standard total nutrient admixture (TNA) formulations.

PART A. CALCULATION WORKSHEET

Patient data needed	Feline example
1. Current body weight in kg	4.1 kg
2. Calculate resting energy requirement (RER) as kcal/day	200 kcal/day
3. Expected fluid volume in ml/kg/day	70 ml/kg
4. Calories from fat as a percent	80%
5. Protein-calorie ratio as g/100 kcal RER	4 g/100 kcal RER
6. Potassium concentration as mEq/l	30 mEq/l

Parenteral solution formula

1. Determine volume of fat and dextrose needed daily

Calculate RER calories from fat	200 x 0.80 = 160 kcal
Calculate volume of 20% lipid needed	160 kcal ÷ 2 kcal/ml = **80 ml/day**
Calculate RER calories from dextrose	200 – 160 = 40 kcal
Calculate volume of 50% dextrose needed	40 kcal ÷ 1.7 kcal/ml = **24 ml/day**

2. Determine volume of amino acid solution needed daily

Calculate g of protein needed	RER x 4 g/100 kcal = 8 g protein/day
Calculate volume of 8.5% amino acid needed	8 g ÷ 0.085 g/ml = **94 ml/day**

3. Determine volume of B vitamins and trace minerals needed daily

Calculate B vitamins needed	RER x 1 ml/100 kcal = **2 ml/day**
Calculate trace minerals needed	RER x 1 ml/100 kcal = **2 ml/day**
Daily parenteral nutrition formula	80 ml of 20% lipid emulsion
	24 ml of 50% dextrose
	94 ml of 8.5% amino acid with electrolytes
	2 ml of vitamin-B complex
	2 ml of trace elements
	Total = 202 ml

4. Determine volume of crystalloid solution needed to meet daily fluid requirement

Daily fluid volume requested	4.1 kg x 70 ml/kg = 287 ml/day
Volume required is daily total – PN total	287 – 202 = 85 ml

5. Determine phosphorus supplementation

Phosphorus from amino acids	94 x 30 mM/l = 2.8 mM
Desired final phosphorus concentration in the TNA	= 10 mM/l x 287 ml = 2.9 mM (no phosphorus is needed)

6. Determine potassium supplementation

K⁺ from lactated Ringer's solution	85 ml x 4 mEq/l = 0.3 mEq
K⁺ from amino acid solution	94 ml x 60 mEq/l = 5.6 mEq
Total K⁺ in TNA solution	0.3 mEq + 5.6 mEq = 5.9 mEq
Desired final K⁺ concentration in TNA	30 mEq/l x 287 ml = 8.6 mEq
KCl (2.0 mEq/ml) required	8.6 mEq – 5.9 mEq = 2.7 mEq ÷ 2.0 = 1.4 ml

PART B. FELINE FORMULA EXAMPLE

Animal data

Body weight	4.1 kg
RER	200 kcal/day
Calories from fat	80%
Calories from glucose	20%
Protein-calorie ratio	4 g/100 kcal (adequate for most cats)
Fluid volume	70 ml/kg (maintenance fluid volume)
Potassium concentration	30 mEq/l

Parenteral solution

50% dextrose	24 ml providing 41 kcal
20% lipid emulsion	80 ml providing 160 kcal
8.5% amino acids with electrolytes	94 ml providing 8 g of amino acids
Potassium chloride	1.4 ml
Vitamin-B complex	2 ml
Trace elements	2 ml
Lactated Ringer's solution	85 ml
Total fluid volume	288 ml

This final solution is a 500-ml bag containing 200 kcal (80% from fat), adequate nitrogen, major B vitamins with the following electrolyte profile

Sodium	61.6 mEq/l
Potassium	29.5 mEq/l
Magnesium	3.3 mEq/l
Phosphorus	9.8 mM/l
Chloride	55.4 mEq/l
Calcium	0.8 mEq/l
Zinc	2 mg
Copper	1 mg
Manganese	0.2 mg
Chromium	8 mg
Final osmolarity	768
Approximate cost = $100 per day	

Table 1. continued

PART C. CANINE FORMULA EXAMPLE
Animal data

Body weight	14 kg
RER	507 kcal/day
Calories from fat	90%
Calories from glucose	10%
Protein-calorie ratio	3 g/100 kcal
Fluid volume	70 ml/kg
Potassium concentration	20 mEq/l

Parenteral solution

50% dextrose	30 ml providing 51 kcal
20% lipid emulsion	227 ml providing 454 kcal
8.5% amino acids with electrolytes	176 ml providing 15 g of amino acids
Potassium phosphate	1.4 ml
Vitamin-B complex	5 ml
Trace elements	5 ml
NormaSol R	543 ml
Total fluid volume	987 ml

This final solution is a 1-liter bag containing 507 kcal (90% from fat), adequate nitrogen, major B vitamins with the following electrolyte profile

Sodium	88.0 mEq/l
Potassium	20.3 mEq/l
Magnesium	3.5 mEq/l
Phosphorus	9.9 mM/l
Chloride	65.5 mEq/l
Calcium	0 mEq/l
Zinc	5 mg
Copper	2 mg
Chromium	20 mg
Manganese	0.5 mg
Final osmolarity	523 mOsm/l
Approximate cost = $100 per day	

Central Veins. The large diameter allows for delivery of high osmolarity PN solutions without the risk of phlebitis. CVCs are preferred for prolonged feeding (>7 days). Cats, because of their smaller size, higher protein requirements and sometimes more restrictive fluid allowances, often receive PN solutions with osmolarities >650 mOsm/l, requiring delivery into a large vein. The right external jugular is the preferred access route for CVCs. Placement is technically difficult and obesity or cachexia can further complicate placement. Infection rates are higher and CVCs require intensive patient monitoring compared to peripheral vein catheters. But there is lower risk of self damage by the patient.

Combined PN and EN. Either central or peripheral vein delivery can be used in combination with EN feeding. Avoid CVC-esophagostomy feeding tube combination; close proximity may increase risk of infection and mechanical problems.

Catheter Complications/Management.

INFECTION. Primarily associated with substandard catheter care. Use meticulous aseptic technique during catheter placement and maintenance. Change the bandage every other day; clean the venipuncture site with an iodine solution and examine for redness, edema or swelling; apply topical povidone iodine ointment to the catheter-skin junction. If problems develop, remove the catheter and obtain culture/sensitivity of the catheter, site and TNA solution. Hot pack to reduce swelling. Initiate systemic antibiotic therapy if indicated. Catheter tunneling helps prevent infection but is a surgical procedure and is more commonly used with long-term CVCs. Other sources of infections include UTI, abscesses, pneumonia and GI bacterial translocation. Contaminated PN fluid is another potential source: minimize by using a closed-circuit fluid system and change the administration set every other day.

THROMBOSIS. Associated complications: loss of vessel patency, septic thrombophlebitis, venous gangrene, extravasation of infusate, pulmonary embolism and death. To minimize thrombus formation use polyurethane or silicone catheters (smooth, pliable and low platelet adhesion). Minimize other risk factors, which include: small peripheral veins, catheter too large for the vein, long-term use, catheter traversing a mobile joint and pre-existing inflammatory diseases. The thrombosis risk associated with a CVC is low but consequences are much more severe than peripheral vein catheter thrombosis.

EXTRAVASATION. Complications with CVC fluid extravasation may not become evident until large volumes have been administered; fluids may accumulate in mediastinal and pleural spaces resulting in labored breathing. Signs of peripheral vein catheter fluid extravasation include swelling and tenderness of the skin overlying the catheter tip. The swelling may feel cool and/or the catheter insertion site may be swollen, red and hot. Left unattended, tissue necrosis and sloughing may occur. Stiff plastic catheters are more likely to perforate vessels during and after placement compared to pliable polyurethane or silicone catheters.

OTHER CATHETER USE. When venous access is limited, PN catheters may be used for blood sampling and administering

Table 2. Metabolic complications of parenteral-nutrition administration, treatment and potential patient considerations.

Complications are listed in descending order of likely occurrence and treatments are listed from immediate to longer term solutions. To minimize complications, patients should be hemodynamically stable and any electrolyte and acid-base abnormalities, severe tachycardia, hypotension and volume deficits should be corrected before starting PN.

Complication	Treatment	Patient considerations

Hyperglycemia	Stop infusion, recheck in two to four hours, decrease PN infusion by 50% until normal, then increase infusion rate slowly
	Subcutaneous insulin therapy
	Change caloric sources:
	    Increase lipid fraction of calories
	    Decrease glucose fraction of calories
		Glucose intolerance

Hypokalemia	Add KCl or KPO_4 to PN bag
	Correct serum magnesium as needed
	Change caloric sources:
	    Increase lipid fraction of calories
	    Decrease glucose fraction of calories
		GI or renal losses
		Drug therapies that increase urinary excretion
		Insulin therapy

Hypophosphatemia	Add $NaPO_4$ or KPO_4 to PN bag	Diabetic ketoacidosis

Hyperlipidemia	Stop infusion, recheck in two to four hours, decrease infusion by 50% until normal, then increase infusion rate slowly
	Change caloric sources:
	    Decrease lipid fraction of calories
	    Increase glucose fraction of calories
		Decreased lipid clearance

Phlebitis	Change catheter and infusion site
	Lower PN osmolality:
	    Increase lipid fraction of calories
	    Decrease glucose fraction of calories
	    Add heparin to PN bag
		Proper hydration
		Endogenous site of infection

Hyperkalemia	Change PN bag and decrease potassium	Acidosis, renal failure, sepsis Drug therapies that decrease urinary excretion
Hyperammonemia	Decrease PN infusion by 50% until normal Change PN bag, decrease amino acid concentration Use branched-chain amino acid sources	Liver dysfunction, GI bleeding
Hypomagnesemia	Add $MgSO_4$ to PN bag	GI or renal losses Drug therapies that increase urinary excretion

Hypoglycemia	Piggyback 50% dextrose drip until normal
	Change caloric sources:
	    Decrease lipid fraction of calories
	    Increase glucose fraction of calories
		Sepsis
		Insulin therapy
		Insulinoma

Infected catheter site	Change catheter and infusion site Culture catheter and PN solution Give antibiotics based on culture and antimicrobial sensitivity tests Hot pack the site	Substandard catheter care Endogenous site of infection Proper hydration

Key: PN = parenteral nutrition, GI = gastrointestinal.

medications if adequately flushed before and after PN administration is interrupted. Proper aseptic technique is imperative.

PN Solutions

Total Nutrient Admixtures. Providing the correct combination of PN constituents is complex and important. Institutions that routinely use PN support have equipment and expertise to mix (compound) their own PN solutions. TNA solutions contain the lipids, dextrose, amino acids and electrolytes combined in a single bag that meet (totally or in part) a patient's fluid, energy, amino acid, electrolyte and vitamin needs for 24 hours. For most practices, purchasing premixed TNA solutions is easier/better than compounding (similar to using prepackaged commercial foods vs. homemade foods). TNA sources include veterinary teaching hospitals (see Miscellaneous below), large referral practices and human hospitals. **Table 1** provides a calculation worksheet and example for

determining typical concentrations for a prescription so a TNA can be ordered; not all sources (see Miscellaneous below) require a prescription. TNA delivery is convenient, requiring only one bag, one infusion pump and one administration set. Any opaque liquid infusion pump can be used. For compounding and feeding information other than PN solutions, see Chapter 26, Small Animal Clinical Nutrition, 5th edition.

Drug Delivery in PN Solutions. Extreme caution should be taken before medications are added to the TNA. The Handbook on Injectable Drugs is updated and published every 2 years and is a good source for current information about drug compatibility with PN solutions. Preferred administration is through a second peripheral catheter (or a multi-lumen central catheter) instead of adding drugs to TNA solutions.

FOLLOWUP

Veterinary Health Care Team Followup

Record body weight and BCS daily. BCS is unlikely to change during the course of a hospital stay. Laboratory tests beyond those routinely performed for critically ill patients are usually unnecessary. **Table 2** lists laboratory findings for potential metabolic complications along with management recommendations. Most patients will show subjective clinical improvement within 36 hours of initiation of PN support.

Potassium. Monitor serum potassium daily. TNAs typically provide maintenance amounts of potassium, not repletion amounts. If necessary, add potassium to the PN regimen using either a 2 mEq/ml potassium chloride solution or a 4.4 mEq/ml potassium phosphate solution. If a patient is hyperkalemic when PN is initiated, do not provide additional potassium.

Transition to Oral Feeding. PN patients should be fed enterally as soon as possible, but may continue to receive TNA as EN intake increases to meet RER. Vomiting and diarrhea are commonly associated with reintroduction of oral food. The transition food may be a recovery-type food (Tables 4 and 5, Chapter 12) or a specific veterinary therapeutic food that may be fed to the patient at home due to an ongoing disease condition. Transition carefully to RER amounts over 2-3 days using small frequent meals; increase the daily amount to maintenance DER (~1.5 RER), as tolerated, over several days. For patients with decreased appetites, initially offer a highly palatable food to stimulate voluntary consumption. After the patient is eating, gradually mix in increasing proportions of the food to be fed long term (Appendix E).

MISCELLANEOUS

For nutrition consultation services and/or purchasing TNA solutions for overnight delivery contact, Dr. Rebecca Remillard, MSPCA Angell Animal Medical Center, Boston, MA, 02130; 617-522-7282. Prescription calculations (**Table 1**) are not required.

See Box 26-3, Small Animal Clinical Nutrition, 5th edition, for potential complications associated with TNA solutions. See Chapters 25 and 26, Small Animal Clinical Nutrition, 5th edition, for more information.

Authors

Condensed from Chapter 26, Small Animal Clinical Nutrition, 5th edition, authored by Korinn E. Saker and Rebecca L. Remillard.

References

See Chapter 26, Small Animal Clinical Nutrition, 5th edition, on the website www.markmorrisinstitute.org for references.

CLINICAL POINTS

- Patients judged to be in ideal body condition have 15-20% body fat.
- Dogs and cats are considered overweight when body fat >20-30% of total weight.
- 42% of dogs and 44% of cats in the U.S. between the ages of 5-11 years are overweight.
- **Table 1** lists detrimental effects associated with obesity; even moderate overweight reduces the lifespan of dogs.
- Obesity assessment should include: 1) reviewing the medical record for associated health issues, 2) conducting a thorough feeding assessment and 3) determining the degree to which the patient is overweight/obese.
- Feeding assessment should include: 1) name of the food, its form and how much is fed, 2) whether treats and/or table foods are fed and if so, how much, and 3) noting feeding methods used and who provides food and treats.
- BCS is a good tool for estimating the degree of overweight/obesity.
- Breed can account for 30-70% of obesity risk in dogs (Table 1, Chapter 5); mixed-breed cats are more likely to be obese than purebred cats.
- Free-choice feeding of highly palatable, energy-dense foods is an obesity risk.
- Neutering greatly increases the obesity risk in dogs and cats (e.g., risk almost doubles in neutered bitches).
- Weight loss is more difficult after body fat is gained and maintained. Postneuter feeding recommendations for dogs and cats: 1) feed low-calorie foods or restricted feeding of regular foods (75% of previous amount) and 2) note body weight and BCS every 2 weeks for 4-5 months after neutering and adjust amount fed accordingly at each recheck (by 10% increments).
- Obesity feeding goals: achieve safe weight loss and prevent regain of lost weight.
- Besides proper food, appropriate feeding methods and timely followup (described below), successful weight-reduction programs include an exercise program and pet owner commitment (see Boxes 27-7 and 27-8, Small Animal Clinical Nutrition, 5th edition).

KEY NUTRITIONAL FACTORS

Detailed descriptions of the KNF recommendations that follow are found in Chapter 27, Small Animal Clinical Nutrition, 5th edition. Water is always a KNF.

Abbreviations
BCS = body condition score (Appendix A)
DER = daily energy requirement
KNF = key nutritional factor
RER = resting energy requirement

Table 1. Diseases associated with or exacerbated by obesity.

Metabolic alterations
Anesthetic complications
Dyslipidemia or hyperlipidemia
Glucose intolerance
Hepatic lipidosis (cats)
Insulin resistance

Endocrinopathies
Diabetes mellitus
Hyperadrenocorticism
Hypopituitarism
Hypothalamic lesions
Hypothyroidism
Insulinoma
Pituitary chromophobe adenoma

Functional alterations
Decreased immune function
Dystocia
Exercise intolerance
Heat intolerance
Hypertension
Osteoarthritis/joint stress/musculoskeletal pain
Respiratory distress or dyspnea

Other diseases
Altered kidney function
Cardiovascular disease
Dermatopathy
Neoplasia
Oral disease
Pancreatitis
Transitional cell carcinoma (bladder)
Urinary tract disease (cats)

KNFs for Calorie-Controlled Foods for Weight Loss and Prevention of Weight Regain in Dogs and Cats

- Calorie-controlled foods: most common food type for weight loss in overweight pets and for weight regain prevention.
- These foods should provide recommended allowances of all required nutrients (nutritional adequacy), but should also contain specific levels of KNFs (certain nutrients and nonnutritional food ingredients or food features that can help manage obesity safely and effectively when fed for weight loss). These foods should be balanced so the patient's essential non-energy nutrient needs are met when the patient consumes less energy. They should minimize loss of lean body mass when fed for weight loss.
- Tables 2 (dogs) and 3 (cats) list KNF recommendations for calorie-controlled foods for weight loss and prevention of weight regain.

Table 2. Key nutritional factors for calorie-restricted dog foods for weight loss and prevention of weight regain.

Factors	Dietary recommendations (dry matter basis)
Energy density	Foods for weight loss and prevention of weight regain should contain ≤3.4 kcal (≤14.2 kJ) metabolizable energy (ME)/g
Fat	Foods for weight loss should contain ≤9% Foods for prevention of weight regain should contain ≤14%
Fiber	Foods for weight loss should contain 12 to 25% Foods for prevention of weight regain should contain 10 to 20%
Protein	Foods for weight loss should contain ≥25% Foods for prevention of weight regain should contain ≥18%
Lysine	Foods for weight loss should contain ≥1.7%
Carbohydrate	Foods for weight loss should contain ≤40% Foods for prevention of weight regain should contain ≤55%
L-carnitine	Foods for weight loss and prevention of weight regain should contain ≥300 ppm
Antioxidants	Foods for weight loss and prevention of weight regain should contain:
Vitamin E	≥400 IU vitamin E/kg
Vitamin C	≥100 mg vitamin C/kg
Selenium	0.5 to 1.3 mg selenium/kg
Sodium	Foods for weight loss and prevention of weight regain should contain between 0.2 to 0.4%
Phosphorus	Foods for weight loss and prevention of weight regain should contain between 0.4 to 0.8%

Table 3. Key nutritional factors for calorie-restricted cat foods for weight loss and prevention of weight regain.

Factors	Dietary recommendations (dry matter basis)
Energy density	Foods for weight loss should contain ≤3.4 kcal (≤14.2 kJ) metabolizable energy (ME)/g Foods for prevention of weight regain should contain ≤3.8 kcal (≤15.9 kJ) ME/g
Fat	Foods for weight loss should contain ≤10% Foods for prevention of weight regain should contain ≤18%
Fiber	Foods for weight loss should contain 15 to 20% Foods for prevention of weight regain should contain between 6 to 15%
Protein	Foods for weight loss and prevention of weight regain should contain ≥35%
Carbohydrate	Foods for weight loss should contain ≤35% Foods for prevention of weight regain should contain ≤40%
L-carnitine	Foods for weight loss and prevention of weight regain should contain ≥500 ppm
Antioxidants	Foods for weight loss and prevention of weight regain should contain:
Vitamin E	≥500 IU vitamin E/kg
Vitamin C	100 to 200 mg vitamin C/kg
Selenium	0.5 to 1.3 mg selenium/kg
Sodium	Foods for weight loss and prevention of weight regain should contain between 0.2 to 0.6%
Phosphorus	Foods for weight loss and prevention of weight regain should contain between 0.5 to 0.8%

KNFs for Metabolic-Control Foods for Weight Loss in Cats

- Metabolic-control foods partition energy to induce ketosis instead of using reduced energy density as their primary

Table 4. Key nutritional factors for metabolic-control cat foods for weight loss.

Factors	Dietary recommendations (dry matter basis)
Carbohydrate	≤20%
Protein	At least 47% but not exceed 55%
Fat	≤25%
Fiber	≥5%
L-carnitine	≥500 ppm
Antioxidants	Foods for weight loss and prevention of weight regain should contain:
Vitamin E	≥500 IU vitamin E/kg
Vitamin C	100 to 200 mg vitamin C/kg
Selenium	0.5 to 1.3 mg selenium/kg
Sodium	Foods for weight loss should contain between 0.2 to 0.6%
Phosphorus	Foods for weight loss should contain between 0.5 to 0.8%

strategy. Most of these foods are equivalent in caloric density to maintenance foods but are formulated to provide all essential nutrients, except calories, when fed in a weight-loss program.

- The use of metabolic-control foods is an alternative to calorie-control foods for weight loss in overweight cats. **Table 4** summarizes KNFs for metabolic-control cat foods for weight loss.

FEEDING PLAN

Weight Reduction

Note that the following food selection and feeding method discussions are for both calorie-controlled foods and metabolic-control foods.

Assess and Select the Food

Ensure the Food's Basic Nutritional Adequacy. AAFCO nutritional adequacy statements are usually found on a product's label. AAFCO approval does not ensure a food will be effective in facilitating healthy weight loss, preventing weight regain or preventing other long-term health problems.

Compare the Food's KNF Content with the Recommended Levels. **Tables 5** and **6** compare the KNF recommendations to the KNF content of selected calorie-controlled commercial veterinary therapeutic foods marketed for weight loss in dogs and cats, respectively. Select a food that is most similar to the KNF recommendations. Contact manufacturers for information for foods not in the table (contact information is listed on product labels). If a calorie-controlled food has been tried in cats, but has not achieved the desired weight loss, a metabolic-control food should be considered. **Table 7** compares the KNF recommendations to the KNF content of veterinary therapeutic cat foods marketed for a metabolic approach to weight loss.

Manage Treats and Snacks. Ideally treats, snacks and human foods should be eliminated from the feeding plan to maximize chances for weight loss. A portion of the total DER for weight loss (<10% of the total diet on a volume, weight or calorie basis) can be reserved if owners insist on feeding treats or snacks. Recommend treats that are specifically formulated for overweight pets (**Table 8**). Treats can also be the dry form of the weight-loss

Table 5. Levels of key nutritional factors in selected commercial foods marketed for calorie-restricted weight loss in dogs compared to recommended levels.* (Numbers in red match optimal KNFs.)

Dry foods	Energy density (kcal/cup)**	Energy density (kcal ME/g)	Fat (%)	Fiber (%)	Prot (%)	Lys (%)	Carb (%)	Carn (ppm)	Vit E (IU/kg)	Vit C (mg/kg)	Se (mg/kg)	Na (%)	P (%)
Recommended levels	-	≤3.4	≤9	12-25	≥25	≥1.7	≤40	≥300	≥400	≥100	0.5-1.3	0.2-0.4	0.4-0.8
Hill's Prescription Diet r/d Canine	242	3.3	8.2	13.5	34.3	1.91	38.7	301.1	618	262	1.37	0.24	0.66
Hill's Prescription Diet r/d with Chicken Canine	241	3.3	8.8	13.6	35.2	1.86	36.0	300.0	620	266	1.49	0.40	0.75
Iams Veterinary Formula Weight Control D/ Optimum Weight Control	209	3.5	9.5	3.0	28.7	na	51.2	na	na	na	na	0.51	1.0
Iams Veterinary Formula Weight Loss/Restricted-Calorie	217	3.7	9.1	2.4	25.0	na	58.0	na	na	na	na	0.24	0.83
Medi-Cal Calorie Control	238	na	10.4	4.1	30.2	na	na	na	na	na	na	0.4	1.4
Medi-Cal Fibre Formula	266	na	10.6	14.3	26.2	na	na	na	na	na	na	0.3	0.9
Purina Veterinary Diets OM Overweight Management	266	3.0	7.2	10.3	31.1	na	44.2	na	na	na	na	0.31	0.89
Royal Canin Veterinary Diet Calorie Control CC 26 High Fiber	232	3.1	10.4	17.6	30.9	1.37	33.7	na	962	na	0.33	0.33	0.77
Royal Canin Veterinary Diet Calorie Control CC 32 High Protein	234	3.9	10.4	3.3	37.4	1.42	38.6	na	962	na	0.38	0.38	1.42

Moist foods	Energy density (kcal/can)**	Energy density (kcal ME/g)	Fat (%)	Fiber (%)	Prot (%)	Lys (%)	Carb (%)	Carn (ppm)	Vit E (IU/kg)	Vit C (mg/kg)	Se (mg/kg)	Na (%)	P (%)
Recommended levels	-	≤3.4	≤9	12-25	≥25	≥1.7	≤40	≥300	≥400	≥100	0.5-1.3	0.2-0.4	0.4-0.8
Hill's Prescription Diet r/d Canine	257/12.3 oz.	3.0	8.6	21.2	25.3	1.39	39.2	370.9	731	131	0.86	0.24	0.53
Iams Veterinary Formula Weight Loss/Restricted-Calorie	397/14 oz.	3.9	14.9	3.2	34.4	na	40.8	na	na	na	na	0.46	0.93
Medi-Cal Calorie Control	212/360 g	na	23.2	1.6	59.2	na	na	na	na	na	na	1.2	1.7
Medi-Cal Fibre Formula	350/396 g	na	9.1	15.0	24.8	na	na	na	na	na	na	0.5	0.8
Purina Veterinary Diets OM Overweight Management	189/12.5 oz.	2.5	8.4	19.2	44.1	na	21.7	na	na	na	na	0.28	1.06
Royal Canin Veterinary Diet Calorie Control CC High Fiber	346/14 oz.	3.6	12.5	8.8	25.9	1.48	46.3	na	271	na	0.41	0.53	0.62
Royal Canin Veterinary Diet Calorie Control CC High Protein in Gel	263/12.7 oz.	4.8	28.5	3.0	51.5	3.1	5.1	na	396	na	na	0.99	1.58

Key: ME = metabolizable energy, na = information not available from manufacturer, Fiber = crude fiber, Prot = protein, Lys = lysine, Carb = digestible carbohydrate, Carn = L-carnitine, Se = selenium, Na = sodium, P = phosphorus, g = grams.
*From manufacturers' published information or calculated from manufacturers' published as-fed values; all values are on a dry matter basis unless otherwise stated.
**Energy density values are listed on an as fed basis and are useful for determining the amount to feed; cup = 8-oz. measuring cup. To convert to kJ, multiply kcal by 4.184.

food, air-popped popcorn and low-fat or low-starch vegetables. Cats in a metabolic weight-loss program should not receive treats unless the treats conform nutritionally to the KNF content of the food and are accounted for in the allotted daily calorie intake.

Assess and Determine the Feeding Method
Determine How Much Food to Feed. Feeding the correct amount of food is essential and is based on the estimate of caloric restriction necessary to achieve safe weight loss. Goals for average weight loss in dogs and cats are 1-2% and 0.5-1% of obese body weight/week, respectively. In dogs, gradual weight loss is more likely to result in maintenance of the target body weight, once

achieved. A weight loss of 0.5%/week for dogs or cats is acceptable as long as owners know how long it will take to achieve the target weight. At 0.5% weight loss/week, it may take ≥1 year. A cautionary reminder about food restriction in cats: be sure they are eating at least 50% of their estimated food dose to mitigate development of hepatic lipidosis.
Estimating the Amount of Food to Feed for Controlled Weight Loss. There are several good methods including using product information, calculations based on ideal weight, calculations based on current food intake and calculations based on obese weight. These are estimates for weight loss and should be considered starting points, which will likely need adjustment over time. This

Table 6. Levels of key nutritional factors in selected commercial foods marketed for calorie-restricted weight loss in cats compared to recommended levels.* (Numbers in red match optimal KNFs.)

Dry foods	Energy density (kcal/cup)**	Energy density (kcal ME/g)	Fat (%)	Fiber (%)	Prot (%)	Carb (%)	Carn (ppm)	Vit E (IU/kg)	Vit C (mg/kg)	Se (mg/kg)	Na (%)	P (%)
Recommended levels	-	≤3.4	≤10	15-20	≥35	≤35	≥500	≥500	100-200	0.5-1.3	0.2-0.6	0.5-0.8
Hill's Prescription Diet r/d Feline	263	3.3	9.3	13.6	36.9	33.5	538.6	614	80	0.66	0.35	0.81
Hill's Prescription Diet r/d with Chicken Feline	266	3.4	9.8	13.8	37.7	32.2	556.3	716	120	0.70	0.35	0.84
Iams Veterinary Formula Weight Control D/ Optimum Weight Control	326	3.8	12.2	1.5	38.6	41.2	na	na	na	na	0.39	1.01
Iams Veterinary Formula Weight Loss/Restricted-Calorie	268	3.7	11.0	2.5	35.2	44.5	na	na	na	na	0.37	0.92
Medi-Cal Calorie Control	230	na	9.7	5.1	43.5	na	na	na	na	na	0.8	1.3
Medi-Cal Fibre Formula	280	na	12.2	14.9	34.2	na	na	na	na	na	0.5	0.8
Medi-Cal Reducing Formula	250	na	9.6	5.2	41.8	na	na	na	na	na	0.3	1.2
Purina Veterinary Diets OM Overweight Management Feline Formula	321	3.6	8.5	5.6	56.2	22.4	na	693	116	na	0.57	1.19
Royal Canin Veterinary Diet Calorie Control CC 29 High Fiber	251	3.3	10.2	14.0	33.5	34.5	na	1,065	na	0.32	0.51	0.81
Royal Canin Veterinary Diet Calorie Control CC 38 High Protein	235	3.7	10.2	4.2	43.5	31.5	na	1,124	na	0.38	0.70	1.40
Moist foods	Energy density (kcal/can)**	Energy density (kcal ME/g)	Fat (%)	Fiber (%)	Prot (%)	Carb (%)	Carn (ppm)	Vit E (IU/kg)	Vit C (mg/kg)	Se (mg/kg)	Na (%)	P (%)
Recommended levels	-	≤3.4	≤10	15-20	≥35	≤35	≥500	≥500	100-200	0.5-1.3	0.2-0.6	0.5-0.8
Hill's Prescription Diet r/d with Liver & Chicken Feline	114/5.5 oz.	3.1	9.2	15.4	37.5	31.3	512.5	746	108	1.67	0.29	0.62
Iams Veterinary Formula Weight Loss/Restricted-Calorie	172/6 oz.	4.3	15.5	1.7	44.2	32.3	na	na	na	na	0.43	0.86
Medi-Cal Calorie Control	99/165 g	na	26.0	1.3	49.6	na	na	na	na	na	1.9	1.6
Medi-Cal Fibre Formula	130/170 g	na	17.1	16.7	40.0	na	na	na	na	na	0.4	0.9
Medi-Cal Reducing Formula	111/170 g	na	27.2	1.3	54.3	na	na	na	na	na	1.0	1.6
Purina Veterinary Diets OM Overweight Management Feline Formula	150/5.5 oz.	3.9	14.6	10.2	44.6	23.2	na	na	na	na	0.31	0.99
Royal Canin Veterinary Diet Calorie Control CC High Fiber	164/6 oz.	4.1	21.3	7.7	33.5	32.5	na	276	na	0.43	0.38	0.81
Royal Canin Veterinary Diet Calorie Control CC High Protein	130/5.8 oz.	4.7	24.4	2.4	53.5	7.0	na	562	na	na	1.50	1.68

Key: ME = metabolizable energy, na = information not available from manufacturer, Fiber = crude fiber, Prot = protein, Carb = digestible carbohydrate, Carn = L-carnitine, Se = selenium, Na = sodium, P = phosphorus, g = grams.
*From manufacturers' published information or calculated from manufacturers' published as-fed values.
**Energy density values are listed on an as fed basis and are useful for determining the amount to feed; cup = 8-oz. measuring cup. To convert to kJ, multiply kcal by 4.184.

chapter uses product information and calculations based on ideal weight for estimating the amount to feed. Chapter 27, Small Animal Clinical Nutrition, 5th edition, reviews other methods. *Product Information.* Simplest and most commonly used method. Obtain the initial food dose estimate from manufacturers' feeding information (product labels, published company literature/websites) or by using "calculators" or proprietary software programs. Some software programs require an estimate of the patient's ideal weight. Free web-based programs are available for estimating ideal weight (**Box 1**) or use **Tables 9** and/or **10**. *Calculation Based on Estimated Ideal Weight.* Assumes RER for the optimal weight and RER for obese weight are the same. As mentioned, **Tables 9** and **10** and **Box 1** provide information for determining ideal body weight and RER. **Table 11** provides an example of using this method for calculating initial food dosage. *Consider How to Offer the Food.* Use food-restricted feeding.

Feed multiple small meals rather than a single large meal to take advantage of increased energy cost for assimilating each meal. Most owners' schedules allow feeding ≥2meals/day. Use portions of practical size (i.e., to the nearest 1/4th cup or can). If the daily amount does not divide evenly into portions, feed larger portions when the owner will be with the pet for the longest time between meals. Free-choice feeding rarely works for weight loss or for maintenance of reduced body weight, even with calorie-restricted foods. To reduce begging and the owner's urge to provide additional food or treats, keep pets out of the kitchen and dining areas when preparing and eating family meals. Ensure that obese patients do not have access to other pets' food. Commercial feeders are available that limit access to food (**Figure 1**). *Manage Food Changes.* As with any food change, it is best to transition the patient to the new weight-loss food gradually over a period of several days (Appendix E); most have good palatability. *Food and Water Receptacle Husbandry.* Food and water bowls should always be washed regularly with warm soapy water and rinsed well. Dishes used for moist foods need daily cleaning. Discard moist or moistened dry foods after 2-4 hours of room temperature exposure to avoid foodborne illnesses (Appendix F).

Box 1. Web-Based Programs for Obesity Management.

www.PetFit.com
This is a commercial pet food company sponsored free program for determining ideal (target) body weight for overweight/obese dogs and cats. The visuals in this program include a profile and dorsal view of a dog and cat with a slide bar beneath. The body condition score of the initial view is 3/5. The patient's current weight is entered and the slide bar is moved to the right (or left) to match the dimensions of the patient. After the operator is satisfied with the match, an ideal body weight is automatically calculated.

Balance IT (info@dvmconsulting.com)
Balance IT is a fee-based program designed to help veterinary health care teams with calculation-based weight-loss feeding plans. The user can select/enter all the foods a patient is currently fed (based on the diet history) and the program will then determine the caloric needs of the patient for weight loss. Users can set the desired weight-loss rates and select the commercial weight-loss food they wish to feed (along with any treats up to 10% of daily calories). The program calculates the amount to feed and enters this information into a report to be printed for clients. Based on weight rechecks, the software adjusts the amount to feed the patient.

Table 7. Levels of key nutritional factors in selected commercial foods marketed for the metabolic approach to weight loss in cats compared to recommended levels.* (Numbers in red match optimal KNFs.)

Dry foods	Energy density (kcal/cup)**	Carb (%)	Prot (%)	Fat (%)	Fiber (%)	Carn (ppm)	Vit E (IU/kg)	Vit C (mg/kg)	Se (mg/kg)	Na (%)	P (%)
Recommended levels	-	≤20	≥47-≤55	≤25	≥5	≥500	≥500	100-200	0.5-1.3	0.2-0.6	0.5-0.8
Hill's Prescription Diet m/d Feline	480	14.7	51.5	22.0	5.9	551.1	946	234	0.79	0.40	0.74
Purina Veterinary Diets DM Dietetic Management Formula	592	15.0	57.8	17.9	1.3	18.0	109	na	1.26	0.60	1.52

Moist foods	Energy density (kcal/can)**	Carb (%)	Prot (%)	Fat (%)	Fiber (%)	Carn (ppm)	Vit E (IU/kg)	Vit C (mg/kg)	Se (mg/kg)	Na (%)	P (%)
Recommended levels	-	≤20	≥47-≤55	≤25	≥5	≥500	≥500	100-200	0.5-1.3	0.2-0.6	0.5-0.8
Hill's Prescription Diet m/d Feline	156/5.5 oz.	15.7	52.8	19.4	6.0	524.2	810	125	1.77	0.36	0.69
Purina Veterinary Diets DM Dietetic Management Formula	194/5.5 oz.	8.1	56.9	23.8	3.7	na	214	na	na	0.39	1.10

Key: na = information not available from manufacturer, Carb = digestible carbohydrate, Prot = protein, Fiber = crude fiber, Carn = L-carnitine, Se = selenium, Na = sodium, P = phosphorus.
*From manufacturers' published information or calculated from manufacturers' published as-fed values; all values are on a dry matter basis unless otherwise stated.
**Energy density values are listed on an as fed basis and are useful for determining the amount to feed; cup = 8-oz. measuring cup. To convert to kJ, multiply kcal by 4.184.

Table 8. Selected commercial treats marketed for weight management in dogs and their respective levels of key nutritional factors (levels for maintenance of target weight [**Table 2**]).* (Numbers in red match optimal KNFs.)

	Energy per treat (kcal)	Energy density (kcal ME/g)	Fat (%)	Protein (%)	Fiber (%)	Phosphorus (%)	Sodium (%)
Recommended levels	na**	≤3.4	≤14	≥18	10-20	0.4-0.8	0.2-0.4
Hill's Prescription Diet Canine Treats	13	2.9	7.3	14.6	17	0.45	0.11
Royal Canin Veterinary Diet Canine Treats	14	3.4	6.3	10.9	6.8	0.47	0.19

Key: na = not applicable, ME = metabolizable energy.
*All values are on a dry matter basis except for energy (kcal)/treat, which is on an as fed basis.
**This information is for feeding purposes only. Treats should not make up more than 10% of the total caloric intake and these calories should be accounted for by reducing the amount of kcal fed as food accordingly.

Table 9. Relationships between body condition score (BCS; 5-point system) and actual body weight, ideal body weight, resting energy requirement (RER; kcal metabolizable energy [ME]/day) and estimated percent body fat (%BF). Actual body weight and BCS can be used to estimate a patient's ideal weight* and associated RER, which can be further used for determining the amount of food to feed for weight loss.

BCS	Body weight (kg)											
5	2	2.5	3	3.5	4	4.5	5	5.5	6	6.5	7	7.5
4	1.7	2.1	2.6	3	3.4	3.9	4.3	4.7	5.1	5.6	6	6.4
3	1.5	1.9	2.3	2.6	3	3.4	3.8	4.1	4.5	4.9	5.3	5.6
RER	95	112	129	144	160	174	189	203	216	230	243	256
BCS	Body weight (kg)											
5	8	8.5	9	9.5	10	10.5	11	11.5	12	12.5	13	13.5
4	6.9	7.3	7.7	8.1	8.6	9	9.4	9.9	10.3	10.7	11.1	11.6
3	6	6.4	6.8	7.1	7.5	7.9	8.3	8.6	9	9.4	9.8	10.1
RER	268	281	293	305	317	329	341	352	364	375	386	397
BCS	Body weight (kg)											
5	14	14.5	15	15.5	16	16.5	17	17.5	18	18.5	19	19.5
4	12	12.4	12.9	13.3	13.7	14.1	14.6	15	15.4	15.9	16.3	16.7
3	10.5	10.9	11.3	11.6	12	12.4	12.8	13.1	13.5	13.9	14.3	14.6
RER	408	419	430	441	451	462	472	483	493	503	513	524
BCS	Body weight (kg)											
5	20	21	22	23	24	25	26	27	28	29	30	31
4	17.1	18	18.9	19.7	20.6	21.4	22.3	23.1	24	24.9	25.7	26.6
3	15	15.8	16.5	17.3	18	18.8	19.5	20.3	21	21.8	22.5	23.3
RER	534	553	573	593	612	631	650	668	687	705	723	741
BCS	Body weight (kg)											
5	32	33	34	35	36	37	38	39	40	41	42	43
4	27.4	28.3	29.1	30	30.9	31.7	32.6	33.4	34.3	35.1	36	36.9
3	24	24.8	25.5	26.3	27	27.8	28.5	29.3	30	30.8	31.5	32.3
RER	759	777	794	812	829	846	863	880	897	914	931	947
BCS	Body weight (kg)											
5	45	47	49	51	53	55	58	61	64	67	70	73
4	38.6	40.3	42	43.7	45.4	47.1	49.7	52.3	54.9	57.4	60	62.6
3	33.8	35.3	36.8	38.3	39.8	41.3	43.5	45.8	48	50.3	52.5	54.8
RER	980	1,013	1,045	1,077	1,108	1,139	1,186	1,231	1,277	1,321	1,365	1,409

BCS	%BF		BCS	%BF		BCS	%BF
5	≥40		4	30		3	20

*Example: A 32-kg dog has a BCS of 4/5. What is its ideal weight and associated RER and approximate %BF?
1. Find the closest value for its current body weight (31.7 kg) in the row for BCS 4/5.
2. Locate the corresponding body weight for BCS 3/5 (ideal weight) in the same number column. In this case it is 27.8 kg.
3. Below the ideal body weight of 27.8 kg, find the RER value for that weight; in this case it is 846 kcal/day (to convert to kJ, multiply kcal by 4.184).
4. At its current BCS (4/5), the dog's approximate %BF is 30.

Table 10. Methods for determining ideal/optimal body weight.

1. Consult the patient's medical record to determine if a body condition score (BCS) of 3/5 was recorded with a simultaneous ideal body weight.
2. Consult the patient's medical record to see if the patient's body weight was recorded at about the time the patient reached one year of age. Such a body weight would likely be near ideal (but not always). Thus, this method might not be as reliable as Method 1 above.
3. Consult **Table 9**.
   a. Determine patient's current BCS and obtain current body weight.
   b. Locate the current BCS and body weight in **Table 9**.
   c. Note the weight in **Table 9** that coincides with a BCS of 3/5 in the same column.
4. Consult web-based programs (**Box 1**).

Table 11. Using ideal body weight to determine initial food dosage for controlled weight loss.

The following steps represent the process for estimating the initial amount to feed for weight loss using ideal body weight:
1. Determine the patient's current weight and BCS.
2. Consult **Table 9**; for current BCS, find current weight and read associated ideal weight (BCS 3/5) from same column.
3. Determine RER for ideal weight (also from **Table 9**, immediately below ideal weight) = initial estimated daily energy intake.
4. Divide RER by the as fed energy density of selected food = initial daily food dose.

An example case follows:
An obese dog weighs 30 kg and has a BCS of 5/5. Consulting **Table 9**, we determine that the dog's ideal body weight (BCS 3/5) is 22.5 kg. In **Table 9**, the RER for a 22.5-kg dog is located immediately below the weight. In this case it is 723 kcal/day.*
The food selected for weight loss provides 220 kcal/cup; 723 kcal/day ÷ 220 kcal/cup = 3.3 cups/day. This amount is a starting point and may need to be modified to achieve the desired weight loss.
Recheck body weight after two to three weeks. The weight-loss target should be between 0.5 and 2% per week of initial obese body weight.
Key: BCS = body condition score (Appendix A), RER = resting energy requirement.
*To convert to kJ, multiply kcal by 4.184.

Table 12. Levels of key nutritional factors in selected commercial foods marketed for weight maintenance in dogs after a weight-loss program compared to recommended levels.* (Numbers in red match optimal KNFs.)

Dry foods	Energy density (kcal/cup)**	Energy density (kcal ME/g)	Fat (%)	Fiber (%)	Prot (%)	Carb (%)	Carn (ppm)	Vit E (IU/kg)	Vit C (mg/kg)	Se (mg/kg)	Na (%)	P (%)
Recommended levels	-	≤3.4	≤14	10-20	≥18	≤55	≥300	≥400	≥100	0.5-1.3	0.2-0.4	0.4-0.8
Hill's Prescription Diet w/d Canine	243	3.3	8.8	16.4	18.9	51.2	349.5	574	274	1.34	0.22	0.56
Hill's Prescription Diet w/d with Chicken Canine	239	3.2	8.7	17.1	19.1	50.1	328.0	611	298	1.52	0.27	0.56
Iams Veterinary Formula Weight Control D/ Optimum Weight Control	209	3.5	9.5	3.0	28.7	51.2	na	na	na	na	0.51	1.00
Medi-Cal Weight Control/ Mature	320	na	8.5	4.0	19.5	na	na	na	na	na	0.2	0.8
Purina Veterinary Diets OM Overweight Management	266	3.0	7.2	10.3	31.1	44.2	na	na	na	na	0.31	0.89

Moist foods	Energy density (kcal/can)**	Energy density (kcal ME/g)	Fat (%)	Fiber (%)	Prot (%)	Carb (%)	Carn (ppm)	Vit E (IU/kg)	Vit C (mg/kg)	Se (mg/kg)	Na (%)	P (%)
Recommended levels	-	≤3.4	≤14	10-20	≥18	≤55	≥300	≥400	≥100	0.5-1.3	0.2-0.4	0.4-0.8
Hill's Prescription Diet w/d Canine	329/13 oz.	3.5	12.7	12.4	17.9	52.6	364.1	614	116	0.72	0.24	0.52
Medi-Cal Weight Control/ Mature	370/396 g	na	10.0	5.5	21.5	na	na	na	na	na	0.3	0.6
Purina Veterinary Diets OM Overweight Management	189/12.5 oz.	2.5	8.4	19.2	44.1	21.7	na	na	na	na	0.28	1.06

Key: ME = metabolizable energy, na = information not available from manufacturer, Fiber = crude fiber, Prot = protein, Carb = digestible carbohydrate, Carn = L-carnitine, Se = selenium, Na = sodium, P = phosphorus, g = grams.
*From manufacturers' published information or calculated from manufacturers' published as-fed values. All values are on a dry matter basis unless otherwise stated.
**Energy density values are listed on an as fed basis and are useful for determining the amount to feed; cup = 8-oz. measuring cup. To convert to kJ, multiply kcal by 4.184.

Table 13. Levels of key nutritional factors in selected commercial foods marketed for weight maintenance in cats after a weight-loss program compared to recommended levels.* (Numbers in red match optimal KNFs.)

Dry foods	Energy density (kcal/cup)**	Energy density (kcal ME/g)	Fat (%)	Fiber (%)	Prot (%)	Carb (%)	Carn (ppm)	Vit E (IU/kg)	Vit C (mg/kg)	Se (mg/kg)	Na (%)	P (%)
Recommended levels	-	≤3.8	≤18	6-15	≥35	≤40	≥500	≥500	100-200	0.5-1.3	0.2-0.6	0.5-0.8
Hill's Prescription Diet w/d Feline	281	3.5	9.8	7.6	39.0	37.4	498.9	692	117	0.85	0.30	0.77
Hill's Prescription Diet w/d with Chicken Feline	278	3.5	9.9	7.6	39.9	35.4	500	721	122	0.70	0.35	0.86
Iams Veterinary Formula Weight Control D/ Optimum Weight Control	326	3.8	12.2	1.5	38.6	41.2	na	na	na	na	0.39	1.01
Medi-Cal Weight Control	325	na	11.8	3.4	34.4	na	na	na	na	na	0.3	1.0
Purina Veterinary Diets OM Overweight Management Feline Formula	321	3.6	8.5	5.6	56.2	22.4	na	693	116	na	0.57	1.19

Moist foods	Energy density (kcal/can)**	Energy density (kcal ME/g)	Fat (%)	Fiber (%)	Prot (%)	Carb (%)	Carn (ppm)	Vit E (IU/kg)	Vit C (mg/kg)	Se (mg/kg)	Na (%)	P (%)
Recommended levels	-	≤3.8	≤18	6-15	≥35	≤40	≥500	≥500	100-200	0.5-1.3	0.2-0.6	0.5-0.8
Hill's Prescription Diet w/d with Chicken Feline	127/5.5 oz.	3.5	16.6	10.6	39.6	26.4	514.9	745	115	1.70	0.38	0.68
Medi-Cal Weight Control	144/170 g	na	22.6	4.2	40.0	na	na	na	na	na	0.5	1.1
Purina Veterinary Diets OM Overweight Management Feline Formula	150/5.5 oz.	3.9	14.6	10.2	44.6	23.2	na	na	na	na	0.31	0.99

Key: ME = metabolizable energy, na = information not available from manufacturer, Fiber = crude fiber, Prot = protein, Carb = digestible carbohydrate, Carn = L-carnitine, Se = selenium, Na = sodium, P = phosphorus, g = grams.
*From manufacturers' published information or calculated from manufacturers' published as-fed values. All values are on a dry matter basis unless otherwise stated.
**Energy density values are listed on an as fed basis and are useful for determining the amount to feed; cup = 8-oz. measuring cup. To convert to kJ, multiply kcal by 4.184.

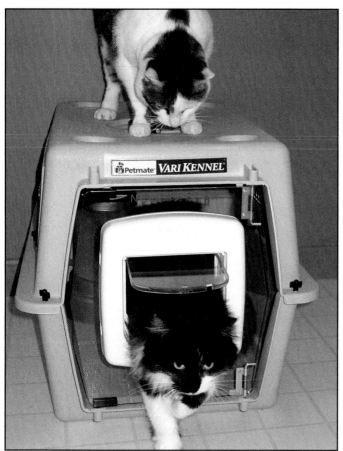

Figure 1. A commercial feeding system for cats and small dogs. Close proximity of a special collar unlocks the feeder door and the pet wearing the collar simply pushes the door open and enters the feeder. More than one pet can have access to one feeder. (Courtesy of NekoFeeder, LLC. www.nekofeeder.com [802-264-6055] 6D Laurette Drive, Essex Junction, VT.)

FOLLOWUP

Owner Followup
Figure 2 is an algorithm for patient monitoring and adjusting the amount to feed during weight loss. When possible, owners can obtain body weights at home and be advised by phone on changing the amount to feed to achieve safe weight loss.

Veterinary Health Care Team Followup
Office rechecks to monitor patient progress are essential to successful weight reduction (equal in importance to diet and exercise). Regular monitoring also helps motivate owners. The most critical times for rechecks are when weight loss slows or stops. Focus on acceptable rates of weight loss instead of specific numbers of days to complete the weight-loss program. Box 27-12, Chapter 27, Small Animal Clinical Nutrition, 5th edition, reviews calculating time to weight loss; realistically, >8-12 months will be required.

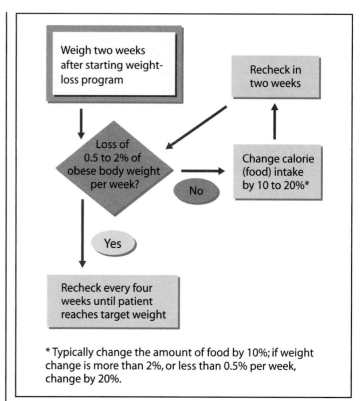

Figure 2. Algorithm for decision making and patient monitoring during weight loss.

FEEDING PLAN

Prevention of Weight Regain
After the patient reaches the target weight, a program should be initiated to ensure that weight regain does not occur. The success of weight-maintenance programs, like weight-loss programs, depends on continued pet owner commitment, proper food and feeding methods, exercise and patient monitoring (followup).

Assess and Select the Food
Ensure the Food's Basic Nutritional Adequacy. The guidelines provided above for weight-loss foods apply to weight-maintenance foods.
Compare the Food's KNF Content with the Recommended Levels. Feeding the original food, even at reduced amounts, may lead to weight regain. The same nutritional principles discussed for calorie-controlled weight loss are valid for weight maintenance, but energy is less restricted. **Tables 12** and **13** compare the KNF recommendations to the KNF content of selected commercial veterinary therapeutic foods for dogs and cats, respectively, marketed for maintenance of ideal weight after weight loss. These foods are also appropriate for prevention of weight gain in patients not previously overweight (see Chapter 1). Select the food that is most similar to the KNF recommendations for weight maintenance. If a metabolic-control food was used for weight loss in an overweight cat, it is appropriate to switch to a calorie-controlled food for maintenance of the recommended weight.

Manage Treats and Snacks. If the owner intends to feed treats or snacks, the same treats (**Table 8**) and snacks recommended for weight loss can be used to prevent weight regain. As with weight loss, calories supplied by treats must be accounted for within the total daily calories allowed in the feeding plan.

Assess and Determine the Feeding Method

Determine How Much Food to Feed. Using the food dose recommendation from the company providing the food is the simplest method. As with foods intended for weight loss, this information may be available on the product label, from product literature, from the company website or by using specially designed "calculators" or proprietary software programs (**Box 1**). Another simple method is to feed 10% more calories than were required for weight loss (Table 27-18, Small Animal Clinical Nutrition, 5th edition).

Consider How to Offer the Food/Manage Food Changes/Food and Water Receptacle Husbandry. See the recommendations for weight loss (above).

FOLLOWUP

Owner Followup

Figure 3 is an algorithm for patient monitoring and adjusting the amount to feed for weight maintenance. When possible, owners can obtain body weights at home and be advised by phone about changing the amount to feed to maintain ideal weight.

Veterinary Health Care Team Followup

Rechecks are essential after the target weight has been attained. More frequent rechecks are needed initially when calories are increased to maintain ideal weight because weight regain can rapidly occur (**Figure 3**). Maintain 2-week rechecks until the patient's body weight has stabilized at the desired weight for at least 3 consecutive weigh-ins. Then, rechecks can occur every 3 months for a year and finally to 6 months thereafter. Office rechecks are equal in importance to diet and exercise; regular monitoring helps keep owners engaged.

MISCELLANEOUS

See Chapters 13, 20 and 27, Small Animal Clinical Nutrition, 5th edition, for more information.

Authors

Condensed from Chapter 27, Small Animal Clinical Nutrition, 5th edition, authored by Philip W. Toll, Ryan M. Yamka, William D. Schoenherr and Michael S. Hand.

References

See Chapter 27, Small Animal Clinical Nutrition, 5th edition, on the website www.markmorrisinstitute.org for references.

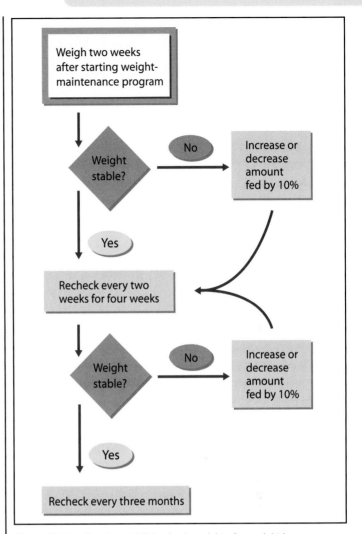

Figure 3. Algorithm for stabilizing body weight after weight loss.

Chapter
15
Disorders of Lipid Metabolism

CLINICAL POINTS

- Hyperlipidemia (hyperlipemia or hyperlipoproteinemia): disturbance of lipid metabolism that results in elevated blood lipids, particularly triglycerides, cholesterol or both.
- Hypertriglyceridemia: most common and most clinically important type of hyperlipidemia.
- Primary hyperlipidemias are familial; secondary hyperlipidemias are associated with underlying primary diseases including protein-losing nephropathy, endocrine disorders (e.g., unregulated diabetes), certain drugs and possibly certain foods.
- **Table 1** lists clinical signs and diseases associated with hypertriglyceridemia.
- Hyperlipidemic patients without clinical signs are considered at risk for future associated disease and should be managed like patients with clinical signs.
- Proper dietary intervention may eliminate/diminish morbidity; concurrent medications are sometime indicated.
- Dietary therapy may eliminate seizures associated with hypertriglyceridemia without concomitant use of anticonvulsant drugs.
- Feeding goals: ameliorate/eliminate clinical signs; maintain laboratory results within normal ranges.

KEY NUTRITIONAL FACTORS

- Foods should provide recommended allowances of all required nutrients (nutritional adequacy), but should also contain specific levels of KNFs (certain nutrients and nonnutritional food ingredients that can assist in the management of hyperlipidemia).
- **Table 2** lists KNF recommendations for foods for dogs and cats with hyperlipidemia. Reduced dietary fat is most important. A detailed determination of these recommendations can be found in Chapter 28, Small Animal Clinical Nutrition, 5th edition. Water is always a KNF.

FEEDING PLAN

Assess and Select the Food
Ensure the Food's Basic Nutritional Adequacy. AAFCO nutritional adequacy statements are usually found on a product's label. AAFCO approval does not ensure a food will be effective in the management of hyperlipidemia or in prevention of long-term health problems.

Table 1. Clinical signs and diseases associated with hypertriglyceridemia in dogs and cats.

Dogs
Abdominal discomfort*
Acute pancreatitis
Behavior (lethargy, inactivity)
Crystalline stromal dystrophy (especially cavalier King Charles spaniels)
Cushing's syndrome
Fasting lipemia (six to 12 hours)
Intermittent diarrhea*
Intermittent vomiting*
Lipemia retinalis
Lipemic aqueous
Lipid corneal dystrophy/arcus lipoides corneae
Seizures
Cats
Cutaneous xanthomata
Lipemia retinalis
Lipid keratopathy
Peripheral nerve paralysis
   Horner's syndrome
   Tibial nerve paralysis
   Radial nerve paralysis
Splenomegaly

*These clinical signs may occur concomitantly in the same patient. The collective term used to describe these signs is "pseudopancreatitis."

Table 2. Key nutritional factors for hyperlipidemia.

Disorder	Factor	Dietary recommendations
Hyperlipidemia	Triglycerides	Feed a food that reduces serum triglycerides Restrict dietary fat (<12% dry matter [DM])
		Feed a food that reduces serum triglycerides and binds cholesterol and bile acids Increase dietary fiber: Dogs: ≥10% DM Cats: ≥7% DM
		Add lipid-reducing drugs (fibrates) if dietary management alone is unsuccessful in controlling hyperlipidemia

Compare the Food's KNF Content with the Recommended Levels. **Tables 3** and **4** list commercially available foods marketed for the management of primary hyperlipidemia for dogs and cats, respectively, and compare their KNF content with the recom-

Table 3. Selected commercial foods used in dogs with hyperlipidemia compared to recommended levels of key nutritional factors.* (Numbers in red match optimal KNFs.)

Dry foods	Energy density (kcal/cup)**	Fat (%)	Crude fiber (%)
Recommended levels	-	<12	≥10
Hill's Prescription Diet r/d Canine	242	8.2	13.5
Hill's Prescription Diet r/d with Chicken Canine	241	8.8	13.6
Iams Veterinary Formula Weight Loss/Restricted Calorie	217	9.1	2.4
Purina Veterinary Diets EN GastroENteric Formula	397	12.6	1.5
Purina Veterinary Diets HA HypoAllergenic Formula	311	10.5	1.6
Purina Veterinary Diets OM Overweight Management Formula	266	7.2	10.3
Royal Canin Veterinary Diets Digestive Low Fat LF	226	6.6	2.3
Moist foods	**Energy density (kcal/can)***	**Fat (%)**	**Crude fiber (%)**
Recommended levels	-	<12	≥10
Hill's Prescription Diet r/d Canine	257 (12.3-oz. can)	8.6	21.2
Iams Veterinary Formula Weight Loss/Restricted Calorie	397 (14-oz. can)	14.9	3.2
Purina Veterinary Diets EN GastroENteric Formula	423 (12.5-oz. can)	13.8	0.9
Purina Veterinary Diets OM Overweight Management Formula	189 (12.5-oz. can)	8.4	19.2
Royal Canin Veterinary Diets Digestive Low Fat LF	442 (13.6-oz. can)	6.9	3.0

*From manufacturers' published information; all values expressed on a dry matter basis unless otherwise stated.
**Energy density values are listed on an as fed basis and are useful for determining the amount to feed (the amount to feed = the daily energy requirement ÷ the energy density [kcal/cup or can]); cup = 8-oz. measuring cup. To convert to kJ, multiply kcal by 4.184.

Table 4. Selected commercial foods used in cats with hyperlipidemia compared to recommended levels of key nutritional factors.* (Numbers in red match optimal KNFs.)

Dry foods	Energy density (kcal/cup)**	Fat (%)	Crude fiber (%)
Recommended levels	-	<12	≥7
Hill's Prescription Diet r/d Feline	263	9.3	13.6
Hill's Prescription Diet r/d with Chicken Feline	266	9.8	13.8
Purina Veterinary Diets OM Overweight Management Formula	321	8.5	5.6
Moist foods	**Energy density (kcal/can)***	**Fat (%)**	**Crude fiber (%)**
Recommended levels	-	<12	≥7
Hill's Prescription Diet r/d with Liver & Chicken Feline	114 (5.5-oz. can)	9.2	15.4
Purina Veterinary Diets OM Overweight Management Formula	150 (5.5-oz. can)	14.6	10.2

*From manufacturers' published information; all values expressed on a dry matter basis unless otherwise stated.
**Energy density values are listed on an as fed basis and are useful for determining the amount to feed (the amount to feed = the daily energy requirement ÷ the energy density [kcal/cup or can]); cup = 8-oz. measuring cup. To convert to kJ, multiply kcal by 4.184.

mended levels. Contact manufacturers for this information for foods not in the tables (manufacturer contact information is listed on product labels). Select a food that best approximates recommended KNF levels. Depending on their primary disease (**Table 1**), patients with secondary hyperlipidemia may also benefit from foods listed in **Tables 3** and **4**, as long as normal body weight is maintained. For these patients, consult the related chapters to see if KNF contraindications exist.

Manage Treats and Snacks. If treats/snacks are fed, commercial treats that match the KNF profiles recommended in **Table 2** (at least in fat content) are best. Table 8, Chapter 14, lists suitable low-fat canine treats for weight management. Treats/snacks should not be fed excessively (<10% of the total diet on a volume, weight or calorie basis).

Assess and Determine the Feeding Method

Determine How Much Food to Feed. The low-fat/increased-fiber foods recommended for hyperlipidemic patients are inherently lower in energy density. Thus, the amount fed may need to be increased accordingly. Initial amounts to feed may be estimated from feeding guides on product labels or by calculation (Appendix C). Feeding guides and calculations are starting points and will likely need to be adjusted over time (see Followup

below). Before initiating feeding of new food, note the patient's BCS and body weight so the appropriateness of the amount fed can be evaluated and changed if necessary.

Consider How to Offer the Food. Generally, if the patient's BCS is normal, use the current feeding method (restricted or free-choice feeding) for the new food. Hyperlipidemic diabetic patients may benefit from feeding protocols that are congruent with their insulin therapy (Chapter 16). To ensure compliance, if the patient is from a household with other dogs or cats, deny access to their food.

Manage Food Changes. Most healthy pets adapt well to new foods, but a transition period to avoid GI upsets and facilitate acceptance of new foods is good practice. Example: to change to a new food, replace 25% of the old food with the new food on Day 1 and continue this incremental change daily until the change is complete on Day 4. Appendix E provides additional information.

Food and Water Receptacle Husbandry.
Food and water bowls should always be washed regularly with warm soapy water and rinsed well. Dishes used for moist foods need daily cleaning. Discard moist or moistened dry foods after 2-4 hours of room temperature exposure to avoid foodborne illnesses (Appendix F).

FOLLOWUP

Veterinary Health Care Team Followup

Initial Assessment. Schedule for 3-4 weeks after initiation of the feeding plan. Evaluate ocular and/or cutaneous lesions for improvement. Positive fasted (>12 hours) lab results include: a clear serum sample, total triglycerides <500 mg/dl and a negative chylomicron test. Acceptable lab results include: slight serum turbidity, triglycerides <1,000 mg/dl and an incomplete cream layer at the top of the sample. Most importantly, review the patient's response: expect amelioration/elimination of clinical signs within 2 weeks (dogs with pseudopancreatitis) to 3 months (cats with cutaneous xanthomata) after initiation of dietary therapy. Note body condition and weight; unless weight loss is desired, the body weight and BCS should be unchanged from the assessment done at initiation of dietary management. For unintended weight loss (>1% of body weight/week), increase the amount fed by 10% and recheck in 1 month. Repeat the cycle as needed until the desired weight is maintained.

Negative Results at First Assessment. Investigate for feeding plan compliance; consumption of high-fat snacks/treats and access to other pet foods, even infrequently, can markedly increase triglyceride levels in affected patients. Note that in some cases, food intake may be inadequate and patients may be seeking additional food. Other patients may remain profoundly hyper-lipidemic despite excellent owner compliance. Continue with the original feeding plan and reassess in 1-2 months. If still no improvement, add appropriate medical management (Box 28-2, Small Animal Clinical Nutrition, 5th edition) to dietary therapy and assess again in 1-2 months.

MISCELLANEOUS

Secondary hyperlipidemia associated with a primary underlying disorder (see Clinical Points above) may result in clinical signs indistinguishable from those caused by primary hyperlipidemias. Resolve via accurate diagnosis and appropriate medical management of the underlying disorder. These patients also benefit from dietary management as long as ideal weight can be maintained.

See Chapters 28 and 29, Small Animal Clinical Nutrition, 5th edition, for more information.

Authors

Condensed from Chapter 28, Small Animal Clinical Nutrition, 5th edition, authored by Richard B. Ford and Chris L. Ludlow.

References

See Chapter 28, Small Animal Clinical Nutrition, 5th edition, on the website www.markmorrisinstitute.org for references.

Chapter

16 Diabetes Mellitus

CLINICAL POINTS

- Most diabetic dogs have IDDM.
- Diabetes in cats is more complex; they may have IDDM or NIDDM at diagnosis and following treatment, NIDDM may progress to IDDM (and vice versa). Dietary management of cats with NIDDM is similar to that for IDDM.
- Common complaints/signs are polydipsia, polyphagia, weight loss and reduced activity. Other signs include unkempt coat (cats), hepatomegaly, cataracts (dogs), rear-limb weakness (cats) and dehydration.
- The most consistent and requisite lab findings are persistent fasting hyperglycemia and glucosuria in the absence of other diseases.
- Dogs and cats may present with concurrent exocrine pancreatic insufficiency or pancreatitis.

Abbreviations
AAFCO = Association of American Feed Control Officials
BCS = body condition score (Appendix A)
DKA = diabetic ketoacidosis
DM = dry matter
IDDM = insulin-dependent diabetes mellitus
KNF = key nutritional factor
NIDDM = non-insulin-dependent diabetes mellitus
RER = resting energy requirement

- Both hypothyroidism and hyperthyroidism may be associated with insulin resistance and can occur in conjunction with diabetes.
- Obesity is a preventable risk factor for development of diabetes in dogs and cats; it increases diabetes risk in cats by fourfold.
- Diabetes treatment usually involves a combination of medical and dietary management.

Table 1. Key nutritional factors for foods for diabetic dogs and cats.*

Factors	Dogs (increased-fiber/ high-carbohydrate food)	Cats (increased-fiber/ high-carbohydrate food)	Cats (low-carbohydrate/ high-protein food)
Water	Fresh, clean water should be available at all times	Fresh, clean water should be available at all times	Fresh, clean water should be available at all times
Digestible carbohydrate	Avoid simple sugars Provide foods with no more than 55% digestible carbohydrate	Avoid simple sugars and starch Provide foods with less than 40% digestible carbohydrate	Avoid simple sugars and starch Provide foods with less than 20% digestible carbohydrate
Fiber	7 to 18%	7 to 18%	–
Fat	<25%	<25%	<25%
Protein	15 to 35% Dogs with renal failure should be fed protein at the low end of the range	28 to 55% Cats with renal failure should be fed protein at the low end of the range	28 to 55% Cats with renal failure should be fed protein at the low end of the range
Food form	Avoid semi-moist foods	Avoid semi-moist foods	Avoid semi-moist foods

*Nutrients expressed on a dry matter basis.

- Treatment with injectable insulin or oral sulfonylurea agents has been the mainstay of medical management for uncomplicated diabetes.
- Dietary management is the primary nonpharmacologic treatment for diabetes and may allow for less, or even preclude, medical intervention.
- Changes in the feeding plan, physiologic status, body weight and exercise may alter insulin requirements and should be accompanied by concurrent monitoring to assess if glycemic control has been affected; e.g., weight loss in overweight patients will improve insulin sensitivity and may lead to hypoglycemia unless the insulin treatment regimen is modified.
- Low-carbohydrate/high-protein foods limit carbohydrate intake in diabetic cats and have the desirable result of causing blood glucose to be maintained primarily by gluconeogenesis, releasing glucose into the circulation at a slow steady rate.
- DKA: affected patients exhibit anorexia, vomiting, diarrhea, weakness and a moribund state.
- DKA may be precipitated by infection, severe stress, hypokalemia, hypomagnesemia, renal failure, drugs that decrease insulin secretion, drugs that cause insulin resistance or inadequate fluid intake. Concurrent disease (e.g., pancreatitis, bacterial infection) accentuates clinical signs, prompting owners to seek veterinary care.
- Feeding goals: achieve ideal body weight, improve glycemic control (and thereby improve clinical signs) and reduce/obviate the need for medical management of uncomplicated NIDDM or IDDM.

KEY NUTRITIONAL FACTORS

- Foods should provide recommended allowances of all required nutrients (nutritional adequacy), but should also contain specific levels of KNFs (certain nutrients and nonnutritional food ingredients that can assist in the management of diabetes).
- **Table 1** lists KNF recommendations for foods for dogs and cats with either IDDM or NIDDM. Water is always a KNF and is particularly important for diabetics. Diabetes in cats is more

Box 1. Feeding Plan for Diabetic Ketoacidosis.

Intensive care and intravenous fluid administration are not required if the patient is bright, alert and well-hydrated. Administration of short- or intermediate-acting insulin can be initiated in conjunction with feeding recommendations similar to those for type I and type II diabetes mellitus. Some patients with diabetic ketoacidosis may require in-hospital intensive care. Goals are to correct dehydration, electrolyte disorders (hypokalemia, hypophosphatemia, hyponatremia, hypochloremia, hypomagnesemia), ketonuria and acidosis while initiating a feeding plan. Nutritional recommendations are similar to those for type I and type II diabetes mellitus after the patient is stabilized (**Table 1**).

complex and may be equally managed by either of 2 different KNF profiles: increased fiber or low carbohydrate/high protein. A detailed description of these KNF recommendations can be found in Chapter 29, Small Animal Clinical Nutrition, 5th edition.

FEEDING PLAN

Adjustments in food and feeding methods (amount fed and timing of feedings) should be considered when insulin therapy is initiated and should be directed at correcting or preventing obesity, maintaining consistency in the timing and caloric content of the meals and furnishing a food that helps minimize postprandial hyperglycemia. **Box 1** provides a feeding plan for DKA.

Assess and Select the Food

Ensure the Food's Basic Nutritional Adequacy. AAFCO nutritional adequacy statements are usually found on a product's label. AAFCO approval does not ensure a food will be effective in the management of diabetes.

Compare the Food's KNF Content with the Recommended Levels. Table 2 lists commercially available increased-fiber foods marketed for the management of IDDM/NIDDM in dogs; Tables 3 and 4 list increased-fiber and low-carbohydrate/high-protein foods, respectively, for cats with IDDM/NIDDM. All 3 tables compare KNF content of the foods with recommended

Table 2. Selected commercial veterinary therapeutic foods marketed for dogs with diabetes mellitus compared to recommended levels of key nutritional factors.* (Numbers in red match optimal KNFs.)

Dry foods	Energy density (kcal/cup)**	Carbohydrate (%)	Fiber (%)	Fat (%)	Protein (%)***
Recommended levels	–	≤55	7-18	<25	15-35
Hill's Prescription Diet r/d Canine	242	38.7	13.5	8.2	34.3
Hill's Prescription Diet r/d with Chicken Canine	241	36	13.6	8.8	35.2
Hill's Prescription Diet w/d Canine	243	51.2	16.4	8.8	18.9
Hill's Prescription Diet w/d with Chicken Canine	239	50.1	17.1	8.7	19.1
Iams Veterinary Formula Weight Control D/Optimum Weight Control	209	51.2	3.0	9.5	28.7
Iams Veterinary Formula Weight Loss/ Restricted-Calorie	217	58.0	2.4	9.1	25.0
Purina Veterinary Diets DCO Dual Fiber Control	320	47.8	7.6	12.4	25.3
Royal Canin Veterinary Diet Diabetic HF 18	186	48.6	12.1	9.9	22.0
Moist foods	**Energy density (kcal/can)****	**Carbohydrate (%)**	**Fiber (%)**	**Fat (%)**	**Protein (%)***
Recommended levels	–	≤55	7-18	<25	15-35
Hill's Prescription Diet r/d Canine	257/12.3 oz.	39.2	21.2	8.6	25.3
Hill's Prescription Diet w/d Canine	329/13 oz.	52.6	12.4	12.7	17.9
Iams Veterinary Formula Weight Loss/Restricted-Calorie	397/14 oz.	40.8	3.2	14.9	34.4

Note: Fresh water should be available at all times; semi-moist foods should be avoided.
*From manufacturers' published information or calculated from manufacturers' published as-fed values; all values are on a dry matter basis unless otherwise stated.
**Energy density values are listed on an as fed basis and are useful for determining the amount to feed; cup = 8-oz. measuring cup. To convert to kJ, multiply kcal by 4.184.
***Dogs with renal failure should be fed protein at the low end of the range.

levels. Contact manufacturers for information for foods not in the table (manufacturer contact information is listed on product labels). For cats, clinician experience is an important factor in selecting the type of food used (increased fiber or low carbohydrate/high protein); both are effective. Select a food that best approximates the recommended KNF levels.

Chronically Underweight Patients. Diabetics may have polyphagia with weight loss. Foods with moderate/high levels of fiber may not have sufficient energy density for weight gain or even maintenance of current weight. If increasing the quantity of food offered (below) does not result in adequate body condition, consider a food with <10% DM crude fiber and/or slightly increased fat content so that energy density is sufficient to increase and/or maintain body weight.

Semi-Moist Foods vs. Moist and Dry Foods. Semi-moist foods tend to have a hyperglycemic effect compared to dry or moist foods because they contain increased levels of simple sugars used as humectants; avoid feeding them to diabetics.

Manage Treats and Snacks. If an owner insists on providing treats, recommend the opposite form of the food being fed; i.e., if a dry food is being fed, offer small amounts of the same food in moist form as a snack and vice versa. Discourage feeding treats/snacks formulated for healthy pets to diabetic patients. Strict compliance is important to achieving good results.

Assess and Determine the Feeding Method
Determine How Much Food to Feed. The amount fed can be estimated either from feeding guides on product labels or by calculation (Appendix C). These estimates are only starting points and will likely need to be adjusted (see Followup below) because of variable effects of diabetes on energy metabolism and potential complicating factors that may require management to help stabilize the patient's RER.

Medical Control of Primary Disease. Before determining the amount to feed, note that the response to dietary management depends on the level of control of the primary disease, e.g., if weight loss or gain is a continuing problem, it may be due to poorly controlled diabetes, rather than incorrect food dosage. Basal metabolic rate and RER may be decreased in patients with poorly controlled diabetes mellitus because of the euthyroid sick syndrome.

Medical Control of Concurrent Disease. Concurrent diseases such as thyroid disorders (dogs and cats), lymphoplasmacytic enteritis (cats) or hyperadrenocorticism (dogs) can affect metabolic rate, RER and counter regulate insulin and insulin action. Management of concurrent illness will facilitate stabilization of diabetes and subsequently RER and food dosage.

Overweight/Obese Patients. Initiate a conservative weight-loss protocol (Chapter 14) after medical problems are managed. Frequent monitoring and readjusting is important because improvement in insulin resistance often occurs with weight loss. Many cats with NIDDM are obese; a carefully controlled weight-loss program is a necessary part of their dietary management.

Underweight Patients. As mentioned, patients with diabetes often are polyphagic with weight loss. If increasing the quantity of food offered does not result in desired effects on body weight

Table 3. Selected commercial fiber-enhanced veterinary therapeutic foods marketed for cats with diabetes mellitus compared to recommended levels of key nutritional factors.[*] (Numbers in red match optimal KNFs.)

Dry foods	Energy density (kcal/cup)[**]	Carbohydrate (%)	Fiber (%)	Fat (%)	Protein (%)[***]
Recommended levels	–	<40	7-18	<25	28-55
Hill's Prescription Diet r/d Feline	263	_33.5_	_13.6_	_9.3_	_36.9_
Hill's Prescription Diet r/d with Chicken Feline	266	_32.2_	_13.8_	_9.8_	_37.7_
Hill's Prescription Diet w/d Feline	281	_37.4_	_7.6_	_9.8_	_39.0_
Hill's Prescription Diet w/d with Chicken Feline	278	_35.4_	_7.6_	_9.9_	_39.9_
Iams Veterinary Formula Weight Control D/Optimum Weight Control	326	41.2	1.5	_12.2_	_38.6_
Iams Veterinary Formula Weight Loss/ Restricted-Calorie	268	44.5	2.5	_11.0_	_35.2_
Purina Veterinary Diets OM Overweight Management	321	_22.4_	5.6	_8.5_	56.2

Moist foods	Energy density (kcal/can)[**]	Carbohydrate (%)	Fiber (%)	Fat (%)	Protein (%)[***]
Recommended levels	–	<40	7-18	<25	28-55
Hill's Prescription Diet r/d with Liver & Chicken Feline	114/5.5 oz.	_31.3_	_15.4_	_9.2_	_37.5_
Hill's Prescription Diet w/d with Chicken Feline	127/5.5 oz.	_26.4_	_10.6_	_16.6_	_39.6_
Iams Veterinary Formula Weight Loss/ Restricted-Calorie	172/6 oz.	_32.3_	1.7	_15.5_	_44.2_
Purina Veterinary Diets OM Overweight Management	150/5.5 oz.	_23.2_	_10.2_	_14.6_	_44.6_

Note: Fresh water should be available at all times; semi-moist foods should be avoided.
[*]From manufacturers' published information or calculated from manufacturers' published as-fed values; all values are on a dry matter basis unless otherwise stated.
[**]Energy density values are listed on an as fed basis and are useful for determining the amount to feed; cup = 8-oz. measuring cup. To convert to kJ, multiply kcal by 4.184.
[***]Cats with renal failure should be fed protein at the low end of the range.

Table 4. Selected commercial low-carbohydrate/high-protein veterinary therapeutic foods marketed for cats with diabetes mellitus compared to recommended levels of key nutritional factors.[*] (Numbers in red match optimal KNFs.)

Dry foods	Energy density (kcal/cup)[**]	Carbohydrate (%)	Fat (%)	Protein (%)[***]
Recommended levels	–	<20	<25	28-55
Hill's Prescription Diet m/d Feline	480	_14.7_	_22.0_	_51.5_
Medi-Cal Diabetic DS 44	247	25.6	_12.9_	_49.5_
Purina Veterinary Diets DM Dietetic Management	592	_15.0_	_17.9_	57.8
Royal Canin Veterinary Diet Diabetic DS 44	239	25.6	_12.9_	_49.5_

Moist foods	Energy density (kcal/can)[**]	Carbohydrate (%)	Fat (%)	Protein (%)[***]
Recommended levels	–	<20	<25	28-55
Hill's Prescription Diet m/d Feline	156/5.5 oz.	_15.7_	_19.4_	_52.8_
Iams Veterinary Formula Stress/Weight Gain Formula	333/6 oz.	_12.2_	37.2	_41.8_
Purina Veterinary Diets DM Dietetic Management	194/5.5 oz.	_8.1_	_23.8_	56.9

Note: Fresh water should be available at all times; semi-moist foods should be avoided.
[*]From manufacturers' published information or calculated from manufacturers' published as-fed values; all values are on a dry matter basis unless otherwise stated.
[**]Energy density values are listed on an as fed basis and are useful for determining the amount to feed; cup = 8-oz. measuring cup. To convert to kJ, multiply kcal by 4.184.
[***]Cats with renal failure should be fed protein at the low end of the range.

and condition, consider a food with increased energy density (above). Neither of these approaches will be effective if there is poor medical management.

Consider How to Offer the Food.

WHEN TO FEED. To minimize glucose dyshomeostasis, the feeding schedule should be designed to enhance the actions of insulin, maximize assimilation of food and minimize postprandial hyperglycemia (Figure 29-4, Small Animal Clinical Nutrition, 5th edition). Several small meals given at regular intervals throughout the day with and after insulin administration should improve hyperglycemia. However, individual eating habits may require modifying how the food is offered.

Patients that "Nibble." Allow them to continue their eating pattern. Make food available at each insulin injection and allow the patient to choose when and how much to eat. The process is repeated at the time of the next insulin injection.

Aggressive Eaters. Feed a set amount of food (calories) at defined times over the course of the day. Generally, for patients receiving once-a-day insulin, feed half the daily amount of food at the time of insulin administration and the other half 8-10 hours later. If insulin is given twice daily, half of the daily food dose should be fed with each injection.

Finicky Eaters. Offer food before insulin administration so that insulin administration can be modified to avoid insulin-induced hypoglycemia, in case the patient does not eat.

FOLLOWUP

Owner Followup
General owner satisfaction and a stable patient body weight indicate the diabetes is adequately controlled. Owner comments suggestive of hyper- or hypoglycemia such as polydipsia, polyuria, lethargy, lack of grooming behavior (cats), weakness, ataxia or changes in jumping ability (cats) are indicative of inadequate control.

Body Weight and BCS. If possible, owners should note body weight every 2 weeks and BCS at least monthly.

Urine Glucose and Ketones. Occasional monitoring/recording for glycosuria and ketonuria at home may be helpful in patients with recurring ketosis or hypoglycemia.

Veterinary Health Care Team Followup
Exam findings suggesting poor control include: unthrifty or thin appearance, poor coat and/or plantigrade stance in cats caused by peripheral neuropathy. Veterinary reassessment should take place every 3-4 months if the patient is stable and doing well. If the patient is symptomatic, reassess and modify the treatment plan every 1-2 weeks until control is attained.

Body Weight and BCS. May indicate the quality of glycemic control or the presence of other diseases, especially when adjustments in food dose do not produce expected changes. It may take several months to achieve weight-loss goals in obese patients. A loss of 10% body weight in already thin patients indicates a need for reassessment of dietary and medical management. When changing the amount to feed, increase or decrease the amount by 10% increments and recheck every 2 weeks for 1 month. At that point, if necessary, the amount fed should be changed again and the cycle repeated.

Food Intake. A decrease, concurrent with maintenance of body weight, indicates a favorable response to insulin administration (more efficient nutrient use). Depressed food intake could be due to inadequate palatability of the food. Try a different food after ruling out potential medical causes. It is important to monitor food intake in cats because prolonged inadequate food intake may result in hepatic lipidosis.

Lab Results.

Urine Glucose and Ketones. Crude indicators of glycemic control. Should be decreased in newly-diagnosed diabetics or DKA; should be negative in well-controlled patients. In cats that have reverted to a non-insulin-requiring state, monitoring helps determine if glycosuria has recurred; in cats treated with oral hypoglycemic drugs, it helps determine if glycosuria has improved or worsened; and in cats with suspected stress-induced hyperglycemia, monitoring helps differentiate transient from persistent hyperglycemia.

Biochemistry Profile. Should return to normal with good control and adequate food intake. The primary exception is hyperglycemia that may/may not be present depending on when the blood sample is obtained in relation to insulin administration. Abnormal results in the face of controlled diabetes suggest separate disease entities.

Serum Fructosamine. Unaffected by acute hyperglycemia, as occurs with stress, but can be affected by hypoalbuminemia (<2.5 g/dl), hyperlipidemia (triglycerides >150 mg/dl) and hyperthyroidism. However, relative hyperglycemia is common, even in well-controlled diabetics. Thus, reasonable serum fructosamine results are 350-450 µmol/l. Values >500 µmol/l indicate inadequate control and a need for insulin adjustments; values >600 µmol/l indicate serious lack of control; check for an underlying problem. Results <300 µmol/l may indicate significant periods of hypoglycemia.

Serial Blood Glucose Curves. Provide valuable information during initial regulation of newly-diagnosed diabetics and whenever insulin therapy is adjusted; however, results are unreliable if obtaining samples causes too much patient stress.

MISCELLANEOUS

Exercise is important for improving/maintaining glycemic control; it helps promote weight loss, eliminates obesity-induced insulin resistance and promotes glucose use by muscles. The amount and timing of exercise should be consistent from day to day to avoid fluctuations in blood glucose that may result in severe hypoglycemia.

See Chapters 27 and 29, Small Animal Clinical Nutrition, 5th edition, for more information.

Authors
Condensed from Chapter 29, Small Animal Clinical Nutrition, 5th edition, authored by Steven C. Zicker, Richard W. Nelson, Claudia A. Kirk and Karen J. Wedekind.

References
See Chapter 29, Small Animal Clinical Nutrition, 5th edition, on the website www.markmorrisinstitute.org for references.

CLINICAL POINTS

Canine Hypothyroidism
- Adult onset hypothyroidism is common in dogs.
- Abnormalities caused by hypothyroidism usually resolve with appropriate thyroid hormone replacement therapy.
- Concurrent with medical treatment, manage overweight canine hypothyroid patients like other overweight/obese dogs (Chapter 14); otherwise, feeding plans for young and mature adult dogs (Chapters 1 and 2) are appropriate.
- Hyperlipidemia associated with hypothyroidism usually resolves with proper medical management; however, lower fat foods are warranted to help manage hyperlipidemia (Chapter 15) and minimize associated health risks and are appropriate for feeding for weight loss.
- The rest of this chapter focuses on the dietary management of feline hyperthyroidism.

Feline Hyperthyroidism
- Hyperthyroidism is the most common endocrine disease affecting cats and is one of the most frequently diagnosed diseases in small animal practice.
- Feline hyperthyroidism is usually caused by adenomatous hyperplasia.
- Hyperthyroidism is a disease of older cats; <5% are younger than 8 years.
- Clinical signs typically include weight loss (which may progress to cachexia), polyphagia and restlessness/hyperactivity. Polyphagia is due to increased metabolism. The most common physical exam/ultrasound findings are discrete thyroid masses in the ventral neck.
- Lab tests may confirm hyperthyroidism (increased serum T_4) as well as screen for concurrent disease, particularly CKD, which is common in older cats and often presents in conjunction with hyperthyroidism.
- Initial treatments are surgical and medical: thyroidectomy and/or long-term antithyroid medication and/or radiation therapy including radioactive iodine.
- Feeding goal: provide nutritional support to return body weight/condition to normal; overall success depends on effectiveness of the initial surgical/medical treatment(s).

KEY NUTRITIONAL FACTORS

- Foods should provide recommended allowances of all required nutrients (nutritional adequacy), but should also contain specific levels of KNFs (certain nutrients and nonnutritional

Abbreviations
AAFCO = Association of American Feed Control Officials
BCS = body condition score (Appendix A)
CKD = chronic kidney disease
DER = daily energy requirement
KNF = key nutritional factor

food ingredients that can assist in managing feline hyperthyroidism).
- Table 2, Chapter 7, and Table 1, Chapter 8, list KNF recommendations for foods for normal young adult and mature adult cats, respectively. KNF recommendations for cats that are normal/underweight and those that are inactive/obese prone are included. These KNFs are suitable for hyperthyroid cats that have been successfully surgically and/or medically treated.
- Untreated hyperthyroid cats are hypermetabolic/catabolic and often present in an underweight or even a severe weight-loss condition. After successful treatment of the primary disease, their metabolic rate usually returns to normal for their age/activity level. During recovery, consider energy density and protein levels at higher ends of recommended ranges for normal/underweight cats (Table 2, Chapter 7, and Table 1, Chapter 8) to facilitate replacement of lost body tissue.
- Rule out CKD in older patients before changing to a higher protein food (see Chapter 37, Small Animal Clinical Nutrition, 5th edition).
- Water is always a KNF and is particularly important for hyperthyroid cats that exhibit polydipsia and polyuria. Detailed descriptions of the KNF recommendations can be found in Chapters 20, 21 and 29, Small Animal Clinical Nutrition, 5th edition.

FEEDING PLAN

Assess and Select the Food
Ensure the Food's Basic Nutritional Adequacy. AAFCO nutritional adequacy statements are usually found on a product's label. AAFCO approval does not ensure a food will be effective in assisting in the management of feline hyperthyroidism or concurrent health problems.
Compare the Food's KNF Content with the Recommended Levels. Table 3, Chapter 7 and Table 2, Chapter 8, compare the KNF profiles for selected commercial foods for normal/underweight young adult and mature adult cats, respectively. Contact manufacturers for information for foods not in the tables (manufacturer contact information is listed on product labels). A new food should be selected if discrepancies are noted and should approximate the recommended KNF levels. During recovery,

consider foods with protein and energy density levels at higher ends of the recommended ranges for normal/underweight cats (Table 3, Chapter 7, and Table 2, Chapter 8) to replenish body fat and protein (assumes concurrent CKD has been ruled out).

Manage Treats and Snacks. If treats/snacks are fed, commercial treats that match nutrient profiles recommended for adult cats (see product label) are best. Otherwise, treats/snacks should not be fed excessively (<10% of the total diet on a volume, weight or calorie basis). See Appendix B for more treats/snack information.

Assess and Determine the Feeding Method

Determine How Much to Feed. Underweight patients: feed an amount that would at least meet the DER for their ideal weight (BCS 3/5) (Appendix C). Ideal weight may be obtained from the medical record or estimated. Using the ideal weight, amounts to feed may be estimated from feeding guides on product labels or by calculation (Appendix C). A viable option is free-choice feeding (below). Feeding guidelines and calculations are estimates and will likely need to be adjusted (see Followup below).

Determine How to Offer the Food. Free-choice feeding is not usually recommended for most situations because it may result in overeating. However, it may be preferred for feeding dry foods to underweight cats to facilitate increased food intake. A combination of dry and moist foods may be used to enhance acceptance. Warming moist foods or adding low-salt broth to dry foods may enhance food and water intake.

Manage Food Changes. Most healthy cats adapt well to new foods but a transition period to avoid GI upsets and food refusal is good practice, particularly in unhealthy older cats. Example: to change to a new food, replace 25% of the old food with the new food on Day 1 and continue this incremental change daily until the change is complete on Day 4. Appendix E provides additional information.

Food and Water Receptacle Husbandry. Food and water bowls should be washed regularly with warm soapy water and rinsed well. Dishes used for moist foods need daily cleaning. Discard moist or moistened dry foods after 2-4 hours of room temperature exposure to avoid foodborne illnesses (Appendix F).

FOLLOWUP

Owner Followup
Owners should chart daily food intake.

Veterinary Health Care Team Followup
Initially, schedule rechecks every 2 weeks. At rechecks, assess owner's food intake data, owner's opinion of changes in clinical signs, patient's body weight, BCS, physical exam findings and lab results. If no improvement and treatment is oral methimazole, consider modifying medical and dietary treatment plans and evaluating owner compliance. If thyroidectomy was performed or radioactive iodine was administered, remnants of hyperfunctioning thyroid tissue could be an issue.

Changing Amount to Feed. Subsequently, if body weight/BCS data indicate a food dose change is in order, change in 10% increments and recheck every 2 weeks for 1 month. At that point, if necessary, the amount fed may be changed again and the cycle repeated.

MISCELLANEOUS

See Chapters 20, 21 and 29, Small Animal Clinical Nutrition, 5th edition, for more information.

Authors
Condensed from Chapter 29, Small Animal Clinical Nutrition, 5th edition, authored by Steven C. Zicker, Richard W. Nelson, Claudia A. Kirk and Karen J. Wedekind.

References
See Chapter 29, Small Animal Clinical Nutrition, 5th edition, on the website www.markmorrisinstitute.org for references.

CLINICAL POINTS

- Cancer is among the most common causes of nonaccidental death in dogs and cats, often ranking 1st or 2nd.
- Increased cancer risk has been associated with retrovirus (FeLV) exposure (cats), obesity (dogs and cats) and overexposure to known carcinogens (e.g., tobacco smoke, insecticides).
- Dog breeds predisposed to certain types/subtypes of cancer include boxers, rottweilers, German shepherd dogs, Scottish terriers and golden retrievers. Siamese cats appear to be at more risk than other feline breeds.
- Progression of metabolic and clinical signs in cancer patients may be divided into 4 phases (**Table 1**). Patients in the "silent" phase may appear clinically normal but gradually lose weight despite a good appetite.
- Cancer cachexia (**Figure 1**) is an adverse paraneoplastic syndrome that manifests as weight loss, reduced food intake and systemic inflammation; contributing factors include tumor-induced metabolic alterations, physical effects of tumors on the GI tract and potent side effects from surgery, chemotherapy and/or radiation therapy (anorexia, nausea or vomiting/diarrhea) (**Tables 2-4**).
- Anticipate the need for nutritional support; place feeding tubes early and feed early to lessen adverse effects.
- Educate owners about the integral role of nutrition in cancer management including its limitations.

Table 1. Phases of clinical and metabolic alterations in cancer patients.

Phase	Clinical changes	Metabolic changes
1	Preclinical, silent phase No obvious clinical signs	Hyperlactatemia Hyperinsulinemia Altered blood amino acid profiles
2	Early clinical signs Anorexia Lethargy Mild weight loss More susceptible to side effects from chemotherapy, etc.	Similar metabolic changes
3	Cachexia Anorexia Lethargy More susceptible to side effects from chemotherapy, etc.	Similar changes but more profound
4	Recovery Remission	Metabolic changes may persist Changes secondary to surgery, chemotherapy or radiation therapy

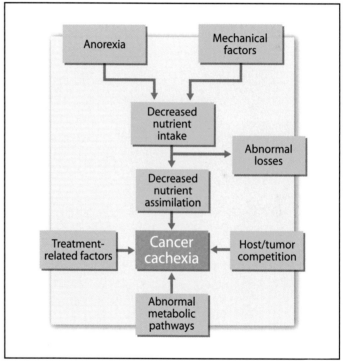

Figure 1. Mechanisms of cancer cachexia.

- Clients may regard supplements as harmless and may not report their use. Unprescribed supplements may have untoward effects on chemotherapy kinetics/dynamics (e.g., antioxidants may squelch free radicals responsible for a drug's anticancer effect).
- Feeding goals: provide nutrient specific support as an adjunct in cancer management to reduce or prevent toxicoses associated with cancer therapies and mitigate metabolic alterations induced by cancer itself, thus increasing quality and length of life.
- BCS and body weight are useful for monitoring cancer progression and treatment; however, in patients with severe malassimilation, which includes hypoalbuminemia and ascites, body weight as an indicator of lean body mass may be confounded by changes in total body water.
- Laboratory evaluation of total lymphocyte count, hematocrit, serum glucose, albumin, urea nitrogen and thyroid hormone levels may be helpful in further evaluating nutritional status.

Table 2. Effects of surgery that may have nutritional implications for cancer patients.

Cancer sites	Surgical procedures	Possible nutritional problems
Head, neck, tongue	Mandibulectomy Maxillectomy Glossectomy	Difficulty prehending, chewing and swallowing food
Esophagus	Esophagectomy, with or without reconstruction	Dysphagia Regurgitation
Stomach	Gastrectomy, partial or complete	Altered gastric emptying Diarrhea
Small intestine	Resection	Malabsorption Diarrhea Intestinal obstruction
Large intestine	Colectomy, partial or complete	Fluid and electrolyte imbalances
Pancreas, liver	Pancreatectomy Cholecystectomy Cholecystoduodenostomy	Diabetes mellitus Maldigestion

Table 3. Effects of chemotherapy that may have nutritional implications for cancer patients.

Alterations in smell or taste	Constipation
Decreased appetite	Diarrhea
Food aversions	Nausea
Stomatitis, glossitis, pharyngitis	Vomiting

Table 4. Effects of radiation therapy that may have nutritional implications for cancer patients.

Treatment areas	Acute effects	Chronic effects
Head and neck	Mucositis of mouth, tongue, esophagus	Dry mouth Dental disease Alterations in smell Alterations in taste
Thorax	Esophagitis	Esophageal fistula Esophageal stricture
Abdomen	Nausea, vomiting Enteritis, diarrhea Malabsorption	Intestinal obstruction Fistula formation Chronic enteritis

- This chapter is directed at nutritional support of patients undergoing cancer treatment rather than cancer prevention.

KEY NUTRITIONAL FACTORS

- Foods should provide recommended allowances of all required nutrients (nutritional adequacy), but should also contain specific levels of KNFs (certain nutrients that can affect cancer management).
- **Table 5** lists KNFs for foods for cancer patients and recommended amounts; they are discussed in detail in Chapter 30, Small Animal Clinical Nutrition, 5th edition.

- Deleterious alterations in carbohydrate, lipid and protein metabolism precede obvious clinical disease in cancer patients and may persist through remission or apparent recovery (**Table 1**).
- Specific levels/types of carbohydrate, fat and protein may help manage these alterations without interfering with drug/radiation treatments. EPA and DHA have inhibitory effects on tumor growth whereas n-6 fatty acids enhance metastases; thus, low n-6:n-3 fatty acid ratios are recommended. Arginine may also slow tumor growth, reduce metastatic rate and increase survival time. Water is always important.

FEEDING PLAN

Cancer and many cancer treatments result in a spectrum of metabolic/nutritional derangements, which are common to most types of cancer and provide the basis for a general feeding plan. The feeding plan also depends on the extent and effects of the disease and consequences of surgical/drug/radiation treatments.

Assess and Select the Food
Ensure the Food's Basic Nutritional Adequacy. AAFCO nutritional adequacy statements are usually found on a product's label. AAFCO approval does not ensure a food will be effective for nutritional support of cancer patients.
Compare the Food's KNF Content with the Recommended Levels. Only one veterinary therapeutic food[a] has been developed for canine cancer patients and shown to improve longevity/quality of life of selected canine cancer patients. However, other veterinary therapeutic foods provide certain KNFs at near recommended levels. **Tables 6** (dogs) and **7** (cats) compare the KNFs for foods for cancer patients to the levels in selected foods. If possible, choose a food that most closely fits the recommended levels.
Assisted Feeding. See Chapters 12 and 13 for feeding patients that cannot or will not eat. Consult Table 6, Chapter 12, for recipes for blenderized foods (such as those in **Tables 6** and **7**) or Tables 4 and 5, Chapter 12, for liquid and moist veterinary foods. If a feeding tube is necessary to provide nutritional support, food selection criteria will include the form of the food (e.g., liquid) as well as its KNF profile.
Other Considerations. Patient condition and owner constraints may affect food selection; feeding goals may have to be modified to simply meet daily water, energy and protein needs for an acceptable quality of life (palliative). Administering glucose- and lactate-containing fluids to critically ill cancer patients may exacerbate hyperglycemia and hyperlactatemia.

Assess and Determine the Feeding Method
Determine How Much Food to Feed. Base the amount to feed hospitalized patients on RER for their current body weight and increase to DER for a more optimal body weight for feeding at home. The DER factor should range from low activity (1.1-1.3 x RER) to normal activity (1.4 x RER for cats and 1.6 x RER for dogs) (Appendix C). These guidelines are starting points; frequent recording of body weight and BCS will help assess

and appropriately modify feeding amounts. Some underweight patients will stabilize at a less than optimal BCS (2/5 rather than 3/5). It may be difficult to achieve weight gain in these patients; consider changing the feeding plan goal to accommodate their leaner body condition.

Consider How to Offer the Food. If the patient has an adequate appetite, the food's form determines how it is offered. For moist foods, divide the daily amount to feed into 2-4 meals/day (depending on the owner's work schedule); dry foods may be fed free choice. A combination of free-choice feeding dry foods and meal-feeding moist foods may also be used.

Methods to Enhance Food Intake. Warming a moist food may improve its aroma and mouth feel. Handfeeding may enhance intake; even the owner's presence may increase interest in food. After chemotherapy, acupuncture appears to have a cumulative positive effect on patients and may increase their interest in eating. Pharmacologic appetite stimulants (e.g., diazepam or oxazepam) may be used to induce food consumption, but voluntary food intake rarely continues and patients' nutrient needs are often unmet (may be contraindicated in patients with reduced hepatic function). B-vitamin complex supplementation may be helpful in patients with B-vitamin deficiencies associated with prolonged inadequate food intake and/or in patients fed unbalanced homemade foods.

Assisted Feeding. Consider if methods to enhance food intake are unproductive and/or the patient has not voluntarily eaten for ≥3 days (Chapters 12 and 13). EN is preferred but PN has shown promise in selected cancer patients. As noted above, anticipate the need for nutritional support; place feeding tubes early and feed early to ensure adequate nutrition.

Manage Food Changes. A transition period to avoid GI upsets is good practice. For patients that are eating on their own, replace 25% of the old food with the new food on Day 1 and continue this incremental change daily until the change is complete on Day 4. If problems occur, feed the previous food for several more days before reattempting the food change. Appendix E provides additional information. See Chapters 12 and 13 for patients receiving assisted feeding.

Manage Treats and Snacks. If treats/snacks are fed, commercial treats that match the nutritional profile recommended for reproduction/growth (see product label) are best. Treats/snacks should not be fed excessively (<10% of the total diet on a volume, weight or calorie basis). See Appendix B for more treats/snacks information.

Food and Water Receptacle Husbandry. Food and water bowls should be washed regularly with warm soapy water and rinsed well. Dishes used for moist foods need daily cleaning. Discard moist or moistened dry foods after 2-4 hours of room temperature exposure to avoid foodborne illnesses (Appendix F).

FOLLOWUP

Owner Followup
Ask owners to record daily food intake. If practical, they should also record body weight and condition (BCS) every 2 weeks.

Table 5. Key nutritional factors for foods for canine and feline cancer patients.

Factors	Dietary recommendations
Digestible carbohydrate	Avoid excess digestible carbohydrate NFE = ≤25% DM or <20% of the food's ME
Fat	Provide a large proportion of energy from fat Fat = 25 to 40% of DM or 50 to 65% of the food's ME
Omega-3 fatty acids	Provide foods with increased levels of omega-3 fatty acids (>5% DM)
Omega-6: omega-3 fatty acid ratio	Provide foods with an omega-6:omega-3 ratio as close to 1:1 as possible
Protein	Avoid protein deficiency Provide protein in excess of adult requirements Dogs: protein = 30 to 45% of DM or 25 to 40% of the food's ME Cats: protein = 40 to 50% of DM or 35 to 45% of the food's ME (Taurine is always a necessary inclusion in feline diets)
Arginine	Provide foods with arginine DM levels >2%

Key: NFE = nitrogen-free extract, DM = dry matter, ME = metabolizable energy.

Veterinary Health Care Team Followup
Monitoring medical/surgical cancer treatments is described elsewhere. The frequency of feeding plan assessment depends on treatment protocols and complexity of the feeding plan. See "Followup" sections in Chapters 12 and 13 if assisted feeding is used. Reassessment may be conducted weekly, monthly or quarterly following discharge until the patient's condition stabilizes. If owners are recording daily food intake and body weight/BCS every 2 weeks (above), correlate findings with the recheck physical exam and lab results to assess treatment and feeding plans. Modify the feeding plan (amount fed, assisted feeding, etc.) as needed.

Food Aversion. Try foods based on novel protein sources (Chapter 19). Another option is to increase a food's fat and/or sodium content. If aversions persist with commercial foods, consider homemade foods.

MISCELLANEOUS

See Chapters 25, 26 and 30, Small Animal Clinical Nutrition, 5th edition, for more information.

Authors
Condensed from Chapter 30, Small Animal Clinical Nutrition, 5th edition, authored by Korinn E. Saker and Kimberly A. Selting.

References
See Chapter 30, Small Animal Clinical Nutrition, 5th edition, on the website www.markmorrisinstitute.org for references.

Endnote
a. Prescription Diet n/d Canine. Hill's Pet Nutrition, Inc., Topeka, KS, USA.

Table 6. Selected commercial foods for canine cancer patients compared to recommended levels of key nutritional factors.* (Numbers in red match optimal KNFs.)

Dry food	Energy density (kcal/cup)**	Carbohydrate (%)	Fat (%)	Omega-3 fatty acids (%)	Omega-6: omega-3 ratio	Protein (%)	Arginine (%)
Recommended levels	-	≤25	25-40	>5	~1:1	30-45	>2
Medi-Cal Development Formula	425	na	17.5	na	na	28.4	na

Moist foods	Energy density (kcal/can)**	Carbohydrate (%)	Fat (%)	Omega-3 fatty acids (%)	Omega-6: omega-3 ratio	Protein (%)	Arginine (%)
Recommended levels	-	≤25	25-40	>5	~1:1	30-45	>2
Hill's Prescription Diet a/d Canine/Feline	180/5.5 oz.	**15.4**	**30.4**	2.62	2.3:1	**44.2**	**2.37**
Hill's Prescription Diet n/d Canine	569/12.7 oz.	**19.9**	**33.2**	**7.29**	**0.3:1**	**38.0**	**2.95**
Iams Veterinary Formula Maximum Calorie/Canine & Feline	333/6 oz.	**12.2**	**37.2**	na	na	**41.8**	na
Medi-Cal Development Formula	445/396 g	na	14.1	na	na	**32.2**	na
Medi-Cal Recovery Formula/ Canine & Feline	185/170 g	na	**32.1**	na	na	53.4	na
Purina Veterinary Diets DM Dietetic Management Feline Formula	194/5.5 oz.	**8.1**	23.8	0.88	3.8:1	56.9	na

Key: na = Information not available from manufacturer; values were obtained from manufacturers' published information, g = grams.
*Nutrients expressed on a % dry matter basis, unless otherwise stated.
**As fed energy density is useful for determining amount to feed; cup = 8-oz. measuring cup; to convert to kJ, multiply by 4.184.

Table 7. Selected commercial foods for feline cancer patients compared to recommended levels of key nutritional factors.* (Numbers in red match optimal KNFs.)

Dry foods	Energy density (kcal/cup)**	Carbohydrate (%)	Fat (%)	Omega-3 fatty acids (%)	Omega-6: omega-3 ratio	Protein (%)	Arginine (%)
Recommended levels	-	≤25	25-40	>5	~1:1	40-50	>2
Medi-Cal Development Formula	425	na	23.9	na	na	34.7	na
Purina Veterinary Diets DM Dietetic Management Feline Formula	592	**15.0**	17.9	0.39	5.6:1	57.8	**3.57**

Moist foods	Energy density (kcal/can)**	Carbohydrate (%)	Fat (%)	Omega-3 fatty acids (%)	Omega-6: omega-3 ratio	Protein (%)	Arginine (%)
Recommended levels	-	≤25	25-40	>5	~1:1	40-50	>2
Hill's Prescription Diet a/d Canine/Feline	180/5.5 oz.	**15.4**	**30.4**	2.62	2.3:1	**44.2**	**2.37**
Iams Veterinary Formula Maximum Calorie/ Canine & Feline	333/6 oz.	**12.2**	**37.2**	na	na	**41.8**	na
Medi-Cal Development Formula	216/170 g	na	**27.5**	na	na	**45.0**	na
Medi-Cal Recovery Formula/Canine & Feline	185/170 g	na	**32.1**	na	na	53.4	na
Purina Veterinary Diets CV Cardiovascular Feline Formula	223/5.5 oz.	**23.1**	**26.8**	na	na	**42.5**	na
Purina Veterinary Diets DM Dietetic Management Feline Formula	194/5.5 oz.	**8.1**	23.8	0.88	3.8:1	56.9	na

Key: na = Information not available from manufacturer; values were obtained from manufacturers' published information, g = grams.
*Nutrients expressed on a % dry matter basis, unless otherwise stated.
**As fed energy density is useful for determining amount to feed; cup = 8-oz. measuring cup; to convert to kJ, multiply by 4.184.

CLINICAL POINTS

- Adverse food reactions are abnormal responses to ingested foods or (more rarely) food additives.
- Classification of adverse food reactions is based on pathomechanisms (**Figure 1**).
- Dietary trials (see Feeding Methods below) are important to confirm or rule out adverse reactions to food but do not define the underlying mechanism (i.e., allergy or intolerance).
- Risk factors include: 1) certain foods/food ingredients (**Table 1**), 2) poorly digestible proteins, 3) diseases that increase intestinal mucosal permeability (e.g., viral enteritis), 4) selective IgA deficiency, 5) genetic predisposition, 6) age (6 months-4 years) and 7) concurrent allergic disease.
- Adverse food reactions can cause a wide variety of dermatologic lesions and should be considered as a cause of any pruritic disease (including otitis externa); accounts for 1-6% of all dermatoses.
- Food allergy is one of the most common causes of hypersensitive skin disease in dogs and cats along with arthropod (flea) hypersensitivity and atopic dermatitis (due to environmental allergens).
- Unusual/atypical dermatoses resulting from adverse food reactions in dogs include erythema multiforme, claw disease and generalized erythematous wheals.
- Up to one-half of patients with cutaneous manifestations of food hypersensitivity may have concurrent GI disturbances.
- Adverse food reactions contribute to idiopathic GI problems and some cases of IBD (Chapter 43). Signs usually relate to gastric and small bowel dysfunction, but colitis can also occur; vomiting and diarrhea are prominent features.
- Patients can develop food allergies after prolonged exposure to one brand, type or form of food. In contrast, adverse reactions attributable to food intolerance can occur after a single exposure to a food ingredient (immune amplification is unnecessary).
- The nutritional history should be reviewed for ingredients associated with adverse food reactions and should include: 1) specific commercial foods, snacks and treats, 2) supplements, 3) chewable medications, 4) chew toys, 5) human foods and 6) access to other food sources (e.g., other pets' foods, garbage).
- Studies support the use of commercial foods containing novel protein sources in the management of adverse food reactions.
- Novel protein sources are protein-containing animal- or vegetable-based ingredients that are not commonly used in pet foods and/or are not commonly associated with adverse food reactions.
- Major food allergens are water-soluble proteins (usually glycosylated) with molecular weights ranging from 10,000-

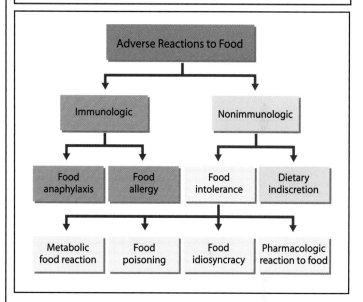

Figure 1. Classification of adverse reactions to food.

Table 1. Ingredients commonly associated with adverse food reactions.*

Dogs Ingredients	% of reported cases
Beef, dairy products, wheat	69
Lamb, chicken egg, chicken, soy	25
Cats Ingredients	**% of reported cases**
Beef, dairy products, fish	80

*Data from cases reported in North America, Europe, Australia, Japan and New Zealand. Common food allergens may differ in other geographic locations.

70,000 daltons.
- Hydrolyzed protein(s) are novel protein sources that may offer advantages over intact proteins; they are less likely to elicit an immune-mediated response when their molecular weights <10,000 daltons.
- Pet food additives rarely cause food allergy or intolerance. Additives are found least often in moist pet foods and most commonly in semi-moist foods, treats, snacks and dry foods.
- Feeding goals: control clinical signs associated with adverse food reactions while concurrently managing unrelated long-term health issues.

KEY NUTRITIONAL FACTORS

- Foods should provide recommended allowances of all required nutrients (nutritional adequacy), but should also contain specific levels of KNFs (certain nutrients and nonnutritional food ingredients that can assist in the management of adverse food reactions and promote long-term health).
- Protein is the nutrient of most concern in patients with suspected food allergy; the number of different proteins, novel protein sources (including hydrolysates) and avoidance of excess protein are KNFs for foods for diagnosis and treatment of adverse food reactions.
- Because of their potential benefit in inflammatory diseases and the treatment phase of the feeding plan (below), n-3 fatty

acids are included as KNFs. However, their inclusion in an elimination food could theoretically confound the diagnostic phase of the feeding method.
- During the treatment phase, elimination foods replace regular foods and are typically fed long term. Thus, several KNFs are included because of their role in preventing common health issues rather than being beneficial for adverse food reactions (Chapters 1, 2, 7 and 8).
- **Table 2** summarizes the KNFs for foods for patients with adverse food reactions. A detailed description of all the KNF recommendations is found in Chapters 13, 14, 20, 21 and 31, Small Animal Clinical Nutrition, 5th edition.

FEEDING PLAN

Unlike most other clinical conditions, the feeding plan for possible adverse food reaction patients includes a diagnostic phase, which determines the food to be fed in the subsequent treatment phase.

Assess and Select the Food
Ensure the Food's Basic Nutritional Adequacy. AAFCO nutritional adequacy statements are usually found on a product's label. AAFCO approval does not ensure a food will be effective for managing adverse food reactions or preventing other long-term health problems.
Compare the Food's KNF Content with Recommended Levels. **Tables 3** and **4** compare KNF recommendations to the KNF content of selected commercial veterinary therapeutic foods intended for dogs and cats (respectively) with adverse food reactions. Select a food for the diagnostic phase of the feeding method (below) that contains only the desired protein ingredient source(s) and is most similar to the KNF recommendations. Contact manufacturers for information for foods not in the tables (contact information is listed on product labels).

PROTEIN INGREDIENT INFORMATION SOURCES. See manufacturers' published information and/or ingredient statements on U.S. commercial pet food labels. Product labels on U.S. foods identify all ingredients; labels on foreign-manufactured foods may not have complete ingredient lists. If necessary, contact manufacturers for ingredient information.

HOMEMADE ELIMINATION FOODS. These foods usually include a single protein source or a single protein source and a single carbohydrate source. Ingredients typically used for foods for cats include lamb baby food, lamb, rice and rabbit. Lamb, rice, potato, fish, rabbit, venison, various beans and tofu are often used in foods for dogs.

Caution. Many homemade foods recommended for initial management of dogs and cats with suspected food allergy are nutritionally imbalanced, lacking calcium sources, essential fatty acids, certain vitamins and other micronutrients while containing excess protein (contraindicated in food allergy cases). Don't feed nutritionally inadequate foods for >3 weeks and don't feed these foods to young dogs (<12 months old).

Table 2. Key nutritional factors for foods for the diagnosis and management of adverse food reactions in dogs and cats.

Factors	Dietary recommendations
Dogs	
Protein	Limit dietary protein to one or two sources
	Use protein hydrolysate or protein sources to which the dog has not been exposed previously
	Avoid excess levels of dietary protein (dermatologic cases only): protein should be 16 to 22% DM
	Use a food that is nutritionally balanced for dogs
	Avoid foods that contain wheat, barley or rye (dogs with diarrhea)
Vasoactive amines	Avoid foods that contain certain fish ingredients (e.g., tuna, mackerel, skipjack, bonito)
Total omega-3 fatty acids	0.35 to 1.8% DM
Phosphorus*	0.4 to 0.8% DM
Sodium*	0.2 to 0.4% DM
Cats	
Protein	Limit dietary protein to one or two sources
	Use protein hydrolysate or protein sources to which the cat has not been exposed previously
	Avoid excess levels of dietary protein (dermatologic cases only): protein should be 30 to 45% DM
	Use a food that is nutritionally balanced for cats
Vasoactive amines	Avoid foods that contain certain fish ingredients (e.g., tuna, mackerel, skipjack, bonito)
Total omega-3 fatty acids	0.35 to 1.8% DM
Phosphorus*	0.5 to 0.8% DM
Sodium*	0.2 to 0.6% DM
Magnesium*	0.04 to 0.1% DM
Urinary pH*	6.2 to 6.4

Key: DM = dry matter.
*Not related to adverse reactions to food but important when elimination foods are used for long-term feeding: phosphorus and sodium are considered key nutritional factors for apparently healthy adult dogs and cats for purposes of ameliorating or slowing the progression of subclinical kidney disease and/or hypertension; magnesium and urinary pH are important for reducing the risk of feline lower urinary tract disease.

Manage Treats and Snacks. During the diagnostic phase (below), it is particularly important to ensure no other substances are ingested including treats, flavored vitamin and/or fatty acid supplements, chewable medications or chew toys. During the treatment phase, providing the opposite form of food as a treat or snack is acceptable as long as it doesn't introduce different protein sources into the food regimen.

Assess and Determine the Feeding Method

Feeding methods for patients suspected of having adverse food reactions have 2 phases.

Diagnostic Phase.

PERFORMING AN ELIMINATION-CHALLENGE TRIAL IN PATIENTS WITH SKIN DISEASE.

Elimination. Discuss potential food allergens with owners to determine protein sources and additives desired in the controlled elimination food (**Tables 2** and **5**, respectively). Feed only the selected food for 6-12 weeks (duration is response dependent); absolutely no other substances should be ingested. Have the owner document the type and amount of food ingested and the occurrence/character of adverse reactions, daily. Make a tentative diagnosis of an adverse food reaction if pruritus markedly decreases. Improvement can be gradual and might take 4-12 weeks to become evident.

Concurrent Yeast Infection, Pyoderma and/or Otitis Externa. If present at initial presentation, treat during the elimination trial (be sure owner is not administering oral drugs in elicit foods). After medical treatment, continue feeding only the elimination food for another 2-3 weeks to ensure improvement, if achieved, is maintained.

Challenge. Diagnosis is confirmed if clinical signs reappear after the former food(s) and other ingested substances are reintroduced as a challenge. Reappearance of signs may occur within hours or take up to 2 weeks. Refeed the elimination food to resolve clinical signs induced by the food challenge. Many owners are satisfied with a presumptive diagnosis of food sensitivity and do not wish to undertake a challenge test; however, failure to challenge a suspected food-sensitive patient can result in misdiagnosis.

Chronic Otitis Externa. If due to adverse food reactions, may require a 4-6 month elimination period for improvement to be noted, especially if proliferative lesions are present.

Concurrent Allergic Skin Disease. Patients may only partially respond to an elimination trial. Flea-allergy and atopic dermatitis triggered by environmental allergens are the most common concurrent diseases and should be eliminated through other diagnostic testing.

PERFORMING AN ELIMINATION-CHALLENGE TRIAL IN PATIENTS WITH GI DISEASE.

The process is similar to that for skin disease (above).

Elimination. Usually a shorter period (2-4 weeks) is satisfactory. In chronic relapsing conditions, the elimination period must be longer than the usual symptom-free period to allow for reliable assessment. As with skin disease, the clinical response during elimination trials will be 100% only if food sensitivity is the sole cause. Resolution of allergies acquired as a result of GI disease will not eliminate clinical signs attributable to an underlying primary disease.

Challenge. GI signs usually recur within 1-3 days after challenge with suspected allergens; it may take up to 7 days if the allergen was removed from the diet for >1 month. As noted above, many owners will forgo challenge trials.

Treatment Phase.

For most patients, avoiding the offending food(s) is the most effective treatment. Thus, after a diagnosis of adverse food reaction is made, feed the elimination food (**Tables 3** and **4**) for long-term maintenance (if using a homemade food, make sure it is nutritionally complete/balanced).

DETERMINE HOW MUCH FOOD TO FEED. When a new food is needed, the amount fed can be estimated from feeding guides on product labels or by calculation (Appendix C). Feeding guidelines and calculations are starting points and may need to be adjusted.

CONSIDER HOW TO OFFER THE FOOD. Both free-choice and restricted-feeding methods have advantages and disadvantages (Appendix D). Food-restricted feeding is best because it is less likely to cause overeating and overweight/obesity conditions. Pet owners often overestimate food needs and feed too much; most people do not recognize overweight/obesity in their pets.

MANAGE FOOD CHANGES. Most dogs and cats adapt well to new foods but a transition period to avoid GI upsets and facilitate acceptance of a new food is good practice. Example: to change to a new food, replace 25% of the old food with the new food on Day 1 and continue this incremental change daily until the change is complete on Day 4. Appendix E provides additional information.

FOOD AND WATER RECEPTACLE HUSBANDRY. Food and water bowls should be washed regularly with warm soapy water and rinsed well. Dishes used for moist foods need daily cleaning. Discard moist or moistened dry foods after 2-4 hours of room temperature exposure to avoid foodborne illnesses (Appendix F).

DRY FOOD STORAGE. Recommend retaining a new food in original packaging; storage in other containers such as previously used plastic bins/buckets risks contamination by fines (small food particles) from previous food(s), house dust or mites.

FOLLOWUP

Owner Followup

Compliance is very important and is patient dependent. Patients can have adverse reactions to even trace quantities of an offending food. If feeding a new food, owners should weigh their pet (if possible) and/or grade its body condition (BCS) monthly. If a trend of increasing or decreasing body weight or BCS is noticed, the amount fed should be changed by 10% increments and rechecked every 2 weeks for 1 month. If necessary, the amount fed should be changed again and the cycle repeated.

Veterinary Health Care Team Followup

Concurrent allergies may influence the threshold level of clinical

Table 3. Selected commercial veterinary therapeutic foods marketed as elimination foods for dogs with adverse food reactions compared to key nutritional factor recommendations.[*] (Numbers in red match optimal KNFs.)

Dry foods	Protein ingredients	Protein (%)[**]	Omega 3 (%)[***]	P (%)[†]	Na (%)[†]
Recommendations	Maximum of 1-2 protein sources Avoid scombroid fish[††] Avoid wheat, barley and rye[†††]	16-22	0.35-1.8	0.4-0.8	0.2-0.4
Hill's Prescription Diet d/d Potato & Duck Formula Canine	Potato, duck	18	0.35	0.58	0.36
Hill's Prescription Diet d/d Potato & Salmon Formula Canine	Potato, salmon	18.4	0.995	0.58	0.37
Hill's Prescription Diet d/d Potato & Venison Formula Canine	Potato, venison	18	0.337	0.57	0.36
Hill's Prescription Diet d/d Rice & Egg Formula Canine	Rice, egg	18.8	0.366	0.5	0.28
Hill's Prescription Diet z/d Low Allergen Canine	Potato, hydrolyzed chicken/chicken liver	19.6	na	0.57	0.36
Hill's Prescription Diet z/d ULTRA Allergen-Free Canine	Hydrolyzed chicken/chicken liver	19	na	0.51	0.29
Iams Veterinary Formula Skin & Coat/ Response FP Canine	Potato, herring meal, beet pulp	25.0	na	0.99	0.35
Iams Veterinary Formula Skin & Coat/ Response KO Canine	Oat flour, kangaroo, canola meal, beet pulp	22.7	na	1.01	0.44
Medi-Cal Hypoallergenic Formula	Oat flour/hulls, rice, duck meal	21.3	0.7	0.8	0.4
Medi-Cal Hypoallergenic HP	Rice, soy protein isolate hydrolysate, beet pulp	23.1	0.4	0.9	0.4
Medi-Cal Sensitivity RC 21	Rice/rice gluten, catfish meal	25.8	na	1.3	0.5
Medi-Cal Vegetarian Formula	Oat flour, rice, potato protein, flax meal, beet pulp, tomato pomace	20.9	na	0.9	0.4
Natural Balance Limited Ingredient Diet Potato & Duck Formula	Potato, duck/duck meal, flaxseed	na	na	na	na
Natural Balance Limited Ingredient Diet Sweet Potato & Fish Formula	Sweet potato, salmon/salmon meal, flaxseed	na	na	na	na
Natural Balance Limited Ingredient Diet Sweet Potato & Venison Formula	Sweet potato, venison/venison meal, potato protein, flaxseed	na	na	na	na
Purina Veterinary Diets DRM Dermatologic Management Canine Formula	Rice, salmon meal, trout, canola meal, brewers yeast	30.2	na	1.16	0.24
Purina Veterinary Diets HA Hypoallergenic Canine Formula	Soy protein isolate	21.3	na	0.87	0.24
Royal Canin Veterinary Diet Canine Hypoallergenic HP 19	Rice, soy protein hydrolysate, beet pulp	23.1	0.901	0.88	0.44
Royal Canin Veterinary Diet Canine Potato & Duck Formula	Potato/potato protein, duck/duck by-product meal	22.2	na	0.68	0.33
Royal Canin Veterinary Diet Canine Potato & Duck Formula Light	Potato/potato protein, duck/duck by-product meal	26.9	na	0.81	0.38
Royal Canin Veterinary Diet Canine Potato & Rabbit Formula	Potato/potato protein, rabbit/rabbit meal	23.1	na	0.67	0.33
Royal Canin Veterinary Diet Canine Potato & Venison Formula	Potato/potato protein, venison/venison meal	22.3	na	1.01	0.24
Royal Canin Veterinary Diet Canine Potato & Venison Formula Large Breed	Potato/potato protein, venison/venison meal	23.6	na	1.08	0.45
Royal Canin Veterinary Diet Canine Potato & Whitefish Formula	Potato, herring meal, whitefish	22.5	na	0.66	0.44
Royal Canin Veterinary Diet Canine Skin Support SS 21	Menhaden fish meal, rice/brown rice, beet pulp	25.3	0.714	1.21	0.44
Royal Canin Veterinary Diet Canine Vegetarian Formula	Oat flour, rice, yeast culture, tomato pomace, beet pulp, flaxseed, carrot pomace	19.1	na	0.56	0.15
Wellness Simple Food Solutions Rice + Duck Formula	Rice/rice protein concentrate, duck, flaxseed	na	na	na	na
Wellness Simple Food Solutions Rice + Venison Formula	Rice/rice protein concentrate, venison, flaxseed	na	na	na	na

Moist foods Recommendations	Protein ingredients Maximum of 1-2 protein sources Avoid scombroid fish[††] Avoid wheat, barley and rye[†††]	Protein (%)** 16-22	Omega 3 (%)*** 0.35-1.8	P (%)[†] 0.4-0.8	Na (%)[†] 0.2-0.4
Hill's Prescription Diet d/d Duck Formula Canine	Duck/duck liver, potato	<u>17.4</u>	<u>0.384</u>	<u>0.69</u>	<u>0.36</u>
Hill's Prescription Diet d/d Lamb Formula Canine	Rice, lamb/lamb liver	15.8	<u>0.395</u>	0.31	<u>0.34</u>
Hill's Prescription Diet d/d Salmon Formula Canine	Salmon, potato	<u>18.9</u>	<u>1.787</u>	<u>0.7</u>	<u>0.33</u>
Hill's Prescription Diet d/d Venison Formula Canine	Venison, potato	<u>18.9</u>	0.328	<u>0.53</u>	<u>0.37</u>
Hill's Prescription Diet z/d ULTRA Allergen-Free Canine	Hydrolyzed chicken liver	<u>19.6</u>	na	<u>0.57</u>	<u>0.2</u>
Iams Veterinary Formula Skin & Coat/Response FP Canine	Catfish, herring meal, potato starch, beet pulp	35.5	na	0.92	0.60
Medi-Cal Hypoallergenic Formula	Pheasant, rice flour, duck meal, oat hulls	<u>20.1</u>	0.006	1.0	0.5
Medi-Cal Sensitivity VR	Venison/venison by-products, rice	35.8	na	2.4	1.2
Medi-Cal Vegetarian Formula	Rice/brown rice, soy protein isolate	26.4	na	<u>0.7</u>	0.5
Natural Balance Duck & Potato Formula	Duck/duck liver, potato	na	na	na	na
Natural Balance Fish & Sweet Potato Formula	Ocean white fish, sweet potato, salmon, potato, fish meal	na	na	na	na
Natural Balance Venison & Sweet Potato Formula	Venison/venison liver, sweet potato, potato	na	na	na	na
Royal Canin Veterinary Diet Canine Duck Formula	Potato, duck/duck by-products	<u>18.5</u>	na	0.86	1.45
Royal Canin Veterinary Diet Canine Venison Formula	Potato, venison/venison by-products	<u>18.5</u>	na	0.86	1.45
Royal Canin Veterinary Diet Canine Whitefish Formula	Potato, whitefish	<u>18.5</u>	na	0.86	1.45
Wysong Duck Au Jus	Duck, animal plasma	na	na	na	na
Wysong Rabbit Au Jus	Rabbit	na	na	na	na
Wysong Turkey Au Jus	Turkey/turkey liver, animal plasma	na	na	na	na
Wysong Venison Au Jus	Venison/venison liver, animal plasma	na	na	na	na

Key: Omega 3 = total omega-3 fatty acids, P = phosphorus, Na = sodium, na = not available from manufacturer.
*Values are on a dry matter basis unless otherwise stated.
**A higher protein level may be necessary to counteract protein losses from the GI tract or impaired absorption in patients with hypoproteinemia and weight loss associated with severe GI disease.
***Omega-3 fatty acids are important for dermatologic cases.
[†]Phosphorus and sodium are not important for adverse food reactions but are important for overall health when feeding these foods long-term.
[††]Fish source ingredients that can be a source of vasoactive amines.
[†††]For dogs with diarrhea.

signs in some patients. Symptomatic therapy for pruritic patients may include corticosteroids and antihistamines. Corticosteroids are often used along with an appropriate feeding plan in cats with IBD (Chapter 43).

MISCELLANEOUS

See Chapters 9, 10, 13, 14, 20, 21 and 31, Small Animal Clinical Nutrition, 5th edition, for more information.

Authors
Condensed from Chapter 31, Small Animal Clinical Nutrition, 5th edition, authored by Philip Roudebush, W. Grant Guilford and Hilary A. Jackson.

References
See Chapter 31, Small Animal Clinical Nutrition, 5th edition, on the website www.markmorrisinstitute.org for references.

Table 4. Selected commercial veterinary therapeutic foods marketed as elimination foods for cats with adverse food reactions compared to key nutritional factor recommendations.* (Numbers in red match optimal KNFs.)

Dry foods	Protein ingredients	Protein (%)** 30-45	Omega 3 (%)*** 0.35-1.8	P (%)† 0.5-0.8	Na (%)† 0.2-0.6	Mg (%)† 0.04-0.1	Urinary pH† 6.2-6.4
Recommendations	Maximum of 1-2 protein sources Avoid scombroid fish††						
Hill's Prescription Diet d/d Duck & Green Pea Formula Feline	Peas, duck/duck meal	32	0.353	0.72	0.4	0.111	6.30
Hill's Prescription Diet d/d Rabbit & Green Pea Formula Feline	Peas, rabbit/rabbit meal	32	0.336	0.73	0.34	0.118	6.38
Hill's Prescription Diet d/d Venison & Green Pea Formula Feline	Peas, venison/venison meal	32	0.34	0.74	0.3	0.116	6.32
Hill's Prescription Diet z/d Low Allergen Feline	Rice, hydrolyzed chicken liver/hydrolyzed chicken	33	0.102	0.67	0.34	0.068	6.30
Medi-Cal Hypoallergenic HP 23	Rice/rice gluten, soy protein isolate hydrolysate	27.4	0.3	0.8	0.5	na	na
Medi-Cal Hypoallergenic/Gastro	Potato meal/potato protein, duck meal, rice	29.8	0.24	0.9	0.4	na	6.2
Medi-Cal Sensitivity RD 30	Rice/rice gluten, duck by-product meal	34.4	na	1.3	0.6	na	na
Natural Balance Limited Ingredient Diets Duck & Green Pea Formula	Peas, duck meal, flaxseed	na	na	na	na	na	na
Royal Canin Veterinary Diet Feline Green Peas & Duck Formula	Peas, duck meal/duck	34.9	na	1.45	0.77	0.118	na
Royal Canin Veterinary Diet Feline Green Peas & Lamb Formula	Peas/pea protein, lamb meal/lamb	34.9	na	1.43	0.76	0.129	na
Royal Canin Veterinary Diet Feline Green Peas & Rabbit Formula	Peas/pea protein, rabbit meal/rabbit	34.9	na	1.13	0.77	0.172	na
Royal Canin Veterinary Diet Feline Green Peas & Venison Formula	Peas/pea protein, venison meal/venison	34.9	na	1.81	0.87	0.129	na

Table 5. Food additives that have been reported as occasional causes of food intolerance in people and that are sometimes present in pet foods or treats.*

Antioxidant preservatives
Butylated hydroxyanisole (BHA)
Butylated hydroxytoluene (BHT)
Antimicrobial preservatives
Sodium nitrite
Humectants
Propylene glycol
Coloring agents/preservatives
Azo dyes
  Tartrazine (FD&C No. 5)
  Sunset yellow (FD&C No. 6)
  Allura red (FD&C No. 40)
Non-azo dyes
  Brilliant blue (FD&C No. 1)
  Indigotin (FD&C No. 2)
Flavors/flavor enhancers
Monosodium glutamate
Spices
Emulsifying agents, stabilizers, thickeners
Seaweed extracts (carrageenan, alginates)
Seed gums (guar gum)

*These additives are frequently incriminated as causing adverse food reactions in dogs and cats, but there are no well-documented case reports to substantiate this perception.

Moist foods Recommendations	Protein ingredients Maximum of 1-2 protein sources Avoid scombroid fish††	Protein (%)** 30-45	Omega 3 (%)*** 0.35-1.8	P (%)† 0.5-0.8	Na (%)† 0.2-0.6	Mg (%)† 0.04-0.1	Urinary pH† 6.2-6.4
Hill's Prescription Diet d/d Duck Formula Feline	Duck/duck liver, peas	38.1	0.479	0.75	0.3	0.083	6.38
Hill's Prescription Diet d/d Rabbit Formula Feline	Rabbit, peas	36	0.594	0.73	0.27	0.08	6.24
Hill's Prescription Diet d/d Venison Formula Feline	Venison/venison liver, peas	37.3	0.654	0.73	0.35	0.088	6.45
Hill's Prescription Diet z/d ULTRA Allergen-Free Feline	Hydrolyzed chicken liver	33.7	na	0.64	0.3	0.064	6.28
Iams Veterinary Formula Skin & Coat/Response LB Feline	Lamb/lamb liver/lamb by-products/lamb meal, barley, beet pulp	43.4	na	1.02	0.34	0.085	na
Medi-Cal Hypoallergenic/Gastro	Duck/duck meal, rice	35.5	0.16	1.7	0.7	na	6.4
Medi-Cal Sensitivity CR	Chicken, rice	34.5	na	1.6	1.1	na	na
Medi-Cal Sensitivity VR	Venison by-products/venison, rice	43.0	na	1.6	1.0	na	na
Natural Balance Limited Ingredient Diets Duck & Green Pea Formula	Duck/duck liver/duck meal, peas/pea protein	na	na	na	na	na	na
Natural Balance Limited Ingredient Diets Venison & Green Pea Formula	Venison/venison liver, venison meal, peas, flax-seed	na	na	na	na	na	na
Royal Canin Veterinary Diet Feline Duck Formula	Duck/duck by-products, peas	44.1	na	0.74	0.47	0.078	na
Royal Canin Veterinary Diet Feline Lamb Formula	Lamb by-products/lamb, peas	44.1	na	0.74	0.47	0.078	na
Royal Canin Veterinary Diet Feline Venison Formula	Venison by-products/venison, peas	44.1	na	0.74	0.47	0.078	na
Wysong Duck Au Jus	Duck, animal plasma	na	na	na	na	na	na
Wysong Rabbit Au Jus	Rabbit	na	na	na	na	na	na
Wysong Turkey Au Jus	Turkey/turkey liver, animal plasma	na	na	na	na	na	na
Wysong Venison Au Jus	Venison/venison liver, animal plasma	na	na	na	na	na	na

Key: Omega 3 = total omega-3 fatty acids, P = phosphorus, Na = sodium, Mg = magnesium, na = not available from manufacturer.
*Values are on a dry matter basis unless otherwise stated.
**A higher protein level may be necessary to counteract protein losses from the GI tract or impaired absorption in patients with hypoproteinemia and weight loss associated with severe GI disease.
***Omega-3 fatty acids are important for dermatologic cases.
†Phosphorus, sodium, magnesium and urinary pH are not important for adverse food reactions but are important for overall health when feeding these foods long-term.
††Fish ingredients that can be a source of vasoactive amines.

Chapter 20

Nutrient-Deficient and Nutrient-Sensitive Dermatoses

CLINICAL POINTS

- This chapter covers a diverse group of nutrient-deficient or nutrient-sensitive skin diseases; Chapter 21 covers n-3 fatty acids for management of skin diseases that have an inflammatory or pruritic component.
- Aside from adverse reactions to food, nutritional skin diseases in pets fed nutritionally adequate commercial pet foods are rare.
- Deficiencies usually occur during growth or reproduction when homemade foods, poor quality commercial foods that contain nutrient excesses or even high quality commercial foods that

Table 1. Breed predilection for non-neoplastic skin diseases often managed by food changes or supplementation.*

Breed	Disease
Airedale terrier	Atopic dermatitis
Akita	Sebaceous adenitis
Basenji	Atopic dermatitis
Basset hound	Atopic dermatitis
Beagle	Atopic dermatitis
Boston terrier	Atopic dermatitis
Boxer	Adverse reactions to food
	Atopic dermatitis
Bull terrier	Acrodermatitis
	Atopic dermatitis
	Zinc-responsive dermatosis
Chesapeake Bay retriever	Atopic dermatitis
Dalmatian	Atopic dermatitis
English bulldog	Atopic dermatitis
German shepherd dog	Adverse reactions to food
	Atopic dermatitis
	Seborrhea, primary
Golden retriever	Atopic dermatitis
Gordon setter	Atopic dermatitis
Irish setter	Atopic dermatitis
	Seborrhea, primary
Labrador retriever	Adverse reactions to food
	Atopic dermatitis
	Seborrhea, primary
Lhasa apso	Atopic dermatitis
Malamute	Zinc-responsive dermatosis
Old English sheepdog	Atopic dermatitis
Poodle, standard	Sebaceous adenitis
Pug	Atopic dermatitis
Schnauzer, miniature	Atopic dermatitis
Shar Pei	Adverse reactions to food
	Atopic dermatitis
Shih Tzu	Atopic dermatitis
Siberian husky	Zinc-responsive dermatosis
Spaniels	Adverse reactions to food
	Atopic dermatitis (American cocker)
	Seborrhea, primary
Terriers	Atopic dermatitis
Vizsla	Sebaceous adenitis

*Atopic dermatitis is often managed with fatty acid supplementation, sebaceous adenitis and primary seborrhea with retinoid supplementation, zinc-responsive dermatosis with zinc supplementation and adverse reactions to food with dietary changes. Specific nutrient deficiencies are usually not breed-specific.

Abbreviations
AAFCO = Association of American Feed Control Officials
BCS = body condition score (Appendix A)
EFA = essential fatty acid
KNF = key nutritional factor

are inappropriately supplemented, are fed.
- Breed predilection can also be a factor (**Table 1**).
- Nutritional history should focus on adequacy of the current food for the patient's lifestage and types and dosages of nutritional supplements; homemade foods should be evaluated for nutritional adequacy by a qualified veterinary nutritionist or a good nutritional software program.
- Physical exam findings suggestive of nutritional problems include: 1) a sparse, dry, dull and brittle coat with hairs that epilate easily, 2) slow hair growth or regrowth from areas that have been clipped, 3) abnormal scale accumulation (seborrhea sicca), 4) loss of hair, erythema or crusting in areas of friction or stretch such as the distal extremities, 5) decubital ulcers and poor wound healing and 6) loss of normal hair color.
- Typical laboratory tests are rarely helpful in evaluating nutritional skin disease; however, they can help rule out potential underlying primary disease causes of cutaneous problems.
- Examination of hair (trichography) and dermatohistopathology are helpful laboratory tests for evaluation of potential nutritional problems.
- **Table 2** lists specific physical exam and laboratory findings and associated underlying nutrient problems.
- **Table 3** lists risk factors for development of zinc-responsive cutaneous disease.
- Poor-quality/inexpensive commercial dry pet foods can be low in total fat and EFAs; EFA deficiency is rapidly reversible (days) if EFA intake is increased.
- Zinc deficiency accelerates development of clinical signs of EFA deficiency; conversely, supplementation with EFAs can reverse signs of zinc deficiency (**Table 2**).
- Vitamin A deficiencies in dogs and cats are seldom encountered clinically.
- **Table 4** lists retinoid dosages for primary keratinization disorders. Common side effects include conjunctivitis, decreased tear production, vomiting, diarrhea, arthralgia/myalgia, elevations in serum triglycerides, elevations in liver enzyme activities and teratogenic effects.
- Naturally occurring vitamin E deficiency has only been reported in cats (steatitis) when sources of highly unsaturated fatty acids (e.g., red meat tuna) were fed without adequate vitamin E.
- Several inflammatory dermatoses are reported to respond to vitamin E (**Table 2**).
- Feeding goals: provide appropriate nutrition to support

Table 2. Key nutritional factors for foods and supplements for dogs and cats with nutrient-responsive dermatoses.

Factors	Associated conditions	Nutritional recommendations

Protein and fat	Keratinization abnormalities
	Loss of normal hair color
	Secondary bacterial or yeast infection
	Impaired wound healing
	Decubital ulcers
	Telogen defluxion
	Anagen defluxion
		Avoid protein and energy deficiency
		Adult maintenance
		  Dogs: Protein = 25 to 30% dry matter (DM)
		           Fat = 10 to 15% DM
		  Cats: Protein = 30 to 45% DM
		           Fat = 10 to 15% DM
		Growth/lactation
		  Dogs: Protein = 30 to 35% DM
		           Fat = 15 to 30% DM
		  Cats: Protein = 35 to 50% DM
		           Fat = 20 to 35% DM
		Phenylalanine + tyrosine >1.3% DM
		Use a food with DM digestibility >80%

Essential fatty acids (EFA)	Excessive scales (seborrhea sicca)
	Alopecia
	Dry, dull coat
	Lack of normal hair growth
	Erythroderma
	Interdigital exudation
		Avoid fatty acid deficiency
		  Dogs: Linoleic acid >1.0% DM
		  Cats: Linoleic acid >0.5% DM
		Some dogs and cats respond to levels in excess of those listed above
		Provide adequate levels and availability of zinc, B-complex
		  vitamins and vitamin E to ensure adequate use of EFA

Zinc	Alopecia
	Skin ulceration
	Dermatitis
	Paronychia
	Footpad disease
	Slow hair growth
	Buccal margin ulceration
	Hyperkeratotic plaques
	Secondary bacterial or yeast infection
		Avoid zinc deficiency
		  Dogs: 100 to 200 mg/kg food DM
		  Cats: 50 to 150 mg/kg food DM
		Avoid excess calcium
		  Higher levels of zinc are required in foods with calcium >1.5% DM
		Avoid excess copper (copper <200 mg/kg food DM)
		Avoid EFA deficiency (see above)
		Zinc supplementation (Do not give with food)
		  Zinc sulfate: 10 mg/kg body weight/day per os
		                   10 to 15 mg/kg body weight/week IV
		  Zinc methionine: 2 mg/kg body weight/day

Copper	Loss of normal color
	Dull or rough coat
	Reduced density of hair
	Alopecia
		Avoid copper deficiency
		  Dogs: >5 to 10 mg/kg food DM
		  Cats: >15 mg/kg food DM
		Avoid excess zinc (zinc <1,000 mg/kg food DM)
		Avoid ingredients that have low copper availability
		  Copper oxide
		  Liver from simple-stomached mammals
		Avoid excess calcium
		  Higher levels of copper are required in foods with
		    calcium >1.5% DM

Vitamin A	Seborrheic skin disease
	  (mainly cocker spaniel breed)
	Keratinization disorders
	Chin acne
	Nasodigital hyperkeratosis
	Ear margin seborrhea/dermatosis
	Callus
	Actinic keratosis
	Cutaneous neoplasms
	Schnauzer comedo syndrome
	Sebaceous adenitis
	Lamellar ichthyosis
		Treatment with retinoids (**Table 4**):
		Vitamin A alcohol
		  625 to 1,000 U/kg body weight, q24h, per os
		  10,000 U q24h, per os (cocker spaniel, miniature schnauzer)
		  50,000 U q24h, per os (Labrador retriever)
		Tretinoin
		  Apply topically q12 to 24h
		Isotretinoin
		  1 to 3 mg/kg body weight, q24h, per os
		Acitretin
		  0.75 to 1.0 mg/kg body weight, q24h, per os

Vitamin E	Discoid lupus erythematosus Systemic lupus erythematosus Pemphigus erythematosus Sterile panniculitis Acanthosis nigricans Dermatomyositis Ear margin vasculitis	Treatment with vitamin E: Dogs: 200 to 800 IU twice daily, per os

healthy skin/hair in patients that have skin disease attributable to genotype, lifestage or inappropriate food type/food supplementation.

KEY NUTRITIONAL FACTORS

• Foods should provide recommended allowances of all required nutrients (nutritional adequacy), but should also contain specific levels of KNFs (certain nutrients that can influence skin and hair health).

• **Table 2** summarizes KNFs for foods and nutritional supplements and recommended amounts and doses for patients with nutrient deficiency dermatoses and are discussed in more detail in Chapter 32, Small Animal Clinical Nutrition, 5th edition.

Table 3. Risk factors for zinc-related skin disease in dogs.

Certain breeds
Siberian husky
Malamute
Bull terrier
Great Dane
Labrador retriever
Other rapidly growing large and giant breeds
Food
High mineral levels (calcium, phosphorus, magnesium)
High phytate levels (high levels of cereal ingredients)
Low essential fatty acid levels
Dietary supplements
Calcium and/or other mineral supplements
Cottage cheese or other dairy products
Small intestinal disease
Viral enteritis
Malassimilation (malabsorption, maldigestion)

Table 4. Indications and dosages for retinoids in primary keratinization disorders.

Vitamin A alcohol (retinol)
Subset of seborrheic skin disease, primarily in cocker spaniels
Dosage: 625 to 1,000 IU/kg q24h per os
   10,000 IU q24h per os in cocker spaniels and miniature
   schnauzers
   50,000 IU q24h per os in Labrador retrievers
Tretinoin (all-trans retinoic acid)
Chin acne of dogs and cats
Nasodigital hyperkeratosis
Ear margin seborrhea/dermatosis
Dosage: Apply topically q12 to 24h to control; then decrease
   frequency for maintenance
Isotretinoin (13-cis retinoic acid)
Lamellar ichthyosis
Schnauzer comedo syndrome
Sebaceous adenitis
Dosage: 1 to 3 mg/kg q24h per os with food for control; then try
   to decrease to alternate-day therapy
Acitretin (analogue of retinoic acid ethyl ester)
Actinic keratosis
Idiopathic seborrhea, especially of cocker spaniels
Lamellar ichthyosis
Sebaceous adenitis
Dosage: 0.75 to 1.0 mg/kg q24h per os for control; then try to
   decrease to alternate-day therapy

FEEDING PLAN

Assess and Select the Food

When to Change Food. Recommend a food change and/or supplementation if one of the following conditions develops: 1) loss of normal hair color, especially lightening, graying or reddish-brown discoloration, 2) brittle/easily broken hair, 3) generalized scaling, crusting, alopecia or loss of hair sheen for which no underlying skin disorder can be readily identified, 4) poor wound healing or decubital ulcers, 5) severe, generalized inflammatory skin diseases, 6) hyperproliferative skin disorders and 7) abnormal hair growth or failure of hair to regrow where clipped or lost.

Ensure the Food's Basic Nutritional Adequacy. AAFCO nutritional adequacy statements are usually found on a product's label and are physiologic-lifestage specific. Example: feed growing or reproducing patients foods that are AAFCO approved for growth/reproduction; feeding maintenance-type foods (usually lower in protein, fat, minerals, vitamins and digestibility than growth/reproduction-type foods) may be a risk factor for nutritional skin disease during these lifestages. AAFCO approval does not ensure a food will be effective in preventing nutritional skin disease in predisposed patients (**Table 1**).

Compare the Food's KNF Content with the Recommended Levels. **Table 2** summarizes KNFs for foods for patients with nutrient-responsive dermatoses. Foods for patients with skin/hair problems should include recommended levels of these nutrients and should be in a form that is readily digested/assimilated. Compare KNFs in **Table 2** to KNF values in food tables for normal dogs and cats (Chapters 1 and 7). Contact manufacturers for information for foods not in the tables (manufacturer contact information is listed on product labels). A new food should be selected if discrepancies are noted; the new food should approximate the recommended KNF levels. Do not supplement poor-quality foods; it is better to change foods.

Supplements. Besides KNFs for foods, **Table 2** also provides information about nutritional supplements for patients with skin/hair disorders. Supplementation with fatty acids, zinc, retinoids and vitamin E usually exceeds levels used to meet nutrient requirements. In these cases, nutrient supplements are being used as therapeutic agents. If supplements are indicated, they can be used with a new or current food.

Assess and Determine the Feeding Method

Determine How Much Food to Feed. If a new food is fed, the amount to feed can be determined from the product label or calculated (Appendix C). The amount fed may need to be changed if the patient's body weight/BCS changes. If the patient's body weight and BCS are not ideal, the initial feeding estimate should take this into account. See Chapter 14 for advice on the amount to feed overweight patients.

Consider How to Offer the Food. If the body weight and BCS are normal, there is no need to change how the food is offered. Both free-choice and restricted-feeding methods have advantages and disadvantages (Appendix D). Free-choice feeding is most popular but is most likely to result in overeating. Food-restricted feeding is best because it is less likely to contribute to overweight/obesity.

Manage Food Changes. A transition period to avoid GI upsets and facilitate acceptance of new foods is good practice. Example: to change to a new food, replace 25% of the old food with the new food on Day 1 and continue this incremental change daily until the change is complete on Day 4. Appendix E provides additional information.

Food and Water Receptacle Husbandry. Food and water bowls should be washed regularly with warm soapy water and rinsed well. Dishes used for moist foods need daily cleaning. Discard moist or moistened dry foods after 2-4 hours of room temperature exposure to avoid foodborne illnesses (Appendix F).

FOLLOWUP

Owner Followup
If a new food is being fed, owners should weigh their pet (if possible) and/or grade its body condition monthly. If a trend of increasing or decreasing body weight or BCS is noticed, the amount fed should be changed by 10% increments and the patient rechecked every 2 weeks for 1 month. At that point, if necessary, the amount fed should be changed again and the cycle repeated until body weight/BCS are at the desired recommendations.

Veterinary Health Care Team Followup
Skin disease attributable to nutrient deficiency will usually respond rapidly (days to weeks) to appropriate nutritional change or supplementation. However, nutrient-sensitive disorders usually respond more slowly to supplements (weeks to months). After a food change or supplementation has been initiated, conduct monthly examinations for changes in skin lesions and hair quality. This includes trichograms for patients that have abnormal hair quality or growth.

Zinc-Supplemented Dogs. Some dogs (e.g., Siberian huskies) do not respond to oral zinc supplementation. Use IV injectable zinc sulfate solutions (10-15 mg/kg). Once weekly injections for at least 4 weeks are necessary to resolve lesions, followed by maintenance injections every 1-6 months, as necessary, to prevent relapses.

MISCELLANEOUS

See Chapter 32, Small Animal Clinical Nutrition, 5th edition, for more information about skin and hair disorders.

Authors
Condensed from Chapter 32, Small Animal Clinical Nutrition, 5th edition, authored by Philip Roudebush and William D. Schoenherr.

References
See Chapter 32, Small Animal Clinical Nutrition, 5th edition, on the website www.markmorrisinstitute.org for references.

Chapter 21

Fatty Acids for Inflammatory Skin Disease

CLINICAL POINTS

- LA and AA are n-6 (omega-6) fatty acids; both LA and AA are essential for cats, whereas only LA is essential for dogs (dogs can convert LA to AA).
- Cell membrane fatty acid composition is influenced by dietary fatty acid intake.
- Amounts of LA and AA in commercial foods usually exceed requirements; thus, AA typically becomes a major constituent of cell membranes.
- Inflammation in response to injury is normally tissue protective; if excessive and/or prolonged it can become pathologic.
- AA-derived eicosanoids are proinflammatory.
- ALA, EPA and DHA are n-3 (omega-3) fatty acids that exhibit antiinflammatory and immunomodulating properties.
- Increased intake of n-3 fatty acids relative to LA and AA increases cell membrane content of ALA, EPA and/or DHA, which reduces synthesis of proinflammatory eicosanoids by interfering with metabolism of AA in various pathways.

Abbreviations
AA = arachidonic acid
AAFCO = Association of American Feed Control Officials
ALA = alpha-linolenic acid
BCS = body condition score (Appendix A)
DHA = docosahexaenioc acid
EPA = eicosapentaenoic acid
GLA = gamma-linolenic acid
KNF = key nutritional factor
LA = linoleic acid

- EPA and DHA are also sources of endogenous mediators (resolvins, protectins) that switch on the resolution phase of an inflammatory response, acting as braking signals to inflammation, thereby reducing inflammatory injury to tissues.
- Antiinflammatory fatty acids also modulate abnormal skin lipid barrier function in patients with inflammatory skin disease.
- Numerous skin diseases have an inflammatory component including: hypersensitivity reactions due to bites from fleas, arachnids and other insects, true food allergies (Chapter 19) and atopic dermatitis.
- Pruritus is the most common clinical complaint associated with allergic skin diseases.

- Skin biopsy and histopathology can be used to confirm the presence of inflammatory skin disease; other methods include intradermal testing and serum-based in vitro allergy tests.
- Up to 50% of patients with allergic skin disease will improve with increased n-3 fatty acid intake if other contributing diseases are controlled.
- Feeding goal: provide nutritional support for resolution of allergic dermatitis so that corticosteroid and other therapies can be reduced or discontinued.

KEY NUTRITIONAL FACTORS

- Foods should provide recommended allowances of all required nutrients (nutritional adequacy), but should also contain specific levels of KNFs (certain nutrients that can affect allergic skin disease).
- Although not listed as KNFs for patients with allergic skin disease, foods fed long term should also take into account KNFs that can influence other important potential health issues (Chapters 1, 2, 7 and 8).
- Table 1 summarizes KNFs for foods and dietary supplements used for n-3 fatty acid-responsive skin diseases. Sources of ALA include flax and flax (linseed) oil; sources of EPA and DHA include fish meal and cold water marine oils.
- GLA (an n-6 fatty acid) can be incorporated into skin, where it is rapidly elongated to DGLA, which is not further metabolized to AA. Eicosanoid metabolites of DGLA are antiinflammatory. Recommendations for food amounts of GLA have not been determined; thus, GLA is currently not a KNF. Evening primrose, borage and black currant oils are used in foods to increase dietary GLA intake.

FEEDING PLAN

Assess and Select the Food and/or Supplement
Ensure the Food's Basic Nutritional Adequacy. AAFCO nutritional adequacy statements are usually found on a product's label. AAFCO approval does not ensure a food will be effective for dietary management of allergic skin disease.

Table 1. Key nutritional factors for foods and supplements for dogs and cats with inflammatory dermatoses.

Factors	Nutritional recommendations
Omega-3 fatty acids (ALA, EPA and/or DHA)	Supplements or foods should initially provide 50 to 300 mg total omega-3 fatty acids/kg body weight/day Foods should contain between 0.35 to 1.8% dry matter

Key: ALA = α-linolenic acid, EPA = eicosapentaenoic acid, DHA = docosahexaenoic acid.

Compare the Food's and/or Supplement's KNF Content with the Recommended Levels. Tables 2 and 3 compare n-6 and n-3 fatty acid intakes of a 10-kg dog and a 4.5-kg cat (respectively) eating equivalent amounts (calorie basis) of each food or the manufacturers' prescribed doses of fatty acid supplements. The recommended dose range for n-3 fatty acid intake for allergic skin disease is 50-300 mg/kg body weight. Compare the total amounts of n-3 fatty acids recommended for a 10-kg dog (500-3,000 mg) or a 4.5-kg cat (225-1,350 mg) to the food/supplement amounts in the tables to determine those providing the best levels.

N-6/N-3 Fatty Acid Ratios. Besides total amounts of dietary n-3 fatty acids, the ratio of dietary n-6 fatty acids to n-3 fatty acids in foods may also influence a food's potential antiinflammatory effect. Though less important than total n-3 fatty acid intake, lower ratios are generally desirable. To obtain ratio estimates for foods in Tables 2 and 3, divide the amount of n-6 fatty acids consumed by the amount of n-3 fatty acids consumed for a given food. Example: total n-6 amount consumed = 4,884 mg and total n-3 amount consumed = 1,548 mg; 4,884/1,548 = 3.1.

Foods or Supplements? Fatty acid supplements at prescribed doses often provide lower levels of fatty acids than the current food (Tables 2 and 3). It may be more convenient to change to a food with higher levels of n-3 fatty acids rather than adding a supplement to the current food.

N-3 and N-6 Fatty Acid Content Information. Specific fatty acid content of commercial pet foods is sometimes difficult to obtain. Such information is not required to be listed on pet food labels nor published by manufacturers. If necessary, contact manufacturers to obtain specific information about the fatty acid content of their products (contact information can be found on product labels). Most supplements marketed to improve skin and coat list fatty acid concentrations on product labels or in published information.

Manage Treats and Snacks. If treats/snacks are fed, commercial treats that match the nutritional profile of the new food (see product labels) are preferred. Otherwise, treats/snacks should not be fed excessively (<10% of the total diet on a volume, weight or calorie basis). See Appendix B for more treats/snacks information.

Assess and Determine the Feeding Method
Determine How Much Food to Feed. If a new food is fed, the amount to feed can be determined from the product label (or other supporting material) or calculated (Appendix C). Food dosage may need to be changed if body weight or the BCS changes. The initial food dosage estimate should be adjusted accordingly if body weight and the BCS are not ideal. Chapter 14 provides advice about determining the amount to feed overweight patients.

Supplements. Prescribed doses should be provided on product labels or other supporting material. The recommended daily dose range for dogs and cats is 50-300 mg/kg body weight.

Consider How to Offer the Food. If body weight and the BCS are normal, there is no need to change how food is offered. Both free-choice and food-restricted feeding methods have advantages and disadvantages (Appendix D). Free-choice feeding is most popular but is most likely to result in overeating. Food-restricted feeding is preferred because it is less likely to result in overweight/obesity.

Table 2. The total essential fatty acid intake for a 10-kg adult dog eating 600 kcal (2,510 kJ) per day of selected commercial foods or being given one of the selected supplements.*

Dry foods	Food consumed (g)	Total omega-6 consumed (mg)	Total omega-3 consumed (mg)**
Hill's Prescription Diet b/d Canine	165	4,884	1,548
Hill's Prescription Diet d/d Potato & Duck Formula Canine	161	4,854	1,164
Hill's Prescription Diet d/d Potato & Salmon Formula Canine	162	4,206	2,100
Hill's Prescription Diet d/d Potato & Venison Formula Canine	161	4,932	1,146
Hill's Prescription Diet d/d Rice & Egg Formula Canine	154	4,692	990
Hill's Prescription Diet j/d Canine	176	4,032	5,688
Hill's Prescription Diet z/d Canine Low Allergen	163	4,812	618
Hill's Prescription Diet z/d ULTRA Allergen Free Canine	161	6,222	804
Hill's Science Diet Canine Active Adult	130	5,976	678
Hill's Science Diet Canine Adult Original	162	5,310	726
Hill's Science Diet Canine Lamb Meal & Rice Recipe Adult	162	4,815	1,002
Hill's Science Diet Canine Light Adult	200	5,988	618
Hill's Science Diet Canine Senior 7+ Original	163	4,590	1,710
Hill's Science Diet Sensitive Skin Dog	158	7,392	2,166
Iams Eukanuba Adult Maintenance Formula	139	4,800	600
Iams Eukanuba Reduced Fat Adult Formula	155	3,600	600
Iams Eukanuba Senior Maintenance Formula	142	3,600	600
Iams Veterinary Formulas Joint/Articulation	142	4,200	600
Iams Veterinary Formulas Response FP	147	1,600	400
Nutro Ultra Adult	166	7,998	1,290
Nutro Ultra Senior	168	7,392	1,380
Purina Veterinary Diets DRM Dermatologic Management Canine Formula	151	1,680	1,680
Royal Canin IVD Limited Ingredient Diets Potato & Duck Canine Formula	175	2,940	1,020
Royal Canin IVD Limited Ingredient Diets Potato & Rabbit Canine Formula	177	3,120	1,380
Royal Canin Veterinary Diet Hypoallergenic HP19	143	7,158	1,158
Royal Canin Veterinary Diet Sensitivity RC21	168	3,354	1,512
Royal Canin Veterinary Diet Skin Support SS21	153	4,884	1,758
Moist foods	**Food consumed (g)**	**Total omega-6 consumed (mg)**	**Total omega-3 consumed (mg)****
Hill's Prescription Diet a/d Canine/Feline	521	6,882	3,126
Hill's Prescription Diet d/d Duck Formula Canine	624	4,932	1,248
Hill's Prescription Diet d/d Lamb Formula Canine	451	3,972	1,488
Hill's Prescription Diet d/d Salmon Formula Canine	613	5,148	4,350
Hill's Prescription Diet d/d Venison Formula Canine	550	4,950	1,098
Hill's Prescription Diet j/d Canine	446	4,104	6,066
Hill's Prescription Diet n/d Canine	380	2,772	8,088
Hill's Prescription Diet z/d ULTRA Allergen Free Canine	617	6,102	738
Iams Veterinary Formulas Response FP	475	9,600	1,200
Royal Canin IVD Limited Ingredient Diets Duck Canine Formula	536	5,340	720
Royal Canin IVD Limited Ingredient Diets Whitefish Canine Formula	522	6,600	3,300
Supplements			
3V Caps for Large & Giant Breeds	1 capsule	0	417
3V Caps for Medium & Large Breeds	1 capsule	0	300
3V Caps for Small & Medium Breeds	1 capsule	0	171
3V Caps Liquid	0.75 ml	0	187
3V Caps Liquid HR	1 ml	0	450
DermCaps 100 lb	1 capsule	402	252
DermCaps ES	1 capsule	368	123
DermCaps ES Liquid	1 ml	375	130
DermCaps Liquid	1 ml	621	65
DermCaps Regular	1 capsule	402	108
Nutrived O.F.A. Granules	1 scoop	539	129
EicosaDerm	1 pump	0	600
Welactin	1 pump	0	330-364
Omegaderm – Small Dogs & Cats	1 packet (4 ml)	1,488	300
Nordic Naturals Omega-3	1 capsule	0	350
Nordic Naturals Arctic Cod Liver Oil	1 capsule	0	280
Nordic Naturals Ultimate Omega	1 capsule	0	700

*Adapted from Roudebush P. Consumption of essential fatty acids in selected commercial dog foods compared to dietary supplementation: An update. In: Proceedings. Annual Members Meeting AAVD & ACVD, Norfolk, VA, 2001: 53-54.
**Laboratory and clinical studies in a number of species have established a daily dosage for total omega-3 fatty acids that seems to be a reasonable starting point in patients with inflammatory disease. An initial dose of 50 to 300 mg of total omega-3 fatty acids/kg body weight/day seems to be effective in a large number of studies.

Manage Food Changes. Most healthy dogs adapt well to new foods but a transition period to avoid GI upsets is good practice. Example: to change to a new food, replace 25% of the old food with the new food on Day 1 and continue this incremental change daily until the change is complete on Day 4. Appendix E provides additional information.

Food and Water Receptacle Husbandry. Food and water bowls should be washed regularly with warm soapy water and rinsed

Table 3. The total essential fatty acid intake for a 4.5-kg cat eating 260 kcal (1,088 kJ) per day of selected commercial foods or being given one of the selected supplements.

Dry foods	Food consumed (g)	Total omega-6 consumed (mg)	Total omega-3 consumed (mg)*
Hill's Prescription Diet d/d Duck & Green Pea Formula Feline	68	2,254	473
Hill's Prescription Diet d/d Rabbit & Green Pea Formula Feline	69	2,304	460
Hill's Prescription Diet d/d Venison & Green Pea Formula Feline	67	2,142	458
Hill's Prescription Diet z/d Low Allergen Feline	69	3,630	419
Hill's Science Diet Adult Original Cat Food	64	2,301	140
Hill's Science Diet Mature Adult 7+ Original Cat Food	66	2,114	146
Hill's Science Diet Sensitive Skin Adult Cat Food	67	3,123	294
Iams Eukanuba Chicken & Rice Formula Cat Food	55	2,158	302
Iams Eukanuba Mature Care Formula for Cats	61	2,049	411
Royal Canin Adult Fit 32 Cat Food	68	2,462	322
Royal Canin Indoor 27 Cat Food	70	2,395	408
Royal Canin IVD Limited Ingredient Diets Green Pea & Venison Feline Formula	73	1,794	624
Royal Canin Persian 30 Cat Food	60	2,889	481
Royal Canin Skin Care 30 Cat Food	63	2,951	499
Royal Canin Veterinary Diet Feline Hypoallergenic HP 23	63	3,003	486
Royal Canin Veterinary Diet Feline Sensitivity RD 30	67	2,140	213
Moist foods	Food consumed (g)	Total omega-6 consumed (mg)	Total omega-3 consumed (mg)*
Hill's Prescription Diet a/d Canine/Feline	226	3,344	1,422
Hill's Prescription Diet d/d Duck Formula Feline	215	3,354	666
Hill's Prescription Diet d/d Rabbit Formula Feline	233	3,403	699
Hill's Prescription Diet d/d Venison Formula Feline	206	4,178	988
Hill's Prescription Diet z/d ULTRA Allergen Free Feline	241	2,574	289
Hill's Science Diet Savory Salmon Entrée Adult Cat Food	250	2,072	1,147
Iams Veterinary Formulas Response LB/Feline	199	2,600	520
Supplements			
3V Caps for Small & Medium Breeds	1 capsule	0	171
3V Caps Liquid HR	1 ml	0	450
DermCaps ES Liquid	1 ml	375	130
DermCaps Liquid	1 ml	621	65
DermCaps Regular	1 capsule	402	108
Nutrived O.F.A. Granules	1 scoop	539	129
EicosaDerm	1/2 pump	0	300
Welactin	1 pump	0	330-364
Nordic Naturals Omega-3	1 capsule	0	350

*Laboratory and clinical studies in a number of species have established a daily dosage for total omega-3 fatty acids that seems to be a reasonable starting point in patients with inflammatory disease. An initial dose of 50 to 300 mg of total omega-3 fatty acids/kg body weight/day seems to be effective in a large number of studies.

well. Dishes used for moist foods need daily cleaning. Discard moist or moistened dry foods after 2-4 hours of room temperature exposure to avoid foodborne illnesses (Appendix F).

FOLLOWUP

Owner Followup
If a new food is fed, owners should record body weight (if possible) and/or grade body condition (BCS) monthly. If a trend of increasing or decreasing body weight or BCS is noticed, change the amount fed by 10% increments and recheck the patient every 2 weeks for 1 month. When necessary, change amount fed again and repeat the cycle to achieve desired body weight/BCS. *Compliance.* Deny access to other pets' food.

Veterinary Health Care Team Followup
Allergic dermatitis patients receiving appropriate n-3 fatty acid intake usually respond within several weeks to several months. After a dietary change or initiation of supplements, reassess every 4 weeks for improvement of pruritus or skin erythema. In some cases a response may not be noted for several months or

the patient may need concurrent therapy with antihistamines, topical agents (medicated shampoo) or corticosteroids. *Side Effects of High Levels of N-3 Fatty Acids.* Soft feces, overt diarrhea, flatulence and oral malodor ("fishy breath") are most commonly noted at levels of fatty acid supplementation used in most patients. However, these side effects are unlikely to occur if there was appropriate transition to a new food or supplements.

MISCELLANEOUS

See Chapters 31 and 32, Small Animal Clinical Nutrition, 5th edition, for more information.

Authors
Condensed from Chapter 32, Small Animal Clinical Nutrition, 5th edition, authored by Philip Roudebush and William D. Schoenherr.

References
See Chapter 32, Small Animal Clinical Nutrition, 5th edition, on the website www.markmorrisinstitute.org for references.

CLINICAL POINTS

- Canine DOD includes a complex and diverse group of musculoskeletal disorders that occur most commonly in fast-growing, large-/giant-breed puppies whose anticipated adult weight >25 kg.
- The most common canine DODs include CHD, osteochondrosis and elbow dysplasia.
- 22% of dogs <1 year of age are affected with musculoskeletal disease; 20% of these are attributed to improper nutrition.
- The skeletal system is most susceptible to nutritional, metabolic and physical insults during growth because of heightened metabolic activity; increased susceptibility of large-/giant-breed puppies may be due in part to their genetic propensity for rapid growth.
- Dysregulation of nutrient supply, bone formation and endocrine regulation may interfere with skeletal maturation, thus increasing the risk for DOD.
- Endocrine dysregulation, whether attributable to nutrition, feeding management or genetics may be responsible for an environment that fosters development of DOD (**Figure 1**).
- High energy intake affects growth velocity directly via nutrient supply and indirectly through changes in GH, IGF-1, T_3, T_4 and insulin (**Figure 1**).
- Excess intake of calcium, calcium and phosphorus or vitamin D is associated with severe disturbances in endochondral ossification, attributable to calcium competing with other minerals and/or by endocrine effects (PTH or calcitonin) or acid-base imbalance (**Figure 1**).
- Increased static forces (weight load) and dynamic forces (muscle pull) may damage immature skeletons, especially in large- and giant-breed puppies (**Figure 1**); counsel owners to be sensible about exercise.
- Growth velocity may be measured in body height/length and weight and is a nutritionally controllable risk factor.
- Fully evaluate all foods, supplements and feeding methods used to ensure that nutritional assessment is comprehensive.
- Differential diagnosis: consider other confounding disease processes that may result in skeletal abnormalities (**Table 1**). Evaluation of serum PTH, ionized calcium and vitamin D may be appropriate in some cases.
- Feeding goals: by means of an appropriate feeding plan, support controlled, healthy growth (reduce/eliminate DOD) while achieving full genetic potential for mature size at adulthood.
- Manage client expectations: proper nutritional management will prevent many, but not all, cases of DOD. Genetic predisposition may still be expressed despite an appropriate and well-executed feeding plan.

Abbreviations

AAFCO = Association of American Feed Control Officials
BCS = body condition score (Appendix A)
CHD = canine hip dysplasia
DHA = docosahexaenioc acid
DM = dry matter
DOD = developmental orthopedic disease
GH = growth hormone
IGF-1 = insulin like growth factor-1
KNF = key nutritional factor
PTH = parathyroid hormone

KEY NUTRITIONAL FACTORS

- Foods should provide recommended allowances of all required nutrients (nutritional adequacy), but should also contain specific levels of KNFs (certain nutrients that support healthy growth in large-/giant-breed puppies).
- KNFs for foods for prevention of DOD affect skeletal growth

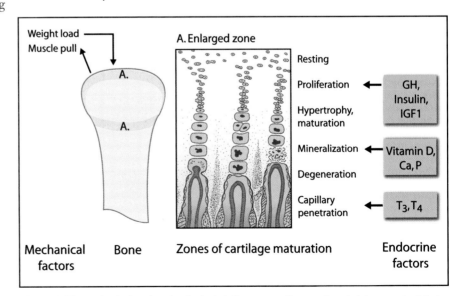

Figure 1. Biomechanical and endocrinologic influences on the growing skeleton are depicted. Biomechanically, excessive static (weight load) and dynamic (muscle pull) forces can damage immature skeletons. Note the various zones of cartilage maturation (resting zone, proliferation, hypertrophy and maturation, mineralization, degeneration and capillary penetration) where hormonal influences are thought to occur.

Table 1. Parathyroid hormone (PTH), ionized calcium and 1,25-dihydroxyvitamin D₃ concentrations in different physiologic/disease states.*

States	PTH	Ionized calcium	1,25-dihydroxyvitamin D₃
Apocrine gland tumors of the anal sacs	Low	High	Low
Chronic renal failure	High	Low/normal	Normal/low
High calcium intake	Low	High	Normal/low
Hypervitaminosis D	Low	High	Normal/high
Hypoparathyroidism	Low	Low	Low
Lymphosarcoma	Low	High	Low
Primary hyperparathyroidism	High	High	Normal/high

*Adapted from Feldman EC, Nelson RW, eds. Canine and Feline Endocrinology and Reproduction, 2nd ed. Philadelphia, PA: WB Saunders Co, 1996; 455-493. Hazewinkel HAW. In: Bojrab MJ, ed. Disease Mechanisms in Small Animal Surgery, 2nd ed. Philadelphia, PA: Lea & Febiger, 1993; 1119-1128. Chastain CB, Ganjam VK, eds. Clinical Endocrinology of Companion Animals. Philadelphia, PA: Lea & Febiger, 1986; 192-217.

Table 2. Key nutritional factors for foods for growth (postweaning) of large- and giant-breed puppies.*

Factors	Dietary recommendations
Energy density	Energy density = 3.2 to 4.1 kcal/g; recommend the lower end of range if clients use free-choice feeding**
Fat	8.5 to 17%
Docosahexaneoic acid***	≥0.02%
Calcium	0.8 to 1.2% calcium
Phosphorus	Phosphorus amount is based on calcium amount to maintain recommended Ca-P ratio (below)
Ca-P ratio	1.1:1 to 2:1 (the lower end of range is preferred)
Supplements	None recommended if a commercial food is fed

Key: Ca = calcium, P = phosphorus.
*Dry matter basis.
**To convert kcal to kJ, multiply kcal by 4.184. Free-choice feeding is not recommended. Energy intake can be better controlled through food-limited feeding.
***For improved learning.

by avoiding overnutrition (i.e., excess energy density/fat, calcium and vitamin D).
- DHA is included as a KNF for normal neural, retinal and auditory development; supports trainability and optimizes special senses.
- **Table 2** lists KNFs for foods for puppies at risk for DOD. Recommended amounts are listed here and discussed in more detail in Chapter 33, Small Animal Clinical Nutrition, 5th edition.

FEEDING PLAN

Assess and Select the Food
Ensure the Food's Basic Nutritional Adequacy. AAFCO nutritional adequacy statements appropriate for growth are usually found on a product's label. AAFCO approval for growth does not ensure a food will be effective for nutritional management of DOD.
Compare the Food's KNF Content with the Recommended Levels. Several commercial growth foods are marketed for management of DOD (**Table 3**). However, other foods may provide

certain KNFs at or near recommended levels. Choose a food that most closely fits recommended levels.
Other Considerations. Other nutrients that may contribute to musculoskeletal disease or growth problems include protein, copper, manganese, zinc, iodine and vitamins A and C; they are more likely to be an issue with improperly formulated home-made foods or if nonprescribed supplements are used. In addition to nutrient imbalances, low digestibility can be a problem in low-quality commercial foods.

Assess and Determine the Feeding Method
In addition to selecting foods with recommended KNF profiles, proper feeding methods are critical to DOD treatment/prevention.
Determine How Much Food to Feed. Appropriate intake levels of KNFs are determined not only by amounts in food, but also by how much food is consumed. If a new food is fed, the amount to feed can be obtained from product labels (or other supporting material) or calculated. To calculate initial amounts use formulas based on age and body weight (Appendix C). If body weight and BCS are not ideal, adjust food dosage estimates appropriately (see Followup below).
Consider How to Offer the Food. How the food is offered can also affect how much is consumed. For controlled feeding, use only meal-restricted feeding of a predetermined food dose (above). Divide the daily amount into 2-4 meals/day. Excess food intake is a risk with free-choice or time-restricted methods of offering foods. If either of these methods must be used, feed foods with lower fat and energy density (<12% DM fat; <3.8 kcal/g [15.9 kJ/g] DM).
Manage Food Changes. A transition period to avoid GI upsets and facilitate acceptance of a new food is good practice. Example: to change to a new food, replace 25% of the old food with the new food on Day 1 and continue this incremental change daily until the change is complete on Day 4. If problems occur, delay the increase or cut back to the previous level of transition for several more days before continuing the food change. Appendix E provides additional information.
Manage Treats and Snacks. If treats/snacks are fed, commercial treats that match the nutritional profile recommended for DOD are best. Treats/snacks should not be fed excessively (<10% of the total diet on a volume, weight or calorie basis). See Appendix B for more treats/snacks information.
SUPPLEMENTS. Vitamin and/or mineral supplements are

Table 3. Recommended levels of key nutritional factors for dogs at risk for developmental orthopedic disease compared to levels in selected dry commercial foods marketed for large- and giant-breed puppies.* (Numbers in red match optimal KNFs.)

Recommended levels	Energy density (kcal/cup)** -	Energy density (kcal/g) DM 3.2-4.1	Fat (%) 8.5-17	DHA (%) ≥0.02	Ca (%) 0.8-1.2	Ca-P ratio 1.1:1–2:1***
Hill's Science Diet Puppy Lamb Meal & Rice Recipe Large Breed	357	3.9	18.0	0.220	1.17	1.1:1
Hill's Science Diet Puppy Large Breed	357	3.9	16.8	0.223	1.20	1.4:1
Iams Eukanuba Large Breed Puppy Formula	362	4.4	17.2	na	0.88	1.2:1
Iams Smart Puppy Large Breed	368	4.5	16.1	na	1.0	1.3:1
Nutro Natural Choice Large Breed Puppy	346	3.9	15.4	0.011	1.32	1.1:1
Purina ONE Large Breed Puppy Formula	404	4.1	16.7	na	1.44	1.1:1
Purina Pro Plan Large Breed Puppy Formula	377	4.0	16.4	na	1.37	1.1:1
Royal Canin Maxi Large Breed Puppy 32	365	4.3	15.6	na	1.12	1.2:1

Key: DM = dry matter, DHA = docosahexaenoic acid, na = not available from manufacturer.
*Nutrients are expressed on dry matter basis except for energy density, which is expressed on an as fed basis.
**Energy density values are as fed and are useful for determining the amount to feed; cup = 8-oz. measuring cup. To convert to kJ, multiply kcal by 4.184.
***The lower end of the range is preferred.

contraindicated when feeding balanced foods, particularly supplements that contain calcium, phosphorus and vitamins A and D.

Food and Water Receptacle Husbandry. Food and water bowls should be washed regularly with warm soapy water and rinsed well. Dishes used for moist foods need daily cleaning. Discard moist or moistened dry foods after 2-4 hours of room temperature exposure to avoid foodborne illnesses (Appendix F).

FOLLOWUP

Owner Followup
Have owners record daily food intake and BCS (and body weight if practical) every 2 weeks.

Veterinary Health Care Team Followup
Regular monitoring is the basis for adjusting the amount to feed for controlled growth. The BCS recommended range for healthy growth is 2/5 to 3/5 (keep puppies lean). **Figure 2** summarizes the entire management plan process and includes details about reassessment and changing the amount to feed through the critical growth phase (before physeal closure), which is approximately 11-12 months of age. After the critical period, feed as adults (Chapter 1), continue with regular reassessment and adjust the amount fed, as necessary.

Use of Owner Data. If owners record daily food intake and BCS/body weight every 2 weeks, correlate their data with a BCS done by a member of the veterinary health care team. If owner data correlate, some rechecks/food adjustments can be done by phone, alternated with in-clinic exams. If skeletal disease occurs despite compliance with a good feeding plan, slow the growth rate by reducing the amount fed by as much as 25%.

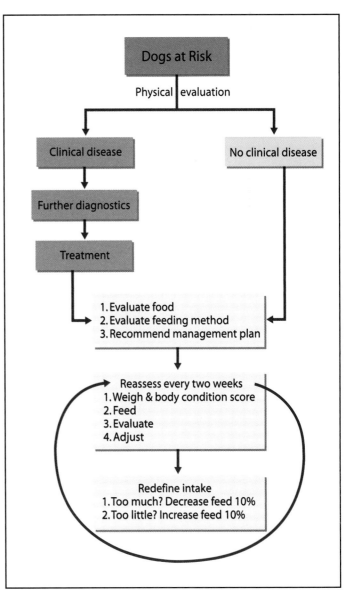

Figure 2. Flowchart for assessing dogs at risk for developmental orthopedic disease.

MISCELLANEOUS

Exercise is healthy for a developing musculoskeletal system but forced/excessive exercise during the critical growth phase may aggravate clinical signs of DOD.

See Chapters 13, 17 and 33, Small Animal Clinical Nutrition, 5th edition, for more information.

Authors
Condensed from Chapter 33, Small Animal Clinical Nutrition, 5th edition, authored by Daniel C. Richardson, Jürgen Zentek, Herman A. W. Hazewinkel, Richard C. Nap, Philip W. Toll and Steven C. Zicker.

References
See Chapter 33, Small Animal Clinical Nutrition, 5th edition, on the website www.markmorrisinstitute.org for references.

Chapter
23
Nutritional Management of Osteoarthritis

CLINICAL POINTS

- OA is a chronic, progressive disease characterized by degeneration of moveable joints and clinical signs of pain and dysfunction.
- OA affects up to 20% of dogs and cats over one year of age in the U.S. and prevalence increases with age; example: in one study, 90% of cats >10 years had radiographic evidence consistent with OA.
- Risk factors include age, breed (large- or giant-breed dogs; Siamese, Persian and Himalayan cats), DOD, trauma and obesity.
- Hip dysplasia and anterior cruciate ligament rupture are common causes of OA in dogs; hip dysplasia and patellar luxation are common causes of OA in cats.
- Diagnosis of OA generally requires a combination of history, known risk factors, physical exam findings and radiographic evidence.
- Table 1 summarizes common clinical signs in dogs and cats.
- OA is associated with degeneration of articular cartilage, loss

Abbreviations
AA = arachidonic acid
AAFCO = Association of American Feed Control Officials
BCS = body condition score (Appendix A)
DER = daily energy requirement (Appendix C)
DHA = docosahexaenoic acid
DOD = developmental orthopedic disease
EPA = eicosapentaenoic acid
KNF = key nutritional factor
NSAID = nonsteroidal antiinflammatory drug
OA = osteoarthritis

of proteoglycan and collagen, proliferation of new bone and inflammation.
- Inflammation in response to injury, if excessive and/or prolonged, can be cyclical and detrimental.
- Intake of n-3 fatty acids above specific levels reduces synthesis of proinflammatory eicosanoids by interfering with metabolism of AA in various pathways. EPA and DHA are precursors of endogenous mediators (resolvins, protectins) that switch on the resolution phase of an inflammatory response, acting as braking signals to inflammation, thereby reducing inflammatory injury to tissues.
- In canine cartilage, EPA inhibits up-regulation of degradative enzymes by blocking the signal at the level of messenger RNA.
- Free radicals are implicated in cartilage aging and the pathogenesis of OA via their damaging effect on cartilage matrix; fortification with dietary antioxidants may have preventive and/or therapeutic value in management of OA.
- OA is usually irreversible but good dietary management can minimize pain and slow progression as exemplified by these possible interventions: 1) mitigating risk factors (e.g., weight loss), 2) controlling clinical signs (e.g., n-3 fatty acids) and 3) slowing progression of the disease (e.g., n-3 fatty acids, antioxidants).

Table 1. Common clinical signs of osteoarthritis (OA).*

Stage	Dogs	Cats
Mild OA	Stiffness, decreased activity, limping	Decreased activity
Moderate OA	Pain, muscle atrophy, difficulty rising	Reluctance to jump, climb stairs, groom
Severe OA	Loss of range of motion, vocalization, crepitus, lethargy, inappetence	Limping, muscle atrophy, inappropriate elimination

*Adapted from Beale B. Orthopedic problems in geriatric dogs and cats. Veterinary Clinics of North America: Small Animal Practice 2005; 35: 655-674.

- Feeding goals: supply specific nutrients that may help reduce inflammation and pain, slow degradative processes, complement prescribed medications and improve clinical signs.

KEY NUTRITIONAL FACTORS

- Foods should provide recommended allowances of all required nutrients (nutritional adequacy), but should also contain specific levels of KNFs (certain nutrients and nonnutritional food ingredients that can affect OA and support long-term health).
- KNFs for foods for OA management help reduce inflammation/pain, slow cartilage degradation, enhance cartilage repair and complement concurrent medications.
- Foods for OA are typically fed long term, replacing maintenance-type foods. Sodium and phosphorus (dog and cat foods) and magnesium and urinary pH (cat foods) are included as KNFs because they can influence important age-related health issues (Chapters 2 and 8).
- Table 2 summarizes KNFs for foods for OA. A detailed description of these recommendations can be found in Chapter 34, Small Animal Clinical Nutrition, 5th edition.

FEEDING PLAN

Assess and Select the Food

Ensure the Food's Basic Nutritional Adequacy. AAFCO nutritional adequacy statements are usually found on a product's label. AAFCO approval does not ensure a food will be effective for dietary management of OA.

Compare the Food's KNF Content with the Recommended Levels. Foods should provide recommended allowances of all required nutrients (nutritional adequacy), but should also contain specific levels of KNFs that can influence OA and long-term health.

Tables 3 and 4 compare KNF recommendations to the KNF content of selected commercial veterinary therapeutic foods intended for dogs and cats (respectively) with OA. Select a food that is most similar to the KNF recommendations. Contact manufacturers for foods not in the tables (contact information is listed on product labels).

Overweight/Obese Patients. Weight reduction alone can result in marked clinical improvement. If a patient's BCS >4/5, consider initiating a weight-loss program, including information about safe weight-loss foods (Chapter 14) before changing to OA foods.

Manage Treats and Snacks. KNFs for OA are usually not included in treats; limit to <10% of the total diet on a volume,

Table 2. Key nutritional factors for foods for canine and feline osteoarthritis patients.*

Factors	Dietary recommendations Dog foods	Cat foods
Total omega-3 fatty acids	3.5-4.0%	1.0-3.0%
Eicosapentaenoic acid	0.4-1.1%	-
Docosahexaenoic acid	-	0.25-0.75%
Omega-6:omega-3 fatty acid ratio	<1:1	2-4:1
L-carnitine	≥300 mg/kg	≥300 mg/kg
Glucosamine HCl	≤0.10%	na
Chondroitin sulfate	≤0.08%	na
Antioxidants		
Vitamin E	≥400 IU/kg	≥400 IU/kg
Vitamin C	≥100 mg/kg	≥100 mg/kg
Selenium	0.5-1.3 mg/kg	0.5-1.3 mg/kg
Phosphorus**	0.3-0.7%	0.5-0.7%
Sodium**	0.2-0.4%	0.2-0.4%
Magnesium***	na	0.05-0.1%
Urinary pH	na	6.4-6.6

Key: na = not applicable.
*All values are expressed on a dry matter basis unless otherwise stated.
**Patients with osteoarthritis are often in age groups at risk for kidney and/or heart disease.
***Middle-aged and older cats for prevention of lower urinary tract disease.

weight or calorie basis (e.g., switch to smaller treats or breakup larger treats). A good option is to offer small amounts of the opposite form (moist or dry) of the selected OA food.

Assess and Determine the Feeding Method

Figure 1 is an overview of the following feeding methods. *Determine How Much Food to Feed.* If a patient's body weight/BCS are normal, the amount to feed can be estimated from the product label (or other supporting material) or calculated (Appendix C). These food dosages are estimates and may need to be changed if body weight or BCS change subsequently (see Followup below).

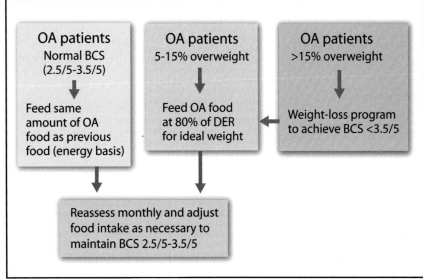

Figure 1. Overview of feeding regimen recommendations for osteoarthritis (OA) patients based on body weight/body condition scores (BCS). See Appendix A for methods for determining BCS. DER = daily energy requirement (Appendix C).

Table 3. Key nutritional factor content of selected veterinary therapeutic foods marketed for osteoarthritis in dogs compared to recommended levels.* (Numbers in red match optimal KNFs.)

Dry foods	Energy density (kcal/cup)**	Energy density (kcal ME/g)	Total omega-3 FAs (%)	EPA (%)	Omega-6:omega-3 ratio	Carn (mg/kg)	Gluc (%)	Chon (%)	Vit E (IU/kg)	Vit C (mg/kg)	Se (mg/kg)	P (%)	Na (%)
Recommended levels	-	-	3.5-4.0	0.4-1.1	<1:1	≥300	≤0.1	≤0.08	≥400	≥100	0.5-1.3	0.3-0.7	0.2-0.4
Hill's Prescription Diet j/d Canine	356	3.9	3.8	0.5	0.7:1	351	0.1	0.07	585	225	0.43	0.54	0.2
Iams Veterinary Formulas Joint	294	3.75	na	na	na	na	0.5	na	na	na	na	1.04	0.47
Medi-Cal Mobility Support	271	na	na	na	na	na	na	na	na	na	na	0.60	0.30
Purina Veterinary Diets JM Joint Mobility	351	4.2	1.07	na	1.8:1	na	0.14	na	1,073	133	na	1.07	0.39
Royal Canin Veterinary Diet Mobility Support JS 21	322	4.2	na	na	na	na	0.1	na	725	na	0.44	0.60	0.29
Royal Canin Veterinary Diet Mobility Support JS 21 Large Breed	332	4.3	na	na	na	na	0.22	na	725	na	0.43	0.60	0.40

Moist food	Energy density (kcal/can)**	Energy density (kcal ME/g)	Total omega-3 FAs (%)	EPA (%)	Omega-6:omega-3 ratio	Carn (mg/kg)	Gluc (%)	Chon (%)	Vit E (IU/kg)	Vit C (mg/kg)	Se (mg/kg)	P (%)	Na (%)
Recommended levels	-	-	3.5-4.0	0.4-1.1	<1:1	≥300	≤0.1	≤0.08	≥400	≥100	0.5-1.3	0.3-0.7	0.2-0.4
Hill's Prescription Diet j/d Canine	498/13 oz.	4.2	4.24	0.85	0.7:1	316.8	0.07	0.04	698	128	0.81	0.56	0.19

Key: ME = metabolizable energy, FAs = fatty acids, EPA = eicosapentaenoic acid, Gluc = glucosamine hydrochloride, Chon = chondroitin sulfate, Se = selenium, Carn = L-carnitine, P = phosphorus, Na = sodium, na = not available from manufacturer.
*Dry matter basis unless otherwise indicated.
**Energy density values are listed on an as fed basis and are useful for determining the amount to feed; cup = 8-oz. measuring cup. To convert to kJ, multiply kcal by 4.184.

Table 4. Key nutritional factor content of selected veterinary therapeutic foods marketed for osteoarthritis in cats compared to recommended levels.* (Numbers in red match optimal KNFs.)

Dry foods	Energy density (kcal/cup)**	Energy density (kcal ME/g)	Total omega-3 FAs (%)	DHA (%)	Omega-6:omega-3 ratio	Carn (mg/kg)	Vit E (IU/kg)	Vit C (mg/kg)	Se (mg/kg)	P (%)	Na (%)	Mg (%)	Urine pH
Recommended levels	-	-	1.0-3.0	0.25-0.75	2-4:1	≥300	≥400	≥100	0.5-1.3	0.5-0.7	0.2-0.4	0.05-0.1	6.4-6.6
Hill's Prescription Diet j/d Feline	506	4.3	1.7	0.33	0.3:1	598.9	841	130	0.83	0.69	0.34	0.077	6.4
Medi-Cal Mobility Support	391	na	na	na	na	na	na	na	na	0.7	0.4	na	na

Moist food	Energy density (kcal/can)**	Energy density (kcal ME/g)	Total omega-3 FAs (%)	DHA (%)	Omega-6:omega-3 ratio	Carn (mg/kg)	Vit E (IU/kg)	Vit C (mg/kg)	Se (mg/kg)	P (%)	Na (%)	Mg (%)	Urine pH
Recommended levels	-	-	1.0-3.0	0.25-0.75	2-4:1	≥300	≥400	≥100	0.5-1.3	0.5-0.7	0.2-0.4	0.05-0.1	6.4-6.6
Hill's Prescription Diet j/d Feline	152/5.5 oz.	4.0	1.20	0.26	0.9:1	719	727	632	0.87	0.79	0.41	0.083	6.3

Key: ME = metabolizable energy, FAs = fatty acids, DHA = docosahexaenoic acid, Carn = L-carnitine, Se = selenium, P = phosphorus, Na = sodium, Mg = magnesium, na = not available from manufacturer.
*Dry matter basis unless otherwise indicated.
**Energy density values are listed on an as fed basis and are useful for determining the amount to feed; cup = 8-oz. measuring cup. To convert to kJ, multiply kcal by 4.184.

Overweight/Obese Patients. If clinical signs are mild and body weight/BCS aren't overly excessive (<15% overweight; BCS 3.5/5 to 4/5), feed the OA food at approximately 80% of DER for ideal weight (Appendix C) until target weight/BCS (<3.5/5) are obtained. If reductions greater than 15% of body weight are indicated, consider a weight-loss program (Chapter 14).

Consider How to Offer the Food. Both free-choice and restricted-feeding methods have advantages and disadvantages (Appendix D). Free-choice feeding is most popular but is more likely to result in overeating. Food-restricted feeding is preferred because it is less likely to result in overweight/obesity.

Manage Food Changes. Most patients adapt well to new foods but a transition period to avoid GI upsets and facilitate acceptance of a new food is good practice. Example: replace 25% of the old food with the new food on Day 1 and continue this incremental change daily until the change is complete on Day 4. Appendix E provides additional information.

Food and Water Receptacle Husbandry. Food and water bowls should be washed regularly with warm soapy water and rinsed well. Dishes used for moist foods need daily cleaning. Discard moist or moistened dry foods after 2-4 hours of room temperature exposure to avoid foodborne illnesses (Appendix F).

FOLLOWUP

Owner Followup
If a new food is fed, the owners should record the patient' body weight (if possible) and/or grade its BCS monthly. If a trend of increasing or decreasing body weight or BCS is noticed, change the amount fed by 10% increments and recheck the patient every 2 weeks for 1-3 months. At that point, if necessary, repeat the cycle until desired body weight/BCS recommendations are achieved.

Compliance. If the pet lives in a multi-pet household, deny access to other pets' foods.

Veterinary Health Care Team Followup
Phone calls within 3 days of initiating a new food and again at 3 weeks improve client and patient acceptance of new foods, and thus, compliance. Evaluate patients after 1 month; include an orthopedic exam, body weight and BCS. Owner quality of life assessments also help determine progress. Increased mobility may occur within 4-6 weeks of appropriate dietary/medical management. Rechecks should be performed at monthly intervals until the patient stabilizes, followed by a semiannual schedule.

Overweight/Obese Patients. If body weight/BCS recommendations have not been achieved and additional weight loss is necessary, further reduce the amount of weight-loss food being offered according to guidelines in Chapter 14. After recommended body weight/BCS are attained, discontinue the weight-loss food and transition to an OA food. Schedule rechecks as described above. Regular monitoring improves compliance and helps prevent weight regain.

ADJUNCTIVE MEDICAL & SURGICAL MANAGEMENT

Concurrent Medical Management
Dosages of concurrent analgesics or supplements should be reevaluated within the first 4-6 weeks. NSAID dose reductions of 25% or more may be possible when used in conjunction with appropriate dietary therapy.

MISCELLANEOUS

Proper rehabilitation practices may protect/promote mobility, assist weight-reduction protocols and reduce joint pain. Box 34-2, Small Animal Clinical Nutrition, 5th edition, provides more information. See Chapters 27 and 34, Small Animal Clinical Nutrition, 5th edition, for more information.

Authors
Condensed from Chapter 34, Small Animal Clinical Nutrition, 5th edition, authored by Todd L. Towell and Daniel C. Richardson.

References
See Chapter 34, Small Animal Clinical Nutrition, 5th edition, on the website www.markmorrisinstitute.org for references.

body weight (if possible) and BCS every 2 weeks to be used for adjusting food intake, if necessary. If a trend of increasing or decreasing body weight or BCS is noticed, the amount fed should be changed by 10% increments and the dog rechecked every 2 weeks for 1 month. If necessary, the amount fed should be changed again and the cycle repeated.

Veterinary Health Care Team Followup

Monitor mature adult dogs with CDS at least twice/year. The frequency of feeding plan assessment depends on treatment protocols, concurrent management of other diseases, if present, and complexity of the feeding plan. If owners are recording daily food intake and body weight/BCS every 2 weeks, correlate their BCS results with recheck physical exam results. Review lab results to further assess treatment and feeding plans. Modify as needed.

MISCELLANEOUS

A program of behavioral enrichment with or without pharmaceutic intervention is recommended because it may also be beneficial. Examples: Walk dog ≥3 times/week (alternate routes; use new routes), rotate play toys ≥ monthly, provide numerous socialization opportunities (e.g., dog parks, visit neighbors).

Authors

Condensed from Chapter 35, Small Animal Clinical Nutrition, 5th edition, authored by Lori-Ann Christie, Viorela Pop, Gary M. Landsberg, Steven C. Zicker and Elizabeth Head.

References

See Chapter 35, Small Animal Clinical Nutrition, 5th edition, on the website www.markmorrisinstitute.org for references.

Endnote

a. Prescription Diet b/d Canine. Hill's Pet Nutrition, Inc., Topeka, KS, USA.

Chapter
25 Cardiovascular Disease

CLINICAL POINTS

- Cardiovascular disease and CHF are common health problems (e.g., they represent the third leading cause of nonaccidental death in dogs).
- Clinical manifestations of CHF are due to reduced cardiac output, pulmonary congestion, systemic fluid retention or a combination of these conditions.
- Systemic fluid retention is due to retention of sodium, chloride and water. Early on, the ability to excrete excess sodium may be diminished, which worsens with progression of CHF. Full expression of sodium-chloride sensitive hypertension depends on intake of both ions and must be offset by reducing intake.
- **Table 1** outlines variability of daily sodium intake of a 15-kg dog and a 4-kg cat fed different foods (i.e., grocery, specialty and veterinary therapeutic foods) and underscores the importance of including dietary management as part of overall management of CHF.
- Foods that avoid excess salt may be helpful in conjunction with other forms of therapy for management of chronic bronchitis

Abbreviations

AAFCO = Association of American Feed Control Officials
ACE = angiotensin-converting enzyme
BCS = body condition score (Appendix A)
CHF = congestive heart failure
CKD = chronic kidney disease
DM = dry matter
KNF = key nutritional factor
RAA = renin-angiotensin-aldosterone

or asthma-like clinical signs.
- Certain myocardial diseases are related to specific nutrient deficiencies (e.g., carnitine- and taurine-associated cardiomyopathies); the association between taurine deficiency and dilated cardiomyopathy in dogs is strongest in American cocker spaniels and golden retrievers.
- Abnormal potassium or magnesium homeostasis is a potential complication of therapy with drugs for cardiac diseases and may result in dysrhythmias, reduced myocardial contractility, profound muscle weakness and potentiation of adverse effects from cardiac glycosides and other drugs.

- Cachexia: anorexia may be attributable to CHF itself (dyspnea, fatigue), concomitant disease (nausea associated with CKD), drugs that cause nausea (e.g., toxic doses of cardiac glycosides) and elevated inflammatory cytokines.
- Obesity occurs frequently in dogs and cats with cardiovascular disease; it not only produces clinical signs that mimic those of early CHF (exercise intolerance, tachypnea, weakness), but also results in cardiovascular changes that can exacerbate underlying cardiovascular disease.
- Besides obesity, risk factors for cardiovascular disease include breed, gender, CKD, drug therapy, endocrinopathies and heartworm infection.
- **Table 2** describes functional classes of CHF. Patients often follow sequential progression through the steps but may change in either direction (e.g., from Class III to II following therapy, or from Class II to Class III following a salty meal).
- Overall treatment objectives for cardiovascular disease and CHF are: prevention (prevent myocardial damage, prevent recurrence of heart failure), relief of clinical signs (eliminate edema and fluid retention, increase exercise capacity, reduce fatigue and respiratory compromise) and improvement of prognosis.
- The treatment plan for CHF often includes: diuretics and salt restriction (reduces preload and venous congestion), pimobendan (increases contractility and dilates vessels to increase contractility and decrease preload and afterload) and ACE inhibitors (arterial and venous dilators to reduce venous congestion, preload and afterload and improve long-term survival due to probable inhibition of the RAA system).
- Feeding goal(s): provide nutritional support to facilitate treatment of amenable cardiovascular diseases, slow progression of CHF and complement actions of commonly used cardiovascular drugs.

KEY NUTRITIONAL FACTORS

- Foods should provide recommended allowances of all required nutrients (nutritional adequacy), but should also contain specific levels of KNFs (certain nutrients that can assist in the management of cardiovascular diseases, CHF and possible concurrent CKD).
- **Table 3** lists KNF recommendations for foods for dogs and cats with cardiovascular disease. KNFs are intended to help manage fluid retention due to chronic CHF (sodium and chloride), hypertension (sodium and chloride), myocardial disease related to a deficiency of taurine or carnitine and cardiac drug-related disorders in potassium and magnesium homeostasis that may cause other untoward cardiovascular problems.
- Along with phosphorus, sodium and chloride restriction are also important for management of potentially concurrent CKD (Chapter 26).
- A detailed description of these KNF recommendations can be found in Chapter 36, Small Animal Clinical Nutrition, 5th edition.

Table 1. Daily sodium intake for a dog and a cat eating various foods.

Daily sodium consumption for a 15-kg dog eating 935 kcal/day

Food	Sodium intake (mg/day)
Grocery moist food[a]	2,338
Grocery dry food[b]	944
Specialty dry food[c]	552
Geriatric dry food[d]	430
Renal moist food[e]	468
Cardiac dry food[f]	159
Cardiac dry food and 1 slice bread	370
Renal moist food and 30 g cheese	700

[a]Pedigree with Chopped Beef
[b]Purina Dog Chow
[c]Hill's Science Diet Adult Original Dog Food
[d]Hill's Science Diet Mature Adult 7+ Original Dog Food
[e]Purina Veterinary Diets NF KidNey Function Canine Formula
[f]Hill's Prescription Diet h/d Canine

Daily sodium consumption for a 4-kg cat eating 270 kcal/day

Food	Sodium intake (mg/day)
Grocery moist food[g]	823
Grocery dry food[h]	405
Specialty dry food[i]	232
Geriatric moist food[j]	184
Renal moist food[k]	135
Renal dry food[l]	151
Renal dry food and 1/2 can tuna	295

[g]Fancy Feast Elegant Medleys White Meat Chicken Florentine
[h]Purina Cat Chow Complete Formula
[i]Hill's Science Diet Adult Original Cat Food
[j]Hill's Science Diet Turkey Entrée Mature Adult 7+ Cat Food
[k]Purina Veterinary Diets NF KidNey Function Feline Formula
[l]Hills Prescription Diet k/d Feline

Table 2. Functional classes of heart failure.*

Class I. The asymptomatic patient
Heart disease is detectable (cardiac murmur, dysrhythmia), but the patient is not overtly affected and does not demonstrate clinical signs of heart failure.
  a. Heart disease is detectable but no signs of compensation are evident, such as volume or pressure overload ventricular hypertrophy.
  b. Heart disease is detectable in conjunction with radiographic or echocardiographic evidence of compensation, such as volume or pressure overload ventricular hypertrophy.

Class II. Mild to moderate heart failure
Clinical signs of heart failure are evident at rest or with mild exercise and adversely affect the quality of life. Typical clinical signs include exercise intolerance, cough, tachypnea, mild respiratory distress and mild to moderate ascites. Hypoperfusion at rest is generally not present.

Class III. Advanced heart failure
Clinical signs of CHF are immediately evident. These clinical signs include respiratory distress (dyspnea), marked ascites, profound exercise intolerance and hypoperfusion at rest. In the most severe cases, the patient is moribund and suffers from cardiogenic shock.

*Adapted from International Small Animal Cardiac Health Council. In: Recommendations for the Diagnosis of Heart Disease and the Treatment of Heart Failure in Small Animals. Academy of Veterinary Cardiology, 1994.

Table 3. Key nutritional factors for foods for dogs and cats with cardiovascular disease.*

Factors	Recommended levels
Sodium	Dogs: Class Ia = 0.15 to 0.25%** Class Ib, II and III = 0.08 to 0.15% Cats: 0.07 to 0.30%
Chloride	Dogs: Class Ia = 1.5 x sodium levels** Class Ib, II and III = 1.5 x sodium levels Cats: 1.5 x sodium levels
Taurine	Dogs: ≥0.1% Cats: ≥0.3%
L-Carnitine	Dogs: ≥0.02%
Phosphorus	Dogs: 0.2 to 0.7% Cats: 0.3 to 0.7%
Potassium	Dogs: ≥0.4% Cats: ≥0.52%
Magnesium	Dogs: ≥0.06% Cats: ≥0.04%

*All values are expressed on a dry matter basis.
**Also appropriate in Class Ib, II and III patients when ACE inhibitors are used, especially when used in combination with diuretics.

FEEDING PLAN

Assess and Select the Food

Ensure the Food's Basic Nutritional Adequacy. AAFCO nutritional adequacy statements are usually found on a product's label. AAFCO approval does not ensure a food will be effective in the management of cardiovascular diseases.

Compare the Food's KNF Content with the Recommended Levels. **Tables 4** and **5** list commercially available foods marketed for management of cardiovascular diseases in dogs and cats (respectively) and compare KNF content with recommended levels. Contact manufacturers for information for foods not in the table (manufacturer contact information is listed on product labels). Select a food that best approximates recommended KNF levels.

Class Ia Patients (Table 2). There is little evidence that foods low in sodium chloride delay disease progression in the initial stages of heart disease in dogs; however, it is prudent to avoid excess sodium chloride early. At the first sign of heart disease without cardiac dilatation, foods with sodium levels in the upper end of the recommended range (0.15-0.25% DM; **Table 4**) should be fed. Early intervention may help a patient accept foods if more restricted sodium chloride levels are necessary later and reminds owners to be vigilant for signs of disease progression. Avoiding excess sodium chloride early in heart disease is not harmful.

Class Ib, II and III Patients (Table 2). When cardiac dilatation becomes evident on radiographs or echocardiograms (Class Ib), sodium chloride-restricted foods are appropriate. Cardiac dilatation implies abnormal sodium chloride handling and intravascular volume expansion and is a prelude to venous congestion. The presence of moderate to severe cardiac dilatation, congestion or

both conditions (Class II or III) indicates that foods lower in sodium chloride are appropriate.

Palatability of Low-Salt Foods. Low-salt foods may be even more palatable than maintenance foods having a higher salt content; communicate this to owners for better compliance (positive bias). However, a few patients might not eat low-salt foods. Also, appetite may be cyclical in patients with advanced CHF. Do not insist on feeding only salt-restricted food if doing so results in inadequate food intake. Consider a trial-and-error approach using different foods (**Tables 4** and **5**). In dogs (but not cats), taste receptors for salt are also stimulated by sugars; try adding sugar or another sweet substance to improve acceptance.

Concurrent ACE Inhibitor Use. Use foods with sodium levels near the upper end of the recommended range (0.15-0.25% DM) when ACE inhibitors are used concurrently, especially in combination with diuretics.

Obese Patients. Because obesity causes profound changes that can complicate cardiovascular disorders, consider initial management with a calorie-restricted food (Chapter 14).

Cachectic Patients. Foods for assisted feeding may need to be considered (Chapters 12 and 13).

Manage Treats and Snacks. Processed human foods are often high in sodium (Appendix I) and should not be provided as treats/snacks. **Table 6** lists selected commercial low-sodium canine treats. Another option is the opposite form of the food being fed; i.e., if a dry food is fed, offer small amounts of the same food in moist form as a snack and vice versa.

Drinking Water. Be familiar with mineral levels in local water supplies; such information can be obtained from municipal water sources or firms that market water conditioning systems. Water samples can be submitted to laboratories for sodium and chloride analyses. Distilled water or water with <150 ppm sodium is recommended for patients with advanced cardiovascular disease.

Assess and Determine the Feeding Method

Determine How Much Food to Feed. The amount to feed can be estimated either from feeding guides on product labels or by calculation (Appendix C). These estimates are only starting points and will likely need to be adjusted (see Followup below).

OBESE PATIENTS. Refer to Chapter 14 for guidelines regarding how to feed weight-loss foods (feeding amount and how to feed). After recommended body weight/BCS are reached, switch to a food for cardiovascular disease (**Tables 4** and **5**). Follow recommendations for amount to feed to prevent weight regain (Chapter 14) and continue to monitor body weight/BCS.

CACHECTIC PATIENTS. Refer to Chapters 12 and 13 for more information.

Determine How to Offer the Food. Free-choice feeding is not recommended for previously overweight patients because it may result in overeating. However, it may be preferred for feeding dry foods to cachectic patients; a combination of dry and moist foods may also be used to enhance intake. Warming moist foods or adding water to dry foods may also increase consumption. Patients with optimal body weight/BCS can usually be fed as before the food change.

Manage Food Changes. A transition period to avoid GI upsets and to facilitate acceptance of a new food is good practice.

Table 4. Levels of key nutritional factors in selected commercial foods for dogs with cardiovascular disease compared to the recommended levels.* (Numbers in red match optimal KNFs.)

Dry foods for Class Ia patients**	Energy density (kcal/cup)***	Na (%)	Taurine (%)[†]	Carnitine (%)[†]	P (%)	K (%)[†]	Mg (%)[†]
Recommended levels	–	0.15-0.25	≥0.1	≥0.02	0.2-0.7	≥0.4	≥0.06
Hill's Prescription Diet g/d Canine	358	0.21	0.1	na	0.41	0.61	0.068
Hill's Prescription Diet j/d Canine	356	0.17	0.13	0.04	0.54	0.83	0.139
Hill's Prescription Diet k/d Canine	396	0.23	0.12	na	0.24	0.67	0.107
Hill's Science Diet Mature Adult Active Longevity Original	363	0.18	0.13	na	0.58	0.83	0.109
Hill's Science Diet Mature Adult Large Breed	357	0.17	0.13	0.03	0.59	0.82	0.108
Hill's Science Diet Mature Adult Small Bites	363	0.18	0.13	na	0.58	0.83	0.109
Medi-Cal Early Cardiac	300	0.3	0.2	0.1	0.8	0.8	0.1
Purina Veterinary Diets NF KidNey Function	459	0.22	na	na	0.29	0.86	0.070
Royal Canin Veterinary Diet Early Cardiac EC 22	291	0.19	0.22	na	0.77	0.82	0.077

Moist foods for Class Ia patients**	Energy density (kcal/can)***	Na (%)	Taurine (%)[†]	Carnitine (%)[†]	P (%)	K (%)[†]	Mg (%)[†]
Recommended levels	–	0.15-0.25	≥0.1	≥0.02	0.2-0.7	≥0.4	≥0.06
Hill's Prescription Diet g/d Canine	377/13 oz.	0.22	0.11	na	0.41	0.78	0.067
Hill's Prescription Diet j/d Canine	498/13 oz.	0.19	0.12	0.03	0.56	0.81	0.112
Hill's Prescription Diet k/d Canine	458/13 oz.	0.19	0.11	na	0.22	0.37	0.141
Hill's Science Diet Mature Adult Active Longevity Gourmet Beef Entrée	164/5.8 oz. 368/13 oz.	0.16	0.12	0.02	0.52	0.76	0.104
Hill's Science Diet Mature Adult Active Longevity Savory Chicken Entrée	155/5.8 oz. 347/13 oz.	0.16	0.12	na	0.57	0.7	0.111
Hills Science Diet Mature Adult Active Longevity Gourmet Turkey Entrée	369/13 oz.	0.17	0.12	na	0.62	0.83	0.107
Iams Veterinary Formula Stress/Weight Gain Formula Maximum-Calorie	333/6 oz.	0.24	0.33	na	0.83	1.01	0.089
Medi-Cal Renal MP	532/380 g	0.2	na	na	0.4	1.5	na
Purina Veterinary Diet NF KidNey Function Formula	498/12.5 oz.	0.24	na	na	0.30	0.72	0.080

Dry foods for Class Ib, II and III patients	Energy density (kcal/cup)***	Na (%)	Taurine (%)[†]	Carnitine (%)[†]	P (%)	K (%)[†]	Mg (%)[†]
Recommended levels	–	0.08-0.15	≥0.1	≥0.02	0.2-0.7	≥0.4	≥0.06
Hill's Prescription Diet h/d Canine	407	0.08	0.14	0.03	0.54	0.8	0.122
Medi-Cal Renal LP	283	0.1	na	na	0.3	0.7	na
Medi-Cal Renal MP	336	0.1	na	na	0.4	0.7	na

Moist foods for Class Ib, II and III patients	Energy density (kcal/can)***	Na (%)	Taurine (%)[†]	Carnitine (%)[†]	P (%)	K (%)[†]	Mg (%)[†]
Recommended levels	–	0.08-0.15	≥0.1	≥0.02	0.2-0.7	≥0.4	≥0.06
Hill's Prescription Diet h/d Canine	480/13 oz.	0.11	0.21	0.03	0.57	0.81	0.131
Medi-Cal Renal LP	643/385 g	0.1	na	na	0.2	1.0	na
Purina Veterinary Diet CV Cardiovascular Formula	638/12.5 oz.	0.12	0.24	na	0.40	1.21	0.060

Key: Na = sodium, P = phosphorus, K = potassium, Mg = magnesium, na = information not available from the manufacturer, g = grams.
*Values are on a dry matter basis unless otherwise stated.
**Also recommended for Class Ib, II and III patients when ACE inhibitors are used, especially when used in combination with diuretics.
***As-fed energy values (kcal/cup or can) are useful for determining the amount to feed; these values can be converted to an amount of food to feed by dividing the energy density of the food (as fed basis) by the patient's daily energy requirement (DER); cup = 8-oz. measuring cup; to convert kcal to kJ, multiply kcal by 4.184. Providing the right amount of food is vital for managing patients with cardiovascular disease. Overweight patients should be fed foods with reduced energy as part of a weight-reduction program (Chapter 14). Patients suffering from cardiac cachexia may need more energy than otherwise normal pets. Body condition scoring should be used frequently to determine the patient's response to the amount of food fed.
[†]See discussion under "Adjunctive Medical & Surgical Management" if additional supplementation is required beyond that present in foods in this table.

Table 5. Levels of key nutritional factors in selected commercial foods for cats with cardiovascular disease compared to the recommended levels.* (Numbers in red match optimal KNFs.)

Dry foods	Energy density (kcal/cup)**	Na (%)	Taurine (%)***	P (%)	K (%)***	Mg (%)***
Recommended levels	–	0.07-0.30	≥0.3	0.3-0.7	≥0.52	≥0.04
Hill's Prescription Diet g/d Feline	297	0.32	0.14	0.54	0.77	0.049
Hill's Prescription Diet k/d Feline	477	0.24	0.16	0.46	0.75	0.058
Hill's Science Diet Mature Adult Active Longevity Original	475	0.32	0.2	0.69	0.88	0.069
Medi-Cal Mature Formula	355	0.4	0.4	0.8	1.0	na
Medi-Cal Reduced Protein	440	0.3	0.4	0.6	0.8	na
Medi-Cal Renal LP	409	0.2	0.2	0.5	1.0	na
Purina Veterinary Diets NF KidNey Function	398	0.2	0.18	0.41	0.88	0.10

Moist foods	Energy density (kcal/can)**	Na (%)	Taurine (%)***	P (%)	K (%)***	Mg (%)***
Recommended levels	–	0.07-0.30	≥0.3	0.3-0.7	≥0.52	≥0.04
Hill's Prescription Diet g/d Feline	165/5.5 oz.	0.32	0.44	0.52	0.72	0.088
Hill's Prescription Diet k/d with Chicken Feline	183/5.5 oz.	0.3	0.42	0.38	1.18	0.049
Hill's Science Diet Mature Adult Active Longevity	87/3 oz.					
Gourmet Turkey Entrée Minced	160/5.5 oz.	0.28	0.48	0.64	0.84	0.072
Iams Veterinary Formula Stress/Weight Gain Formula Maximum-Calorie	333/6 oz.	0.24	0.33	0.83	1.01	0.089
Medi-Cal Mature Formula	205/170 g	0.3	0.3	0.6	0.7	na
Medi-Cal Reduced Protein	265/170 g	0.2	0.3	0.5	0.7	na
Medi-Cal Renal LP	125/85 g pouch	0.6	0.8	0.5	1.1	na
Purina Veterinary Diets CV Cardiovascular Formula	223/5.5 oz.	0.2	0.31	0.92	1.33	0.07
Purina Veterinary Diets NF KidNey Function	234/5.5 oz.	0.16	0.45	0.52	0.96	0.10

Key: Na = sodium, P = phosphorus, K = potassium, Mg = magnesium, na = information not available from the manufacturer.
*Values are on a dry matter basis unless otherwise stated.
**As-fed energy values (kcal/cup or can) are useful for determining amount to feed; These values can be converted to an amount of food to feed by dividing the energy density of the food (as fed basis) by the patient's daily energy requirement (DER); cup = 8-oz. measuring cup; to convert kcal to kJ, multiply kcal by 4.184. Providing the right amount of food is vital for managing patients with cardiovascular disease. Overweight patients should be fed foods with reduced energy as part of a weight-reduction program (Chapter 14). Patients suffering from cardiac cachexia may need more energy than otherwise normal pets. Body condition scoring should be used frequently to determine the patient's response to the amount of food fed.
***See discussion under "Adjunctive Medical & Surgical Management" if additional supplementation is required beyond that present in foods in this table.

Table 6. Low sodium commercial treats for dogs with cardiovascular disease. (Numbers in red match optimal KNFs.)

Treats	Sodium (%DM)
Recommended sodium range for dogs with cardiac disease	0.08 to 0.25
Hill's Science Diet Adult Treats Medium/Large Bone with Real Chicken	0.23
Hill's Science Diet Adult Light Treats Medium/Large Bone with Real Chicken	0.24
Hill's Science Diet Jerky Plus with Real Beef and Vegetables	0.29
Medi-Cal Medi-Treats	0.1
Purina Veterinary Diets Lite Snackers Canine Formula	0.21
Royal Canin Veterinary Diet Treats for Dogs	0.21

Key: DM = dry matter.

Example: to change to a new food, replace 25% of the old food with the new food on Day 1 and continue this incremental change daily until the change is complete on Day 4. Appendix E provides more information.

Food and Water Receptacle Husbandry. Food and water bowls should be washed regularly with warm soapy water and rinsed well. Dishes used for moist foods need daily cleaning. Discard moist or moistened dry foods after 2-4 hours of room temperature exposure to avoid foodborne illnesses (Appendix F).

FOLLOWUP

Owner Followup

Initially, owners should note daily food consumption and, if possible, body weight/BCS every 2 weeks in case feeding amount needs to be adjusted.

Compliance. Deny access to other pets' food in a multi-pet household. Inform all family members of the high salt content of human food snacks to ensure these snacks are not fed to CHF patients.

Veterinary Health Care Team Followup

Monitor frequently (weekly for the first 4-6 weeks), including body weight/BCS, serum electrolyte and magnesium levels and renal function. If body weight/BCS data indicate a change in food dose is warranted, increase or decrease the amount by 10% increments and recheck every 2 weeks for 1 month. At that point, the amount fed should be changed again and the cycle repeated, if necessary.

ADJUNCTIVE MEDICAL & SURGICAL MANAGEMENT

Because many cardiovascular patients are treated with a combination of dietary management and drugs, potential nutrient-drug interactions are important.

Medications

Diuretics. Via stimulation of the RAA system, diuretics may play a role in the progressive self-perpetuating cycle of CHF. Currently, diuretic monotherapy is not recommended early in the management of symptomatic CHF. Reserve this therapy for management of more advanced CHF in patients already receiving moderately sodium chloride-restricted foods, ACE inhibitors, pimobendan or combination therapy. Feeding patients foods without excess sodium chloride may allow lower dosages of diuretics to be used for control of clinical signs of CHF.

ACE Inhibitors. Although clinically significant hyperkalemia (6.5 mEq/l) is uncommon, use of ACE inhibitors in dogs with CHF or CKD fed foods with high potassium content may increase the risk for hyperkalemia. Drug-induced azotemia in CHF patients is treated by reducing the diuretic dose (usually at least by half–skip a dose if there is not active pulmonary edema); if no resolution occurs, reduce the ACE inhibitor dose by half as well or sodium intake can be increased to the next level (**Table 4**) or use a combination of these methods.

Pimobendan. Dietary influences apparently do not affect pimobendan's pharmacodynamics. Its use may dramatically stimulate appetite.

Cardiac Glycosides. Absorption is influenced by the formulation of the drug and its administration in relation to meals (see Chapter 69, Small Animal Clinical Nutrition, 5th edition). Because administering digoxin or digitoxin with food may result in up to a 50% reduction in serum concentrations, these drugs are best given between meals. Body condition may also influence pharmacokinetics of these drugs. Reduce digoxin dose by 1/3 in cats receiving concomitant furosemide, aspirin and sodium-restricted food.

Supplements

Potassium and/or Magnesium Supplementation. Hypokalemia, hyperkalemia and hypomagnesemia are potential complications of drug therapy in heart disease patients.

DIURETICS. Patients should receive adequate amounts of potassium and magnesium.

ACE INHIBITORS. Patients may be predisposed to mild hyperkalemia; therefore, food should not contain excess potassium. If hyperkalemia develops, discontinue supplementation, if provided, and switch to a food with lower potassium levels. Consider loop or thiazide diuretics rather than potassium-sparing diuretics.

CKD. Often concomitant with cardiovascular disorders. If hypokalemia develops, feed a food with more potassium or supplement with 3-5 mEq (or mmol) potassium/kg/day. If hypomagnesemia develops, feed a food with a higher magnesium content or supplement (magnesium oxide, 20-40 mg/kg/day).

Taurine Supplementation. Taurine deficiency is more likely to respond favorably to oral supplementation (250-500 mg/day for cats; 500-1,000 mg t.i.d. for dogs). Foods properly formulated for nutritional management of cardiovascular disease contain increased taurine (**Tables 4** and **5**); patients eating these foods usually do not require additional taurine. Discontinue supplementation of cat foods after 12-16 weeks if clinical signs of CHF have resolved, echocardiographic values are near normal and the cat will eat a food known to support normal whole blood taurine concentrations. The length of time needed for taurine supplementation of dog foods is unknown. Appendix I provides taurine levels in various meats.

L-Carnitine Supplementation. The oral dose for dogs with myocardial L-carnitine deficiency is 50-100 mg L-carnitine/kg body weight t.i.d. For 25- to 40-kg dogs, mix 2 g of L-carnitine with food 3 times daily. The high dose may increase plasma concentrations 10-20 times above usual pretreatment values, which will usually raise myocardial levels into the normal range. Supplementation cost is approximately $80 (U.S.)/month for a large-breed dog. L-carnitine is usually available in human health food stores. Dogs that respond dramatically usually experience improved clinical signs in 1-4 weeks and echocardiographic improvement after 8-12 weeks. Improvement may continue for 6-8 months and plateau, at which time patients appear clinically normal but echocardiography often indicates depressed ventricular function.

MISCELLANEOUS

See Chapters 25-27, 36 and 37, Small Animal Clinical Nutrition, 5th edition, for more information.

Authors

Condensed from Chapter 36, Small Animal Clinical Nutrition, 5th edition, authored by Philip Roudebush and Bruce W. Keene.

References

See Chapter 36, Small Animal Clinical Nutrition, 5th edition, on the website www.markmorrisinstitute.org for references.

CLINICAL POINTS

- CKD ranks just behind cancer as a leading cause of nonaccidental death in dogs and cats.
- In addition to familial associations (Appendix J), increasing age is a risk for CKD.
- Causes of acquired kidney diseases that could lead to CKD include infections, inflammatory/immune-mediated conditions, neoplasia, drugs, antimicrobials, antifungals, analgesics, immunosuppressive agents and chemotherapeutics.
- Clinical signs of CKD may include polyuria/polydipsia (less frequent in cats than dogs), lethargy, inappetence, vomiting, weight loss, nocturia, constipation, diarrhea, acute blindness (associated with hypertension) and seizures or coma (terminal uremia). Cats also may exhibit ptyalism and muscle weakness with cervical ventriflexion due to hypokalemic myopathy.
- Routine laboratory evaluation includes CBCs, serum biochemistry profiles and urinalyses; other useful diagnostic tests include blood pressure measurement and diagnostic imaging.
- The IRIS scheme for staging CKD in dogs and cats identifies stages, based on creatinine, and substages based on proteinuria and magnitude of hypertension, a risk for end-organ damage (Appendix J).
- Most routine tests for CKD do not reveal abnormal findings until there is advanced disease (stage 2 or higher). Example: generally, azotemia doesn't occur until 75% of nephrons are nonfunctional. Patients in stage 1 do not have azotemia.
- A variety of compensatory and adaptive responses are involved in the pathogenesis and progression of naturally occurring CKD. Certain of these factors are the basis for nutritional therapy (KNFs) and recommendations for medical management (**Table 1**).
- Feeding an appropriately formulated commercial veterinary therapeutic renal food is the only treatment shown (randomized, controlled clinical studies) to prolong survival time and improve quality of life in patients with CKD.
- Feeding goals: improve quality and length of life through appropriate nutritional management that reduces signs of uremia, slows progression to later stages of disease and complements medical treatments.

KEY NUTRITIONAL FACTORS

- Foods should provide recommended allowances of all required nutrients (nutritional adequacy), but should also contain

specific levels of KNFs (certain nutrients proven to assist in the management of CKD).
- Etiopathogenesis of CKD (**Table 1**) is the basis for the KNF recommendations.
- **Table 2** lists KNF recommendations for foods for dogs and cats with CKD. A detailed review of these recommendations can be found in Chapter 37, Small Animal Clinical Nutrition, 5th edition.
- Dogs with protein-losing glomerulonephropathy should also be fed reduced-protein foods designed for patients with CKD, whether azotemic or not.

FEEDING PLAN

Consider feeding a food for CKD when the earliest stages are documented (e.g., persistent renal proteinuria, loss of urine concentrating ability or mild azotemia), although the general guideline is to institute the feeding plan when serum creatinine >2 mg/dl (≥ stage 2).

Before initiating a feeding plan for patients with stage 3 or 4 CKD that have uremic signs (e.g., anorexia, vomiting and diarrhea), provide aggressive fluid and electrolyte therapy to ameliorate azotemia, uremia, electrolyte abnormalities and acidosis.

Assess and Select the Food

Ensure the Food's Basic Nutritional Adequacy. AAFCO nutritional adequacy statements are usually found on a product's label. AAFCO approval does not ensure a food will be effective in the management of CKD.

Compare the Food's KNF Content with the Recommended Levels. Tables **3** and **4** list commercially available foods marketed for the management of CKD in dogs and cats (respectively) and compare the KNF content of these foods with recommended levels. Contact manufacturers for information for foods not in the tables (manufacturer contact information is listed on product labels). Select a food that best approximates the recommended KNF levels.

FOOD FORM. Adequate water intake in CKD patients is particularly important. If readily consumed, moist foods are preferred; their consumption results in increased total water intake compared to dry foods.

PALATABILITY. Commercial veterinary therapeutic foods for CKD are as palatable, or more so, than regular maintenance foods. However, CKD may affect taste preferences. Feeding plans may be more successful if owners are informed of the palatability of renal foods (positive bias).

Manage Treats and Snacks. Many commercial treats and human foods (Appendix I) contain sodium, chloride and phosphorus far in excess of KNF levels. If treats/snacks are fed, commercial treats that most closely match the KNF profile recommended for foods for CKD are best. Limit treats to <5% of the total diet on a volume, weight or calorie basis. Options: 1) use the opposite form of the food being fed; i.e., if a dry food is fed, offer small amounts of the same food in moist form as a snack and vice versa, 2) keep kibbles of a dry food for CKD patients in a separate container away from the usual feeding area and use as treats.

Assess and Determine the Feeding Method

Determine How Much Food to Feed. The amount fed can be estimated from feeding guides on product labels or by calculation (Appendix C). These estimates are only starting points and will likely need to be adjusted (see Followup below). Food intake tends to decrease as renal function declines because of progressive anorexia and reduced activity.

Consider How to Offer the Food. Method(s) of offering the previous food (e.g., free-choice feeding or multiple offerings per day of a prescribed amount) can be continued if the food form is unchanged.

Free-choice feeding of dry foods or a combination of dry and moist foods for CKD may also be used to enhance intake. Appendix J provides other tips for increasing acceptance of foods for CKD patients.

Manage Food Changes. Gradual transition to a new food improves acceptance and also decreases the likelihood of problems in patients that cannot rapidly adjust urinary sodium levels because of their renal dysfunction. Dogs with CKD usually tolerate a dietary change over 7-10 days; cats may need 3-4 weeks (or longer). Manage owner's expectations; both patience and persistence are required. Appendix J provides additional suggestions.

Food and Water Receptacle Husbandry. Food and water bowls should be washed regularly with warm soapy water and rinsed well. Dishes used for moist foods need daily cleaning. Discard moist or moistened dry foods after 2-4 hours of room temperature exposure to avoid foodborne illnesses (Appendix F).

FOLLOWUP

Owner Followup

Initially, owners should note daily food consumption and, if possible, record body weight/BCS every 2 weeks in case the feeding amount/method needs to be adjusted.

Compliance. Deny access to other pets' food in multi-pet households. Also, studies indicate that owners of cats with CKD often

---

Table 1. Potential etiopathogenic mechanisms in chronic kidney disease and therapeutic approaches for each.

Factors	Therapeutic approaches
Chronic renal hypoxia	Maintain hydration (increased water intake)
	Avoid excessive sodium intake
	ACE inhibitors
	Control anemia (erythropoietin)
Glomerular hypertension and hyperfiltration	Avoid excessive dietary protein and sodium
	Increased dietary omega-3 fatty acids
	ACE inhibitors
Hyperphosphatemia and secondary renal hyperparathyroidism	Limit dietary phosphorus
	Intestinal phosphate binders
	Calcitriol (after normophosphatemia is achieved)
Hypokalemia	Potassium supplementation
Metabolic acidosis	Avoid excessive dietary protein
	Alkalinizing foods (therapeutic renal foods)
	Alkalinizing agents (bicarbonate, potassium citrate)
Proteinuria	Avoid excessive dietary protein
	Increased dietary omega-3 fatty acids
	ACE inhibitors
Renal oxidative stress	Avoid excessive dietary protein, phosphorus and sodium
	Increased dietary antioxidants
	Omega-3 fatty acid supplementation
Systemic hypertension	Avoid excessive dietary sodium
	ACE inhibitors
	Calcium-channel antagonists (amlodipine)
Tubulointerstitial inflammation/fibrosis	Increased dietary omega-3 fatty acids
	Avoid excessive dietary phosphorus and protein

Key: ACE = angiotensin-converting enzyme.

Table 2. Key nutritional factors for dogs and cats with chronic kidney disease.*

Factors	Dietary recommendations
Water	Parenteral fluid therapy if dehydration, blood volume contraction or renal hypoperfusion is clinically significant
	Offer water free choice at all times
	Recommend moist foods
Protein	14 to 20% in foods for dogs
	28 to 35% in foods for cats
Phosphorus	0.2 to 0.5% in foods for dogs
	0.3 to 0.6% in foods for cats
Sodium	≤0.3% in foods for dogs
	≤0.4% in foods for cats
Chloride	1.5 x sodium levels in foods for dogs
	1.5 x sodium levels in foods for cats
Potassium	0.4 to 0.8% in foods for dogs
	0.7 to 1.2% in foods for cats
	If patient becomes hyperkalemic, switch to a lower potassium food
Omega-3 fatty acids	0.4 to 2.5% in foods for dogs and cats
	Omega-6:omega-3 fatty acid ratio of 1:1 to 7:1
Antioxidants	
Vitamin E	≥400 IU vitamin E/kg of food for dogs
	≥500 IU vitamin E/kg of food for cats
Vitamin C	≥100 mg vitamin C/kg of food for dogs
	100 to 200 mg vitamin C/kg of food for cats

*All values expressed on a dry matter basis, unless otherwise indicated.

Table 3. Key nutritional factors in selected commercial veterinary therapeutic foods for dogs with chronic kidney disease compared to recommended levels.* (Numbers in red match optimal KNFs.)

Moist foods	Energy density (kcal/can)**	Protein (%)	P (%)	Na (%)	K (%)	Omega-3 fatty acids (%)	Omega-6: omega-3	Vit. E (IU/kg)	Vit. C (mg/kg)
Recommended levels	–	14-20	0.2-0.5	≤0.3	0.4-0.8	0.4-2.5	1:1-7:1	≥400	≥100
Hill's Prescription Diet g/d Canine	377 kcal/13 oz.	18.1	0.41	0.22	0.78	0.67	3.7:1	719	107
Hill's Prescription Diet k/d Canine	458 kcal/13 oz.	14.8	0.22	0.19	0.37	1.93	2.3:1	844	130
Hill's Prescription Diet u/d Canine	489 kcal/13 oz.	13.3	0.17	0.28	0.45	0.38	13.5:1	643	na
Medi-Cal Reduced Protein	525 kcal/396 g	16.5	0.5	0.2	0.5	na	na	na	na
Medi-Cal Renal LP	643 kcal/385 g	16.8	0.2	0.1	1.0	na	na	na	na
Medi-Cal Renal MP	532 kcal/380 g	28.2	0.4	0.2	1.5	na	na	na	na
Medi-Cal Weight Control/Mature	370 kcal/396 g	21.5	0.6	0.3	0.6	na	na	na	na
Purina Veterinary Diets NF KidNey Function Canine Formula	498 kcal/12.5 oz.	16.5	0.30	0.24	0.72	0.59	6.9:1	na	na
Royal Canin Veterinary Diet Renal LP	785 kcal/13.6 oz.	16.1	0.24	0.08	0.84	na	na	1,034	na
Royal Canin Veterinary Diet Renal MP	670 kcal/13.4 oz.	26.2	0.42	0.19	1.17	na	na	552	na

Dry foods	Energy density (kcal/cup)**	Protein (%)	P (%)	Na (%)	K (%)	Omega-3 fatty acids (%)	Omega-6: omega-3	Vit. E (IU/kg)	Vit. C (mg/kg)
Recommended levels	–	14-20	0.2-0.5	≤0.3	0.4-0.8	0.4-2.5	1:1-7:1	≥400	≥100
Hill's Prescription Diet g/d Canine	358	18.7	0.41	0.21	0.61	0.78	3.5:1	263	na
Hill's Prescription Diet k/d Canine	396	14.7	0.24	0.23	0.67	1.54	1.9:1	679	344
Hill's Prescription Diet u/d Canine	396	11.2	0.15	0.23	0.54	0.74	4.4:1	856	na
Iams Veterinary Formula Renal Early Stage	245	21.0	0.46	0.41	0.63	na	5:1	na	na
Medi-Cal Reduced Protein	360	13.7	0.4	0.2	0.7	na	na	na	na
Medi-Cal Renal LP	283	14.7	0.3	0.1	0.7	na	na	na	na
Medi-Cal Renal MP	336	18.4	0.4	0.1	0.7	na	na	na	na
Medi-Cal Weight Control/Mature	320	19.5	0.8	0.2	0.8	na	na	na	na
Purina Veterinary Diets NF KidNey Function Canine Formula	459	15.9	0.29	0.22	0.86	0.30	9.3:1	na	na
Royal Canin Veterinary Diet Renal LP 11	275	14.7	0.30	0.08	0.66	na	na	302	na
Royal Canin Veterinary Diet Renal MP 14	327	18.4	0.40	0.10	0.66	na	na	302	na

Key: P = phosphorus, Na = sodium, K = potassium, omega-6:omega-3 = omega-6 to omega-3 fatty acid ratio, Vit. E = vitamin E, Vit. C = vitamin C, na = information not available from manufacturer, g = grams.
*All values are reported on a dry matter basis unless otherwise indicated. Moist foods are best. All values were obtained from manufacturers' published information.
**Energy density as-fed (per can or cup) is useful for determining the amount to feed; cup = 8-oz. measuring cup; to convert kcal to kJ, multiply kcal by 4.184.

augment dry veterinary therapeutic renal foods with unprescribed regular moist foods. Feeding an over-the-counter moist food that contains increased sodium, chloride and phosphorus could decrease/negate the effectiveness of the prescribed food for CKD.

Veterinary Health Care Team Followup

Table 5 lists recommended parameters for reassessment. Hematocrit and serum albumin are laboratory indices for malnutrition. Recheck azotemic patients every 2-3 months and uremic patients as often as every 2-4 weeks. The time between evaluations may be longer in patients with stable disease.

Loss of Body Weight/BCS. Gradual weight loss is not uncommon and increasing the amount of food offered typically does not help anorectic patients. Ensure other causes have been corrected including dehydration, GI hemorrhage, metabolic acidosis, hypokalemia, anemia, UTI, dental disease and drug-associated anorexia. See Appendix J for tips on getting CKD patients to eat.

Table 4. Key nutritional factors in selected commercial veterinary therapeutic foods for cats with chronic kidney disease compared to recommended levels.* (Numbers in red match optimal KNFs.)

Moist foods	Energy density (kcal/can)**	Protein (%)	P (%)	Na (%)	K (%)	Omega-3 fatty acids (%)	Omega-6: omega-3 1:1-7:1	Vit. E (IU/kg)	Vit. C (mg/kg)
Recommended levels	–	28-35	0.3-0.6	≤0.4	0.7-1.2	0.4-2.5	1:1-7:1	≥500	100-200
Hill's Prescription Diet g/d Feline	165 kcal/5.5 oz.	34.3	0.52	0.32	0.72	0.64	6.1:1	817	104
Hill's Prescription Diet k/d with Chicken Feline	183 kcal/5.5 oz.	28.9	0.38	0.30	1.18	0.72	6.1:1	814	103
Iams Veterinary Formula Multi Stage Renal	199 kcal/6 oz.	33.6	0.60	0.40	1.03	na	5:1	na	na
Medi-Cal Reduced Protein	265 kcal/170 g	33.9	0.5	0.2	0.7	na	na	na	na
Medi-Cal Renal LP	125 kcal/85-g pouch	29.3	0.5	0.6	1.1	na	na	na	na
Purina Veterinary Diets NF KidNey Function	234 kcal/5.5 oz.	31.1	0.52	0.16	0.96	0.85	3.7:1	na	na
Royal Canin Veterinary Diet Modified Formula	256 kcal/6 oz.	34.7	0.65	0.28	0.81	na	na	178	na
Royal Canin Veterinary Diet Renal LP	126 kcal/3-oz. pouch	34.1	0.55	0.47	1.10	na	na	437	na

Dry foods	Energy density (kcal/cup)**	Protein (%)	P (%)	Na (%)	K (%)	Omega-3 fatty acids (%)	Omega-6: omega-3 1:1-7:1	Vit. E (IU/kg)	Vit. C (mg/kg)
Recommended levels	–	28-35	0.3-0.6	≤0.4	0.7-1.2	0.4-2.5	1:1-7:1	≥500	100-200
Hill's Prescription Diet g/d Feline	297	33.5	0.54	0.32	0.77	0.19	15.5:1	232	na
Hill's Prescription Diet k/d Feline	477	28.8	0.46	0.24	0.75	0.25	15.1:1	952	229
Iams Veterinary Formula Multi Stage Renal	514	32.1	0.42	0.39	0.65	na	5:1	na	na
Medi-Cal Reduced Protein	440	28.1	0.6	0.3	0.8	na	na	na	na
Medi-Cal Renal LP	409	24.7	0.5	0.2	1.0	na	na	na	na
Purina Veterinary Diets NF KidNey Function	398	30.8	0.41	0.20	0.88	0.31	6.4:1	na	na
Royal Canin Veterinary Diet Modified Formula	432	27.1	0.49	0.23	1.07	na	na	380	na
Royal Canin Veterinary Diet Renal LP 21	395	24.7	0.49	0.16	1.02	na	na	355	na

Key: P = phosphorus, Na = sodium, K = potassium, omega-6:omega-3 = omega-6 to omega-3 fatty acid ratio, Vit. E = vitamin E, Vit. C = vitamin C, na = information not available from manufacturer, g = grams.
*All values are reported on a dry matter basis unless otherwise indicated. Moist foods are best. All values were obtained from manufacturers' published information.
**Energy density as fed (per can or cup) is useful for determining the amount to feed; cup = 8-oz. measuring cup; to convert kcal to kJ, multiply kcal by 4.184.

Medical Management of CKD-Induced Anorexia. Options that may be effective include recombinant human erythropoietin and ACE inhibitors (benazepril); H₂-antagonists (ranitidine, famotidine) may help by managing uremic gastroenteritis.
Assisted Feeding. If food intake remains inadequate for >3-5 days, consider feeding via percutaneous gastrostomy or esophagostomy tubes (Chapter 12 and Appendix H). Feeding using these routes can be done at home and may reverse progressive weight loss and result in extended periods of improved quality of life.
Proteinuric Dogs: Dietary Protein Reassessment. Monitor every 2-4 weeks initially to determine optimal intake of dietary protein. Continue to feed the selected reduced protein food if proteinuria (UPC ratios) declines and there is no evidence of protein malnutrition (i.e., stable or increasing body weight/BCS,

serum albumin and total protein). If evidence develops, gradually increase protein intake (e.g., supplement with hard-boiled eggs) in stepwise fashion while closely monitoring the patient.

MISCELLANEOUS

See Chapters 13, 14, 20 and 21, Small Animal Clinical Nutrition, 5th edition, for nutritional measures recommended for prevention of CKD. See Chapters 25, 26 and 37, Small Animal Clinical Nutrition, 5th edition, for more information about feeding patients with CKD.

Table 5. Reassessment of patients with chronic kidney disease.

Physical examination
Abdominal palpation (size and contour of kidneys, presence of ascites)
Blood pressure measurement
Body condition/muscle mass
Body weight
Fundic examination (retinal hemorrhage, detached retina)
Hair and coat quality
Hydration status
Oral examination (uremic odor, ulcers, mucous membrane color)

Laboratory evaluation
Serum biochemistries (urea nitrogen, creatinine, albumin, phosphorus)
Serum electrolytes (calcium, potassium, chloride, sodium, magnesium)
Total serum carbon dioxide or venous blood gases (blood pH, bicarbonate, base excess) to evaluate acid-base status
Urinalysis
    Microscopic sediment exam (pyuria or bacteriuria may indicate urinary tract infection)
    Urine specific gravity (crude index of tubulointerstitial function)
    pH (very crude index of acid-base status)
Urine protein-creatinine ratio (assess proteinuria and response to treatment)

Diagnostic imaging
Abdominal radiographs (assess kidney shape and size, reference L_2 vertebra on ventrodorsal view)
Excretory urogram (assess obstruction due to nephroliths)
Ultrasound (assess kidney and prostate gland, presence of hydronephrosis, hydroureter, uroliths)

Authors
Condensed from Chapter 37, Small Animal Clinical Nutrition, 5th edition, authored by S. Dru Forrester, Larry G. Adams and Timothy A. Allen.

References
See Chapter 37, Small Animal Clinical Nutrition, 5th edition, on the website www.markmorrisinstitute.org for references.

Chapter
27 Canine Purine Urolithiasis

CLINICAL POINTS

- Purines are catabolites of DNA and RNA and are further metabolized to xanthine, uric acid and allantoin for excretion in urine (**Figure 1**). Allantoin is the major end product in most dogs and is more soluble than xanthine or uric acid. Uroliths composed of uric acid salts, xanthine or uric acid form when urine is oversaturated with these substances.
- Out of >350,000 canine uroliths analyzed (Appendix K), purine uroliths accounted for 5-6% of all uroliths and ~13% of nephroliths. More than 95% were urates (salts of uric acid); the rest were uric acid, xanthine and uric acid monohydrate; in this chapter, "urate" is often used interchangeably with "purine."
- Mean age at diagnosis is 4 years; **Table 1** summarizes other risks.
- Dalmatian dogs are predisposed to urate urolithiasis because of

Abbreviations
AAFCO = Association of American Feed Control Officials
BCS = body condition score (Appendix A)
CKD = chronic kidney disease
DM = dry matter
KNF = key nutritional factor
UTI = urinary tract infection

their reduced ability to convert uric acid to allantoin. Thus, they excrete relatively high quantities of uric acid; however, only a small percentage form urate uroliths.
- Increased dietary purines (**Tables 1** and **2**) may promote urate urolithiasis in predisposed dogs because they are incorporated into the purine pool and eventually excreted in the urine (**Figure 1**).
- High-protein foods increase urine uric acid excretion and increase urine saturation with uric acid, sodium urate and ammonium urate compared to low-protein foods.

- Low-protein, low-purine foods, in combination with appropriate medical therapy, can result in urate urolith dissolution.
- Concentrations of lithogenic substances in urine also depend on urine volume; consumption of dry foods is a risk factor for urate urolith formation because they produce more concentrated urine than moist foods (**Table 1**). Moderate protein restriction can increase urine volume by decreasing renal medullary urea concentration and urine concentrating ability.
- Urine acidity is a risk factor for urate lithogenesis because the solubility of most purines, especially ammonium urate, is pH-dependent; consumption of foods that promote aciduria (e.g., high-protein foods or those with other acidifying ingredients) may be a risk factor (**Table 1**).
- Recommendations for urolith dissolution and prevention are based on mineral composition of uroliths; therefore, it is important to analyze uroliths whenever possible. Appendix K lists clinical signs, urologic diagnostic laboratories and other diagnostic aids.
- Recurrence of urate uroliths may be influenced by several factors including: 1) persistence of underlying causes, 2) incomplete removal of all uroliths by surgery or lithotripsy, 3) persistence/recurrence of UTI with urease-producing bacteria and/or 4) failure to comply with preventive recommendations.
- Feeding goals: by use of appropriate foods, feeding methods and medical management, dissolve urate uroliths and reduce their recurrence.

KEY NUTRITIONAL FACTORS

- Foods should provide recommended allowances of all required nutrients (nutritional adequacy), but should also contain specific levels of KNFs (certain nutrients that can assist in the management of purine urolithiasis).
- **Table 3** summarizes KNFs for foods intended for dissolution and prevention of urate uroliths in dogs and includes restriction of purines, moderate restriction of protein and sodium and production of an alkaline urinary pH.
- Water is always a KNF but is particularly important for

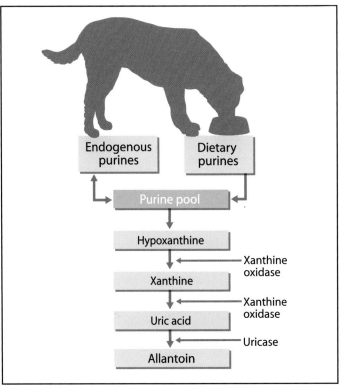

Figure 1. Diagram of normal canine purine degradation.

management of urolithiasis. Increased water intake augments urine volume, thereby decreasing urine uric acid and ammonium concentrations; it also enhances urine flow through the urinary tract.

- A detailed review of these recommendations can be found in Chapter 39, Small Animal Clinical Nutrition, 5th edition.

FEEDING PLAN

Typically, medical and sometimes surgical interventions are used in concert with dietary management (below).

Assess and Select the Food
Ensure the Food's Basic Nutritional Adequacy. AAFCO nutritional adequacy statements are usually found on a product's label.

Table 1. Some potential risk factors for canine purine urolithiasis.

Food	Urine	Metabolic	Drugs
High purine content (**Table 2**)	Hyperuricuria	Males	Urine acidifiers
Acidifying potential	Hyperammonuria	Breed	Salicylates
Low moisture content	Acidic pH	Dalmatians	Chemotherapeutic agents
Ascorbic acid?	Urine concentration	English bulldogs	(especially 6-mercaptopurine)
	Urine retention	Miniature schnauzers	
	Urease-producing microburia	Yorkshire terriers	
	Increased promoters?	Shih Tzus	
	Decreased inhibitors?	Hyperuricemia	
		Hyperammonuria	
		Hepatic dysfunction	
		Neoplasia with rapid cell destruction	

Table 2. Purine content of selected foods.

Foods to avoid (high purine concentration)	Foods to use sparingly (moderately high purine concentration)	Foods that can be fed (negligible purine concentration)
Anchovies	Asparagus	Breads (whole grain cereal products)
Brain	Cauliflower	Butter and fats
Clams	Fish*	Cheese
Goose	Legumes (beans and peas)	Eggs
Gravies	Lentils	Fruits and fruit juices
Heart	Meats	Gelatin
Kidney	Mushrooms	Milk
Liver	Spinach	Nuts
Mackerel		Refined cereals
Meat extracts including bouillon		Sugars
Mussels		Vegetable soups
Oysters		Cream soups
Salmon		Vegetables**
Sardines		Water
Scallops		
Shrimp		
Sweetbreads		
Tuna		
Yeast (baker's and brewer's)		

*Except those listed in the first column.
**Except those listed in the second column.

Table 3. Key nutritional factors for foods for dissolution and prevention of canine purine uroliths.

Factors	Dietary recommendations
Water	Water intake should be encouraged to achieve a urine specific gravity <1.020
Protein and purines	Restrict dietary protein to 10 to 18% dry matter (DM)
	Restrict dietary purines: the first three non-water ingredients on the product label ingredient panel should be low in purines (**Table 2**)
Sodium	Moderate sodium restriction (<0.3% DM)
	Avoid sodium supplements
Urinary pH	Feed a food that maintains an alkaline urine (urinary pH = 7.1 to 7.5)

AAFCO approval does not ensure a food will be effective in the management of purine urolithiasis.

Compare the Food's KNF Content with the Recommended Levels. **Table 4** lists commercially available foods marketed for dissolution and prevention of canine purine urolithiasis and compares KNF content of the foods with recommended levels. Contact manufacturers for information for foods not in the table (manufacturer contact information is listed on product labels). Select a food that best approximates the recommended KNF levels.

NEED FOR DIURETICS. Because properly formulated low-protein urate litholytic foods impair urine-concentrating capacity by decreasing renal medullary urea concentration, additional diuretic agents are unnecessary.

URINE ALKALINIZING INGREDIENTS. The recommended urinary pH range for urate dissolution is 7.1-7.5. Properly formulated urate litholytic foods should contain potassium citrate (check ingredient labels) as an alkalinizing ingredient (also a good source of potassium).

FOOD FORM. Adequate water intake in urolithiasis patients is particularly important. If readily consumed, moist foods are preferred; their consumption results in increased total water intake compared to dry foods. If dry foods are fed, consider adding liberal amounts of water. Do not leave moist foods or moistened dry foods at room temperature for prolonged intervals (>2-4 hours, see below).

INCREASING WATER INTAKE. 1) Provide water bowls in multiple locations (e.g., several bowls outside in a large enclosure or a bowl on each level of the house). 2) Be sure water bowls are clean and filled regularly with fresh water. 3) Offer ice cubes as treats or snacks. 4) Do not use even small amounts of salt-free bouillon as a flavoring substance in drinking water to increase consumption; meat extracts contain increased levels of purines (**Table 2**).

ESTIMATED RELATIVE FOOD PURINE CONTENT. Use foods with relatively low purine content. At least the first 3 non-water ingredients (see the ingredient panel on the food label) should be low in purines (**Table 2**).

Dogs with Portal Vascular Anomalies. Successful urolith dissolutions have been reported to occur with foods designed for CKD (Chapter 26) following surgical correction of portal vascular anomalies. Additional studies are needed to evaluate litholytic foods and medical management for dissolution of ammonium urate uroliths in dogs with portal vascular anomalies. Allopurinol efficacy may be altered because its biotransformation requires adequate hepatic function.

Puppies. Safety and efficacy of litholytic foods in growing puppies with urate uroliths are unknown. Appendix K provides recipes for adding non-purine-containing protein to litholytic foods. Surgical removal of large uroliths has the most predictable short-term outcome.

Manage Treats and Snacks. Many commercial treats and human foods (Appendix I and **Table 2**) contain sodium, protein and purines far in excess of KNF levels. If treats/snacks are fed, commercial treats that most closely match the KNF profile rec-

Table 4. Levels of key nutritional factors in selected veterinary therapeutic foods used for dissolution and to minimize recurrence of urate urolithiasis in dogs compared to recommended levels.* (Numbers in red match optimal KNFs.)

Dry foods	Protein (%)	Restricted purines (Yes/No)**	Sodium (%)	Urinary pH***
Recommended levels	10-18	Yes	<0.3	7.1-7.5
Hill's Prescription Diet u/d Canine	11.2	Yes	0.23	7.70
Medi-Cal Reduced Protein	13.7	Yes	0.2	na
Medi-Cal Renal LP	14.7	Yes	0.1	na
Medi-Cal Renal MP	18.4	Yes	0.1	na
Medi-Cal Vegetarian Formula	20.9	Yes	0.4	na
Purina Veterinary Diets NF KidNey Function	15.9	Yes	0.22	6.7-7.5
Purina Veterinary Diets HA HypoAllergenic	21.3	Yes	0.24	na
Royal Canin Veterinary Diets Vegetarian Formula	19.1	Yes	0.15	6.78

Moist foods	Protein (%)	Restricted purines (Yes/No)**	Sodium (%)	Urinary pH***
Recommended levels	10-18	Yes	<0.3	7.1-7.5
Hill's Prescription Diet u/d Canine	13.3	Yes	0.28	7.4
Medi-Cal Reduced Protein	16.5	No	0.2	na
Medi-Cal Renal LP	16.8	No	0.1	na
Medi-Cal Renal MP	28.2	No	0.2	na
Medi-Cal Vegetarian Formula	26.4	Yes	0.5	na
Purina Veterinary Diets NF KidNey Function	16.5	No	0.24	6.7-7.5

Key: na = information not available from manufacturer.
*Manufacturers' published values; nutrients expressed as % dry matter; moist foods are best.
Restricted purines = products having low-purine ingredients (Table 2**) as the first three non-water ingredients on the ingredient panel of the product label.
***Protocols for measuring urinary pH may vary.

ommended for foods for urate urolithiasis are best. Limit treats to <10% of the total diet on a volume, weight or calorie basis. Options: 1) use the opposite form of the food fed; i.e., if a dry food is fed, offer small amounts of the same food in moist form as a snack and vice versa, 2) keep kibbles of a dry food for urate urolithiasis in a separate container away from the usual feeding area and use as treats.

Assess and Determine the Feeding Method

Determine How Much Food to Feed. The amount to feed can be estimated either from feeding guides on product labels or by calculation (Appendix C). These estimates are only starting points and will likely need to be adjusted (see Followup below).
Consider How to Offer the Food. Maintaining an alkaline urinary pH is important for urate urolith dissolution. Free-choice feeding is associated with more persistent aciduria compared to meal feeding. Thus, meal feeding (2 meals/day) is recommended whether using dry and/or moist foods.
Manage Food Changes. A transition period to avoid GI upsets and to facilitate acceptance of a new food is good practice. Example: to change to a urate litholytic food, replace 25% of the old food with the litholytic food on Day 1 and continue this incremental change daily until the change is complete on Day 4. Appendix E provides additional information.
Food and Water Receptacle Husbandry. Food and water bowls should be washed regularly with warm soapy water and rinsed well. Dishes used for moist foods need daily cleaning. Discard moist or moistened dry foods after 2-4 hours of room temperature exposure to avoid foodborne illnesses (Appendix F).

Table 5. Expected changes associated with dietary and medical therapy of purine uroliths.

Factors	Pre-therapy	During therapy	Prevention therapy
Polyuria	±	1+ to 3+	1+ to 3+
Pollakiuria	0 to 4+	↑ then ↓	0
Hematuria	0 to 4+	↓	0
Urine specific gravity	Variable	1.004 to 1.015	1.004 to 1.015
Urinary pH	<7.0	>7.0	>7.0
Pyuria	0 to 4+	↓	0
Purine (urate) crystals	0 to 4+	0	Variable
Bacteriuria	0 to 4+	0	0
Bacterial culture of urine	0 to 4+	0	0
Urea nitrogen (mg/dl)	Variable	≤15	≤15
Urolith size and number	Small to large	↓	0

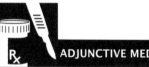

ADJUNCTIVE MEDICAL & SURGICAL MANAGEMENT

Medical Management
Xanthine Oxidase Inhibitors. Allopurinol inhibits the action of xanthine oxidase, and thereby decreases production of uric acid by inhibiting conversion of hypoxanthine to xanthine, and xanthine to uric acid (**Figure 1**). Food does not affect the availability of allopurinol; thus, it can be administered with meals.

CONTRAINDICATIONS. Only administer allopurinol to patients consuming purine-restricted foods; otherwise a layer of xanthine many form around ammonium urate uroliths.

Allopurinol is not recommended for puppies or dogs with portal vascular anomalies. Azotemic patients require a lower dose. *Eradication/Control of UTIs.* UTIs may be due to altered local host defenses associated with urolith-induced trauma and/or catheterization. Prevent, eradicate or control infections because they may cause problems of equal or greater severity as uroliths. Antimicrobial dosages should consider that litholytic foods induce diuresis, which reduces urine concentration of antimicrobial agents.

Surgery

Indications include uroliths obstructing urine outflow. Lithotripsy is effective in removing uroliths that obstruct the urethra. Initiation of dietary and medical dissolution protocols are indicated if such patients have multiple uroliths in several locations and if circumstances preclude surgical removal when the obstructing urolith is removed. Certain patients with portal vascular anomalies and urate uroliths may benefit from a combination of surgical, dietary and medical urolith dissolution protocols (Chapter 39, Small Animal Clinical Nutrition, 5th edition).

FOLLOWUP

Owner Followup

Monitor for development of urethroliths in male dogs during dissolution. Owners should weigh their dog (if possible) and/or grade its BCS monthly. If a trend of increasing or decreasing body weight or condition is noticed, the amount fed should be changed by 10% increments and the dog rechecked every 2 weeks for 1 month. Then, if necessary, the amount fed should be changed again and the cycle repeated. Water intake should be encouraged to achieve a urine specific gravity <1.020.
Compliance. If the dog lives in a multi-pet household, deny access to other pets' foods. Counsel owners to adhere strictly to feeding only the litholytic food. Dogs consuming a high-purine food, while receiving allopurinol, may form a xanthine shell around urate uroliths or form xanthine uroliths.

Veterinary Health Care Team Followup

Monitor urolith size/location (radiography, ultrasonography), urinary pH, urine sediment, serum urea nitrogen and serum uric acid monthly. **Table 5** lists expected changes of these and other parameters. Decreased serum urea nitrogen (<10 mg/dl) suggests compliance. Mean time for urate urolith dissolution is 3.5 months (1-18 months). Continue feeding the litholytic food and administering allopurinol (and alkalinizing therapy if used) for 1 month following radiographic disappearance of uroliths.
Urine Alkalinizers. If urinary pH is <7.1 when feeding a litholytic food and no UTI is present, supplement with potassium citrate (wax matrix tablets[a] or liquid[b]). Dose is 40-75 mg/kg q12h. Divided doses help maintain a consistently non-acidic

urine. Avoid sodium bicarbonate (potential risk for sodium urate uroliths) and do not exceed a urinary pH of 7.5 (potential risk for calcium phosphate uroliths).
Partial Urolith Dissolution. Partial dissolution may occur even with appropriate dietary and medical intervention. In some dogs, the remaining uroliths can be retrieved using voiding urohydropropulsion or catheter-assisted retrieval (Appendix K).
Dissolution Failure. Reevaluation of the diagnosis and/or alternate methods of management should be considered if uroliths enlarge during therapy or do not begin to decrease in size after ~8 weeks of appropriate medical and dietary therapy.
Urethroliths. Ammonium urate urocystoliths have a propensity to move into the urethra. If small enough, they readily pass through but often lodge behind the os penis of male dogs. Owners should be informed of this possibility and given a list of associated clinical signs.

Urethroliths may be returned to the bladder lumen by urohydropropulsion (Appendix K) or removed by lithotripsy. The physical characteristics that permit passage of these uroliths into the urethra also facilitate their removal from the urethra.
Prevention of Recurrence. Dalmatian dogs have high recurrence rates (also consider preventive measures for non-Dalmatian dogs). First choice: continue to feed urate litholytic foods (**Table 4**). If dry foods are fed, water should be added with the goal of maintaining a urine specific gravity <1.025. Use the same feeding methods described above.
Persistent Urate Crystalluria or Hyperuricuria. Serial urinary pH measurements are indicated to ensure alkalinization (7.1-7.5). If necessary, add potassium citrate (above). If difficulties persist, give low doses of allopurinol (~10-20 mg/kg/day), cautiously. Prolonged high doses (30 mg/kg/day) may result in formation of xanthine uroliths.

MISCELLANEOUS

See Appendix K for information about canine compound urolithiasis. See Chapters 38 and 39, Small Animal Clinical Nutrition, 5th edition, for more information.

Authors

Condensed from Chapter 39, Small Animal Clinical Nutrition, 5th edition, authored by Carl A. Osborne, Joseph W. Bartges, Jody P. Lulich, Hasan Albasan and Carroll Weiss.

References

See Chapter 39, Small Animal Clinical Nutrition, 5th edition, on the website www.markmorrisinstitute.org for references.

Endnotes
a. Urocit-K. Mission Pharmacal, San Antonio, TX, USA.
b. Polycitra-K. Willen Drug Co., Baltimore, MD, USA.

Chapter 28

Canine Calcium Oxalate Urolithiasis

CLINICAL POINTS

- Uroliths composed of calcium oxalate monohydrate and calcium oxalate dihydrate form as a result of interactions of several environmental and demographic risk factors and several metabolic disturbances.
- Out of >350,000 canine uroliths analyzed, calcium oxalate accounted for 38% of all uroliths with percentages appearing to increase with time (Appendix K).
- Mean age at diagnosis is 8-9 years; **Table 1** summarizes other risks.
- Calcium oxalate uroliths are nearly always found in the lower urinary tract.
- For calcium oxalate uroliths to form, urine must be super-saturated with calcium and oxalic acid.
- Dietary ingredients that promote hypercalciuria or hyper-oxaluria are nutritional risk factors for calcium oxalate urolith formation (**Tables 1 and 2**). Dogs with calcium oxalate urolithiasis frequently consume human food.
- Calcium oxalate urolithiasis is also associated with consumption of commercial dog treats. The high sodium content of some treats may explain this association; excessive sodium intake promotes hypercalciuria.
- Reducing both dietary calcium and oxalate is important; reducing consumption of only calcium may increase the availability of oxalic acid for intestinal absorption and subsequent urinary excretion.
- Dietary phosphorus should not be overly restricted in patients with calcium oxalate urolithiasis; reduced dietary phosphorus may augment intestinal calcium absorption and hypercalciuria.
- Urinary pH reflects the acidifying effects of a food. Foods that promote acidic urine promote hypercalciuria and hypocitraturia and increase the risk of calcium oxalate urolithiasis in

susceptible dogs. On the other hand, metabolic alkalosis enhances tubular reabsorption of calcium.
- Ingestion of foods that contain high quantities of animal protein may contribute to calcium oxalate urolithiasis by increasing urine calcium excretion and decreasing urine citrate excretion; an obligatory acid excretion is associated with protein metabolism.
- Pyridoxine (vitamin B_6) deficiency can cause oxalate crystalluria in cats. Supplemental B_6 is sometimes recommended to help decrease oxalate crystalluria in dogs (see Followup below).
- Hyperparathyroidism, hyperadrenocorticism, paraneoplastic hypercalcemia and furosemide administration promote hypercalciuria.
- Naturally occurring macromolecular crystal growth inhibitors such as nephrocalcin, Tamm-Horsfall glycoprotein and glycosaminoglycans normally inhibit calcium oxalate crystal aggregation.
- Recommendations for urolith dissolution and prevention are based on mineral composition of uroliths; therefore, it is important to analyze uroliths whenever possible. Appendix K lists clinical signs, urolith analytical laboratories and other diagnostic aids.
- Surgery is the time-honored method to remove calcium oxalate uroliths from the urinary tract; small urocystoliths may be aspirated through a transurethral catheter or removed by voiding urohydropropulsion (Appendix K).
- Rate of recurrence of calcium oxalate uroliths increases with time: in 1 study, 3% recurred after 3 months, 9% after 6 months, 36% after 1 year, 42% after 2 years and 48% after 3 years.

Abbreviations
AAFCO = Association of American Feed Control Officials
BCS = body condition score (Appendix A)
DM = dry matter
KNF = key nutritional factor

Table 1. Some potential risk factors for canine calcium oxalate urolithiasis.

Diet	Urine	Metabolic status	Drugs
Acidifying potential	Hypercalciuria	Chronic metabolic acidosis	Urine acidifiers
High protein content	Hyperoxaluria	Males	Furosemide
High sodium content	Hypocitraturia?	Breed	Glucocorticoids
Excessive calcium content	Hypomagnesuria?	Miniature schnauzers	Sodium chloride
Excessive restriction of calcium	Hyperuricuria?	Miniature poodles	Vitamin D
Low moisture content	Increased crystal promoters	Lhasa apsos	Ascorbic acid
Excessive phosphorus restriction	Decreased crystal inhibitors	Yorkshire terriers	
Excessive magnesium content	Urine concentration	Shih Tzus	
Excessive magnesium restriction	Urine retention	Bichon Frises	
Excessive vitamin D content		Older age	
Excessive vitamin C content		Hypercalcemia	
Deficient pyridoxine?		Glucocorticoid excess	
High oxalate content		Hypophosphatemia	
		Hyperoxalemia?	
		Osteolysis?	

Table 2. Selected human foods to limit or avoid feeding to dogs with calcium oxalate uroliths.*

Moderate/high-calcium foods	Moderate/high-oxalate foods	
Food items	**Food items**	
Meats	**Meats**	
Bologna (M)	Sardines (M)	Oranges (M)
Herring (M)	**Vegetables**	Peaches (M)
Oysters (M)	Asparagus (M)	Pears (M)
Salmon (H)	Broccoli (M)	Peel of lemon, lime or orange (H)
Sardines (H)	Carrots (M)	Pineapple (M)
Vegetables	Celery (H)	Tangerine (H)
Baked beans (M)	Corn (M)	**Breads, grains, nuts**
Broccoli (H)	Cucumber (H)	Cornbread (M)
Collards (H)	Eggplant (H)	Fruitcake (H)
Lima beans (M)	Green beans (H)	Grits (H)
Spinach (M)	Green peppers (H)	Peanuts (H)
Tofu (soybean curd) (M)	Lettuce (H)	Pecans (H)
Milk and dairy products	Spinach (H)	Soybeans (H)
Cheese (H)	Summer squash (H)	Wheat germ (H)
Ice cream (H)	Sweet potatoes (H)	**Miscellaneous**
Milk (H)	Tofu (H)	Beer (H)
Yogurt (H)	Tomatoes (M)	Chocolate (H)
Breads, grains, nuts	**Fruits**	Cocoa (H)
Brazil nuts (M)	Apples (H)	Coffee (M)
Miscellaneous	Apricots (H)	Tea (H)
Cocoa (M)	Cherries (M)	Tomato soup (H)
Hot chocolate (M)	Most berries (H)	Vegetable soup (H)

Key: M = moderate; feed in limited amounts. H = high; avoid feeding.
*Adapted from Wainer L, Resnick VA, Resnick MI. Nutritional aspects of stone disease. In: Pak CYC, ed. Renal Stone Disease, Pathogenesis, Prevention, and Treatment. Boston, MA: Martinus Nihoff Publishing, 1987; 85-120. Burroughs M. Renal diseases and disorders. In: Nelson JK, Moxness KE, Jensen MD, et al, eds. Mayo Clinic Diet Manual, 7th ed. St. Louis, MO: Mosby, 1994; 208-209.

Table 3. Key nutritional factors for foods for prevention of calcium oxalate uroliths.

Factors	Recommended levels
Water	Water intake should be encouraged to achieve a urine specific gravity <1.020
	Moist food will increase water consumption and formation of less concentrated urine
Protein	Avoid excess dietary protein
	Restrict dietary protein to 10 to 18% dry matter (DM)
Calcium	Avoid excess dietary calcium, especially dietary supplements given independent of diet
	Restrict dietary calcium to 0.4 to 0.7% DM
Oxalate	Avoid foods high in oxalic acid (**Table 2**)
Phosphorus	Avoid phosphorus deficiency and maintain a normal Ca:P ratio (1.1:1 to 2:1)
	Dietary phosphorus should be in the range of 0.3 to 0.6% DM
Sodium	Recommend moderate dietary sodium restriction
	Dietary sodium should be <0.3% DM
Magnesium	Avoid excess or deficient dietary magnesium
	Dietary magnesium should be in the range of 0.04 to 0.15% DM
Ascorbic acid (vitamin C)	Avoid pet foods, supplements or human foods that contain ascorbic acid
Urinary pH	Avoid acidifying foods
	Foods should produce a urinary pH 7.1-7.5

- To prevent recurrence, dietary/medical management need to reduce urinary calcium and oxalic acid concentrations, promote high concentration and activity of inhibitors of calcium oxalate crystal growth/aggregation and reduce urine concentration.

- Dissolution of calcium oxalate uroliths in dogs has not been reported; the goal of dietary management is to prevent recurrence by use of appropriate foods, feeding methods and medical management.

KEY NUTRITIONAL FACTORS

- Foods should provide recommended allowances of all required nutrients (nutritional adequacy), but should also contain specific levels of KNFs (certain nutrients that can assist in the prevention of recurrence of calcium oxalate urolithiasis).
- **Table 3** summarizes KNFs for foods intended for prevention of calcium oxalate uroliths in dogs and includes moderate restriction of protein, calcium, oxalic and ascorbic acids and sodium and adequate phosphorus and magnesium and production of an alkaline urinary pH.
- Water is always a KNF but is particularly important for management of urolithiasis. Increased water intake increases urine volume and decreases urinary calcium and oxalate concentrations; it also enhances urine flow through the urinary tract.
- A detailed review of recommendations can be found in Chapter 40, Small Animal Clinical Nutrition, 5th edition.

Table 4. Levels of key nutritional factors in selected veterinary therapeutic foods used to minimize recurrence of calcium oxalate urolithiasis in dogs compared to recommended levels.* (Numbers in red match optimal KNFs.)

Dry foods	Protein (%)	Calcium (%)**	Phosphorus (%)**	Sodium (%)	Magnesium (%)	Urinary pH***
Recommended levels	10-18	0.4-0.7	0.3-0.6	<0.3	0.04-0.15	7.1-7.5
Hill's Prescription Diet u/d Canine	<u>11.2</u>	0.34	0.15	<u>0.23</u>	<u>0.046</u>	7.70
Medi-Cal Urinary SO 13	<u>16.7</u>	1.0	<u>0.6</u>	1.3	0.2	5.5-6.0
Purina Veterinary Diets NF KidNey Function	<u>15.9</u>	0.76	0.29	<u>0.22</u>	<u>0.07</u>	6.7-7.5
Royal Canin Veterinary Diet Urinary SO 14	<u>17.0</u>	0.80	0.63	1.38	<u>0.066</u>	5.5-6.0

Moist foods	Protein (%)	Calcium (%)**	Phosphorus (%)**	Sodium (%)	Magnesium (%)	Urinary pH***
Recommended levels	10-18	0.4-0.7	0.3-0.6	<0.3	0.04-0.15	7.1-7.5
Hill's Prescription Diet u/d Canine	<u>13.3</u>	0.35	0.17	<u>0.28</u>	<u>0.049</u>	<u>7.4</u>
Medi-Cal Urinary SO	18.7	1.0	0.8	1.1	<u>0.10</u>	5.5-6.0
Purina Veterinary Diets NF KidNey Function	<u>16.5</u>	<u>0.50</u>	<u>0.30</u>	<u>0.24</u>	<u>0.08</u>	6.7-7.5
Royal Canin Veterinary Diet Urinary SO	18.5	0.97	0.86	1.45	<u>0.059</u>	5.5-6.0

*Manufacturers' published values. Nutrients expressed as % dry matter, unless otherwise stated; moist foods are best; avoid foods with added vitamin C (ascorbic acid); avoid foods with high oxalate ingredients (**Table 2**).
**Calcium-phosphorus ratio should be in the range of 1.1:1 to 2:1.
***Protocols for measuring urinary pH may vary.

FEEDING PLAN

Assess and Select the Food

Ensure the Food's Basic Nutritional Adequacy. AAFCO nutritional adequacy statements are usually found on a product's label. AAFCO approval does not ensure a food will be effective in the prevention of recurrence of calcium oxalate urolithiasis.

Compare the Food's KNF Content with the Recommended Levels. **Table 4** lists selected commercially available foods marketed for prevention of recurrence of canine calcium oxalate urolithiasis and compares the KNF content of these foods with recommended levels. Contact manufacturers for information for foods not in the table (manufacturer contact information is listed on product labels). Select a food that best approximates the recommended KNF levels.

Supplements. Avoid supplemental ascorbic acid and vitamin D.

Urine Alkalinizing Ingredients. The recommended urinary pH range for calcium oxalate prevention is 7.1-7.5. Properly formulated foods should contain potassium citrate (check ingredient labels) as an alkalinizing ingredient. Additional citric acid has other benefits (See Adjunctive Medical & Surgical Management below).

Food Form. Adequate water intake in urolithiasis patients is particularly important. If readily consumed, moist foods are preferred; their consumption increases total water intake compared to dry foods. Consider adding liberal amounts of water to dry foods. Do not leave moist foods or moistened dry foods at room temperature for prolonged intervals (>2-4 hours, below).

Increasing Water Intake. 1) Provide water bowls in multiple locations (e.g., several bowls outside in a large enclosure or a bowl on each level of the house). 2) Be sure water bowls are clean and filled regularly with fresh water. 3) Offer ice cubes as treats or snacks.

Manage Treats and Snacks. Many commercial treats and human foods (Appendix I and **Table 2**) contain protein, calcium,

Table 5. Selected human foods with minimal calcium or oxalate content.

Food items	Low-calcium foods	Low-oxalate foods
Meats and eggs	Eggs	Beef
	Poultry	Eggs
		Fish and shellfish*
		Lamb
		Pork
		Poultry
Vegetables		Cabbage
		Cauliflower
		Mushrooms
		Peas, green
		Radishes
		Potatoes, white
Milk and dairy products		Cheese*
		Milk*
		Yogurt*
Fruits		Apple
		Avocado
		Banana
		Bing cherries
		Grapefruit
		Grapes, green
		Mangos
		Melons
		Cantaloupe
		Casaba
		Honeydew
		Watermelon
		Plums, green or yellow
Breads, grains, nuts	Almonds	Bread, white
	Macaroni	Macaroni
	Pretzels	Noodles
	Rice	Rice
	Spaghetti	Spaghetti
	Walnuts	
Miscellaneous	Popcorn	Jellies
		Preserves
		Soups with allowed ingredients

*Low in oxalate, but not low in calcium content.

Table 6. Expected changes associated with dietary and medical therapy to minimize recurrence of calcium oxalate uroliths.

Factors	Pre-therapy	Prevention therapy
Polyuria	±	Variable
Pollakiuria	0 to 4+	0
Hematuria	0 to 4+	0
Urine specific gravity	Variable	1.004-1.015
Urinary pH	<7.0	>7.0
Pyuria	0 to 4+	0
Calcium oxalate crystals	0 to 4+	0
Bacteriuria	0 to 4+	0
Bacterial culture of urine	0 to 4+	0
Urea nitrogen (mg/dl)	>15	<15
Urolith size and number	Small to large	0

sodium, oxalic acid and/or ascorbic acid in excess of KNF levels. If treats/snacks are fed, commercial treats that most closely match KNF profiles recommended for foods for calcium oxalate urolithiasis prevention are best. Limit to <10% of the total diet on a volume, weight or calorie basis. Options: 1) use the opposite form of the food being fed; i.e., if a dry food is fed, offer small amounts of the same food in moist form as a snack and vice versa, 2) keep kibbles of a dry food for calcium oxalate urolithiasis prevention in a separate container away from the usual feeding area and use as treats. **Table 5** lists human foods with minimal calcium and oxalic acid content.

Assess and Determine the Feeding Method
Determine How Much Food to Feed. The amount to feed can be estimated either from feeding guides on product labels or by calculation (Appendix C). These estimates are only starting points and will likely need to be adjusted (see Followup below).
Consider How to Offer the Food. Maintaining an alkaline urinary pH is important for calcium oxalate urolith prevention. Free-choice feeding is associated with more persistent aciduria compared to meal feeding. Thus, meal feeding (2 times/day) is recommended whether using dry and/or moist foods.
Manage Food Changes. A transition period to avoid GI upsets and to facilitate acceptance of a new food is good practice. Example: to change to a calcium oxalate urolith prevention food, replace 25% of the old food with the new food on Day 1 and continue this incremental change daily until the change is complete on Day 4. Appendix E provides additional information.
Food and Water Receptacle Husbandry. Food and water bowls should be washed regularly with warm soapy water and rinsed well. Dishes used for moist foods need daily cleaning. Discard moist or moistened dry foods after 2-4 hours of room temperature exposure to avoid foodborne illnesses (Appendix F).

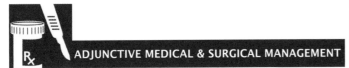

ADJUNCTIVE MEDICAL & SURGICAL MANAGEMENT

Urine Alkalinizers
Potassium citrate in aqueous solution ionizes and the citrate anion may form soluble salts with calcium (reduces calcium oxa-

late crystal formation), promotes formation of alkaline urine and, via metabolic alkalosis, enhances tubular reabsorption of calcium. If necessary (see Followup below) supplement with potassium citrate (wax matrix tablets[a] or liquid[b]). Chewable treats[c] are also available. Dose is 40-75 mg/kg q12h. Divided doses help maintain a consistently non-acidic urine. Avoid sodium bicarbonate (sodium increases urinary calcium excretion) and do not exceed a pH of 7.5. Potassium citrate should be administered with meals to reduce gastric irritation. Additional supplementation may not be needed when feeding foods with adequate potassium citrate.

Thiazide Diuretics
Thiazide diuretics reduce recurrence of calcium-containing uroliths because of their ability to reduce urine calcium excretion, especially when used concurrently with a urolith prevention food. Thiazide diuretics are not recommended as first-line therapy. Use should be accompanied by owner informed consent and appropriate clinical and laboratory monitoring for early detection of adverse effects (dehydration, hypokalemia, hypercalcemia).

FOLLOWUP

Owner Followup
Owners should weigh their dog (if possible) and/or grade its body condition (BCS) monthly. If a trend of increasing or decreasing body weight or condition is noticed, the amount fed should be changed by 10% increments and the patient rechecked every 2 weeks for 1 month. At that point, if necessary, the amount fed should be changed again and the cycle repeated. Water intake should be encouraged to achieve a urine specific gravity <1.020.
Compliance. If the dog lives in a multi-pet household, deny access to other pets' food.

Veterinary Health Care Team Followup
Immediately postsurgery or after voiding urohydropropulsion, obtain data (radiography, complete urinalysis, serum concentrations of calcium, urea nitrogen and creatinine) to evaluate effectiveness of renal function and calcium homeostasis. If hypercalcemia is present, correct the underlying cause; if normocalcemia exists, initiate the above feeding plan.
1st Reevaluation (2-4 Weeks). **Table 6** lists expected changes. Decreased serum urea nitrogen (<10 mg/dl) suggests compliance. Consider additional potassium citrate if calcium oxalate crystals and aciduria persist and do 2nd reevaluation (otherwise, go to last step, below).
2nd Reevaluation (2-4 Weeks). Consider vitamin B$_6$ supplementation (2-4 mg/kg q24-48 hours) if calcium oxalate crystalluria persists perform the 3rd reevaluation (otherwise, go to last step, below).
3rd Reevaluation (2-4 Weeks). Consider administration of hydrochlorothiazide (2 mg/kg q24-48 hours) if calcium oxalate crystalluria persists.
Last Step. After 3-6 months, reevaluate to verify compliance and amelioration of crystalluria. Check for urolith recurrence by

radiography. If no uroliths are present, continue current therapy and reevaluate in 3-6 months. If uroliths have recurred, consider voiding urohydropropulsion (Appendix K) or lithotripsy. If unsuccessful and clinical signs referable to urocystoliths are persistent, consider surgery. Continue therapy to minimize urolith growth if clinical signs are not present.

MISCELLANEOUS

See Appendix K for information about canine compound urolithiasis. For more information, see Chapters 38 and 40, Small Animal Clinical Nutrition, 5the edition.

Authors

Condensed from Chapter 40, Small Animal Clinical Nutrition, 5th edition, authored by Jody P. Lulich, Carl A. Osborne and Lori A. Koehler.

References

See Chapter 40, Small Animal Clinical Nutrition, 5th edition, on the website www.markmorrisinstitute.org for references.

Endnotes

a. Urocit-K. Mission Pharmacal, San Antonio, TX, USA.
b. Polycitra-K. Willen Drug Co., Baltimore, MD, USA.
c. K-CIT-V. V.E.T. Pharmaceuticals, Inc., Fenton, MO, USA.

Chapter 29

Canine Calcium Phosphate Urolithiasis

CLINICAL POINTS

> ### Abbreviations
>
> AAFCO = Association of American Feed Control Officials
> BCS = body condition score (Appendix A)
> DM = dry matter
> KNF = key nutritional factor
> RTA = renal tubular acidosis

- At least 4 mineral types have been identified in calcium phosphate uroliths; the most common is hydroxyapatite, followed by brushite.
- Uroliths composed predominantly of calcium phosphate are uncommon; out of >350,000 canine uroliths analyzed, calcium phosphate accounted for 0.5% (Appendix K).
- Calcium phosphate is usually found as a minor component in naturally occurring struvite and calcium oxalate uroliths.
- More than 80% of hydroxyapatite uroliths were removed from the lower urinary tract.
- 40 different breeds were affected including mixed breeds, cocker spaniels, miniature schnauzers, Yorkshire terriers, Shih Tzus and springer spaniels.
- Calcium phosphate uroliths may occur in patients with: 1) primary hyperparathyroidism, 2) other hypercalcemic disorders, 3) distal RTA and 4) idiopathic hypercalciuria.
- Calcium phosphate solubility depends on: 1) urinary pH, 2) urine calcium ion concentration, 3) total urine inorganic phosphate concentration, 4) urine concentration of inhibitors of calcium crystallization and 5) urine concentration of potentiators of crystallization.
- With the exception of brushite, calcium phosphate solubility decreases in alkaline urine and increases in acidic urine. Moderate urinary acidification is recommended for prevention of recurrent calcium phosphate uroliths in most patients, except for those with distal RTA, where long-term alkalinization therapy is beneficial.
- Hypercalciuria may result in oversaturation with calcium

phosphate and can result from: 1) excessive resorption of calcium from bone, 2) enhanced intestinal absorption of calcium, 3) impaired renal tubular reabsorption of calcium or 4) combinations of these factors.
- Reduction of dietary calcium may be important because intestinal hyperabsorption of calcium has been identified as one mechanism promoting hypercalciuria in dogs with calcium oxalate uroliths.
- Dietary phosphorus should not be excessive but should not be overly restricted; excess restriction of dietary phosphorus may augment intestinal calcium absorption and promote hypercalciuria. Overrestriction may also enhance production of 1,25-vitamin D, thereby further promoting hypercalciuria.
- Dry and moist grocery brand dog foods may contain 3-4 times the recommended allowance of calcium and phosphorus.
- Feeding foods high in vitamin D or excessive supplementation with vitamin D may promote hypercalciuria (Table 1).
- Excess sodium intake may promote hypercalciuria and enhance the risk of calcium phosphate urolith formation. Oral sodium chloride therapy is not recommended to promote diuresis in dogs with uroliths containing calcium salts.
- Foods with high protein content tend to contribute to hypocitraturia. Citric acid ions inhibit calcium phosphate crystallization. High-protein foods also contribute to hypercalciuria and hyperphosphaturia.

Table 1. Some potential risk factors for canine calcium phosphate urolithiasis.

Food	Urine	Metabolic	Drugs
Alkalinizing potential	Alkaline pH	Hypercalcemia	Urine alkalinizing drugs
High calcium content	Hypercalciuria	Distal renal tubular acidosis	Furosemide
High sodium content	High phosphate ion concentration		Glucocorticoids
High phosphorus content?	Increased concentration of promoters		Sodium chloride
Low-moisture content	Decreased concentration of inhibitors		Vitamin D
Excessive vitamin D content	Hypocitraturia		
High protein content	Hypomagnesuria		
Low magnesium content	Blood clots in renal pelvis or bladder lumen		
	Urine concentration		
	Urine retention		

Table 2. Key nutritional factors for foods for the prevention of recurrence of calcium phosphate urolithiasis in dogs.[*]

Factors	Recommended levels
Water	Water intake should be encouraged to achieve a urine specific gravity <1.020. Moist food will increase water consumption and formation of less concentrated urine
Protein	10 to 25%
Calcium	0.4 to 0.7%
Phosphorus	0.3 to 0.6%
Ca:P ratio	1.1:1 to 2:1
Sodium	<0.3%
Magnesium	0.06 to 0.15%
Vitamin D	500 to 1,500 IU/kg
Urinary pH	6.2 to 6.6[**]

Key: Ca:P ratio = calcium-phosphorus ratio.
[*]Nutrients expressed on a dry matter basis.
[**]Alkaline urine is recommended for patients with distal renal tubular acidosis.

- Formation of calcium phosphate uroliths may be promoted by epitaxy. Calcium phosphate precipitation may be stimulated by calcium oxalate and monosodium urate crystals.
- Inhibitors of calcium phosphate crystallization include nephrocalcin, inorganic pyrophosphates, citric acid ions and magnesium ions. Magnesium can replace calcium on the surfaces of growing crystals, blocking epitaxial growth.
- **Table 1** lists these and other risk factors.
- Recommendations for urolith dissolution and prevention are based on mineral composition of uroliths; therefore, it is important to analyze uroliths whenever possible. Appendix K lists clinical signs, urolith diagnostic laboratories and other diagnostic aids.
- Dietary dissolution of calcium phosphate uroliths has not been successful. Depending on size, calcium phosphate uroliths are readily removed by surgery, lithotripsy, voiding urohydropropulsion or aspiration through a urinary catheter (Appendix K).
- Feeding goal: minimize recurrence by use of appropriate foods, feeding methods and medical management.

KEY NUTRITIONAL FACTORS

- Foods should provide recommended allowances of all required nutrients (nutritional adequacy), but should also contain specific levels of KNFs (certain nutrients that can help minimize recurrence of calcium phosphate urolithiasis).
- **Table 2** summarizes KNFs for foods intended for prevention of calcium phosphate uroliths in dogs. Excessive dietary protein consumption should be avoided in dogs at risk for recurrence of calcium phosphate urolithiasis; the lower end of the recommended range is probably better. Moderate to lower calcium, phosphorus, Ca:P ratio, sodium and magnesium and production of acidic urinary pH are also KNFs.
- Water is always a KNF and is particularly important for management of urolithiasis. Increased water intake increases urine volume and decreases urinary calcium and phosphate concentrations; it also enhances urine flow through the urinary tract.
- A detailed review of these recommendations can be found in Chapter 41, Small Animal Clinical Nutrition, 5th edition.

FEEDING PLAN

Assess and Select the Food
Ensure the Food's Basic Nutritional Adequacy. AAFCO nutritional adequacy statements are usually found on a product's label. AAFCO approval does not ensure a food will be effective in the prevention of recurrence of calcium phosphate urolithiasis.
Compare the Food's KNF Content with the Recommended Levels. **Table 3** lists selected commercially available foods that can be considered for prevention of recurrence of canine calcium phosphate urolithiasis and compares KNF content of these foods with recommended levels. Contact manufacturers for information for foods not in the table (manufacturer contact information is listed on product labels). Select a food that best approximates the recommended KNF levels.
Supplements. Avoid supplemental vitamin D.
Food Form. If readily consumed, moist foods are preferred; their consumption results in increased total water intake compared to

Table 3. Levels of key nutritional factors in selected commercial veterinary therapeutic foods used to minimize recurrence of calcium phosphate urolithiasis in dogs compared to recommended levels.* (Numbers in red match optimal KNFs.)

Dry foods	Protein (%)	Calcium (%)	Phosphorus (%)	Ca:P ratio	Sodium (%)	Magnesium (%)	Vitamin D (IU/kg)	Urinary pH
Recommended levels	10-25	0.4-0.7	0.3-0.6	1.1:1-2:1	<0.3	0.06-0.15	500-1,500	6.2-6.6**
Hill's Prescription Diet c/d Canine	22.3	0.82	0.59	1.4:1	0.28	0.111	618	6.22
Hill's Prescription Diet w/d Canine	18.9	0.66	0.56	1.2:1	0.22	0.088	632	6.40
Hill's Prescription Diet w/d with Chicken Canine	19.1	0.66	0.56	1.2:1	0.27	0.080	677	6.30
Medi-Cal Urinary SO 13	16.7	1.0	0.6	na	1.3	0.2	na	5.5-6.0

Moist foods	Protein (%)	Calcium (%)	Phosphorus (%)	Ca:P ratio	Sodium (%)	Magnesium (%)	Vitamin D (IU/kg)	Urinary pH
Recommended levels	10-25	0.4-0.7	0.3-0.6	1.1:1-2:1	<0.3	0.06-0.15	500-1,500	6.2-6.6**
Hill's Prescription Diet c/d Canine	23.6	0.68	0.51	1.3:1	0.27	0.079	1,370	6.16
Hill's Prescription Diet w/d Canine	17.9	0.64	0.52	1.2:1	0.24	0.088	1,745	6.40
Medi-Cal Urinary SO	18.7	1.0	0.8	na	1.1	0.1	na	5.5-6.0

Key: na = information not available from the manufacturer.
*This list represents products with the largest market share for which published information is available. Nutrient levels expressed on a dry matter basis. Moist foods are best.
**Alkaline urine recommended for patients with distal renal tubular acidosis.

dry foods. If feeding dry foods, consider adding liberal amounts of water. Do not leave moist foods or moistened dry foods at room temperature for prolonged intervals (below).

Increasing Water Intake. 1) Provide water bowls in multiple locations (e.g., several bowls outside in a large enclosure or a bowl on each level of the house). 2) Be sure water bowls are clean and filled regularly with fresh water. 3) Offer ice cubes as treats or snacks.

Manage Treats and Snacks. Many commercial treats and human foods (Appendix I) contain sodium in excess of KNF levels. If treats/snacks are fed, commercial treats that most closely match the KNF profile recommended for foods for calcium phosphate urolithiasis prevention are best. Limit consumption to <10% of the total diet on a volume, weight or calorie basis. Options: 1) use the opposite form of the food being fed; i.e., if a dry food is fed, offer small amounts of the same food in moist form as a snack and vice versa, 2) store kibbles of a dry food for prevention of calcium phosphate urolithiasis in a separate container away from the usual feeding area and use as treats.

Assess and Determine the Feeding Method

Determine How Much Food to Feed. The amount to feed can be estimated either from feeding guides on product labels or by calculation (Appendix C). These estimates are only starting points and will likely need to be adjusted (see Followup below). Consider How to Offer the Food. Maintaining a moderately acidic urinary pH is important for calcium phosphate urolith prevention, except for patients with distal RTA. Free-choice feeding is associated with more persistent aciduria compared to meal feeding. If moist foods are fed, provide multiple portions (≥3/day). Feeding a specific amount/day is recommended for

dogs that tend to be overweight.

Manage Food Changes. A transition period to avoid GI upsets and to facilitate acceptance of a new food is good practice. Example: to change to a calcium phosphate urolith prevention food, replace 25% of the old food with the new food on Day 1 and continue this incremental change daily until the change is complete on Day 4. Appendix E provides additional information.

Food and Water Receptacle Husbandry. Food and water bowls should be washed regularly with warm soapy water and rinsed well. Dishes used for moist foods need daily cleaning. Discard moist or moistened dry foods after 2-4 hours of room temperature exposure to avoid foodborne illnesses (Appendix F).

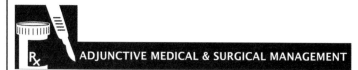

ADJUNCTIVE MEDICAL & SURGICAL MANAGEMENT

Urine Acidifying and Alkalinizing Agents

Because of potential problems with calcium oxalate urolith formation, routine use of urine acidifiers with urine acidifying foods for patients with calcium phosphate urolithiasis is not recommended.

Brushite is less soluble in acidic urine. However, brushite may be converted to other insoluble forms of calcium phosphate in alkaline urine. Use of potassium citrate, an alkalinizing agent, might be considered to minimize acidosis-induced hypercalciuria and formation of soluble calcium citrate rather than insoluble calcium phosphate, especially if concurrent distal RTA is present.

Thiazide Diuretics

Thiazide diuretics reduce urine calcium excretion; they may be considered for minimizing renal-leak hypercalciuria but are not recommended as first-line therapy. Use should be accompanied by owner informed consent and appropriate clinical and laboratory monitoring for early detection of adverse effects (dehydration, hypokalemia, hypercalcemia). Thiazide diuretic therapy is not recommended to treat absorptive hypercalciuria because it does not correct the hyperabsorptive state. Also, positive systemic calcium balance may result that could predispose to soft-tissue calcification. The hydrochlorothiazide trial dose is 2-4 mg/kg q12h.

FOLLOWUP

Owner Followup
Owners should weigh their dog (if possible) and/or grade its body condition (BCS) monthly. If a trend of increasing or decreasing body weight or condition is noticed, the amount fed should be changed by 10% increments and the patient rechecked every 2 weeks for 1 month. At that point, if necessary, the amount fed should be changed again and the cycle repeated. Water intake should be encouraged (above) to achieve a urine specific gravity <1.020.

Veterinary Health Care Team Followup
Immediately postsurgery or following voiding urohydropropulsion, obtain data (radiography, complete urinalysis, serum concentrations of calcium, urea nitrogen and creatinine) to evaluate effectiveness of renal function and calcium homeostasis. If the patient is hypercalcemic, correct the underlying cause; if the dog is normocalcemic, initiate the above feeding plan. Patients should be monitored periodically (3-6 months) by urinalyses, radiographic or ultrasonographic procedures and other hematologic and urologic laboratory tests, as indicated. If necessary, consider thiazide therapy (above).

MISCELLANEOUS

See Appendix K for information about canine compound uroliths. For more information, see Chapters 38 and 41, Small Animal Clinical Nutrition, 5th edition.

Authors
Condensed from Chapter 41, Small Animal Clinical Nutrition, 5th edition, authored by Carl A. Osborne, Jody P. Lulich, John M. Kruger and Amy Cokley.

References
See Chapter 41, Small Animal Clinical Nutrition, 5th edition, on the website www.markmorrisinstitute.org for references.

Chapter
30 Canine Cystine Urolithiasis

CLINICAL POINTS

- Cystine (also called dicysteine) is a nonessential sulfur-containing amino acid composed of two molecules of cysteine.
- Prevalence of cystine uroliths varies geographically; as high as 39% in some European centers to just under 1% in the U.S.
- Numerous breeds affected including English bulldogs, mixed breeds, dachshunds, mastiffs, basset hounds and Newfoundlands; 98% occur in males.
- Mean age at time of cystine urolith retrieval is approximately 6 years. Cystine uroliths are often detected at <1 year of age in Newfoundlands. Compared to other breeds, the magnitude of the renal tubular transport defect for cystine in Newfoundlands is more severe.
- Most cystine uroliths are pure; a few contain ammonium urate, calcium oxalate and/or silica (Appendix K).
- More than 98% are removed from the lower urinary tract;

Abbreviations
AAFCO = Association of American Feed Control Officials
BCS = body condition score (Appendix A)
KNF = key nutritional factor
UTI = urinary tract infection

however, a relatively high incidence of cystine nephroliths has been observed in Newfoundlands.
- The main cause of uroliths is attributable to a genetic inborn error of metabolism resulting in cystinuria. Cystinuria is characterized by impaired absorption of dibasic amino acids (e.g., cystine, ornithine, lysine and arginine) by the intestine and proximal renal tubules. Amino acids other than cystine are soluble at normal physiologic urinary pH and are not lithogenic.
- Unless protein intake is severely restricted, abnormalities associated with loss of amino acids has not resulted in recognizable disorders, with the exception of formation of cystine uroliths.

- Impaired intestinal absorption of these amino acids is apparently harmless because they are nonessential and their dipeptide forms are still absorbed; thus, the major causes of morbidity and mortality associated with this disorder are sequelae of urolith formation.
- Newfoundlands and possibly other breeds (excluding mastiffs and English bulldogs) that form cystine uroliths before one year of age have a severe form of cystinuria caused by a homozygous mutation of the rBAT gene. Breeds in which cystine uroliths are recognized after the first year of life probably do not have this mutation. The quantity of cystine and other amino acids excreted in the urine of these dogs is not as great as that observed in Newfoundlands.
- High-protein foods increase the risk for cystine urolithiasis, including high-protein dry foods, especially those rich in methionine (a precursor of cysteine). Besides most meats, other food ingredients high in methionine include eggs, wheat and peanuts. Also, decreased protein intake reduces concentration of urea in the renal medulla; the associated reduction in urine concentrating ability is an important indirect benefit.
- Increased dietary sodium may enhance cystinuria.
- Cystine is relatively insoluble in acidic urine but becomes more soluble in alkaline urine; the solubility of cystine at a urinary pH of 7.8 is approximately double that at a pH of 5.0.
- Recommendations for urolith dissolution and prevention are based on mineral composition of uroliths; therefore, it is important to analyze uroliths whenever possible. Appendix K lists clinical signs, urologic diagnostic laboratories and other diagnostic aids.
- Detection of flat, colorless, hexagonal cystine crystals provides strong support for a diagnosis of cystinuria.
- Cystine urolith dissolution requires reducing urine cystine concentration and increasing cystine solubility through: 1) dietary modification, 2) administration of thiol-containing drugs and 3) alkalinization of urine (if necessary). Small cystine urocystoliths may be removed by voiding urohydropropulsion or retrieval with a urinary catheter (Appendix K). Urethroliths can be removed by lithotripsy.
- Recurrence is high, typically within 2-12 months without preventive therapy in most breeds; recurrence in Newfoundlands appears to be more rapid. Consider prevention in all cases.
- Feeding goals: use of appropriate foods, feeding methods and medical management can dissolve cystine uroliths and reduce their recurrence.

KEY NUTRITIONAL FACTORS

- Foods should provide recommended allowances of all required nutrients (nutritional adequacy), but should also contain specific levels of KNFs (certain nutrients that can assist in dissolution and prevention of recurrence of cystine urolithiasis).
- **Table 1** summarizes KNFs for foods intended for dissolution/prevention of cystine uroliths in dogs. They include moderate

Table 1. Key nutritional factors for foods for canine cystine urolith dissolution and prevention.

Factors	Dietary recommendations
Water	Water intake should be encouraged to achieve a urine specific gravity <1.020 Moist food will increase water consumption and formation of less concentrated urine
Protein	Avoid excess dietary protein Restrict high quality dietary protein to 10 to 18% dry matter
Sodium	Restrict sodium to <0.3% dry matter
Urinary pH	Feed a food that maintains an alkaline urine (urinary pH = 7.1 to 7.7)

restriction of protein and sodium and production of alkaline urine.
- Water is always a KNF and is particularly important for management of urolithiasis. Increased water intake increases urine volume and decreases urinary cystine concentration; it also enhances urine flow through the urinary tract.
- A detailed review of these recommendations can be found in Chapter 42, Small Animal Clinical Nutrition, 5th edition.

FEEDING PLAN

Assess and Select the Food
Ensure the Food's Basic Nutritional Adequacy. AAFCO nutritional adequacy statements are usually found on a product's label. AAFCO approval does not ensure a food will be effective in the dissolution and prevention of cystine uroliths.
Compare the Food's KNF Content with the Recommended Levels. **Table 2** lists commercially available foods used for dissolution and prevention of canine cystine uroliths and compares KNF content with recommended levels. Contact manufacturers for information for foods not in the table (manufacturer contact information is listed on product labels). Select a food that best approximates the recommended KNF levels.
Food Form. If readily consumed, moist foods are preferred; their consumption increases total water intake compared to dry foods. Also, high-protein dry foods are often associated with higher urine concentrations of urolith constituents such as sulfur amino acids. If dry foods are fed, consider adding liberal amounts of water. Do not leave moist foods or moistened dry foods at room temperature for prolonged intervals (below).
Increasing Water Intake. 1) Provide water bowls in multiple locations (e.g., several bowls outside in a large enclosure or a bowl on each level of the house). 2) Be sure water bowls are clean and filled regularly with fresh water. 3) Offer ice cubes as treats or snacks.
Manage Treats and Snacks. Many commercial treats and human foods (Appendix I) contain sodium in excess of KNF levels. If treats/snacks are fed, commercial treats that most closely match the KNF profile recommended for foods for cystine

Table 2. Levels of key nutritional factors in selected commercial veterinary therapeutic foods used for dissolution and to minimize recurrence of cystine uroliths in dogs compared to recommended levels.* (Numbers in red match optimal KNFs.)

Dry foods	Protein (%)	Sodium (%)	Urinary pH**
Recommended levels	10-18	<0.3	7.1-7.7
Hill's Prescription Diet u/d Canine	11.2	0.23	7.70
Medi-Cal Reduced Protein	13.7	0.2	na
Medi-Cal Renal LP 11	14.7	0.1	na
Medi-Cal Renal MP 14	18.4	0.1	na
Medi-Cal Vegetarian Formula	20.9	0.4	na
Royal Canin Veterinary Diet Hypoallergenic HP 19	23.1	0.44	na
Royal Canin Veterinary Diet Vegetarian Formula	19.1	0.15	6.78
Moist foods	**Protein (%)**	**Sodium (%)**	**Urinary pH****
Recommended levels	10-18	<0.3	7.1-7.7
Hill's Prescription Diet u/d Canine	13.3	0.28	7.40
Medi-Cal Reduced Protein	16.5	0.2	na
Medi-Cal Renal LP	16.8	0.1	na
Medi-Cal Renal MP	28.2	0.2	na
Medi-Cal Vegetarian Formula	26.4	0.5	na

Key: na = information not available from the manufacturer.
*Manufacturers' published values; protein and sodium expressed as % dry matter; when possible chose moist foods.
**Protocols for measuring urinary pH may vary.

urolithiasis management are best. Limit consumption to <10% of the total diet on a volume, weight or calorie basis. Options: 1) use the opposite form of the food being fed; i.e., if a dry food is fed, offer small amounts of the same food in moist form as a snack and vice versa, 2) keep kibbles of a dry food for cystine urolithiasis prevention/dissolution in a separate container away from the usual feeding area and use as treats.

Assess and Determine the Feeding Method

Determine How Much Food to Feed. The amount to feed can be estimated either from feeding guides on product labels or by calculation (Appendix C). These estimates are only starting points and will likely need to be adjusted (see Followup below).
Consider How to Offer the Food. Maintaining an alkaline urinary pH is important for cystine urolith dissolution and prevention. Free-choice feeding is associated with more persistent aciduria compared to meal feeding. Thus, meal feeding (2 times/day) is recommended whether using dry and/or moist foods. Feeding a specific amount/day is recommended for dogs that have a tendency to be overweight.
Manage Food Changes. A transition period to avoid GI upsets and to facilitate acceptance of a new food is good practice. Example: to change to a cystine urolith dissolution/prevention food, replace 25% of the old food with the new food on Day 1 and continue this incremental change daily until the change is complete on Day 4. Appendix E provides additional information.
Food and Water Receptacle Husbandry. Food and water bowls should be washed regularly with warm soapy water and rinsed well. Dishes used for moist foods need daily cleaning. Discard moist or moistened dry foods after 2-4 hours of room temperature exposure to avoid foodborne illnesses (Appendix F).

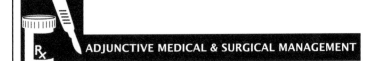

ADJUNCTIVE MEDICAL & SURGICAL MANAGEMENT

Thiol-Containing Drugs

2-MPG (tiopronin[a]). 2-MPG decreases urine concentration of cystine by combining with cysteine to form cysteine-2-MPG, which is more soluble than cystine. Oral 2-MPG at 30 mg/kg (divided in two equal doses) is effective for dissolution of cystine urocystoliths. A cystine litholytic food and 2-MPG are more effective for dissolution of uroliths than either alone. The mean time required to dissolve cystine uroliths with combined therapy is ~2.5 months (range 11-211 days).

POTENTIAL SIDE EFFECTS. Nonpruritic vesicular skin lesions, thrombocytopenia, anemia, elevated hepatic enzyme activity and protein-losing glomerular disease may occur. Dogs that become hypersensitive to D-penicillamine (below) may also become hypersensitive to 2-MPG. The beneficial action of both drugs is dose dependent as are the side effects.
D-Penicillamine (and Other Thiol-Containing Drugs). D-penicillamine[b] is effective in reducing urine cystine concentrations but adverse side effects limit its use; 2-MPG is a better option. For more information about this and other thiol-containing drugs, see Chapter 42, Small Animal Clinical Nutrition, 5th edition.

Urine Alkalinizing Agents

Cystine solubility increases in alkaline urine. If an increase in urinary pH is required (see Followup below), supplemental potassium citrate (wax matrix tablets[c] or liquid[d]) should be considered. Chewable treats[e] are also available. Dose is 40-75 mg/kg q12h. Divided doses help maintain a consistently non-acidic urine. Avoid sodium bicarbonate (sodium may enhance cystinuria) and do not exceed pH 7.7 (a potential risk for development of calcium phosphate uroliths).

FOLLOWUP

Owner Followup

Owners should weigh their dog (if possible) and/or grade its condition (BCS) monthly. If a trend of increasing or decreasing body weight or BCS is noticed, the amount fed should be changed by 10% increments and the patient rechecked every 2 weeks for 1 month. At that point, if necessary, the amount fed should be changed again and the cycle repeated. Water intake should be encouraged to achieve a urine specific gravity <1.020. *Compliance.* If the dog lives in a multi-pet household, deny access to other pets' food. Counsel owners to adhere strictly to feeding only the litholytic food.

Veterinary Health Care Team Followup

Urolith Dissolution. Monitor urolith size/location (radiography, ultrasonography), urinary pH, urine sediment and serum urea nitrogen monthly. **Table 3** lists expected changes. Decreased serum urea nitrogen (<10 mg/dl) suggests compliance. If necessary, administer potassium citrate orally to eliminate aciduria; the recommended pH is 7.5 (range 7.1-7.7). Treat UTI if present. Continue litholytic food, 2-MPG and alkalinizing therapy for 1 month after disappearance of uroliths as detected by radiography. If slow/no response, consider increasing the 2-MPG dose to 20 mg/kg q12h.

Prevention of Recurrence. Continue the dissolution feeding plan. The objectives are minimization of cystine crystalluria and negative cyanide-nitroprusside test results (below). Monitor regularly; **Table 3** lists expected changes. If necessary, urine alkalinization and/or 2-MPG therapy may be included to maintain urine cystine levels <200 mg/liter. If the dosage cannot be titrated by measuring urine cystine, 2-MPG may be given at the prescribed dose (above).

MISCELLANEOUS

For more information, see Chapters 38 and 42, Small Animal Clinical Nutrition, 5th edition.

Table 3. Expected changes associated with combined dietary and medical therapy of cystine uroliths.

Factors	Pre-therapy	During therapy	Prevention therapy
Polyuria	±	1+ to 3+	1+ to 3+
Pollakiuria	0 to 4+	↑ then ↓	0
Hematuria	0 to 4+	↓	0
Urine specific gravity	Variable	1.004-1.020	1.004-1.020
Urinary pH	<7.0	>7.0	>7.0
Pyuria	0 to 4+	↓	0
Cystine crystals	0 to 4+	0	Variable
Bacteriuria	0 to 4+	0	0
Bacterial culture of urine	0 to 4+	0	0
Urea nitrogen (mg/dl)	Variable	<15	≤15
Urolith size and number	Small to large	↓	0

Screening Patients for Cystinuria with the Nitroprusside Test

Submit fresh urine or urine allowed to dry on 3-mm filter paper to the Metabolic Screening Laboratory, Section of Medical Genetics, Veterinary Hospital, University of Pennsylvania, Philadelphia 19104-6010 (fax number 215-573-2162). Contact this center for specific instructions about DNA testing, urine and blood sample preservation and sample submission. Their website address is www.vet.upenn.edu/penngen/research.

Canine Compound Urolithiasis

See Appendix K for more information.

Authors

Condensed from Chapter 42, Small Animal Clinical Nutrition, 5th edition, authored by Carl A. Osborne, Jody P. Lulich and Michelle Buettner.

References

See Chapter 42, Small Animal Clinical Nutrition, 5th edition, on the website www.markmorrisinstitute.org for references.

Endnotes

a. Thiola. Mission Pharmacal, San Antonio, TX, USA.
b. Cuprimine. Merck and Co., Rahway, NJ, USA.
c. Urocit-K. Mission Pharmacal, San Antonio, TX, USA.
d. Polycitra-K. Willen Drug Co., Baltimore, MD, USA.
e. K-CIT-V. V.E.T. Pharmaceuticals, Inc., Fenton, MO, USA.

CLINICAL POINTS

- Struvite is composed of MAP hexahydrate.
- For years, struvite was the most common urolith type in dogs but the relative percentage appears to be decreasing; in 2007 the prevalence of struvite uroliths fell below that of calcium oxalate.
- Numerous breeds are affected including mixed breeds, Shih Tzus, miniature schnauzers, Bichon Frises, pugs, dachshunds, Labrador retrievers, miniature poodles, Pekingese, cocker spaniels and Lhasa apsos.
- Mean age at time of struvite urolith retrieval is 6 years.
- 99% are removed from the lower urinary tract; **Table 1** lists these and other risk factors.
- Urine must be supersaturated with MAP hexahydrate for struvite uroliths to form and may be associated with: UTIs caused by urease-producing microbes, genetic predisposition, alkaline urine and/or food.
- Metabolic and anatomic abnormalities may indirectly induce struvite urolithiasis by predisposing to UTIs.
- Dietary and metabolic factors may be involved in the development of sterile struvite uroliths; microbial urease is not involved.
- 85% occur in females; possibly associated with increased frequency of UTI.
- Struvite uroliths can form within 2-8 weeks after infection with urease-producing bacteria.
- Microbial urease in the presence of adequate urea increases urinary pH and concentrations of ammonium, phosphate and carbonate, which favor formation of struvite (also calcium apatite and carbonate apatite). The degree of hyperammonuria, hypercarbonaturia and alkaluria depends on the availability of urea, which in turn depends on dietary protein intake and acid-base status. Excess protein intake results in increased urinary excretion of urea or ammonium derived from catabolism of amino acids for energy.
- Dietary protein restriction can also increase urine volume by contributing to obligatory polyuria via a decrease in renal medullary urea concentration resulting from a reduction of hepatic urea production.
- Foods high in protein are generally high in phosphorus unless special ingredients are used in formulation.
- Abnormal urinary excretion of phosphorus or magnesium is not required for initiation and growth of infection-induced struvite uroliths. However, foods high in phosphorus and magnesium may predispose susceptible dogs to sterile struvite urolith formation. Also, pH reversibly influences urinary concentration of anionic phosphate.
- Avoiding excessive dietary magnesium and phosphorus may

reduce the urinary concentration of these minerals.
- Continued production of ammonia as a consequence of urease-induced ureolysis may cause an inflammatory response in the urothelium. The associated increase in urinary proteinaceous inflammatory products may act as a form of matrix and contribute to lithogenesis.
- UTIs may also reduce urine concentration of citrate, a crystallization inhibitor. Citrate can combine with cations such as calcium and magnesium to increase their solubility and decrease struvite formation.
- Recommendations for urolith dissolution and prevention are based on the mineral composition of uroliths; therefore, it is important to analyze uroliths whenever possible. Appendix K lists clinical signs, urologic diagnostic laboratories and other diagnostic aids.
- Recommendations for dissolution of struvite include: eradication/control of UTIs due to urease-producing microbes is the most important factor in preventing recurrence of most infection-induced struvite uroliths, use of litholytic foods and administration of urease inhibitors, if necessary.
- The rate of recurrence after dietary and medical dissolution is less frequent than that associated with surgery, attributable to the inability to remove all uroliths, especially those located in inaccessible sites or those that are small or subvisual.
- Feeding goals: dissolve struvite uroliths and minimize their recurrence through the use of appropriate foods, feeding methods and medical management.

KEY NUTRITIONAL FACTORS

- Foods should provide recommended allowances of all required nutrients (nutritional adequacy), but should also contain specific levels of KNFs (certain nutrients that can assist in dissolution or prevention of recurrence of struvite urolithiasis).
- **Table 2** summarizes KNFs for foods intended for dissolution or prevention of recurrence of struvite uroliths in dogs. They include restriction of protein, phosphorus and magnesium and production of acidic urine.
- Water is always a KNF and is particularly important for management of urolithiasis. Increased water intake increases urine volume and decreases urinary struvite concentration; it

Table 1. Some potential risk factors for canine infection-induced struvite urolithiasis.

Diet	Urine	Patient/metabolic	Drugs
High protein content (source of urea)	Urease-positive UTI	Females	Glucocorticoid-associated bacterial UTI
Urine alkalinizing potential	High urea concentration	Breeds	
High phosphorus content	Hyperammonuria	Miniature schnauzers	
High magnesium content	High-ionic phosphorus concentration	Bichon Frises	
	High magnesium levels	Shih Tzus	
	High pH	Pugs	
	Urine retention	Dachshunds	
	Concentration of urine and thus lithogenic substances	Hyperadrenocorticism associated with bacterial UTI	

Key: UTI = urinary tract infection.

Table 2. Key nutritional factors for dissolution and prevention of canine struvite urolithiasis.

Factors	Dietary recommendations
Water	Water intake should be encouraged to achieve urine specific gravity <1.020
	Moist food will increase water consumption and formation of less concentrated urine
Protein	Avoid excess dietary protein
	Dissolution: restrict dietary protein to ≤8%, dry matter (DM)
	Prevention: restrict dietary protein to <25% DM
Phosphorus	Avoid excess dietary phosphorus
	Dissolution: restrict dietary phosphorus to ≤0.1% DM
	Prevention: restrict dietary phosphorus to <0.6% DM
Magnesium	Avoid excess dietary magnesium
	Dissolution: restrict dietary magnesium to <0.02% DM
	Prevention: restrict dietary magnesium to 0.04 to 0.1% DM
Urinary pH	Feed a food that maintains an acidic urine
	Dissolution: urinary pH = 5.9 to 6.1
	Prevention: urinary pH = 6.2 to 6.4

Table 3. Key nutritional factors in selected commercial veterinary therapeutic foods used for dissolution of struvite uroliths in dogs compared to recommended levels.* (Numbers in red match optimal KNFs.)

Dry foods	Protein (%)	Phosphorus (%)	Magnesium (%)	Urinary pH**
Recommended levels	≤8	≤0.1	<0.02	5.9-6.1
Royal Canin Veterinary Diet Control Formula	23.9	0.84	0.130	6.0-6.3
Royal Canin Veterinary Diet Urinary SO 14	17.0	0.63	0.066	5.5-6.0
Moist foods	**Protein (%)**	**Phosphorus (%)**	**Magnesium (%)**	**Urinary pH****
Recommended levels	≤8	≤0.1	<0.02	5.9-6.1
Hill's Prescription Diet s/d Canine	_7.9_	_0.10_	0.024	_5.935_
Royal Canin Veterinary Diet Control Formula	22.8	0.66	0.078	6.0-6.3
Royal Canin Veterinary Diet Urinary SO	18.5	0.86	0.059	5.5-6.0

*Manufacturers' published values; nutrients expressed on a dry matter basis; moist foods are best.
**Protocols for measuring urinary pH may vary.

also enhances urine flow through the urinary tract.
- A detailed review of these recommendations can be found in Chapter 43, Small Animal Clinical Nutrition, 5th edition.

FEEDING PLAN

Struvite Dissolution
Assess and Select the Food.
COMPARE THE FOOD'S KNF CONTENT WITH THE RECOMMENDED LEVELS. Table 3 lists selected commercially available foods used for dissolution of canine struvite uroliths

and compares KNF content with recommended levels. Contact manufacturers for information for foods not in the table (manufacturer contact information is listed on product labels).

FOOD FORM. If readily consumed, moist foods are preferred; their consumption increases total water intake compared to dry foods. If feeding dry foods, consider adding liberal amounts of water. Do not leave moist foods or moistened dry foods at room temperature for prolonged intervals (below).
Increasing Water Intake. 1) Provide water bowls in multiple locations (e.g., several bowls outside in a large enclosure or a bowl on each level of the house). 2) Be sure water bowls are clean and filled regularly with fresh water. 3) Offer ice cubes as treats or snacks.

Table 4. Characteristic clinical findings before and after initiation of dietary and medical therapy, or dietary therapy alone, to dissolve struvite uroliths in nonazotemic dogs.*

Factors	Pre-therapy	During therapy	After successful therapy**
Polyuria	±	1+ to 3+	Negative
Pollakiuria	1+ to 4+	Transient ↑; subsequent ↓	Negative
Gross hematuria	0 to 4+	↓ by 5 to 10 days	Negative
Abnormal urine odor	0 to 4+	↓ by 5 to 10 days	Negative
Small uroliths voided	±	Common in females	Negative
Urine specific gravity	Variable	1.004 to 1.014	Normal
Urinary pH	≥7	Decreased (usually acidic)	Variable
Urine protein	1+ to 4+	Decreased to absent	Negative
Urine RBC	1+ to 4+	Decreased to absent	Negative
Urine WBC	1+ to 4+	Decreased to absent	Negative
Struvite crystals	0 to 4+	Usually absent	Variable
Other crystals	Variable	May persist	May persist
Bacteriuria	0 to 4+	Decreased to absent	Negative
Quantitative bacterial urine culture	0 to 4+	Decreased to absent	Negative
Serum urea nitrogen	>15 mg/dl	<10 mg/dl	Dependent on food
Serum creatinine	Normal	Normal	Normal
Serum alkaline phosphatase	Normal	↑ by 2 to 5 times	Normal
Serum albumin	Normal	↓ by 0.5 to 1 g/dl	Normal
Serum phosphorus	Normal	Slight decrease	Normal
Urolith size (radiographic)	Small to large	Progressive decrease	Negative
Hemogram	Normal	Normal	Normal

*For dogs with urinary tract infection, therapy consists of a litholytic food and antimicrobial agents. For dogs without urinary tract infection, therapy consists of a litholytic food.
**All forms of therapy withdrawn.

Table 5. Mean times for struvite urolith dissolution.

Urolith location and infective status	Mean time for dissolution	Comments and precautions
Infection-induced urocystoliths	Approximately 2.5 months (range two weeks to seven months)	Use appropriate caution in dogs at increased risk for pancreatitis, dogs with renal failure and dogs with hypoalbuminemic edema
Sterile urocystoliths	Three to four weeks	If idiopathic, appropriately monitor for recurrence
Infection-induced struvite urocystoliths in immature dogs	Less than two weeks	If circumstances warrant feeding for a longer period, monitor body weight, body condition, serum albumin concentration and packed cell volume for evidence of protein-calorie malnutrition
Infection-induced nephroliths	Approximately 184 days (range 67 to 300 days)	Contraindicated in dogs with concomitant obstruction to urine outflow

Manage Treats and Snacks. If owners insist on feeding treats/ snacks, suggest small portions of the food being fed, or if available, the opposite form of the food fed; i.e., if a dry food is fed, offer small amounts of the same food in moist form and vice versa; keep kibbles of a dry food for struvite urolithiasis for use as treats in a separate container away from the usual feeding area.

Precautions.

LONG-TERM FEEDING. KNFs for properly formulated canine litholytic foods are restricted to near minimum requirements and are designed for short-term (weeks-months) dissolution therapy. These foods may be marginally adequate for some patients if feed long-term (months-years).

PUPPIES. Struvite urocystoliths can be successfully dissolved in puppies, often in a few days. Recommend limiting feeding duration >2 times/week. If the food needs to be fed for longer periods, monitor body weight, BCS, serum albumin and PCV for evidence of protein-calorie malnutrition and adjust dietary management as necessary. The urocystoliths may be removed by voiding urohydropropulsion (Appendix K) or lithotripsy, if their size has been reduced enough to permit passage through a distended urethra.

ABNORMAL FLUID RETENTION. Properly formulated struvite litholytic foods are restricted in protein and supplemented with sodium chloride. Both could affect fluid balance. Therefore, the food should not be routinely fed to patients with comorbid diseases associated with positive fluid balance (e.g., heart failure, nephrotic syndrome) or hypertension.

RENAL FAILURE.

Obstruction of Urine Outflow. Regard complete obstruction of urine outflow caused by uroliths in patients with a concomitant UTI as an emergency. Obstruction and pyelonephritis caused by rapid spread of infection throughout the kidneys is likely to induce acute renal failure and septicemia. Dietary dissolution of struvite uroliths located in the upper urinary tract should not be considered until adequate urine flow has been restored and

Table 6. Key nutritional factors in selected commercial veterinary therapeutic foods used to minimize recurrence of struvite urolithiasis in dogs compared to recommended levels.* (Numbers in red match optimal KNFs.)

Dry foods	Protein (%)	Phosphorus (%)	Magnesium (%)	Urinary pH**
Recommended levels	<25	<0.6	0.04-0.1	6.2-6.4
Hill's Prescription Diet c/d Canine	22.3	0.59	0.111	6.22
Hill's Prescription Diet w/d Canine	18.9	0.56	0.088	6.40
Hill's Prescription Diet w/d with Chicken Canine	19.1	0.56	0.080	6.30
Medi-Cal Preventive Formula	23.9	0.8	na	na
Medi-Cal Urinary SO	16.7	0.6	0.2	5.5-6.0
Medi-Cal Weight Control/Mature	19.5	0.8	na	6.4
Purina Veterinary Diet DCO Dual Fiber Control	25.3	0.93	0.130	6.0-6.2
Purina Veterinary Diet OM Overweight Management	31.1	0.89	0.130	6.2-6.4
Royal Canin Veterinary Diet Control Formula	23.9	0.84	0.130	6.0-6.3
Royal Canin Veterinary Diet Urinary SO 14	17.0	0.63	0.066	5.5-6.0

Moist foods	Protein (%)	Phosphorus (%)	Magnesium (%)	Urinary pH**
Recommended levels	<25	<0.6	0.04-0.1	6.2-6.4
Hill's Prescription Diet c/d Canine	23.6	0.51	0.079	6.16
Hill's Prescription Diet w/d Canine	17.9	0.52	0.088	6.40
Medi-Cal Preventive Formula	23.8	0.7	na	na
Medi-Cal Urinary SO	18.7	0.8	0.1	5.5-6.0
Medi-Cal Weight Control/Mature	21.5	0.6	na	6.6
Purina Veterinary Diet OM Overweight Management	44.1	1.06	0.190	6.2-6.4
Royal Canin Veterinary Diet Control Formula	22.8	0.66	0.078	6.0-6.3
Royal Canin Veterinary Diet Urinary SO	18.5	0.86	0.059	5.5-6.0

Key: na = information not available from the manufacturer.
*Manufacturers' published values; nutrients expressed on a dry matter basis; moist foods are best.
**Protocols for measuring urinary pH may vary.

deficits/excesses in fluid, electrolyte, acid-base and endocrine balance have been corrected.

Nonobstructing Struvite Nephroliths. Struvite uroliths in nonazotemic renal failure patients (caused by ascending pyelonephritis) may be amenable to dietary dissolution. Use litholytic foods cautiously in patients with moderate azotemic primary renal failure because they may induce protein malnutrition if fed for prolonged periods and some litholytic foods contain increased sodium to promote diuresis.

PATIENTS AT RISK FOR PANCREATITIS. Approximately 1 dog/250 is affected by pancreatitis; ~1 dog/40 fed a struvite litholytic food may develop pancreatitis. Litholytic foods may be high in fat so that restriction of nutrient KNFs is more readily accomplished. Increased dietary fat is a risk factor for pancreatitis; monitor serum activity of pancreatic enzymes (amylase, lipase, trypsin-like immunoreactivity) before initiating therapy in patients at risk for pancreatitis. Repeat if clinical signs of pancreatitis develop during treatment with litholytic foods. Consider other signs as well.

Pancreatitis Risk Factors. Age (5-8 years) is a risk. Breeds at risk include miniature schnauzers, Bichon Frises, Yorkshire terriers, Chihuahuas, Jack Russell terriers, Japanese spaniels, Labrador retrievers, Maltese and Shetland sheepdogs. Female miniature schnauzers are also at risk for infection-induced struvite urolithiasis. Hyperadrenocorticism is a risk for UTIs and pancreatitis. Advise clients of these associations and how to respond to possible adverse events.

Assess and Determine the Feeding Method
Determine How Much Food to Feed. The amount to feed can be estimated either from feeding guides on product labels or by calculation (Appendix C). These estimates are only starting points and will likely need to be adjusted (See Followup below).

Consider How to Offer the Food. Maintaining an acidic urinary pH is important for struvite urolith dissolution and prevention. Free-choice feeding is associated with more persistent aciduria compared to meal feeding. For moist foods (recommended, above), use meal feeding (>3 times/day). Limit feed either form if patient has a tendency to be overweight.

Manage Food Changes. A transition period to avoid GI upsets and to facilitate acceptance of a new food is good practice. Example: to change to a new food, replace 25% of the old food with the new food on Day 1 and continue this incremental change daily until the change is complete on Day 4. Appendix E provides additional information.

Food and Water Receptacle Husbandry. Food and water bowls should be washed regularly with warm soapy water and rinsed well. Dishes used for moist foods need daily cleaning. Discard moist or moistened dry foods after 2-4 hours of room temperature exposure to avoid foodborne illnesses (Appendix F).

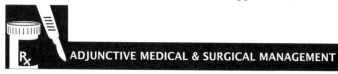

ADJUNCTIVE MEDICAL & SURGICAL MANAGEMENT

Eradication or Control of UTIs
Sterilization of urine is an important component in the overall management of struvite urolithiasis (not necessary for patients with persistently sterile urine). Select oral antimicrobial agents based on quantitative bacterial culture and antimicrobial susceptibility tests. Diuresis induced by concurrent dietary management reduces urine concentration of antimicrobial agents. To prevent relapse of bacteriuria and infection, continue therapy as long as uroliths can be identified by radiography.

Urease Inhibitors

Consider including AHA in the therapeutic regimen if infection-induced struvite uroliths do not dissolve after a trial with diet modification and antimicrobial agents. Dosage is 12.5 mg/kg PO q12h. Higher dosages may cause reversible hemolytic anemia and abnormalities in bilirubin metabolism. Do not administer to pregnant dogs (teratogenic); this drug has not been evaluated in puppies. It is not necessary for patients with persistently sterile urine.

Surgery and Other Procedures

Nephroliths and Obstructive Ureteroliths. Manage by surgical intervention or, if possible, by percutaneous nephropyelolithotomy, especially if associated with concomitant bacterial infection. Prolonged dietary and medical therapy is unlikely to be effective in patients with poorly functioning kidneys; uroliths must be completely surrounded by urine that is undersaturated with struvite for prolonged periods to be dissolved.

Obstructive Urethroliths. Manage by lithotripsy or surgery.

Anatomic Abnormalities. Consider surgery if correctable abnormalities predisposing the patient to recurrent UTIs are identified by diagnostic imaging or other means.

Small Urocystoliths and Urethroliths. Remove by voiding urohydropropulsion (Appendix K) or lithotripsy.

FOLLOWUP

Owner Followup

Owners should weigh their dog (if possible) and/or grade its body condition (BCS) monthly. If a trend of increasing or decreasing body weight or BCS is noticed, the amount fed should be changed by 10% increments and the patient rechecked every 2 weeks for 1 month. At that point, if necessary, the amount fed should be changed again and the cycle repeated. Water intake should be encouraged to achieve a urine specific gravity <1.020.

Compliance. If the dog comes from a multi-pet household, deny access to other pets' food. Counsel owners to adhere strictly to feeding only the litholytic food.

Veterinary Health Care Team Followup

Table 4 lists characteristic clinical findings before and after combined dietary and medical therapy. Monitor monthly. Decreased serum urea nitrogen (<10 mg/dl) suggests compliance. Continue feeding the litholytic food for 1 month after disappearance of uroliths as detected by radiography. **Table 5** lists mean times for struvite urolith dissolution.

Dissolution Failure. If uroliths increase in size, or do not begin to decrease in size after 4-8 weeks of appropriate dietary and medical management, possible problems include: 1) wrong mineral component identified, 2) nucleus is different from other portions of the urolith (compound urolith) and/or 3) client or patient is not complying. Consider concurrent AHA (above) for patients with persistent uroliths and persistent urease-producing microburia despite proper dietary and antibiotic therapies.

FEEDING PLAN

Prevention of Struvite Urolith Recurrence

After urolith dissolution, initiate a program to ensure that urolithogenesis does not recur. The success of urolith preventive programs depends on continued pet owner commitment, proper food and feeding methods and patient monitoring (followup). Also, consider concurrent or alternative medical management.

Assess and Select the Food.

ENSURE THE FOOD'S BASIC NUTRITIONAL ADEQUACY. AAFCO nutritional adequacy statements are usually found on a product's label. AAFCO approval does not ensure a food will be effective in minimizing recurrence of struvite uroliths or in preventing other long-term health problems.

COMPARE THE FOOD'S KNF CONTENT WITH THE RECOMMENDED LEVELS. **Table 6** lists selected commercially available foods used to minimize recurrence of canine struvite uroliths and compares KNF content with recommended levels. Contact manufacturers for information for foods not in the table (manufacturer contact information is listed on product labels).

FOOD FORM. If readily consumed, moist foods are preferred; their consumption increases total water intake compared to dry foods. Consider adding water if dry foods are fed. Do not leave moist foods or moistened dry foods at room temperature for prolonged intervals (below).

Increasing Water Intake. 1) Provide water bowls in multiple locations (e.g., several bowls outside in a large enclosure or a bowl on each level of the house). 2) Be sure water bowls are clean and filled regularly with fresh water. 3) Offer ice cubes as treats or snacks.

Precautions. Prolonged use of this type of food has been associated with calcium oxalate crystalluria and/or calcium oxalate uroliths, especially in dogs predisposed to calcium oxalate uroliths.

Urolith Dissolution Foods for Prevention. Recommend long-term use of low-protein litholytic foods only if patients frequently develop recurrent urolithiasis despite attempts to control infection, increase diuresis and acidify the urine. Use if the benefits of therapy outweigh the risks and monitor regularly.

Manage Treats and Snacks. If owners insist on feeding treats/snacks, suggest small portions of the food being fed, or if available, the opposite form of the food fed; i.e., if a dry food is fed, offer small amounts of the same food in moist form and vice versa; another option is to store kibbles of a dry food for struvite urolithiasis prevention for use as treats in a separate container away from the usual feeding area.

Assess and Determine the Feeding Method.

CONSIDER HOW TO OFFER THE FOOD/MANAGE FOOD CHANGES/FOOD AND WATER RECEPTACLE HUSBANDRY. See recommendations for struvite urolith dissolution (above).

induced by recurrent UTI. Although formation of less concentrated urine tends to minimize the supersaturation of urine with lithogenic crystalloids (a benefit), it tends to counteract innate antimicrobial properties of urine (a risk).

FOLLOWUP

Owner Followup
Owners should weigh their dog (if possible) and/or grade its body condition (BCS) monthly. If a trend of increasing or decreasing body weight or BCS is noticed, the amount fed should be changed by 10% increments and the patient rechecked every 2 weeks for 1 month. At that point, if necessary, the amount fed should be changed again and the cycle repeated. Instruct owners to observe for signs of recurrent UTIs.

Veterinary Health Care Team Followup
Regular clinical examinations should include a complete urinalysis (**Table 4**).
Medical Management of UTI. Eradication/control of UTIs due to urease-producing bacteria is most important in minimizing recurrence of infection-induced struvite uroliths. If UTI persists or is recurrent, indefinite therapy is indicated with prophylactic dosages of appropriate antimicrobials. If UTI persists, consider concurrent AHA therapy. Reconsider whether or not to induce prophylactic diuresis in patients with a history of struvite uroliths

MISCELLANEOUS

See Appendix K for information about canine compound urolithiasis. For more information about struvite urolithiasis, see Chapters 38 and 43, Small Animal Clinical Nutrition, 5th edition.

Authors
Condensed from Chapter 43, Small Animal Clinical Nutrition, 5th edition, authored by Carl A. Osborne, Jody P. Lulich, Hasan Albasan and Laurie L. Swanson.

References
See Chapter 43, Small Animal Clinical Nutrition, 5th edition, on the website www.markmorrisinstitute.org for references.

Chapter 32

Canine Silica Urolithiasis

CLINICAL POINTS

- Silicon (Si) is a naturally occurring nonmetallic element. When combined with oxygen, silicon forms SiO_2 and is called silica or silicon dioxide.
- Out of >350,000 canine uroliths analyzed, silica accounted for 0.4%. Silica uroliths may contain varying quantities of other minerals, especially calcium oxalate.
- Most canine silica uroliths have a jackstone configuration and occur in multiples with some patients having more than 30.
- 99% of silica uroliths were removed from the lower urinary tract.
- The mean age of dogs at the time of urolith retrieval was ~7-8 years. Males are affected (95%) much more often than females. Females may void small silica uroliths before they cause clinical signs, thereby reducing the detection rate.
- 82 different breeds were affected including mixed breeds, German shepherd dogs, golden retrievers, Shih Tzus, black Labrador retrievers, rottweilers, miniature schnauzers, cocker

Abbreviations
AAFCO = Association of American Feed Control Officials
BCS = body condition score (Appendix A)
KNF = key nutritional factor
UTI = urinary tract infection

spaniels, Yorkshire terriers, Lhasa apsos and old English sheep dogs.
- Silicic acid is readily absorbed across the intestinal wall. Animal tissues contain very low concentrations of silica whereas plants contain much larger quantities, particularly plant hulls. Thus, certain plant-based ingredients in foods are risks for silica urolithiasis.
- Rice and soybean hulls and corn gluten feed (not corn gluten meal) are examples of ingredients high in silica; foods containing them increase the risk in susceptible dogs. Corn gluten meal is an unlikely source of silica in pet foods.
- Another possible risk is consumption of soil, usually secondary to food-associated pica.
- Prolonged consumption of large doses of antacids containing magnesium trisilicate is a risk factor.

- Note that the type of silica compound ingested influences its absorption from the GI tract. Thus, large quantities of silica in food may be absorbed and excreted in urine.
- Moderate restriction of dietary protein contributes to obligatory polyuria by decreasing renal medullary urea concentration.
- Silica is less soluble in acidic than alkaline biologic environments, such as urine.
- Recommendations for urolith dissolution and prevention are based on mineral composition of uroliths; therefore, it is important to analyze uroliths whenever possible. Appendix K lists clinical signs, urologic diagnostic laboratories and other diagnostic aids.
- Surgery is the only practical method to remove large silica uroliths; small uroliths may be removed by voiding urohydropropulsion (Appendix K). Consider lithotripsy to remove urethroliths.
- The goal of dietary management is to prevent recurrence by use of appropriate foods, feeding methods and medical management.

KEY NUTRITIONAL FACTORS

- Foods should provide recommended allowances of all required nutrients (nutritional adequacy), but should also contain specific levels of KNFs (certain nutrients that can assist in the prevention of recurrence of silica urolithiasis).
- Table 1 summarizes KNFs for foods intended for prevention of recurrence of silica uroliths; these include moderate restriction of protein, avoiding foods containing ingredients high in silica and promoting production of alkaline urinary pH.
- Water is always a KNF but is particularly important for management of urolithiasis. Increased water intake increases urine volume and decreases urinary silica concentrations; it also enhances urine flow through the urinary tract.
- A detailed review of these recommendations can be found in Chapter 44, Small Animal Clinical Nutrition, 5th edition.

FEEDING PLAN

Assess and Select the Food
Ensure the Food's Basic Nutritional Adequacy. AAFCO nutritional adequacy statements are usually found on a product's label. AAFCO approval does not ensure a food will be effective in minimizing the recurrence of silica urolithiasis.
Compare the Food's KNF Content with the Recommended Levels. Table 2 lists commercially available foods used to minimize recurrence of silica urolithiasis and compares KNF content with recommended levels. Contact manufacturers for information for foods not in the table (manufacturer contact information is listed on product labels). Select a food that best approximates the recommended KNF levels.

Food Ingredients. Check the ingredient list on product labels; avoid foods listing "corn gluten feed" (corn gluten meal is an acceptable ingredient), "rice hulls" or "soybean hulls" as one of the first 4 non-water ingredients.

Food Form. Adequate water intake in urolithiasis patients is particularly important. If readily consumed, moist foods are preferred; their consumption increases total water intake compared to dry foods. Consider adding liberal amounts of water if dry foods are fed. Do not leave moist foods or moistened dry foods at room temperature for prolonged intervals (>2-4 hours, below).

Increase Water Intake. 1) Provide water bowls in multiple locations (e.g., several bowls outside in a large enclosure or a bowl on each level of the house). 2) Be sure water bowls are clean and filled regularly with fresh water. 3) Offer ice cubes as treats.

Manage Treats and Snacks. Treats/snacks should not be fed excessively; limit consumption to <10% of the total diet on a volume, weight or calorie basis. The same recommendations regarding avoiding certain food ingredients (above) apply.

Assess and Determine the Feeding Method
Determine How Much Food to Feed. The amount to feed can be estimated either from feeding guides on product labels or by calculation (Appendix C). These estimates are only starting points and will likely need to be adjusted (see Followup below).

Consider How to Offer the Food. Maintaining an alkaline urinary pH is recommended for silica urolith prevention. Free-choice feeding is associated with more persistent aciduria compared to meal feeding. Thus, meal feeding (2 times/day) is recommended whether using dry and/or moist foods.

Manage Food Changes. A transition period to avoid GI upsets and to facilitate acceptance of a new food is good practice. Example: to change to a new food, replace 25% of the old food with the new food on Day 1 and continue this incremental change daily until the change is complete on Day 4. Appendix E provides additional information.

Food and Water Receptacle Husbandry. Food and water bowls should be washed regularly with warm soapy water and rinsed well. Dishes used for moist foods need daily cleaning. Discard moist or moistened dry foods after 2-4 hours of room temperature exposure to avoid foodborne illnesses (Appendix F).

FOLLOWUP

Owner Followup
Owners should weigh their dog (if possible) and/or grade its body condition (BCS) monthly. The amount fed should be changed by 10% increments and the patient rechecked every 2 weeks for 1 month if a trend of increasing or decreasing body weight or BCS is noticed. At that point, if necessary, the amount fed should be changed again and the cycle repeated. Water intake should be encouraged to achieve a urine specific gravity <1.020.

Compliance. If the dog lives in a multi-pet household deny access to other pets' food.

Veterinary Health Care Team Followup

Immediately postsurgery or after voiding urohydropropulsion, obtain baseline data (radiography, complete urinalysis). Reevaluate every 3-4 months, initially. Depending on the results, the interval may subsequently be increased or decreased. Detect recurrent uroliths while they are still small enough to be removed by voiding urohydropropulsion (Appendix K). If necessary, eradicate or control UTIs should they occur.

Urinary pH. Avoid efforts to deliberately acidify the urine; rather, consider mild alkalinization (pH range 7.1 to 7.7) of urine for dogs affected by frequently recurring silica uroliths. Potassium citrate can be used. Wax matrix tablets,[a] liquid[b] or chewable treats[c] are available. Dose is 40-75 mg/kg q12h. Divided doses help maintain a consistently non-acidic urine.

MISCELLANEOUS

For more information, see Chapters 38 and 44, Small Animal Clinical Nutrition, 5th edition. For information about canine compound urolithiasis, see Appendix K.

Authors

Condensed from Chapter 44, Small Animal Clinical Nutrition, 5th edition, authored by Carl A. Osborne, Jody P. Lulich and Lisa K. Ulrich.

References

See Chapter 44, Small Animal Clinical Nutrition, 5th edition, on the website www.markmorrisinstitute.org for references.

Endnotes

a. Urocit-K. Mission Pharmacal, San Antonio, TX, USA.
b. Polycitra-K. Willen Drug Co., Baltimore, MD, USA.
c. K-CIT-V. V.E.T. Pharmaceuticals, Inc., Fenton, MO, USA.

Table 1. Key nutritional factors for foods for canine silica urolithiasis prevention.

Factors	Dietary recommendations
Water	Water intake should be encouraged to achieve a urine specific gravity <1.020
	Moist food will increase water consumption and formation of less concentrated urine
Protein	Restrict high quality dietary protein to 10 to 18% dry matter
Silica	Avoid foods with corn gluten feed, rice hulls and soybean hulls listed on the ingredient panel of the product label
Urinary pH	Feed a food that maintains an alkaline urine (urinary pH = 7.1 to 7.7)

Table 2. Levels of key nutritional factors in selected commercial foods used to minimize recurrence of silica uroliths in dogs compared to recommended levels.* (Numbers in red match optimal KNFs.)

Dry food	Protein (%)	Urinary pH**
Recommended levels	10-18	7.1-7.7
Hill's Prescription Diet u/d Canine	11.2	7.70
Moist food		
Hill's Prescription Diet u/d Canine	13.3	7.40

*Manufacturer's published values; protein expressed as % dry matter; when possible recommend moist foods; where possible, check the ingredient panel of the product label and avoid foods that list corn gluten feed, rice hulls or soybean hulls.
**Protocols for measuring urinary pH may vary.

Chapter 33
Feline Idiopathic Cystitis

CLINICAL POINTS

- Cat owners' top 3 feline health concerns are urinary disease, followed by, dental disease and cancer.
- FIC is the most common cause of FLUTD, followed by urolithiasis and urethral plugs.
- Risk factors for FLUTD include patient characteristics, environmental conditions and various nutritional factors; Appendix L summarizes risks for FIC compared to those for struvite and calcium oxalate uroliths.
- Overweight/obesity conditions are a risk factor for lower urinary tract diseases in general.
- Periuria (urinating in inappropriate locations) often accompanies FLUTD and is the most common behavioral problem for which pet owners seek professional counsel. It is also the primary behavioral reason owners relinquish cats to shelters. Correct diagnosis and management of periuria are important for maintaining the pet-family bond.
- It is helpful to categorize patients into 1 of 4 clinical presentations, realizing that some cats may have features of multiple presentations (Appendix L). A thorough history, physical exam and diagnostic evaluation including urinalysis and diagnostic imaging (radiology or ultrasonography) are indicated for every patient.
- Radiography: patients with FIC may appear normal or have abnormalities including focal or diffuse thickening of the urinary bladder wall, irregularities of the urinary bladder mucosa or filling defects.
- Urethrocystoscopy may be the method of choice for evaluating female cats with signs of periuria, pollakiuria, dysuria or stranguria. Submucosal petechial hemorrhages (glomerulations), in the absence of other lesions, support a diagnosis of FIC.
- If clinical signs of FLUTD are present and a specific cause is not identified after appropriate evaluation, FIC is the most likely diagnosis.

Abbreviations
AAFCO = Association of American Feed Control Officials
BCS = body condition score (Appendix A)
DHA = docosahexaenoic acid
EPA = eicosapentaenoic acid
FCV = feline calicivirus
FIC = feline idiopathic cystitis
FLUTD = feline lower urinary tract disease
KNF = key nutritional factor
UTI = urinary tract infection

- UTI is the most common cause of lower urinary tract signs in cats older than 10 years.
- The clinical course of FIC is characterized by episodes of lower urinary tract signs that usually resolve spontaneously within 3-5 days, with or without treatment. Signs recur in 40-65% of cats with FIC within 6-12-months.
- Despite increasing evidence that FCV invades the urinary system, and that cats with FIC have increased exposure to FCV, FCV as a cause of FIC has not been proven.
- Although there are many risk factors for patients with FIC, additional evaluation is likely needed to identify definitive cause(s). Abnormalities are not limited to the urinary bladder; interactions between other systems (e.g., nervous and endocrine) may be involved. Consider this possibility when formulating a treatment plan.
- Nutritional management plays a key role in the treatment of patients with FIC; the modification proven most beneficial is feeding moist foods. Moist foods increase urine volume (**Table 1**).
- Urinary bladder inflammation is characteristic of FIC. Dietary n-3 fatty acids such as EPA and DHA have antiinflammatory properties and are incorporated into cell membranes, including those of the urinary bladder, where they may beneficially limit production of inflammatory mediators.
- Environmental enrichment (e.g., stress reduction, litter box management) also should be implemented in patients with FIC (Appendix L).
- Other treatments such as pain management may be needed for some cats, especially during acute episodes (Appendix L).
- Feeding goals: through proper foods and feeding methods (in combination with decreasing environmental stress, behavioral modification and appropriate pain management) improve the quality of life by decreasing frequency of episodes and their severity. Because of the nature of FIC, complete elimination of episodes is unlikely.

Table 1. Water intake and urine volume in cats fed dry or moist food.*

Volume (ml/day)	Moist food	Dry food
Water (in food)	246	6
Water (in addition to food)	32	221
Total water intake	278	227
Fecal water	27	44
Urine	166	79

*Adapted from Burger IH, Smith PM. Effects of diet on the urine characteristics of the cat. In: Proceedings. International Symposium on Nutrition, Malnutrition and Dietetics in the Dog and Cat, 1987: 71-73.

KEY NUTRITIONAL FACTORS

- Foods should provide recommended allowances of all required nutrients (nutritional adequacy), but should also contain specific levels of KNFs (certain nutrients that can assist in the management of FIC).
- Table 2 summarizes KNFs for foods intended for prevention of recurrence of FIC and includes increased water and n-3 fatty acids.
- A detailed review of these recommendations can be found in Chapter 46, Small Animal Clinical Nutrition, 5th edition.

FEEDING PLAN

Assess and Select the Food

Ensure the Food's Basic Nutritional Adequacy. AAFCO nutritional adequacy statements are usually found on a product's label. AAFCO approval does not ensure a food will be effective in the management of FIC.

Compare the Food's KNF Content with the Recommended Levels. Table 3 lists commercial foods marketed for management of FIC and compares their KNF content with recommended levels. Several foods have been developed that are intended to manage the combination of risk factors associated with FIC-, struvite- and/or calcium oxalate-based FLUTD. Table 4 lists these foods and compares them to the composite KNFs for these 3 forms of FLUTD. Contact manufacturers for information for foods not in the tables (manufacturer contact information is listed on product labels). Select a food that best approximates the recommended KNF levels.

Food Form. Adequate water intake in FIC patients is particularly important. If readily consumed, moist foods are preferred; their consumption results in a 2X increase in urine volume compared to dry foods. Appendix L provides tips for increasing water intake.

Manage Treats and Snacks. If treats/snacks are fed, consider commercial treats that most closely match the KNF profile recommended for foods for adult cats. Limit to <10% of the total diet on a volume, weight or calorie basis.

Assess and Determine the Feeding Method

Determine How Much Food to Feed. The amount to feed can be estimated either from feeding guides on product labels or by calculation (Appendix C). These estimates are only starting points and will likely need to be adjusted (see Followup below).

Consider How to Offer the Food. Feeding moist foods is important in the management of FIC; moist foods require meal feeding. A combination of dry and moist foods can be used. Water (warm may be better) can be added to dry foods. Dividing the daily amount of food into several meals increases daily water intake. Do not leave moist foods or moistened dry foods at room temperature for prolonged intervals (>2-4 hours below).

Table 2. Key nutritional factors and recommended levels for managing cats with common lower urinary tract diseases.*

Factors	Dietary recommendations	
	FIC	Combined FIC, struvite and calcium oxalate prevention
Water	Moist foods are best	Moist foods are best
Magnesium (%)	–	0.07 to 0.14
Phosphorus (%)	–	0.5 to 0.9
Calcium (%)	–	0.6 to 1.0
Protein (%)	–	32 to 45
Sodium (%)	–	0.3 to 0.6
Urinary pH	–	6.2 to 6.4
Total omega 3 (%)	0.35 to 1.0	0.35 to 1.0

Key: FIC = feline idiopathic cystitis, Total omega 3 = total omega-3 fatty acids.
*Nutrients expressed on a dry matter basis unless otherwise stated.

Table 3. Comparison of key nutritional factors in selected commercial veterinary therapeutic foods for reducing the recurrence of feline idiopathic cystitis.* (Numbers in red match optimal KNFs.)

Moist foods**	Omega 3 (%)
Recommended levels	**0.35-1.00**
Hill's Prescription Diet c/d Multicare with Chicken Feline	0.96
Hill's Prescription Diet c/d Multicare with Seafood Feline	0.62
Iams Veterinary Formula Urinary S Low pH/S Feline	na
Medi-Cal Veterinary Diet Urinary SO	na
Purina Veterinary Diets UR Urinary St/Ox Feline Formula	na
Royal Canin Veterinary Diet Feline Urinary SO in Gel	na
Dry foods	**Omega 3 (%)**
Recommended levels	**0.35-1.00**
Hill's Prescription Diet c/d Multicare Feline	0.65
Hill's Prescription Diet c/d Multicare with Chicken Feline	0.64
Medi-Cal Veterinary Diet Urinary SO	na
Purina Veterinary Diets UR Urinary St/Ox Feline Formula	na

Key: Omega 3 = total omega-3 fatty acids, na = not available from manufacturer.
*Nutrients expressed on a dry matter basis.
**Moist foods are best because increased water intake is considered important in the management of feline idiopathic cystitis.

Manage Food Changes. Some owners believe that their cats will not eat moist food. However, switching to moist food is usually possible if done gradually, over several days to weeks. Encourage owners to take the time. Failure to gradually transition a cat to a moist food may result in refusal to eat the food and increase stress, with subsequent recurrence of clinical signs. Offer moist food initially as an option in a second dish next to the usual dry food. As the cat consumes the moist food, gradually increase the amount of moist food while decreasing the amount of dry food correspondingly.

Food and Water Receptacle Husbandry. Food and water bowls should be washed regularly with warm soapy water and rinsed well. Dishes used for moist foods need daily cleaning. Discard moist or moistened dry foods after 2-4 hours of room temperature exposure to avoid foodborne illnesses (Appendix F).

Table 4. Comparison of key nutritional factors in selected commercial veterinary therapeutic foods for reducing the recurrence of feline idiopathic cystitis, struvite disease (uroliths or urethral plugs) and/or calcium oxalate uroliths in cats.* (Numbers in red match optimal KNFs.)

Moist foods** Recommended levels	Mg (%) 0.07-0.14	P (%) 0.5-0.9	Ca (%) 0.6-1.0	Protein (%) 32-45	Na (%) 0.3-0.6	Urinary pH 6.2-6.4	Total omega 3 (%) 0.35-1.0
Hill's Prescription Diet c/d Multicare with Chicken Feline	0.052	0.68	0.72	43.8	0.32	6.35	0.96
Hill's Prescription Diet c/d Multicare with Seafood Feline	0.054	0.71	0.62	44.8	0.33	6.4	0.62
Medi-Cal Urinary SO	na	1.20	1.20	43.5	1.1	6.4	na
Purina Veterinary Diets UR Urinary St/Ox Feline Formula	0.07	0.97	0.96	50.6	0.62	6.0-6.4	na
Royal Canin Veterinary Diet Urinary SO in gel	0.10	1.36	1.02	41.3	1.02	6.0-6.3	na

Dry foods Recommended levels	Mg (%) 0.07-0.14	P (%) 0.5-0.9	Ca (%) 0.6-1.0	Protein (%) 32-45	Na (%) 0.3-0.6	Urinary pH 6.2-6.4	Total omega 3 (%) 0.35-1.0
Hill's Prescription Diet c/d Multicare Feline	0.06	0.65	0.74	36.1	0.35	6.3	0.65
Hill's Prescription Diet c/d Multicare with Chicken Feline	0.06	0.65	0.76	34.6	0.33	6.3	0.64
Purina Veterinary Diets UR Urinary St/Ox Feline Formula	0.07	1.08	1.1	44.9	1.17	6.0-6.4	na

Key: Mg = magnesium, P = phosphorus, Ca = calcium, Na = sodium, total omega 3 = total omega-3 fatty acids, na = not available from manufacturer.
*Nutrients expressed on a dry matter basis unless otherwise stated.
**In general, it is recommended that moist foods be fed to cats with lower urinary tract disorders, especially those with feline idiopathic cystitis or calcium oxalate uroliths.

FOLLOWUP

Owner Followup

Note the severity/frequency of episodes and trends in water and food intake. Owners should weigh their cat and/or grade its body condition (BCS) monthly. If a trend of increasing or decreasing body weight or BCS is noticed, the amount fed should be changed by 10% increments and the patient rechecked every 2 weeks for 1 month. At that point, if necessary, the amount fed should be changed again and the cycle repeated. *Ancillary Management.* Ensure environmental enrichment, stress reduction and appropriate litter box maintenance.

Veterinary Health Care Team Followup

Because of stress associated with hospital visits, it may be preferable to conduct followup evaluations by phone rather than direct examination of the patient. If episodes increase in severity/frequency or other clinical signs are reported despite appropriate treatment, patient evaluation including urinalysis, urine culture and diagnostic imaging is indicated to detect other disorders (e.g., uroliths, UTI). Beneficial effects may be observed when urine specific gravity is in the range of 1.030 to 1.040.

Ancillary Management. Appendix L provides information for advising clients about methods for environmental enrichment, stress reduction, appropriate litter box maintenance and behavioral management as well as pain management and recommendations for use of feline facial pheromone, glycosaminoglycans and amitriptyline therapy.

MISCELLANEOUS

See Chapter 34 for dietary management of struvite urolithiasis and Chapter 35 for dietary management of calcium oxalate urolithiasis. See Appendix L for information about other uroliths. See Chapter 46, Small Animal Clinical Nutrition, 5th edition, for more information about FLUTD.

Authors

Condensed from Chapter 46, Small Animal Clinical Nutrition, 5th edition, authored by S. Dru Forrester, John M. Kruger and Timothy A. Allen.

References

See Chapter 46, Small Animal Clinical Nutrition, 5th edition, on the website www.markmorrisinstitute.org for references.

CLINICAL POINTS

- Cat owners' top 3 feline health concerns are urinary disease, followed by dental disease and cancer.
- FIC is the most common cause of FLUTD; next is uroliths and urethral plugs. In cats >10 years, UTI and uroliths are the most common causes.
- Risk factors for FLUTD include patient characteristics, environmental conditions and various nutritional factors; Appendix L summarizes risks for struvite uroliths and compares them to those for FIC and calcium oxalate uroliths.
- Periuria (urinating in inappropriate locations) often accompanies FLUTD and is the most common behavioral problem for which pet owners seek professional counsel. It is also the primary behavioral reason owners relinquish cats to shelters. Correct diagnosis and management of periuria are important for maintaining the pet-family bond.
- In 2008, struvite was the most common feline urolith (49%), followed by calcium oxalate (39%) and urate (~5%). Struvite is also the most common mineral type identified in urethral plugs.
- In general, overweight/obesity conditions are risk factors for lower urinary tract disease.
- It is helpful to categorize patients into 1 of 4 clinical presentations, realizing that some cats may have features of multiple presentations (Appendix L). A thorough history, physical exam and diagnostic evaluation including urinalysis and diagnostic imaging (radiology or ultrasonography) are indicated for every patient.
- A nutritional history includes: specific brand(s) of food fed, form (dry, moist, semi-moist, combination), method of feeding (meal fed, free choice) and whether table food, supplements or treats are offered. Note access to other foods (e.g., multi-pet household, other households or from the outdoors). Water consumption (i.e., increased, decreased or unchanged) should also be noted.
- Appendix L lists clinical and diagnostic findings associated with struvite urolithiasis.
- Urolith formation occurs in 2 phases: initiation of a crystal nidus and subsequent growth to form a urolith. Growth requires: 1) oversaturation of urine with calculogenic crystalloids (MAP), which may result from increased urinary excretion or increased urine concentration (due to decreased water intake), 2) decreased solubility of crystalloids (e.g., struvite is less soluble in alkaline urine), 3) presence/absence of crystallization inhibiters or promoters and 4) retention of crystals/uroliths within the urinary tract.
- Formation of matrix-crystalline urethral plugs requires 2 simultaneous but unrelated events (**Figure 1**): formation of matrix that may result from some inflammatory process (e.g.,

Abbreviations

AAFCO = Association of American Feed Control Officials
BCS = body condition score (Appendix A)
CHF = congestive heart failure
CKD = chronic kidney disease
FIC = feline idiopathic cystitis
FLUTD = feline lower urinary tract disease
KNF = key nutritional factor
MAP = magnesium ammonium phosphate (struvite)
UTI = urinary tract infection

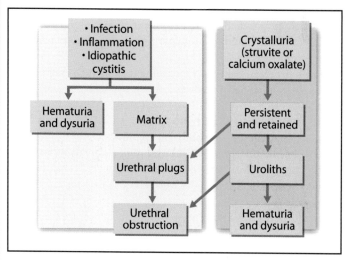

Figure 1. Unifying concept for pathogenesis of feline lower urinary tract disease. Infection or inflammation (e.g., idiopathic cystitis) results in clinical signs of lower urinary tract disease and production of excess matrix. Persistent crystalluria can combine with matrix to form urethral plugs or contribute to urolith formation and typical clinical signs. (Adapted from Osborne CA, Kruger JM, Lulich JP. Feline lower urinary tract disorders: Definition of terms and concepts. Veterinary Clinics of North America: Small Animal Practice 1996; 76: 169-179.)

idiopathic, bacterial or viral UTI) and formation of crystalline precipitates (MAP).
- Compared to dry foods, moist foods double urine volume (Table 1, Chapter 33). However, increasing urine volume may have less effect on struvite urolith formation than on calcium oxalate or FIC.
- Urinary magnesium excretion increases linearly with increases in dietary magnesium intake; the risk of struvite urolithiasis increases in cats fed foods high in magnesium.
- Varying dietary phosphorus can alter urinary phosphate concentrations in cats. High-phosphorus foods have been associated with increased risk of struvite urolithiasis.
- Urinary phosphate can exist in several states; anionic phosphate (PO_4^{-3}) is the important form in struvite. As urine becomes more acidic, PO_4^{-3} is converted to monobasic and

dibasic hydrogen phosphate. As urine becomes more alkaline, the reaction proceeds in the opposite direction and the concentration of PO_4^{-3} increases.

- Cats fed foods formulated to produce urinary pH values between 6.5-6.9 are twice as likely to develop struvite uroliths as cats fed foods formulated to produce a urinary pH between 5.99-6.15.
- Excessive dietary protein intake provides additional urea and glutamine, which are metabolized to ammonia and ammonium (respectively) and excreted in urine where they are more available for combining with magnesium and PO_4^{-3} to form struvite crystals and uroliths. Also, foods that have increased amounts of protein also tend to have increased phosphorus.
- Although most cats do not have UTI, infection with urease-producing organisms may cause struvite urolithiasis in some cats and other bacteria may cause UTI secondary to uroliths in others.
- Treatment options for cats with struvite uroliths include dissolution by nutritional management and physical removal (e.g., cystotomy, voiding urohydropropulsion, catheter retrieval, laser lithotripsy).
- Dissolution by nutritional management is rapid (average = 28 days; but may be as early as 7 days), cost effective and noninvasive.
- In one study in a veterinary teaching hospital, 14% of cats had incomplete removal of uroliths by cystotomy.
- Recommendations for urolith dissolution and prevention are based on mineral composition of uroliths; analyze uroliths whenever possible. Appendix K lists urolith diagnostic laboratories.
- The rate of urolith recurrence is ~3% with an average time of 27 months. Recurrence is higher in females than males.
- Generally, appropriate nutritional management is the most important consideration for prevention of recurrence of struvite uroliths and urethral plugs.
- Feeding goals: by using appropriate foods and feeding methods (and if necessary, medical management), dissolve struvite uroliths and minimize recurrence.
- Environmental enrichment (e.g., stress reduction, litter box management) may be helpful for cats with lower urinary tract

disorders (Appendix L).

KEY NUTRITIONAL FACTORS

- Foods should provide recommended allowances of all required nutrients (nutritional adequacy), but should also contain specific levels of KNFs (certain nutrients that can assist in the management of struvite urolithiasis).
- **Table 1** summarizes KNFs for foods intended for struvite dissolution and prevention of recurrence and includes increased water and decreased protein, phosphorus, sodium, magnesium and urinary pH. **Table 1** also includes composite KNFs for foods for management of struvite-, FIC- and/or calcium oxalate-based FLUTD.
- A detailed review of these recommendations can be found in Chapter 46, Small Animal Clinical Nutrition, 5th edition.

FEEDING PLAN

Struvite Urolith Dissolution
Assess and Select the Food.
COMPARE THE FOOD'S KNF CONTENT WITH THE RECOMMENDED LEVELS. Table 2 lists commercial foods marketed for struvite urolith dissolution and compares KNF content of these foods with recommended levels. Contact manufacturers for information for foods not in the tables (manufacturer contact information is listed on product labels). Select a food that best approximates the recommended KNF levels.

FOOD FORM. If readily consumed, moist foods are preferred; their consumption results in a 2-fold increase in urine volume compared to dry foods.

INCREASING WATER INTAKE. Appendix L provides tips for increasing water intake.

PRECAUTIONS.

Long-Term Feeding. Some KNFs for properly formulated struvite litholytic foods are restricted to near minimum requirements and are designed for short-term (weeks-months) dissolution therapy. These foods may be marginally adequate for some patients if fed long term (months-years).

Kittens and Reproducing Queens. Contraindicated.

Concomitant Conditions. Contraindicated in patients with metabolic acidosis or hypokalemia; foods with increased amounts of sodium (**Table 2**) are not recommended for patients with CKD, hypertension or CHF.

Manage Treats and Snacks. Avoid treats/snacks during struvite dissolution. Otherwise, suggest small portions of the food being fed or the opposite form of the food fed; i.e., if a dry food is fed, offer small amounts of the same food in

Table 1. Key nutritional factors and recommended levels for managing cats with common lower urinary tract diseases.*

Factors	Dietary recommendations		
	Struvite dissolution	Struvite prevention	Combined FIC, struvite and calcium oxalate prevention
Water	Moist foods may be best	Moist foods may be best	Moist foods are best
Magnesium (%)	0.04 to 0.09	0.04 to 0.14	0.07 to 0.14
Phosphorus (%)	0.45 to 1.1	0.5 to 0.9	0.5 to 0.9
Calcium (%)	–	–	0.6 to 1.0
Protein (%)	30 to 45	30 to 45	32 to 45
Sodium (%)	0.3 to 0.6	0.3 to 0.6	0.3 to 0.6
Urinary pH	5.8 to 6.2	6.0 to 6.4	6.2 to 6.4
Total omega 3 (%)	–	–	0.35 to 1.0

Key: FIC = feline idiopathic cystitis, Total omega 3 = total omega-3 fatty acids.
*Nutrients expressed on a dry matter basis unless otherwise stated.

Table 2. Comparison of key nutritional factors in selected commercial veterinary therapeutic foods for dissolution of struvite uroliths in cats.* (Numbers in red match optimal KNFs.)

Moist foods	Mg (%)	P (%)	Protein (%)	Na (%)	Urinary pH
Recommended levels	0.04-0.09	0.45-1.1	30-45	0.3-0.6	5.8-6.2
Hill's Prescription Diet s/d Feline	0.056	0.56	39.9	0.37	6.08
Medi-Cal Veterinary Diets Dissolution Formula	na	1.1	46.5	1.1	6.2
Purina Veterinary Diets UR Urinary St/Ox Feline Formula	0.07	0.97	50.6	0.62	6.0-6.4
Royal Canin Veterinary Diet Dissolution Formula	0.052	1.0	49.9	1.21	5.9
Royal Canin Veterinary Diet Urinary SO in Gel	0.097	1.36	41.3	1.02	6.0-6.3
Dry foods	**Mg (%)**	**P (%)**	**Protein (%)**	**Na (%)**	**Urinary pH**
Recommended levels	0.04-0.09	0.45-1.1	30-45	0.3-0.6	5.8-6.2
Hill's Prescription Diet s/d Feline	0.059	0.77	34.4	0.4	5.9
Medi-Cal Veterinary Diets Feline Dissolution Formula	na	1.0	35.7	0.4	5.8
Purina Veterinary Diets UR Urinary St/Ox Feline Formula	0.07	1.08	44.9	1.17	6.0-6.4
Royal Canin Veterinary Diet Urinary SO 33	0.065	0.88	37.1	1.45	6.0-6.3

Key: Mg = magnesium, P = phosphorus, Na = sodium, na = not available from manufacturer.
*Nutrients expressed on a dry matter basis unless otherwise stated.
**In general, moist foods should be fed to cats with FLUTD.

moist form and vice versa; keep kibbles of a dry food for struvite urolith dissolution for use as treats in a separate container away from the usual feeding area.

Assess and Determine the Feeding Method.

Determine How Much Food to Feed. The amount to feed can be estimated either from feeding guides on product labels or by calculation (Appendix C). These estimates are only starting points and will likely need to be adjusted (see Followup below).

Consider How to Offer the Food. Maintaining an acidic urinary pH within a defined range is important for struvite urolith management. Free-choice feeding is associated with more persistent aciduria compared to meal feeding. For moist foods (recommended above), use meal feeding (>3 times/day). A combination of dry and moist foods can be used. Provide measured/limited amounts of either form if patient has a tendency to be overweight. Dividing the daily amount into several meals also increases daily water intake. Do not leave moist foods or moistened dry foods at room temperature for prolonged intervals (>2-4 hours, see below).

Manage Food Changes. A transition period to avoid GI upsets and to facilitate acceptance of a new food is good practice. Example: to change to a new food, replace 10-15% of the old food with the new food on Day 1 and continue this incremental change daily until the change is complete on Day 7. Appendix E provides additional information. Chapter 33 provides suggestions for transitioning from dry to moist foods.

Food and Water Receptacle Husbandry. Food and water bowls should be washed regularly with warm soapy water and rinsed well. Dishes used for moist foods need daily cleaning. Discard moist or moistened dry foods after 2-4 hours of room temperature exposure to avoid foodborne illnesses (Appendix F).

FOLLOWUP

Owner Followup

Ask owners to note the presence/absence of clinical signs (gross hematuria and dysuria/pollakiuria) daily and have them weigh their cat and/or grade its body condition (BCS) monthly. If a trend of increasing or decreasing body weight or BCS is noticed, the amount fed should be changed by 10% increments and the patient rechecked every 2 weeks for 1 month. Then, if necessary, the amount fed should be changed again and the cycle repeated. *Compliance.* If the cat comes from a multi-pet household, deny access to other pets' foods. Adhere strictly to feeding only the prescribed foods/treats/supplements.

Veterinary Health Care Team Followup

Figure 2 is an algorithm to assist in managing patients with struvite urolithiasis. Typical clinical signs (gross hematuria and dysuria/pollakiuria) present before nutritional management is initiated, and are usually absent by the first reevaluation in 2 weeks. Time to resolution of clinical signs or urolith dissolution does not differ significantly with urolith numbers.

Sterile Struvite Uroliths. The average time for dissolution is 3-4 weeks.

Struvite Uroliths with Concurrent UTI. The average time for dissolution is about 6 weeks (range, 14-92 days). Appropriate antimicrobial therapy should continue for 2-3 weeks beyond removal or radiographic disappearance of uroliths.

Urinary pH Measurements. Note when the urine sample was collected relative to the time of eating. Samples obtained before food is offered tend to be more acidic; samples obtained within several hours of eating tend to be more alkaline (postprandial alkaline tide). Standardize the time of collection relative to the time of eating when evaluating effects of a food change on urinary pH. For most accurate results, measure the sample using a pH meter.

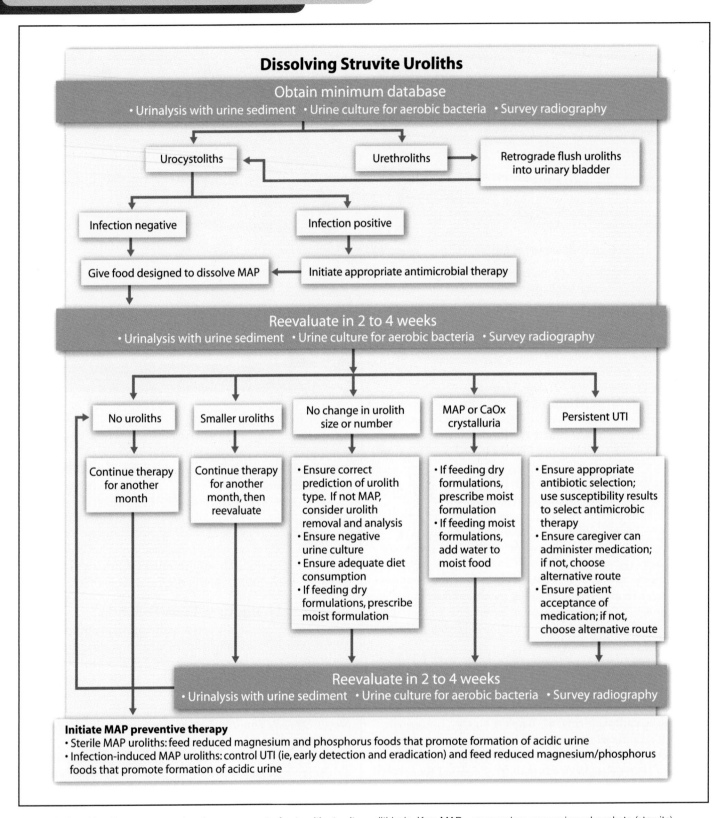

Figure 2. Algorithm for management and reassessment of cats with struvite urolithiasis. Key: MAP = magnesium ammonium phosphate (struvite), CaOx = calcium oxalate, UTI = urinary tract infection. (Adapted from Lulich JP. FLUTD: Are you choosing the right therapy? Part 1. Urolithiasis. In: Proceedings. Hill's Symposium on Feline Lower Urinary Tract Disease, 2007a: 29-36).

Table 3. Comparison of key nutritional factors in selected commercial veterinary therapeutic foods for decreasing risk of recurrence of struvite disease (uroliths or urethral plugs) in cats.* (Numbers in red match optimal KNFs.)

Moist foods** Recommended levels	Mg (%) 0.04-0.14	P (%) 0.5-0.9	Protein (%) 30-45	Na (%) 0.3-0.6	Urinary pH 6.0-6.4
Hill's Prescription Diet c/d Multicare with Chicken Feline	0.052	0.68	43.8	0.32	6.35
Hill's Prescription Diet c/d Multicare with Seafood Feline	0.054	0.71	44.8	0.33	6.4
Hill's Prescription Diet r/d with Liver & Chicken Feline	0.075	0.62	37.5	0.29	6.25
Hill's Prescription Diet w/d with Chicken Feline	0.064	0.68	39.6	0.38	6.26
Iams Veterinary Formula Urinary S Low pH/S/Feline	0.088	0.75	41.8	0.26	na
Medi-Cal Veterinary Diets Feline Dissolution Formula	na	1.1	46.5	1.1	6.2
Medi-Cal Veterinary Diets Feline Preventive Formula	na	0.9	47.1	0.4	6.3
Medi-Cal Veterinary Diets Feline Reducing Formula	na	1.6	54.3	1.0	6.5
Medi-Cal Veterinary Diets Feline Urinary SO in Gel	na	1.2	43.5	1.1	6.4
Medi-Cal Veterinary Diets Feline Weight Control	na	1.1	40.0	0.5	6.6
Purina Veterinary Diets UR Urinary St/Ox Feline Formula	0.07	0.97	50.6	0.62	6.0-6.4
Royal Canin Veterinary Diet Feline Control Formula	0.082	1.03	43.0	0.45	6.0-6.3
Royal Canin Veterinary Diet Feline Urinary SO in Gel	0.097	1.36	41.3	1.02	6.0-6.3
Dry foods Recommended levels	Mg (%) 0.04-0.14	P (%) 0.5-0.9	Protein (%) 30-45	Na (%) 0.3-0.6	Urinary pH 6.0-6.4
Hill's Prescription Diet c/d Multicare Feline	0.06	0.65	36.1	0.35	6.30
Hill's Prescription Diet c/d Multicare with Chicken Feline	0.061	0.65	34.6	0.33	6.35
Hill's Prescription Diet r/d Feline	0.073	0.81	36.9	0.35	6.38
Hill's Prescription Diet r/d with Chicken Feline	0.067	0.84	37.7	0.35	6.33
Hill's Prescription Diet w/d Feline	0.059	0.77	39.0	0.3	6.27
Hill's Prescription Diet w/d with Chicken Feline	0.068	0.86	39.9	0.35	6.22
Iams Veterinary Formula Urinary S Low pH/S/Feline	0.096	0.93	36.5	0.45	na
Medi-Cal Veterinary Diets Feline Dissolution Formula	na	1.0	35.7	0.4	5.8
Medi-Cal Veterinary Diets Feline Preventive Formula	na	0.9	33.4	0.4	6.1
Medi-Cal Veterinary Diets Feline Reducing Formula	na	1.2	41.8	0.3	6.1
Medi-Cal Veterinary Diets Feline Urinary SO 30	na	0.9	34.6	1.4	6.2
Medi-Cal Veterinary Diets Feline Weight Control	na	1.0	34.4	0.3	6.0
Purina Veterinary Diets UR Urinary St/Ox Feline Formula	0.07	1.08	44.9	1.17	6.0-6.4
Royal Canin Veterinary Diet Feline Control Formula	0.065	0.65	33.7	0.71	6.0-6.3
Royal Canin Veterinary Diet Feline Urinary SO 33	0.065	0.88	37.1	1.45	6.0-6.3

Key: Mg = magnesium, P = phosphorus, Na = sodium, na = not available from manufacturer.
*Nutrients expressed on a dry matter basis unless otherwise stated.
**In general, moist foods should be fed to cats with FLUTD.

FEEDING PLAN

Prevention of Recurrence of Struvite Urolithiasis and Urethral Plugs

Assess and Select the Food.

ENSURE THE FOOD'S BASIC NUTRITIONAL ADEQUACY. AAFCO nutritional adequacy statements are usually found on a product's label. AAFCO approval does not ensure a food will be effective in preventing struvite recurrence or other long-term health problems.

COMPARE THE FOOD'S KNF CONTENT WITH THE RECOMMENDED LEVELS. Table 3 lists commercial foods marketed for struvite urolith prevention and compares KNF content of these foods with recommended levels. Several foods have been developed to manage the combination of risk factors associated with struvite-, calcium oxalate- and/or FIC-based FLUTD. These foods are listed in **Table 4** and are compared to the composite KNFs for these 3 forms of FLUTD. Contact manufacturers for information for foods not in the tables (manufacturer contact information is listed on product labels). Select a food that best approximates the recommended KNF levels.

FOOD FORM. If readily consumed, moist foods are preferred.

INCREASING WATER INTAKE. Appendix L provides tips for increasing water intake.

Manage Treats and Snacks. If treats/snacks are fed, commercial treats that most closely match the KNF profile recommended for foods for struvite prevention are best. Limit to <10% of the total diet on a volume, weight or calorie basis. Suggest small portions of the food being fed or the opposite form of the food fed; i.e., if a dry food is fed, offer small amounts of the same food in moist form and vice versa; consider kibbles of the dry struvite prevention food for use as treats (keep in a separate container away from the usual feeding area).

Assess and Determine the Feeding Method.

CONSIDER HOW TO OFFER THE FOOD/MANAGE FOOD CHANGES/FOOD AND WATER RECEPTACLE HUSBANDRY. See recommendations for struvite urolith dissolution (above).

FOLLOWUP

Struvite uroliths may recur months to years after removal or dissolution, particularly if preventive measures are not implemented.

Table 4. Comparison of key nutritional factors in selected commercial veterinary therapeutic foods for reducing the recurrence of feline idiopathic cystitis, struvite disease (uroliths or urethral plugs) and/or calcium oxalate uroliths in cats.* (Numbers in red match optimal KNFs.)

Moist foods** Recommended levels	Mg (%) 0.07-0.14	P (%) 0.5-0.9	Ca (%) 0.6-1.0	Protein (%) 32-45	Na (%) 0.3-0.6	Urinary pH 6.2-6.4	Total omega 3 (%) 0.35-1.0
Hill's Prescription Diet c/d Multicare with Chicken Feline	0.052	0.68	0.72	43.8	0.32	6.35	0.96
Hill's Prescription Diet c/d Multicare with Seafood Feline	0.054	0.71	0.62	44.8	0.33	6.4	0.62
Medi-Cal Urinary SO	na	1.20	1.20	43.5	1.1	6.4	na
Purina Veterinary Diets UR Urinary St/Ox Feline Formula	0.07	0.97	0.96	50.6	0.62	6.0-6.4	na
Royal Canin Veterinary Diet Urinary SO in gel	0.10	1.36	1.02	41.3	1.02	6.0-6.3	na
Dry foods Recommended levels	Mg (%) 0.07-0.14	P (%) 0.5-0.9	Ca (%) 0.6-1.0	Protein (%) 32-45	Na (%) 0.3-0.6	Urinary pH 6.2-6.4	Total omega 3 (%) 0.35-1.0
Hill's Prescription Diet c/d Multicare Feline	0.06	0.65	0.74	36.1	0.35	6.3	0.65
Hill's Prescription Diet c/d Multicare with Chicken Feline	0.06	0.65	0.76	34.6	0.33	6.3	0.64
Purina Veterinary Diets UR Urinary St/Ox Feline Formula	0.07	1.08	1.1	44.9	1.17	6.0-6.4	na

Key: Mg = magnesium, P = phosphorus, Ca = calcium, Na = sodium, total omega 3 = total omega-3 fatty acids, na = not available from manufacturer.
*Nutrients expressed on a dry matter basis unless otherwise stated.
**In general, it is recommended that moist foods be fed to cats with lower urinary tract disorders, especially those with feline idiopathic cystitis or calcium oxalate uroliths.

Owner Followup

Ask owners to monitor for recurrence of clinical signs. After switching to the prevention food, have them weigh their cat and/or grade its body condition (BCS) monthly. If a trend of increasing or decreasing body weight or BCS is noticed, the amount fed should be changed by 10% increments and the patient rechecked every 2 weeks for 1 month. At that point, if necessary, the amount fed should be changed again and the cycle repeated. *Compliance.* If the cat lives in a multi-pet household deny access to other pets' food. Adhere strictly to feeding only the prescribed foods/treats/supplements.

Veterinary Health Care Team Followup

Monitor cats eating struvite preventive foods periodically for urinary pH and crystalluria. Detection of large aggregates of struvite crystals is an important finding when monitoring effectiveness of preventive measures. If no episodes of struvite uroliths occur for several years, consider recommending a high-quality wellness food (Chapter 7); continue to monitor periodically for occurrence of alkaline urinary pH, struvite crystalluria and urolith recurrence.

Struvite Uroliths with Concurrent UTI. If UTI due to urease-producing bacteria was the cause of uroliths, controlling infection may prevent urolith recurrence.

If Uroliths Recur. Consider: 1) Were all uroliths removed from the urinary tract at the time of surgery or other procedure? 2)

Did nonabsorbable suture materials left exposed in the lumen of the urinary bladder provide a nidus for precipitation of crystalline material? 3) What diagnostic methods were used to detect recurrence? 4) How often was the patient evaluated for recurrence? 5) Were recommendations to decrease likelihood of recurrence given and did the owner follow them? 6) Has infection with a urease-producing microorganism persisted or recurred? 7) Was an underlying anatomic defect corrected?

MISCELLANEOUS

See Chapters 33 and 35 for dietary management of FIC and calcium oxalate precipitates. See Appendix L for information about less common uroliths.

Authors

Condensed from Chapter 46, Small Animal Clinical Nutrition, 5th edition, authored by S. Dru Forrester, John M. Kruger and Timothy A. Allen.

References

See Chapter 46, Small Animal Clinical Nutrition, 5th edition, on the website www.markmorrisinstitute.org for references.

CLINICAL POINTS

- Cat owners' top 3 feline health concerns are urinary disease, dental disease and cancer.
- FIC is the most common cause of FLUTD; next is uroliths and urethral plugs. In cats >10 years, UTI and uroliths are the most common causes.
- Risk factors for FLUTD include patient characteristics, environmental conditions and various nutritional factors; Appendix L summarizes risks for calcium oxalate and compares them to those for FIC and struvite.
- Periuria (urinating in inappropriate locations) often accompanies FLUTD and is the most common behavioral problem for which pet owners seek professional counsel. It is also the primary behavioral reason owners relinquish cats to shelters. Correct diagnosis and management of periuria are important for maintaining the pet-family bond.
- In 2008, struvite was the most common feline urolith analyzed (49%), followed by calcium oxalate (39%) and urate (~5%). Struvite is also by far the most common mineral type (~84%) identified in urethral plugs with calcium oxalate a distant second (~1%).
- Overweight/obesity conditions are a risk factor for lower urinary tract diseases in general.
- It is helpful to categorize patients into 1 of 4 clinical presentations, realizing that some cats may have features of multiple presentations (Appendix L). A thorough history, physical exam and diagnostic evaluation including urinalysis and diagnostic imaging (radiology or ultrasonography) are indicated for every patient.
- A nutritional history includes: specific brand(s) of food fed, form (dry, moist, semi-moist, combination), method of feeding (meal fed, free choice) and whether table food, supplements or treats are offered. Note access to other foods (multi-pet household, at other households, in the outdoor environment). Water consumption (increased, decreased, unchanged) should also be noted.
- Clinical and diagnostic findings associated with calcium oxalate urolithiasis are listed in Appendix L. In general, cats with calcium oxalate uroliths tend to be older than those with struvite uroliths (**Figure 1**).
- Urolith formation occurs in 2 phases: initiation of a crystal nidus and subsequent growth to form a urolith. Growth requires: 1) oversaturation of urine with calculogenic crystalloids (calcium and oxalate), which may result from increased urinary excretion or increased urine concentration (due to decreased water intake), 2) decreased solubility of crystalloids (e.g., calcium oxalate is somewhat less soluble at lower urinary pH), 3) presence/absence of crystallization

Abbreviations
AAFCO = Association of American Feed Control Officials
BCS = body condition score (Appendix A)
FIC = feline idiopathic cystitis
FLUTD = feline lower urinary tract disease
KNF = key nutritional factor
UTI = urinary tract infection

inhibiters or promoters and 4) retention of crystals/uroliths within the urinary tract.
- Compared to dry foods, eating moist foods doubles urine volume (Table 1, Chapter 33). Cats fed moist foods are about a third as likely to develop calcium oxalate uroliths as cats fed dry foods.
- Hypercalcemia has been reported to occur in 14-35% of cats with calcium oxalate uroliths; these patients should be evaluated for underlying causes (e.g., hyperparathyroidism, neoplasia and hypervitaminosis D). When possible, manage underlying causative diseases; however, a cause is usually not evident and idiopathic hypercalcemia is diagnosed.
- Avoid excessive dietary calcium to prevent recurrence of calcium oxalate uroliths. The most important sources are commercial foods and mineral supplements containing high calcium levels.
- Compared to foods containing moderate amounts of phosphorus, both low- and high-phosphorus foods are associated with increased risk of calcium oxalate formation. Low phosphorus may activate vitamin D, promoting intestinal calcium absorption and subsequent urinary calcium excretion.
- Excessive intake of oxalate is unlikely in cats eating commercial foods but could occur if they receive excessive amounts of

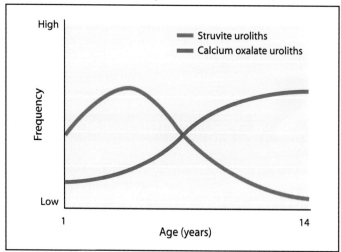

Figure 1. Relationship between urolith mineral type and age in cats. Note that struvite urolithiasis occurs more frequently in younger cats, whereas calcium oxalate urolithiasis occurs more frequently in older cats.

certain human foods as treats (see Manage Treats and Snacks below).

- Crystallization inhibitors such as citrate and magnesium form soluble complexes with calcium or oxalic acid, making them unavailable to form insoluble calcium oxalate; urinary magnesium excretion increases linearly with increases in dietary magnesium intake. Moderate dietary magnesium may be protective but excessive dietary magnesium can result in hypercalciuria.
- Cats fed foods formulated to produce urinary pH values between 5.99 and 6.15 were 3 times as likely to develop calcium oxalate uroliths as cats fed foods formulated to produce urinary pH values ranging from 6.5-6.9.
- Metabolic acidosis may contribute to formation of calcium-containing uroliths by mobilizing bone calcium resulting in increased urinary calcium excretion. Acidosis also decreases urinary citrate excretion. In one study, 64% of nonazotemic cats and 92% of azotemic cats with calcium oxalate uroliths were acidemic (serum total CO_2 <18 mEq/l).
- Increasing intake of sodium chloride should be done cautiously and with careful monitoring because of the potential for increased risk of calcium oxalate urolith formation in some patients.
- Treatment options for cats with calcium oxalate uroliths include surgery, voiding urohydropropulsion (females or males with previously performed perineal urethrostomies), catheter retrieval and laser lithotripsy.
- Recommendations for urolith prevention are based on mineral composition of uroliths; analyze uroliths whenever possible. Appendix K lists urolith diagnostic laboratories
- Rate of urolith recurrence is ~7% with an average time of 23 months. Recurrence is not different between males and females.
- Generally, appropriate nutritional management is the most important consideration for prevention of recurrence of calcium oxalate uroliths.
- The goal of dietary management is to prevent recurrence by use of appropriate foods, feeding methods and, if necessary, medical management.
- Environmental enrichment (e.g., stress reduction, litter box management) may be helpful for cats with lower urinary tract disorders (Appendix L).

KEY NUTRITIONAL FACTORS

- Foods should provide recommended allowances of all required nutrients (nutritional adequacy), but should also contain specific levels of KNFs (certain nutrients that can assist in the management of calcium oxalate urolithiasis).
- KNFs for foods intended for minimizing recurrence of calcium oxalated urolithiasis are summarized in **Table 1** and include increased water and urinary pH and moderate protein, calcium, phosphorus, sodium and magnesium. Composite KNFs for foods for management of calcium oxalate-, FIC- and/or struvite-based FLUTD are also included in **Table 1**.

- A detailed review of these recommendations can be found in Chapter 46, Small Animal Clinical Nutrition, 5th edition.

FEEDING PLAN

Assess and Select the Food

Ensure the Food's Basic Nutritional Adequacy. AAFCO nutritional adequacy statements are usually found on a product's label. AAFCO approval does not ensure a food will be effective in preventing calcium oxalate recurrence or other long-term health problems.

Compare the Food's KNF Content with the Recommended Levels. **Table 2** lists commercial foods marketed for calcium oxalate urolith prevention and compares KNF content of these foods with recommended levels. Several foods have been developed that are intended to manage the combination of risk factors associated with calcium oxalate-, struvite- and/or FIC-based FLUTD. These foods are listed in **Table 3** and are compared to the composite KNFs for these 3 forms of FLUTD. Contact manufacturers for information for foods not in the tables (manufacturer contact information is listed on product labels). Select a food that best approximates the recommended KNF levels.

Supplements. Avoid supplemental calcium, ascorbic acid and vitamin D.

Urine Alkalinizing Ingredients. The recommended urinary pH range for calcium oxalate prevention is ≥6.2. Properly formulated foods should contain potassium citrate (see label ingredient panel) as an alkalinizing ingredient. Additional citric acid has other benefits (see Adjunctive Medical & Surgical Management below).

Food Form. If readily consumed, moist foods are preferred.

Increasing Water Intake. Appendix L provides tips for increasing water intake.

Manage Treats and Snacks. If treats/snacks are fed, commercial treats that most closely match the KNF profile recommended for foods for calcium oxalate prevention are best. Limit to <10% of the total diet on a volume, weight or calorie basis. Suggest small portions of the food being fed or the opposite form of the food fed; i.e., if a dry food is fed, offer small amounts of the same food in moist form and vice versa; consider kibbles of the dry calcium oxalate prevention food for use as treats (keep in a separate container away from the usual feeding area).

Human Foods as Snacks. Avoid calcium-rich human foods (Table 1, Chapter 28) or foods high in oxalates (Tables 1 and 5, Chapter 28).

Assess and Determine the Feeding Method

Determine How Much Food to Feed. The amount to feed can be estimated from feeding guides on product labels or by calculation (Appendix C). These estimates are only starting points and will likely need to be adjusted (see Followup below).

Consider How to Offer the Food. Although calcium oxalate crystalluria is not as pH dependent as struvite, management of urinary pH is still important. Free-choice feeding is associated with more persistent aciduria compared with meal feeding. Thus, meal feeding (2 times/day [dry or moist foods]), rather than feeding multiple small meals per day (as would happen with free-choice feeding), might lower the risk of calcium oxalate urolith formation because of the production of a more alkaline urinary pH.

Manage Food Changes. A transition period to avoid GI upsets and to facilitate acceptance of a new food is good practice. Example: to change to a new food, replace 10-15% of the old food with the new food on Day 1 and continue this incremental change daily until the change is complete on Day 7. Appendix E provides additional information. Chapter 33 contains suggestions for transitioning from dry to moist foods, which may require several weeks or more in some cats.

Food and Water Receptacle Husbandry. Food and water bowls should be washed regularly with warm soapy water and rinsed

Table 1. Key nutritional factors and recommended levels for managing cats with common lower urinary tract diseases.*

Factors	Dietary recommendations	
	Calcium oxalate uroliths	Combined FIC, struvite and calcium oxalate prevention
Water	Moist foods are best	Moist foods are best
Magnesium (%)	0.07 to 0.14	0.07 to 0.14
Phosphorus (%)	0.5 to 1.0	0.5 to 0.9
Calcium (%)	0.6 to 1.0	0.6 to 1.0
Protein (%)	≥32	32 to 45
Sodium (%)	0.3 to 0.6	0.3 to 0.6
Urinary pH	≥6.2	6.2 to 6.4
Total omega 3 (%)	–	0.35 to 1.0

Key: FIC = feline idiopathic cystitis, Total omega 3 = total omega-3 fatty acids.
*Nutrients expressed on a dry matter basis unless otherwise stated.

Table 2. Comparison of key nutritional factors in selected commercial veterinary therapeutic foods for decreasing risk of recurrence of calcium oxalate uroliths in cats.* (Numbers in red match optimal KNFs.)

Moist foods**	Mg (%)	P (%)	Ca (%)	Protein (%)	Na (%)	Urinary pH
Recommended levels	0.07-0.14	0.5-1.0	0.6-1.0	≥32	0.3-0.6	≥6.2
Hill's Prescription Diet c/d Multicare with Chicken Feline	0.052	0.68	0.72	43.8	0.32	6.35
Hill's Prescription Diet c/d Multicare with Seafood Feline	0.054	0.71	0.62	44.8	0.33	6.4
Iams Veterinary Formula Urinary O - Moderate pH/O	0.085	0.77	1.11	43.4	0.34	na
Medi-Cal Urinary SO in Gel	na	1.2	1.2	43.5	1.1	6.4
Purina Veterinary Diets UR Urinary St/Ox Feline Formula	0.07	0.97	0.96	50.6	0.62	6.0-6.4
Royal Canin Veterinary Diet Urinary SO in Gel	0.097	1.36	1.02	41.3	1.02	6.0-6.3
Dry foods	Mg (%)	P (%)	Ca (%)	Protein (%)	Na (%)	Urinary pH
Recommended levels	0.07-0.14	0.5-1.0	0.6-1.0	≥32	0.3-0.6	≥6.2
Hill's Prescription Diet c/d Multicare Feline	0.06	0.65	0.74	36.1	0.35	6.3
Hill's Prescription Diet c/d Multicare with Chicken Feline	0.061	0.65	0.76	34.6	0.33	6.3
Iams Veterinary Formula Urinary O - Moderate pH/O	0.098	0.91	1.24	36.5	0.46	na
Medi-Cal Urinary SO	na	0.9	1.1	34.6	1.4	6.2
Purina Veterinary Diets UR Urinary St/Ox Feline Formula	0.07	1.08	1.1	44.9	1.17	6.0-6.4
Royal Canin Veterinary Diet Urinary SO 33	0.065	0.88	0.96	37.1	1.45	6.0-6.3

Key: Mg = magnesium, P = phosphorus, Ca = calcium, Na = sodium, na = not available from manufacturer.
*Nutrients expressed on a dry matter basis unless otherwise stated.
**In general, moist foods should be fed to cats with FLUTD.

Table 3. Comparison of key nutritional factors in selected commercial veterinary therapeutic foods for reducing the recurrence of feline idiopathic cystitis, struvite disease (uroliths or urethral plugs) and/or calcium oxalate uroliths in cats.* (Numbers in red match optimal KNFs.)

Moist foods**	Mg (%)	P (%)	Ca (%)	Protein (%)	Na (%)	Urinary pH	Total omega 3 (%)
Recommended levels	0.07-0.14	0.5-0.9	0.6-1.0	32-45	0.3-0.6	6.2-6.4	0.35-1.0
Hill's Prescription Diet c/d Multicare with Chicken Feline	0.052	0.68	0.72	43.8	0.32	6.35	0.96
Hill's Prescription Diet c/d Multicare with Seafood Feline	0.054	0.71	0.62	44.8	0.33	6.4	0.62
Medi-Cal Urinary SO	na	1.20	1.20	43.5	1.1	6.4	na
Purina Veterinary Diets UR Urinary St/Ox Feline Formula	0.07	0.97	0.96	50.6	0.62	6.0-6.4	na
Royal Canin Veterinary Diet Urinary SO in gel	0.10	1.36	1.02	41.3	1.02	6.0-6.3	na
Dry foods	Mg (%)	P (%)	Ca (%)	Protein (%)	Na (%)	Urinary pH	Total omega 3 (%)
Recommended levels	0.07-0.14	0.5-0.9	0.6-1.0	32-45	0.3-0.6	6.2-6.4	0.35-1.0
Hill's Prescription Diet c/d Multicare Feline	0.06	0.65	0.74	36.1	0.35	6.3	0.65
Hill's Prescription Diet c/d Multicare with Chicken Feline	0.06	0.65	0.76	34.6	0.33	6.3	0.64
Purina Veterinary Diets UR Urinary St/Ox Feline Formula	0.07	1.08	1.1	44.9	1.17	6.0-6.4	na

Key: Mg = magnesium, P = phosphorus, Ca = calcium, Na = sodium, total omega 3 = total omega-3 fatty acids, na = not available from manufacturer.
*Nutrients expressed on a dry matter basis unless otherwise stated.
**In general, moist foods should be fed to cats with lower urinary tract disorders, especially those with feline idiopathic cystitis or calcium oxalate uroliths.

well. Dishes used for moist foods need daily cleaning. Discard moist or moistened dry foods after 2-4 hours of room temperature exposure to avoid foodborne illnesses (Appendix F).

ADJUNCTIVE MEDICAL & SURGICAL MANAGEMENT

Urine Alkalinizers

Potassium citrate in aqueous solution ionizes and the citrate anion may form soluble salts with calcium (reduces calcium oxalate crystal formation), promote formation of alkaline urine and, via metabolic alkalosis, enhance tubular reabsorption of calcium. If necessary (see Followup below), supplement with potassium citrate (wax matrix tablets[a] or liquid[b]). Chewable treats[c] are also available. Dose is 40-75 mg/kg q12h. Divided doses may help maintain consistently non-acidic urine. Potassium citrate should be administered with meals to reduce gastric irritation. Additional supplementation may not be needed when feeding foods with adequate potassium citrate (see label ingredient panel).

Thiazide Diuretics

Thiazide diuretics reduce recurrence of calcium-containing uroliths because of their ability to reduce urine calcium excretion, especially when used concurrently with a urolith prevention diet. Thiazide diuretics are not recommended as first-line therapy. Use should be accompanied by owner informed consent and appropriate clinical and laboratory monitoring for early detection of adverse effects (dehydration, hypokalemia, hypercalcemia).

FOLLOWUP

Owner Followup

Have owners observe for signs of recurrence. After the food change, ask owners to weigh their cat and/or grade its body condition (BCS) monthly. If a trend of increasing or decreasing body weight or BCS is noticed, the amount fed should be changed by 10% increments and the patient rechecked every 2 weeks for 1 month. At that point, if necessary, the amount fed should be changed again and the cycle repeated. Encourage increased water intake.

Compliance. If the cat lives in a multi-pet household, deny access to other pets' foods. Adhere strictly to feeding only the prescribed foods/treats/supplements.

Grocery Brand Foods with Urinary Health Claims. Caution owners not to feed these foods. They are formulated for healthy cats to avoid struvite crystals and uroliths. Feeding such foods may actually increase the risk of developing calcium oxalate uroliths.

Veterinary Health Care Team Followup

Immediately postsurgery, obtain data (radiography, complete urinalysis, serum concentrations of calcium, urea nitrogen and creatinine) to evaluate effectiveness of renal function and calcium homeostasis. If the cat is hypercalcemic, correct the underlying cause; if normocalcemic, initiate feeding plan (above).

1st Reevaluation (2-4 Weeks). Consider adding potassium citrate if calcium oxalate crystals and aciduria persist and perform the 2nd reevaluation (otherwise, go to last step, below). Detection of large aggregates of crystals is an important finding when monitoring effectiveness of preventive measures.

2nd Reevaluation (2-4 Weeks). Consider vitamin B_6 supplementation (2-4 mg/kg q24-48 hours). If calcium oxalate crystalluria persists do 3rd reevaluation (otherwise, go to last step, below).

3rd Reevaluation (2-4 Weeks). Consider administration of hydrochlorothiazide (2 mg/kg q24-48 hours) if calcium oxalate crystalluria persists.

Last Step. After 3-6 months, reevaluate to verify compliance and amelioration of crystalluria. Check for urolith recurrence by radiography. If no uroliths are present, continue current therapy and reevaluate in 3-6 months. If uroliths have recurred, consider voiding urohydropropulsion in females or males with previously performed perineal urethrostomy. Consider surgery if clinical signs of urocystolithiasis persist.

MISCELLANEOUS

See Chapter 33 for dietary management of FIC and Chapter 34 for dietary management of struvite urolithiasis. See Appendix L for information about other uroliths. See Chapter 46, Small Animal Clinical, 5th edition, for more detailed information.

Authors

Condensed from Chapter 46, Small Animal Clinical Nutrition, 5th edition, authored by S. Dru Forrester, John M. Kruger and Timothy A. Allen.

References

See Chapter 46, Small Animal Clinical Nutrition, 5th edition, on the website www.markmorrisinstitute.org for references.

Endnotes

a. Urocit-K. Mission Pharmacal, San Antonio, TX, USA.
b. Polycitra-K. Willen Drug Co., Baltimore, MD, USA.
c. K-CIT-V. V.E.T. Pharmaceuticals, Inc., Fenton, MO, USA.

CLINICAL POINTS

- Periodontal disease is common in dogs and cats (60-80%) and is the primary cause of tooth loss.
- Periodontal infections are associated with increased levels of C-reactive protein, proinflammatory cytokines, cholesterol, plasma fibrinogen, white blood cells and blood glucose.
- Correlation between the severity of periodontal disease and histopathologic changes in the kidneys, myocardium and liver suggest systemic complications.
- Small, toy and brachycephalic breeds are more prone to malocclusion, a risk for plaque accumulation. Brachycephalic breeds are also predisposed to mouth breathing, which may dry and irritate oral tissues.
- Periodontal disease, tooth resorption and gingivostomatitis are more common in purebred cats, especially Asian breeds.
- Immunocompetence may be a risk: an overexaggerated immune response can cause severe local periodontal destruction; an inadequate response may predispose pets to opportunistic/overwhelming systemic infection.
- Age increases the risk for periodontal disease in dogs and cats.
- Plaque accumulation may be influenced by food form and ingredients; calcium deficiency may result in loss of alveolar bone and is most likely to occur in pets fed improperly formulated homemade foods. Soft sticky foods fed to patients with occlusal abnormalities may result in excessive retained food debris.
- There is no significant difference in plaque accumulation between regular commercial moist and dry foods.
- **Table 1** lists clinical signs associated with periodontal disease.
- Plaque forms from enamel pellicle, a thin film composed of proteins and glycoproteins deposited from saliva and gingival crevicular fluid. Initially pellicle protects and lubricates, but bacterial components become incorporated and existing constituents are modified forming plaque. Plaque forms within minutes after a dental prophylaxis.
- Initially plaque is supragingival but eventually colonizes subgingival surfaces. The subsequent inflammation and destruction of periodontal tissues result from direct action of bacteria and indirect action of host inflammatory responses.
- Calculus (tartar) is mineralized plaque and provides a roughened surface that enhances plaque attachment and chronically irritates gingival tissue; however, calculus control in the absence of plaque control is cosmetic only.
- Plaque is very adherent and not easily removed by normal tongue activity or drinking water; it can be affected by chemical and mechanical means.
- Control of plaque, the cause of periodontal disease, is the primary goal of an oral health program; good oral health may positively affect systemic health.

- Brushing done correctly and regularly is an effective method of plaque control.
- Control of plaque by brushing may be difficult and compliance is low; properly formulated dental foods can effectively control plaque and gingivitis (**Figure 1**).
- Fed daily, foods with certain mechanical aspects can control plaque (and calculus and stain) in dogs and cats; an appropriate combination of shape, size and texture is important. Certain dietary fibers may be used to affect texture of dry foods; proper orientation of fibers within kibbles can maximize tooth contact time and plaque removal (**Figure 2**).
- Antioxidants (vitamins E and C and selenium) may lessen oxidative stress associated with subgingival/periodontal infection and inflammation.
- HMP is a polyphosphate calcium chelator that can be applied topically to foods or treats for calculus control in dogs; however, polyphosphates have no known direct effect on plaque or oral microflora.
- A good way to assess whether specific foods or treats are effective in preventing plaque is the VOHC Seal of Acceptance on the product's label. The VOHC is similar to the ADA and is recognized worldwide. There are 2 claim categories: "helps control plaque" and "helps control tartar." Products may qualify for either or both as indicated on product labels.
- Complete clinical and nutritional histories and thorough oral examinations are important to evaluate the types of intervention needed for a comprehensive oral health program.
- Feeding goal: provide a sufficient level of plaque control to prevent gingivitis and periodontal disease.

Table 1. Clinical signs associated with periodontal disease.

Anorexia	Red, swollen or bleeding gingivae
Behavioral changes	Substrate accumulation (plaque,
Difficulty eating	calculus, stain)
Halitosis	Tooth mobility
Head shaking	Ulcerations on gingivae or oral mucosa
Ptyalism	

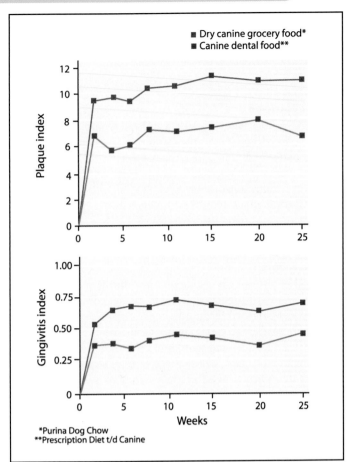

Figure 1. The effects of commercial dog foods on plaque accumulation and gingival health in dogs. These graphs compare plaque accumulation and gingival inflammation in dogs fed two different foods for six months. Each group of dogs began the study with a plaque index of zero and clinically healthy gingivae. At all time points, the dogs consuming the test food (Prescription Diet t/d Canine) had significantly lower scores for plaque accumulation and gingival inflammation than the dogs consuming the control food (Purina Dog Chow).

Table 2. Key nutritional factors for foods for dogs and cats for prevention of periodontal disease and maintenance of overall health.*

Factors	Dogs	Cats
Food texture	VOHC Seal for plaque control	VOHC Seal for plaque control
Antioxidants		
Vitamin E (IU/kg)	≥400	≥500
Vitamin C (mg/kg)	≥100	100-200
Selenium (mg/kg)	0.5-1.3	0.5-1.3
Phosphorus (%)	0.4-0.8	0.5-0.8
Sodium (%)	0.2-0.4	0.2-0.5
Magnesium (%)	-	0.04-0.1
Average urinary pH	-	6.2-6.4

Key: VOHC = Veterinary Oral Health Council Seal of Acceptance for plaque control.
*All values are amounts in food on a dry matter basis unless otherwise stated.

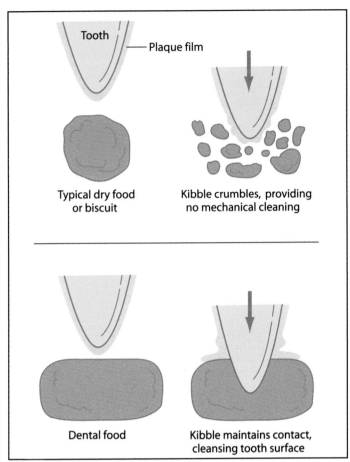

Figure 2. This illustration depicts the mechanical cleansing properties of commercial dog and cat foods. The top illustration demonstrates what occurs when a dog or cat chews a typical dry food. The kibble crumbles providing little to no mechanical cleansing. The bottom illustration demonstrates what happens when a dog or cat chews a dental food. The kibble stays together, maintaining contact with the tooth surface and providing mechanical cleansing.

KEY NUTRITIONAL FACTORS

- Foods should provide recommended allowances of all required nutrients (nutritional adequacy), but should also contain specific KNFs appropriate for reduction of plaque and promotion of long-term health.
- KNFs for foods for cats and dogs intended to control plaque and recommended amounts are listed in **Table 2** and discussed in more detail in Chapter 47, Small Animal Clinical Nutrition, 5th edition.
- Dental foods replace regular foods and are typically fed long term. Thus, several KNFs (phosphorus and sodium for dogs and cats and magnesium and urinary pH for cats) are included because of their role in preventing common health issues rather than being beneficial for plaque control (Chapters 1, 2, 7 and 8).
- If concurrent disease is present, KNFs for that disease should also be taken into consideration.
- Nutrient balance should be evaluated in all homemade foods; especially calcium and vitamins.

Table 3. Key nutritional factor content of selected dry commercial dog foods marketed for dental health compared to recommended levels.*
(Numbers in red match optimal KNFs.)

Factors	VOHC Seal for plaque control (Yes/No)	Vitamin E (IU/kg)	Vitamin C (mg/kg)	Selenium (mg/kg)	Phosphorus (%)	Sodium (%)
Recommended levels	Yes	≥400	≥100	0.5-1.3	0.4-0.8	0.2-0.4
Hill's Prescription Diet t/d Canine	Yes	652	79	0.50	0.40	0.22
Hill's Prescription Diet t/d Small Bites Canine	Yes	652	79	0.50	0.40	0.22
Hill's Science Diet Adult Oral Care	Yes	564	175	0.62	0.65	0.24
Medi-Cal Dental Formula	No	na	na	na	0.90	0.40
Purina Veterinary Diet DH Dental Health	No	1,171	na	na	1.25	0.57
Purina Veterinary Diet DH Dental Health Small Bites	No	1,169	na	na	1.24	0.61
Royal Canin Veterinary Diet Dental DD 20	No	604	na	0.44	0.66	0.38
Royal Canin Veterinary Diet Dental DS 23 Small Breed	No	725	na	0.44	0.66	0.77

Key: VOHC = Veterinary Oral Health Council Seal of Acceptance for plaque control, na = information not available from manufacturer.
*All values are amounts in food on a dry matter basis unless otherwise stated.

Table 4. Key nutritional factor content of selected dry commercial cat foods marketed for dental health compared to recommended levels.*
(Numbers in red match optimal KNFs.)

Factors	VOHC Seal for plaque control (Yes/No)	Vitamin E (IU/kg)	Vitamin C (mg/kg)	Selenium (mg/kg)	Phosphorus (%)	Sodium (%)	Magnesium (%)	Urinary pH
Recommended levels	Yes	≥500	100-200	0.5-1.3	0.5-0.8	0.2-0.5	0.04-0.1	6.2-6.4
Hill's Prescription Diet t/d Feline	Yes	811	83	0.59	0.80	0.33	0.065	6.34
Hill's Science Diet Adult Oral Care	Yes	670	171	0.55	0.75	0.37	0.058	6.30
Medi-Cal Dental Formula	No	na	na	na	0.70	0.60	na	na
Purina Veterinary Diets DH Dental Health	Yes	722	na	na	1.50	0.63	0.10	na
Royal Canin Veterinary Diet Dental DD 27	No	710	na	0.34	0.81	0.65	0.097	na

Key: VOHC = Veterinary Oral Health Council Seal of Acceptance for plaque control, na = information not available from manufacturer.
*All values are amounts in food on a dry matter basis unless otherwise stated.

FEEDING PLAN

Assess and Select the Food

Ensure the Food's Basic Nutritional Adequacy. AAFCO nutritional adequacy statements appropriate for maintenance are usually found on a product's label. AAFCO acceptance for maintenance does not ensure a food will be effective for plaque control.

Compare the Food's KNF Content with the Recommended Levels. Tables 3 and 4 list several commercial dry foods marketed for management of dental health in dogs and cats, respectively, and are compared to the corresponding KNFs. However, other foods may provide KNFs at or near recommended levels. Choose a food that most closely fits recommended levels. The VOHC Seal of Acceptance for plaque is the most important KNF for plaque control (see product labels).

MOISTENING DRY FOODS. Moistening dry dental foods to improve acceptance will likely negate dental benefits.

Assess and Determine the Feeding Method

Determine How Much Food to Feed. If a new food is fed, the amount to feed can be obtained from product labels (or other supporting material) or calculated. To calculate initial amounts, use formulas that factor in age and body weight (Appendix C). If body weight and BCS are not ideal, adjust food dosage estimates appropriately (see Followup below).

Consider How to Offer the Food. Both free-choice and restricted-feeding methods have advantages and disadvantages (Appendix D). Although free-choice feeding is most popular, it is most likely to result in overeating. Food-restricted feeding is best because it is less likely to cause overweight/obesity.

Manage Food Changes. A transition period to avoid GI upsets and facilitate acceptance of a new food is good practice. If the patient is eating a nonpreferred food, replace 25% of the old food with the new food on Day 1 and continue this incremental change daily until the change is complete on Day 4. If problems occur, delay the increase or cut back to the previous level of transition for several more days before continuing the food change. Appendix E provides additional information.

Manage Treats and Snacks. Commercial treats are often marketed to provide dental health benefits; documentation is important to verify dental claims and should be the same as for foods; thus, VOHC approved treats are recommended. An option is VOHC approved foods (as small amounts fed separately) provided as treats. Treats/snacks should not be fed excessively (<10% of the total diet on a volume, weight or calorie basis). See Appendix B for more treats/snacks information. Miscellaneous, below, provides information about dental chews and chew toys. *Food and Water Receptacle Husbandry.* Food and water bowls should be washed regularly with warm soapy water and rinsed well. Dishes used for moist foods need daily cleaning. Discard moist or moistened dry foods after 2-4 hours of room temperature exposure to avoid foodborne illnesses (Appendix F).

FOLLOWUP

Owner Followup

Have owners weigh their dog or cat (if possible) and/or grade its body condition (BCS) monthly. If a trend of increasing or decreasing body weight or BCS is noticed, the amount fed should be changed by 10% increments and the patient rechecked every 2 weeks for 1 month. At that point, if necessary, the amount fed should be changed again and the cycle repeated. Instruct owners to be aware of signs of recurrence of excessive plaque buildup by visual inspection (if possible) and/or presence of halitosis.

Veterinary Health Care Team Followup

Monitoring schedules depend on: 1) the degree of oral pathology, 2) level of periodontal therapy and 3) owner ability to provide routine oral hygiene.
Patients with Good Oral Health and Normal Occlusion. Annual oral exams are usually adequate.
Patients with Invasive or Advanced Procedures. Consider offering soft food during the initial healing phase. Reassess weekly until healing and plaque control are verified, then extend the schedule to 3-month intervals. Eventually, intervals between further followup visits will be dictated by the degree of plaque retention by the patient and/or the ability of the owner to provide plaque control.

MISCELLANEOUS

For more information about periodontal disease, see Chapter 47, Small Animal Clinical Nutrition, 5th edition.

Chews and Chew Toys

In most cases, dental benefits of chews and chew toys have not been substantiated; some practitioners have reported safety issues.
Potential Safety Issues with Chews.
RAWHIDE CHEWS. If chewed aggressively or used as "catch" toys, compacted hard rawhide treats formed as balls or bones may cause tooth fractures. Softer strips and wafers may be safer.
FORMED RICE AND WHEY TREATS. These products are available in various shapes (e.g., bones, toothbrushes). Some have effectively controlled plaque and/or tartar as indicated by the VOHC Seal of Acceptance on their packaging/product information. However, there are reports of serious GI side effects associated with their use, even after reformulation.

Authors

Condensed from Chapter 47, Small Animal Clinical Nutrition, 5th edition, authored by Ellen I. Logan, Robert B. Wiggs, Dale Scherl and Paul Cleland.

References

See Chapter 47, Small Animal Clinical Nutrition, 5th edition, on the website www.markmorrisinstitute.org for references.

CLINICAL POINTS

- The oral cavity is susceptible to several acquired and congenital disorders but in comparison to the high incidence of periodontal disease (Chapter 36), these conditions are relatively uncommon.
- The more common conditions affecting the oral cavity include inflammatory lesions and physical abnormalities such as neoplasia, trauma and congenital malformations (e.g., cleft palate).
- Approximately 50% of cats with FIV infection and 60% of cats with calicivirus infection have chronic oral lesions; other infectious oral disorders (e.g., candidiasis or fusospirochetal infections) are rare and usually occur in immunocompromised animals.
- Patients with oral disease have variable clinical signs depending on the type and location of the lesions; signs include dysphagia or pain associated with eating, excessive salivation, oral hemorrhage, halitosis and reluctance to eat resulting in loss of body weight and condition.
- A history may exist of ingestion of foreign bodies, caustic materials or trauma. Neonates with congenital anomalies such as cleft palate may be presented because of ineffectual suckling, poor weight gain and coughing or gagging following attempts to nurse.
- Laboratory values are often unremarkable and generally reflect underlying conditions, if present. Leukocytosis and a polyclonal hyperglobulinemia are frequent findings in cats with lymphoplasmacytic stomatitis.
- Radiography is often of value in cases with suspected trauma to assess the extent of bony injury.
- Diagnosis of lesions within the oral cavity often requires biopsy and histopathologic examination.
- Young patients are more likely to present with congenital and traumatic lesions, whereas older patients are more likely to suffer from oral neoplasia and inflammatory disorders.
- Patients undergoing radiation therapy of the head and neck for cancer are susceptible to radiation-induced mucositis.
- Certain breeds are predisposed to various oral disorders (**Table 1**).
- Dehydration is a frequent problem in dogs and cats with oral disorders that interfere with water intake.
- High energy density foods may be helpful in meeting the patient's caloric requirement in a small volume.
- Feeding goals are to provide adequate nutrition via whatever feeding route is necessary while minimizing discomfort to the patient and enhancing resolution of the oral lesions.

KEY NUTRITIONAL FACTORS

- Foods should provide recommended allowances of all required nutrients (nutritional adequacy), but should also contain specific KNFs appropriate for patients with oral diseases.
- **Table 2** lists KNFs for foods for cats and dogs with oral diseases and recommended amounts; these KNFs are discussed in more detail in Chapter 49, Small Animal Clinical Nutrition, 5th edition.
- Patients with extensive oral injuries or inflammation of the oral cavity may benefit from foods having KNFs for assisted feeding or recovery (Chapter 12). Patients with oral neoplasia may benefit from foods with KNFs for patients with cancer (Chapter 18).
- If concurrent disease is present, KNFs for that disease should also be taken into consideration.

FEEDING PLAN

Assess and Select the Food
Ensure the Food's Basic Nutritional Adequacy. If long-term (weeks-months) feeding is anticipated, check product labels for AAFCO nutritional adequacy statements. AAFCO approval does not ensure a food will be effective in the management of oral diseases.
Compare the Food's KNF Content with the Recommended Levels. KNFs for foods for patients with oral diseases should be compared with levels in foods under consideration for feeding.

FOOD FORM. Experiment with foods of different consistencies. Often, liquid foods or slurries made from moist foods and water are more readily accepted. Also, a food with a dilute consistency may be less likely to accumulate in oral lesions and adhere to surgical sites.

UNDERWEIGHT PATIENTS. Consider a nutrient profile similar to that found in growth (Chapters 5 and 11) or recovery-type formulas (Chapter 12).

PATIENTS WITH EXTENSIVE ORAL INJURIES OR ORAL CAVITY INFLAMMATION. Consider foods designed for assisted feeding or recovery (Chapter 12) combined with tube feeding

Table 1. Breed-associated oral disorders.

Disorders	Breeds
Cleft palate	Brachycephalic dogs and cats
Epulides	Boxer
Gingivitis/stomatitis	Maltese dog
	Siberian husky
Lymphoplasmacytic	Abyssinian cat
stomatitis	Burmese cat
	Himalayan cat
	Maltese cat
	Persian cat
	Siamese cat
Neoplasia	Cocker spaniel
	German shepherd dog
	German shorthaired pointer
	Golden retriever
	Weimaraner

Table 2. Key nutritional factors for foods for patients with oral diseases.

Factors	Dietary recommendations
Water	Maintain fluid balance with oral, and if necessary, parenteral fluids
Energy	For dogs: >4.5 kcal/g (>18.8 kJ/g) dry matter For cats: >5 kcal/g (>20.9 kJ/g) dry matter
Food form	Liquid foods and slurries made from moist food are often more readily accepted

(see Feeding Methods below).

ORAL NEOPLASIA. Consider foods specifically formulated for cancer (Chapter 18).

Assess and Determine the Feeding Method

Determine How Much Food to Feed. The amount to feed can be obtained from the product label or it can be calculated (Appendix C). If using enteral-assisted feeding methods, see Chapter 12.

Consider How to Offer the Food. Initially feed several small meals daily if the patient is able and willing to consume food voluntarily. After each meal, flush the oral cavity with water to remove particulate matter adhered to oral mucous membranes.

ASSISTED FEEDING. In many cases, tube-feeding methods are preferred until oral discomfort is reduced, oral lesions are healed and voluntary food consumption resumes (Chapter 12). Some patients may require nasoesophageal, esophageal or pharyngostomy feeding rather than orogastric feeding. Consider preplacement in surgical patients with these requirements.

Manage Food Changes.

INITIATION OF ORAL DISEASE FOOD. Based on feeding recommendations from product labels/information or calculations (Appendix C) feed 25-33% of the recommended/calculated

amount on Day 1, with a goal to meet the patient's total need by the end of Days 2 or 3.

RETURN TO REGULAR FOOD. Patients that have recovered and are eating on their own can be fed their regular food. Replace 25% of the oral disease food with the regular food on Day 1 and continue this incremental change daily until the change is complete on Day 4. If problems occur, feed the previous food for several more days before repeating the food change. Appendix E provides additional information.

FOLLOWUP

Owner Followup

After recovery, owners should obtain body weight (if possible) and/or grade body condition (BCS) monthly. For patients that had normal body condition before the development of oral disease, the amount fed previously should be appropriate. If the patient is underweight, the amount fed should be increased by 10% increments and the patient rechecked every 2 weeks for 1 month. At that point, if necessary, the amount fed should be increased again and the cycle repeated until normal body weight/BCS are achieved.

Veterinary Health Care Team Followup

During hospitalization, monitor BCS and hydration status regularly to determine adequacy of food and water intake. Institute assisted feeding if necessary (Chapter 12). Mucositis associated with radiation therapy usually occurs during Week 3 of a 4-5 week protocol and typically resolves in 3-4 days.

MISCELLANEOUS

See Chapters 25, 47 and 49, Small Animal Clinical Nutrition, 5th edition, for more information.

Authors

Condensed from Chapter 49, Small Animal Clinical Nutrition, 5th edition, authored by Deborah J. Davenport, Rebecca L. Remillard and Ellen I. Logan.

References

See Chapter 49, Small Animal Clinical Nutrition, 5th edition, on the website www.markmorrisinstute.org for references.

CLINICAL POINTS

- Relative to vomiting and diarrhea, swallowing disorders are uncommon. However, they are often profoundly debilitating due to inadequate food intake and recurrent pulmonary infections resulting from aspiration.
- Pharyngeal and esophageal disorders can generally be grouped into 3 categories: aberrant motility, obstructive lesions or inflammatory degenerative conditions (**Table 1**).
- Congenital pharyngeal and esophageal disorders are typically diagnosed after weaning. In some puppies, clinical/subclinical esophageal dysmotility may improve with age, whereas it progresses in others.
- Acquired pharyngeal and esophageal disease can occur at any age and may be related to: 1) esophageal foreign bodies (dental chew treats, bones or bone and raw food diets), 2) recent anesthetic procedures (reflux esophagitis) 3), in cats, recent oral antibiotic (tetracycline, doxycycline and clindamycin) therapy and 4) neuromuscular diseases.
- Dogs with dysphagia due to pharyngeal disease typically cough or gag as they chew and swallow food.
- The hallmark clinical sign of esophageal disease is regurgitation (Appendix M). Additional signs include ptyalism, frequent swallowing, gurgling esophageal noises, halitosis and apparent pain on swallowing. Affected cats may vocalize in conjunction with gagging or regurgitation. Frequency of regurgitation and temporal relation to eating are variable.
- Patients with noninflammatory oral disorders often have a voracious appetite despite regurgitation unless they have secondary aspiration pneumonia. Poor body condition is often evident.
- Young patients with congenital megaesophagus, vascular ring anomalies or cricopharyngeal dysphagia are often stunted.
- Auscultatory findings often indicate secondary aspiration pneumonia and may include crackles and prominent bronchovesicular sounds. Dogs with aspiration pneumonia may be febrile and have a mucopurulent nasal discharge.
- A complete neurologic examination should be performed on adult dogs with swallowing disorders because acquired megaesophagus is often associated with neuromuscular disorders.
- Lab findings: CBC may indicate aspiration pneumonia. In chronically affected patients, serum protein and albumin may reflect nutritional status. Other serum biochemical abnormalities may point to an underlying disorder (e.g., hypoadrenocorticism, hypothyroidism).
- Use routine and specialized radiography in patients with suspected swallowing disorders.
- Esophagoscopy is useful for evaluating patients with suspected

Abbreviations
AAFCO = Association of American Feed Control Officials
BCS = body condition score (Appendix A)
KNF = key nutritional factor

Table 1. Mechanisms of pharyngeal and esophageal disorders.

Mechanisms	Disorders
Aberrant motility	Congenital megaesophagus
	Cricopharyngeal dysphagia
	Dysautonomia
	Endocrinopathies (hypothyroidism, hypoadrenocorticism)
	Esophageal dysmotility in young dogs
	Extraluminal obstruction (mediastinal or hilar lymphadenopathy)
	Idiopathic megaesophagus
	Infectious diseases (canine distemper)
	Myasthenia gravis
	Paraneoplastic syndromes (lymphosarcoma, thymoma)
	Polymyopathies
	Polyneuropathies
	Secondary megaesophagus
	Toxin ingestion (lead)
Inflammatory conditions	Foreign body esophagitis
	Pharyngitis
	Reflux esophagitis
Obstructive lesions	Foreign bodies
	Neoplasia
	Spirocerca lupi granulomas
	Strictures
	Vascular ring anomalies

Table 2. Breed-associated disorders of the pharynx and esophagus.

Conditions	Breeds
Cricopharyngeal dysphagia	Cocker spaniel
Congenital esophageal dysmotility and/or megaesophagus	Bouvier des Flandres
	Chinese Shar-Pei
	Fox terrier and other terrier breeds
	German shepherd dog
	Great Dane
	Irish setter
	Labrador retriever
	Miniature schnauzer
	Newfoundland
	Siamese cat
Idiopathic acquired megaesophagus	German shepherd dog
	Golden retriever
	Great Dane
	Irish setter
Vascular ring anomalies	Boston terrier
	English bulldog
	German shepherd dog
	Irish setter
	Labrador retriever
	Poodle

obstructive, neoplastic or inflammatory lesions of the esophagus and pharynx.

- Certain breeds are more at risk for swallowing disorders than others (**Table 2**).
- Although several different medical, procedural and/or surgical approaches exist for managing swallowing disorders, there are basically 2 nutritional approaches based on whether the patient has: 1) motility/obstructive disorders or 2) an inflammatory condition (**Table 1**).
- For patients with motility/obstructive disorders, a relatively high energy/nutrient density (including high dietary fat) is helpful in meeting requirements in a small volume of food.
- Foods with lower levels of dietary fat are recommended for managing patients with inflammatory conditions; higher levels of dietary fat may precipitate gastroesophageal reflux by delaying gastric emptying and reducing gastroesophageal sphincter tone.
- Increased dietary protein is needed for tissue repair and, in young patients, for growth. Additionally, protein may play an important role in reducing gastric reflux because protein stimulates an increase in gastroesophageal sphincter tone.
- Food form and proper feeding methods (below) are important for the management of swallowing disorders; usually moist foods and gruels are recommended. Occasionally foods containing more bulk or prepared in larger boluses may stimulate esophageal motility in patients with a mild aberrant motility defect.
- Feeding goal: minimize regurgitation, avoid secondary aspiration and provide adequate nutrition to regain or maintain body condition (or support growth in puppies/kittens) and promote healing.

Table 3. Key nutritional factors for foods for patients with swallowing disorders due to obstructive lesions or aberrant motility.*

Factors	Recommended levels
Energy density	≥4.5 kcal/g (≥18.8 kJ/g)
Fat	≥25%
Protein	≥25% for dog foods
	≥35% for cat foods

*Nutrients expressed on a dry matter basis; food form is also a key nutritional factor but varies with individual patients (see text).

Table 4. Key nutritional factors for foods for dogs and cats with esophagitis/gastroesophageal reflux.*

Factors	Recommended levels
Energy density	≥4 kcal/g (≥16.7 kJ/g)
Fat	≤15% for dog foods
	≤20% for cat foods
Protein	≥25% for dog foods
	≥35% for cat foods

*Nutrients expressed on a dry matter basis; food form is also a key nutritional factor, but varies with the disease and individual patients (see text).

KEY NUTRITIONAL FACTORS

- Foods should provide recommended allowances of all required nutrients (nutritional adequacy), but should also contain specific levels of KNFs (certain nutrients and food features that may assist in the management of pharyngeal and esophageal disorders).
- **Table 3** lists KNF recommendations for foods for patients with swallowing disorders due to obstructive lesions or aberrant motility; **Table 4** lists KNF recommendations for foods for patients with inflammatory swallowing disorders. A detailed review of these recommendations can be found in Chapter 50, Small Animal Clinical Nutrition, 5th edition. In addition to KNFs in **Tables 3** and **4**, other KNFs may be important depending on the patient's lifestage (e.g., growth; Chapters 5 and 11).

FEEDING PLAN

Assess and Select the Food

Ensure the Food's Basic Nutritional Adequacy. AAFCO nutritional adequacy statements are usually found on a product's label. AAFCO approval does not ensure a food will be effective in the management of pharyngeal/esophageal disorders.

Compare the Food's KNF Content with the Recommended Levels.

Obstructive Lesions and Aberrant Motility. Feeding an energy/nutrient-dense, highly digestible growth or recuperative food or a working/sporting food for dogs is appropriate for most patients. Compare KNFs of the food being considered with the recommendations in **Table 3**. Depending on lifestage and feeding methods, consider foods in Tables 17-4, 18-12, 24-3, 25-8 and 25-9, in Small Animal Clinical Nutrition, 5th fifth edition.

Food Form. Food consistency that best promotes flow through the esophagus to the stomach is determined by trial and error.

Gruels. Gruels often work well. Moist foods typically blenderize easily with water. Nutrient-dense, highly digestible foods meet requirements in the smallest volume possible. Consider larger cans of nutrient-dense cat food to help reduce volume and cost of feeding a large dog.

Larger Boluses. Esophageal performance may improve in megaesophagus patients when the swallowing reflex is maximally stimulated by the texture of dry foods or moist foods formed into large boluses. In these patients, gruels/liquids may not stimulate secondary peristalsis, thereby increasing the risk of aspiration pneumonia.

Inflammatory Conditions. Tables 5 and 6 compare KNF content of selected veterinary therapeutic foods to recommended levels for canine and feline patients, respectively.

Food Form. As noted above, moist foods are usually more readily liquefied.

Table 5. Key nutritional factor content of selected commercial veterinary therapeutic foods for dogs with esophagitis/gastroesophageal reflux compared to recommended levels.* (Numbers in red match optimal KNFs.)

Dry foods	Energy density (kcal/cup)**	Energy density (kcal/g)	Fat (%)	Protein (%)
Recommended levels	–	≥4	≤15	≥25
Hill's Prescription Diet i/d Canine	379	4.2	14.1	26.2
Iams Veterinary Formula Intestinal Low-Residue	257	3.8	10.7	24.6
Medi-Cal Gastro Formula	330	na	13.9	22.9
Purina Veterinary Diets EN GastroENteric Formula	397	4.2	12.6	27.0
Royal Canin Veterinary Diet Intestinal HE	389	4.5	22.0	33.0
Moist foods	Energy density (kcal/can)**	Energy density (kcal/g)	Fat (%)	Protein (%)
Recommended levels	–	≥4	≤15	≥25
Hill's Prescription Diet i/d Canine	485/13 oz.	4.4	14.9	25.0
Iams Veterinary Formula Intestinal Low-Residue	413/14 oz.	4.6	13.2	35.9
Medi-Cal Gastro Formula	455/396 g	na	11.7	22.1
Purina Veterinary Diets EN GastroENteric Formula	423/354 g	4.0	13.8	30.5
Royal Canin Veterinary Diet Intestinal HE	446/396 g	4.3	11.8	23.1

Key: na = information not available from manufacturer.
*From manufacturers' published information or calculated from manufacturers' published as-fed values; all values are on a dry matter basis unless otherwise stated.
**Energy density values are listed on an as fed basis and are useful for determining the amount to feed; cup = 8-oz. measuring cup. To convert to kJ, multiply kcal by 4.184.

Table 6. Key nutritional factor content of selected commercial veterinary therapeutic foods for cats with esophagitis/gastroesophageal reflux compared to recommended levels.* (Numbers in red match optimal KNFs.)

Dry foods	Energy density (kcal/cup)**	Energy density (kcal/g)	Fat (%)	Protein (%)
Recommended levels	–	≥4	≤20	≥35
Hill's Prescription Diet i/d Feline	483	4.3	20.2	40.3
Iams Veterinary Formula Intestinal Low-Residue	348	3.9	13.7	35.8
Medi-Cal Hypoallergenic/Gastro	350	na	11.5	29.8
Purina Veterinary Diets EN GastroENteric Formula	572	4.4	18.4	56.2
Royal Canin Veterinary Diet Intestinal HE 30	396	4.4	23.7	34.4
Moist foods	Energy density (kcal/can)**	Energy density (kcal/g)	Fat (%)	Protein (%)
Recommended levels	–	≥4	≤20	≥35
Hill's Prescription Diet i/d Feline	161/5.5 oz.	4.2	24.1	37.6
Iams Veterinary Formula Intestinal Low-Residue	169/6 oz.	4.0	11.7	38.4
Medi-Cal Hypoallergenic/Gastro	184/170 g	na	35.9	35.5
Medi-Cal Sensitivity CR	162/165 g	na	35.1	34.5

Key: na = information not available from manufacturer.
*From manufacturers' published information or calculated from manufacturers' published as-fed values; all values are on a dry matter basis unless otherwise stated.
**Energy density values are listed on an as fed basis and are useful for determining the amount to feed; cup = 8-oz. measuring cup. To convert to kJ, multiply kcal by 4.184.

Assess and Determine the Feeding Method

Determine How Much Food to Feed. The amount fed can be estimated from feeding guides on product labels or by calculation (Appendix C). These estimates are only starting points and will likely need to be adjusted (see Followup below).

Consider How to Offer the Food. Small-volume, frequent meals of a gruel/liquid form are recommended. During feeding, position the patient in an upright position and maintain this position for 20-30 minutes after feeding to provide ample time for gravitational flow of the food through the esophagus to the stomach. Other patients may need assisted feeding.

UPRIGHT FEEDING METHODS. Use elevated food bowls so the patient has to sit or stand on its hind legs to eat. Pets can be trained to eat on stairs or from a counter or stool. Owners can cradle small dogs and cats in an upright position while eating

(Chapter 50, Small Animal Clinical Nutrition, 5th edition). Large dogs can be trained to sit after eating or lie in sternal recumbency on an inclined board for the required period of time.

ASSISTED FEEDING. If upright feeding is inadequate to control regurgitation or is impractical because of the pet's temperament or owner's schedule, consider gastrostomy or jejunostomy tubes to bypass the esophagus (Chapter 12). Nasoesophageal, pharyngostomy and esophagostomy tubes are not recommended because they deliver food into the esophagus where it can be regurgitated. Nasogastric tubes may promote esophagitis. Inform owners that regurgitation might not completely cease even if food and water are provided through a gastrostomy tube. Many patients will continue to regurgitate salivary fluid. However, the likelihood of aspiration pneumonia is greatly reduced. Consider tube placement at the time of initial endoscopic examination.

Manage Food Changes. To transition to the GI food, provide 25-33% of the patient's estimated total daily amount of food on Day 1, with a goal to feed 100% of the total amount by the end of Days 3 or 4.

Food and Water Receptacle Husbandry. Food and water bowls should be washed regularly with warm soapy water and rinsed well. Dishes used for gruels and moist foods need daily cleaning. Discard moist or moistened dry foods after 2-4 hours of room temperature exposure to avoid foodborne illnesses (Appendix F).

ADJUNCTIVE MEDICAL & SURGICAL MANAGEMENT

The feeding plan is often used in conjunction with other treatments: 1) surgery (e.g., cricopharyngeal myotomy, esophageal stricture, vascular ring anomaly and esophageal foreign bodies), 2) bougienage (e.g., esophageal stricture), 3) endoscopy (e.g., foreign body removal) and 4) drugs (e.g., antibiotics, prokinetic agents, corticosteroids, antacids, H_2-receptor blockers, mucosal protective agents).

FOLLOWUP

Owner Followup
Note episodes of dysphagia or regurgitation. Obtain body weight (if possible) and/or grade body condition (BCS) monthly. If the patient is underweight, the amount fed should be increased by 10% and the patient rechecked every 2 weeks for 1 month.

At that point, if necessary, the amount fed should be increased again and the cycle repeated until normal body weight/BCS are achieved.

Veterinary Health Care Team Followup
Monitor changes in body weight and BCS. Evaluate owner compliance regarding feeding the proper amount of food. Determine the extent of ongoing dysphagia or regurgitation and monitor resolution of other concurrent disease processes (e.g., pneumonia, myopathies, endocrinopathies). Assist owner with food dosage and necessary adjustments as indicated by the patient's body weight and BCS.

MISCELLANEOUS

For information about hairballs see Appendix M. For more information, see Chapters 17, 18, 24, 25 and 50, Small Animal Clinical Nutrition, 5th edition.

Authors
Condensed from Chapter 50, Small Animal Clinical Nutrition, 5th edition, authored by Deborah J. Davenport, Michael S. Leib and Rebecca L. Remillard.

References
See Chapter 50, Small Animal Clinical Nutrition, 5th edition, on the website www.markmorrisinstitute.org for references.

CLINICAL POINTS

- Acute gastroenteritis is covered in Chapter 42.
- The prevalence of gastritis is thought to be high because many different insults can result in gastric mucosal inflammation (**Table 1**). Gastritis has been diagnosed in 35% of dogs presented for chronic vomiting and has been identified in 26-48% of asymptomatic dogs. The prevalence in cats is unknown.
- Previously, the prevalence of gastroduodenal ulcers in pets was thought to be low. However, it is now diagnosed more frequently possibly due to increased use of NSAIDs.
- Gastritis is one of the most common causes of vomiting in dogs and cats. It is important to differentiate vomiting from regurgitation (Appendix M).
- Chronic gastritis generally is defined as intermittent vomiting that occurs for more than 1-2 weeks.
- Younger and/or unsupervised pets are more likely to develop gastritis secondary to foreign bodies or dietary indiscretion. Older pets are more likely to suffer from metabolic or neoplastic causes of gastritis.
- Dogs of any age receiving NSAIDs, corticosteroids, or both, for management of osteoarthritis are at risk for gastritis and gastroduodenal ulceration.
- Several breeds are at risk for gastritis (Appendix M).
- Dogs with liver or kidney disease, hypoadrenocorticism, spinal cord disease, shock, stress, neoplasia, mastocytosis and systemic disease are at increased risk for gastroduodenal ulceration.
- Racing sled dogs in competition are at risk for gastroduodenal erosions and ulceration although dogs in training are not. Nearly 50% of dogs completing the Iditarod were found to have gastric lesions.
- Hematemesis usually indicates that gastroduodenal ulcers are present. Although some patients are asymptomatic, vomiting is the most common presenting complaint for both acute and chronic gastritis.
- Other signs may include diarrhea, abdominal pain and melena. Some owners report that their dog assumes a "praying posture" (considered a sign of upper abdominal pain). Anorexia is the presenting sign in many patients.
- Physical examination is often unremarkable. Check for dehydration. Abdominal pain may indicate peritonitis due to a perforated ulcer. Pallor and weakness may be present with significant GI blood loss.
- Routine hematology, serum biochemistry and urinalyses help assess severity and chronicity and rule out possible underlying diseases (e.g., renal disease, hepatopathies, hypoadrenocorticism, neoplasia).
- Abdominal radiographs are often normal but may be useful for diagnosis of radiopaque foreign bodies.

Abbreviations
AAFCO = Association of American Feed Control Officials
BCS = body condition score (Appendix A)
IBD = inflammatory bowel disease
KNF = key nutritional factor
NPO = nothing per os
NSAID = nonsteroidal antiinflammatory drug

Table 1. Potential causes of gastritis and/or gastroduodenal ulceration.

Adverse reactions to food
Food allergy (hypersensitivity)
Food intolerance
Dietary indiscretion
Chemicals
Foreign bodies
Garbage toxicosis
Gluttony
Heavy metal toxicosis
Plants
Drug administration
Corticosteroids
Nonsteroidal antiinflammatory agents
Idiopathic gastritis
Infectious agents
Fungi
Parasites
Spiral bacteria
Inflammatory bowel disease
Neoplasia
Gastrinoma
Mastocytosis
Primary gastric neoplasia
Reduced gastric blood flow
Disseminated intravascular coagulopathy
Neurologic disorders
Sepsis
Shock
Reflux gastritis
Systemic disease
Hypoadrenocorticism
Kidney disease
Liver disease
Pancreatitis

- Endoscopy is the most sensitive diagnostic tool for either gastritis or gastroduodenal ulceration. Chronic gastritis is diagnosed based on histopathologic examination of biopsy specimens.
- Chronic idiopathic gastritis may be a subset of IBD or may be due to an adverse reaction to food. It can be localized or occur with more diffuse IBD of the small or large bowel (Chapters 19 and 43 and Chapters 31 and 57, Small Animal Clinical Nutrition, 5th edition).
- Elimination foods are sometimes recommended for patients with chronic idiopathic gastritis because dietary antigens are

Table 2. Key nutritional factors for dogs and cats with gastritis and/or gastroduodenal ulceration.*

Factors	Recommended levels
Potassium	0.8 to 1.1%
Chloride	0.5 to 1.3%
Sodium	0.3 to 0.5%
Protein	***Highly digestible food approach:*** ≤30% for dogs and ≤40% for cats ***Elimination food approach:*** Limit dietary protein to one or two sources Use protein sources that the patient has not been exposed to previously or feed a protein hydrolysate (Chapter 19) 16 to 26% for dogs 30 to 40% for cats
Fat	<15% for dogs <25% for cats
Fiber	≤5% crude fiber; avoid foods with gel-forming fiber sources such as pectins and gums (e.g., gum arabic, guar gum, carrageenan, psyllium gum, xanthan gum, carob gum, gum ghatti and gum tragacanth)
Food form and temperature	Moist foods are best; warm foods to between 70 to 100°F (21 to 38°C)

*Nutrients expressed on a dry matter basis.

suspected to play a role in etiopathogenesis.
- Water is the most important nutrient for patients with acute vomiting because of the potential for life-threatening dehydration due to excessive fluid loss and inability of the patient to replace those losses.
- Mild hypokalemia, hypochloremia and either hypernatremia or hyponatremia are electrolyte abnormalities most commonly associated with acute vomiting (and diarrhea). Foods for patients with acute gastritis should contain levels of potassium, chloride and sodium above minimum recommended allowances.
- Besides interfering with gastric motility and reservoir function (which leads to vomiting), gastric mucosal inflammation results in protein loss. However, foods for patients with acute gastritis/gastroduodenal ulcers should not provide excess protein. Products of protein digestion (peptides, amino acids and amines) increase gastrin and gastric acid secretion.
- Higher fat foods are emptied more slowly from the stomach than foods with less fat. Fat in the duodenum stimulates cholecystokinin release, which delays gastric emptying.
- Foods containing gel-forming soluble fibers increase viscosity of ingesta and slow gastric emptying; these include pectins and gums (e.g., gum arabic, guar gum, carrageenan, psyllium gum, xanthan gum, carob gum, gum ghatti and gum tragacanth).
- Moist foods, warm foods and smaller meals reduce gastric retention time and promote gastric emptying.
- Beneficial effects of "feeding through vomiting" (see Feeding Methods below) may be due to the physical presence of food and nutrients serving as mechanical and chemical stimuli to normalize bowel motility and function.
- Feeding goals: provide a food that meets the patient's nutrient requirements, allows normalization of gastric motility and function and helps control vomiting.

KEY NUTRITIONAL FACTORS

- Foods should provide recommended allowances of all required nutrients (nutritional adequacy), but should also contain specific levels of KNFs (certain nutrients and food features that may assist in the management of gastritis and gastroduodenal ulcers).
- **Table 2** lists KNF recommendations for foods for patients with gastritis and gastroduodenal ulcerations. Included are KNFs for a highly-digestible food approach or an elimination food approach (for chronic gastritis). A detailed review of these recommendations can be found in Chapter 52, Small Animal Clinical Nutrition, 5th edition. In addition to KNFs in **Table 2**, other KNFs may be important depending on the patient's lifestage (e.g., growth; Chapters 5 and 11).

FEEDING PLAN

The first objective in managing vomiting patients should be to correct dehydration and electrolyte/acid-base imbalances, if present. In most cases of acute vomiting, NPO for 24-48 hours with parenteral fluid administration reduces/resolves vomiting by removing effects of undigested food and offending agents from the stomach and duodenum. Patients with chronic vomiting generally require a more detailed diagnostic and therapeutic (i.e., combined medical and nutritional) approach.

Assess and Select the Food
Ensure the Food's Basic Nutritional Adequacy. AAFCO nutritional adequacy statements are usually found on a product's label. AAFCO approval does not ensure a food will be effective in the management of gastritis/gastroduodenal ulcers.
Compare the Food's KNF Content with the Recommended Levels. **Tables 3** and **4** include the KNF content of selected commercial foods marketed for GI diseases and compare them to the recommended levels for vomiting patients (dogs and cats, respectively). Tables 3 and 4, Chapter 19, include KNF content of selected elimination foods; consider these for use in patients with chronic vomiting. Select foods that most closely match KNF target levels.

FOOD FORM. Liquids are emptied from the stomach more quickly than solids due to lower digesta osmolality. Consider gruels based on blenderized moist GI foods. For feeding through vomiting in cats (see Consider How to Offer the Food below), use liquid foods (Tables 5 and 6, Chapter 12).

FOOD TEMPERATURE. Cold meals slow gastric emptying; food should be between room and body temperature (70 to 100°F [21 to 38°C]).

FLUIDS. Patients with persistent nausea and vomiting and/or moderate to severe dehydration should receive parenteral rather than oral fluids. Moderate to severe dehydration should also be

Table 3. Key nutritional factors in selected commercial veterinary therapeutic foods compared to recommended levels for dogs with gastritis and/or gastroduodenal ulceration.* (Numbers in red match optimal KNFs.)

Moist foods**	Potassium (%)	Chloride (%)	Sodium (%)	Protein (%)***	Fat (%)	Crude fiber (%)
Recommended levels	0.8-1.1	0.5-1.3	0.3-0.5	≤30	<15	≤5
Hill's Prescription Diet i/d Canine	0.95	1.22	0.44	25.0	14.9	1.0
Iams Veterinary Formula						
Intestinal Low-Residue	0.84	0.84	0.53	35.9	13.2	3.9
Medi-Cal Gastro Formula	0.6	na	0.6	22.1	11.7	1.0
Purina Veterinary Diets						
EN GastroENteric Formula	0.61	0.78	0.37	30.5	13.8	0.9
Royal Canin Veterinary Diet						
Digestive Low Fat LF	0.74	1.06	0.39	31.9	6.9	3.0
Royal Canin Veterinary Diet Intestinal HE	0.80	0.92	0.57	23.1	11.8	1.4
Dry foods	Potassium (%)	Chloride (%)	Sodium (%)	Protein (%)***	Fat (%)	Crude fiber (%)
Recommended levels	0.8-1.1	0.5-1.3	0.3-0.5	≤30	<15	≤5
Hill's Prescription Diet i/d Canine	0.92	1.04	0.45	26.2	14.1	2.7
Iams Veterinary Formula						
Intestinal Low-Residue	0.90	0.66	0.35	24.6	10.7	2.1
Medi-Cal Gastro Formula	0.8	na	0.5	22.9	13.9	1.9
Purina Veterinary Diets						
EN GastroENteric Formula	0.66	0.85	0.60	27.0	12.6	1.5
Royal Canin Veterinary Diet						
Digestive Low Fat LF 20	0.88	1.10	0.49	24.2	6.6	2.3
Royal Canin Veterinary Diet Intestinal HE 28	0.88	0.99	0.55	33.0	22.0	1.6

Key: na = information not available from manufacturer.
*From manufacturers' published information or calculated from manufacturers' published as-fed values; all values are on a dry matter basis unless otherwise stated.
**Moist foods are best and ideally they should be offered at temperatures between 70 to 100°F (21 to 38°C).
***Dietary protein may need to be limited to one or two sources that the patient has not been exposed to previously. Table 3, Chapter 19, contains foods with these characteristics.

Table 4. Key nutritional factors in selected commercial veterinary therapeutic foods compared with recommended levels for cats with gastritis and/or gastroduodenal ulceration.* (Numbers in red match optimal KNFs.)

Moist foods**	Potassium (%)	Chloride (%)	Sodium (%)	Protein (%)***	Fat (%)	Crude fiber (%)
Recommended levels	0.8-1.1	0.5-1.3	0.3-0.5	≤40	<25	≤5
Hill's Prescription Diet i/d Feline	1.06	1.18	0.33	37.6	24.1	2.4
Iams Veterinary Formula Intestinal Low-Residue	0.93	0.69	0.40	38.4	11.7	3.7
Medi-Cal Hypoallergenic/Gastro	1.1	na	0.7	35.5	35.9	1.2
Medi-Cal Sensitivity CR	1.1	na	1.1	34.5	35.1	2.5
Dry foods	Potassium (%)	Chloride (%)	Sodium (%)	Protein (%)***	Fat (%)	Crude fiber (%)
Recommended levels	0.8-1.1	0.5-1.3	0.3-0.5	≤40	<25	≤5
Hill's Prescription Diet i/d Feline	1.07	1.11	0.37	40.3	20.2	2.8
Iams Veterinary Formula Intestinal Low-Residue	0.66	0.63	0.25	35.8	13.7	1.8
Medi-Cal Hypoallergenic/Gastro	0.8	na	0.4	29.8	11.5	3.1
Purina Veterinary Diets EN GastroENteric	0.99	0.58	0.64	56.2	18.4	1.3
Royal Canin Veterinary Diet Intestinal HE 30	0.97	0.97	0.65	34.4	23.7	5.8

Key: na = information not available from manufacturer.
*From manufacturers' published information or calculated from manufacturers' published as-fed values; all values are on a dry matter basis unless otherwise stated.
**Moist foods are best and ideally they should be offered at temperatures between 70 to 100°F (21 to 38°C).
***Dietary protein may need to be limited to one or two sources that the patient has not been exposed to previously. Table 4, Chapter 19, contains foods with these characteristics.

corrected with appropriate parenteral fluid therapy.

Assess and Determine the Feeding Method
Determine How Much Food to Feed. Estimate from feeding guides on product labels or by calculation (Appendix C). These estimates are only starting points and will likely need to be adjusted (see Followup below).
Consider How to Offer the Food. Two feeding methods have

been described for patients with acute gastric disorders: "NPO" and "feeding through vomiting."

NPO. Withhold food and water for 24-48 hours followed by small amounts of water/ice cubes every few hours. If water is tolerated, provide small amounts of a GI food 6-8 times/day. If no vomiting occurs, the amount fed can be increased gradually over 3-4 days until the patient is receiving its estimated daily food dose in 2-3 meals/day. If the patient begins to vomit during this period, withdraw food and offer it again in a few hours. Transition to the original food after the patient has stabilized on the GI food (see Manage Food Changes below).

Feeding Through Vomiting. An alternative to NPO therapy in patients with persistent vomiting. Simply refeeding dogs (orally) and cats (via nasoesophageal tube) has stopped protracted vomiting (lasting >7 days) successfully without using antiemetic drugs. Feedings are continued although the patient may vomit. Most vomiting ceases within 24 hours of administering gruel or liquid food (Tables 5 and 6, Chapter 12). Then offer small frequent meals of a GI food (**Tables 3** and **4**) 24 hours after the last episode of vomiting.

Metoclopramide. In some cases, persistent vomiting may complicate refeeding. If so, metoclopramide or other antiemetic agents are recommended after GI obstruction has been ruled out (Appendix M). Rarely, some patients may require parenteral feeding (Chapter 13).

Manage Food Changes.

Initiation of GI Food. For transition feeding to GI or elimination foods, see NPO, above.

Return to Regular Food. For patients suspected of having food hypersensitivity, consider lifetime feeding of the elimination food. For other patients, following recovery, gradually change back to the original food. Example: to change to the original food, replace 25% of the GI food with the original food on Day 1 and continue this incremental change daily until the change is complete on Day 4. Appendix E provides additional information.

Food and Water Receptacle Husbandry. Food and water bowls should be washed regularly with warm soapy water and rinsed well. Dishes used for gruels and moist foods need daily cleaning. Discard gruels, moist or moistened dry foods after 2-4 hours of room temperature exposure to avoid foodborne illnesses (Appendix F).

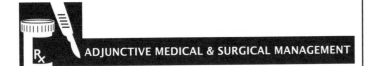

ADJUNCTIVE MEDICAL & SURGICAL MANAGEMENT

Nutritional management is often augmented with other treatments including parenteral fluids, antacids, histamine (H$_2$)-receptor antagonists, cytoprotective drugs, PGE$_2$ analogs, antibiotics and anthelmintics (Appendix M).

FOLLOWUP

Owner Followup
Following a clinic visit for uncomplicated gastritis, some owners can manage dietary treatment at home (NPO above).

Veterinary Health Care Team Followup
Nutritional reassessment of patients with gastritis or gastroduodenal ulcers includes monitoring changes in body weight and BCS and determining the extent of vomiting. Daily food dosage should be adjusted as indicated by changes in body weight, BCS and patient tolerance.

Persistent Vomiting. If vomiting persists in the face of appropriate medical and nutritional therapy (described above), further diagnostics are warranted. Additionally, different foods could be tried (**Tables 3** and **4**).

Anemia. If anemia was identified as a problem in pets with GI ulcers, obtain a followup hemogram to ensure adequate repletion of iron and copper. In addition, frequently monitor for fecal occult blood loss.

MISCELLANEOUS

See Appendix M for information about hairballs.
See Chapters 17, 24, 26, 31, 50, 52 and 56, Small Animal Clinical Nutrition, 5th edition, for more information.

Authors
Condensed from Chapter 52, Small Animal Clinical Nutrition, 5th edition, authored by Deborah J. Davenport, Rebecca L. Remillard and Christine Jenkins.

References
See Chapter 52, Small Animal Clinical Nutrition, 5th edition, on the website www.markmorrisinstitute.org for references.

Gastric Dilatation and Gastric Dilatation-Volvulus in Dogs

CLINICAL POINTS

- GD is distention of the stomach with a mixture of air, food and fluid. GD often occurs intermittently, usually in young, large-breed, deep-chested dogs, particularly as a result of overeating or some other dietary indiscretion.
- GDV is characterized by rotation of the stomach on its mesenteric axis, entrapping gastric contents and compromising vascular supply to the stomach, spleen and pancreas. Acute GDV is an emergency with high morbidity and mortality. Rarely, chronic, intermittent GDV may occur associated with a partial (i.e., <90°) rotation of the stomach.
- GDV most commonly affects large-breed, deep-chested dogs and is estimated to affect 40,000-60,000 dogs/year. Risk typically increases with age.
- GDV accounted for 3.4% of deaths of military dogs in one study and has been reported to occur at a monthly rate of 2.5 cases/1,000 military dogs.
- GDV is usually acute and often occurs at night or in the early morning, commonly associated with some precipitating stressful event (**Table 1**).
- Clinical signs of GD include nausea, belching and vomiting. Conversely, there may be no effort to vomit, but instead lethargy, reluctance to move and grunting sounds with respiratory effort.
- GDV patients exhibit restlessness, progressive abdominal distention with tympany, abdominal pain, hypersalivation and repeated, nonproductive attempts to vomit. Occasionally, owners find affected dogs dead or in shock.
- CBC often reflects stress and can provide early evidence of disseminated intravascular coagulopathy (thrombocytopenia). Hypokalemia is common. Metabolic acidosis, metabolic alkalosis, respiratory acidosis and mixed acid-base disorders have been reported to occur in dogs with GDV.
- Radiography is critical for diagnosis of GD/GDV.
- Dysrhythmias occur in approximately half of patients; generally, they are ventricular and can be life-threatening. Monitor electrocardiographic data in patients with GDV pre- and postoperatively.
- No definitive cause for GD/GDV has been identified. Previously, consumption of dry dog food, nutritional supplements and cereal- or soy-based foods was incriminated as a risk factor for GDV. More recent epidemiologic studies have not found these factors to increase GDV risk but other factors, including elevated food bowls and small particle size (<30 mm), have been implicated (**Table 1**).
- Delayed gastric emptying (Chapter 41) may be involved in the etiopathogenesis of GDV.
- GD/GDV appears not to have an age predisposition, but both

Abbreviations
AAFCO = Association of American Feed Control Officials
BCS = body condition score (Appendix A)
GD = gastric dilatation
GDV = gastric dilatation-volvulus
KNF = key nutritional factor

Table 1. Risk factors for canine gastric dilatation-volvulus.

Consuming a food with vegetable oil or animal fat listed as one of the first four ingredients
Eating a large volume of food per meal
Eating from an elevated food bowl
Eating only one meal per day
Excluding moist food, table food and treats from the diet
Exclusive feeding of one food type
Exercising more than two hours per day
Fearful, nervous or aggressive temperament
Feeding food with a mean particle size <5 mm
Having an affected first-degree relative
Increased adult weight, based on breed standards
Increased chest or abdominal depth:width ratio
Increasing age
Large- or giant-breed status
   Great Danes, Weimaraners, Saint Bernards, Gordon setters, Irish setters, standard poodles, basset hounds, Doberman pinschers, Old English sheepdogs, German shorthaired pointers
Lean body condition (body condition score ≤2/5)
Male gender
Purebred status
Rapid eating
Stressful events (boarding in kennel or travel)

are more common in middle-aged dogs.
- Without early treatment, GDV is usually fatal. Initial management includes cardiovascular stabilization, gastric decompression, surgery (i.e., gastric repositioning and permanent gastropexy) and postsurgical care.
- If a permanent gastropexy is not performed after gastric repositioning, recurrence approaches 80%.
- Feeding goals: use appropriate foods and feeding methods to facilitate recovery from emergency management of GDV and to help prevent occurrence/recurrence of GD/GDV.

KEY NUTRITIONAL FACTORS

- Foods should provide recommended allowances of all required nutrients (nutritional adequacy), but should also contain a specific KNF (a food feature that may assist in the management of GD/GDV).
- KNFs for postoperative patients are similar to those for patients with acute gastritis (Chapter 39).

- **Table 2** lists the KNF recommendation (kibble size) for dry foods to help prevent GD/GDV. Low dietary fat levels may be desirable but data are inconclusive. A detailed review of KNF recommendations can be found in Chapter 53, Small Animal Clinical Nutrition, 5th edition.

FEEDING PLAN

The feeding plan includes dietary management recommendations after emergency treatment and dietary management as part of a preventive strategy.

Assess and Select the Food

Ensure the Food's Basic Nutritional Adequacy. AAFCO nutritional adequacy statements are usually found on a product's label. AAFCO approval does not ensure a food will be effective in the management of GD/GDV.

Compare the Food's KNF Content with the Recommended Levels.

POSTOPERATIVE PERIOD. Use foods that provide KNF levels for acute gastritis (Chapter 39). Moist foods are preferred. Initially, consider gruels made from moist foods.

Table 2. Key nutritional factor for dry foods for dogs for the prevention of gastric dilatation and volvulus.

Factor	Recommendation
Kibble size	Large particle size: >30 mm was protective against GDV in giant-breed dogs (Great Danes). Somewhat smaller kibble dimensions may be effective in medium- and large-breed dogs as long as the size of the kibble is sufficiently large to prevent rapid eating.

Table 3. Kibble size comparison of selected large-kibble dry commercial foods to consider for feeding medium-, large- and giant-breed dogs to reduce the risk of gastric dilatation and volvulus.*

Factor	Kibble cross sectional dimension(s)**
Recommendation	>30 mm for giant-breed dogs Somewhat smaller kibbles (<30 mm) may be effective in medium- and large-breed dogs as long as the kibble is sufficiently large to prevent rapid eating.
Hill's Prescription Diet t/d Canine	28.3 x 26.4 mm
Medi-Cal Dental Formula	23.3 x 20.3 mm
Purina Veterinary Diets DH Dental Health	21.9 x 21.2 mm
Royal Canin Giant Adult 28	29.72 x 28.88 mm

*For additional key nutritional factors of importance for canine maintenance, see appropriate lifestage recommendations (Chapters 1 through 5).
**Kibble size represents the mean of measurements (diameter or width X thickness) made on three randomly selected kibbles from one bag of each product listed.

PREVENTION. Table 3 includes the KNF content (kibble dimensions) of selected large kibble dry commercial dog foods and compares them to the recommended dimensions (note: none of these specific products have been shown to prevent/reduce the risk of GDV). Select foods that most closely match the KNF recommendation and that slow eating (subjective feeding trials at home). Feeding a mixture of moist and dry foods may reduce the risk.

PUPPIES. Because these foods are intended for adult maintenance, consider KNFs for growth as well if feeding puppies at risk for GD (Chapter 5).

Manage Treats and Snacks. If treats/snacks are fed, commercial treats that match the nutritional profile recommended for the patient (see product label) are best. Treats/snacks should not be fed excessively (<10% of the total diet on a volume, weight or calorie basis). See Appendix B for more information about treats/snacks.

Assess and Determine the Feeding Method

Determine How Much Food to Feed. Estimate either from feeding guides on product labels or by calculation (Appendix C). Feeding guidelines and calculations are based on population averages and may need to be adjusted for individual dogs (see Followup below).

Consider How to Offer the Food.

POSTOPERATIVELY. Provide small amounts of water/ice cubes every few hours on Day 1. If water is tolerated, provide small amounts of food with KNFs appropriate for GI disease (Chapter 39) 6-8 times/day (initially, consider providing as a gruel). If no vomiting occurs, the amount fed can be increased gradually over 3-4 days until the patient is receiving its estimated daily food dose in 2-3 meals/day. If the patient vomits, withdraw food and begin the process over again in a few hours. Transition to the original food after the patient has stabilized on the GI food (see Manage Food Changes: Postrecovery and Prevention below).

PREVENTION. Meal feed a specific amount at least 2-3 times/day. Do not feed from an elevated platform or feeder. Susceptible dogs should be fed individually and in a quiet location.

RAPID EATERS. Place large balls or rocks in the food bowl or feed from a muffin tin to slow consumption and reduce aerophagia. Specially made food bowls[a] with 3 large vertical cylinders protruding from the bottom to slow food consumption are available.

EXERCISE. Avoid vigorous exercise 1 hour before and 2 hours after feeding.

Manage Food Changes.

POSTOPERATIVELY. See Consider How to Offer the Food above.

POSTRECOVERY AND PREVENTION. Replace 25% of the previous food with the new food on Day 1 and continue this incremental change daily until the change is complete on Day 4 or 5. Appendix E provides additional information.

Food and Water Receptacle Husbandry. Food and water bowls should be washed regularly with warm soapy water and rinsed well. Dishes used for gruels and moist foods need daily cleaning. Discard moist or moistened foods after 2-4 hours of room temperature exposure to avoid foodborne illnesses (Appendix F).

FOLLOWUP

Owner Followup
Provide a low-stress feeding environment and manage exercise in relation to feeding (above). Report suspected episodes of GD/GDV and possible precipitating factors. Monitor appetite, activity level and attitude. Weigh the dog (if possible) and/or grade its body condition (BCS) monthly. If a trend of increasing or decreasing body weight or BCS is noted, change the amount fed by 10% increments and recheck the patient every 2 weeks for 1 month. Then, if necessary, change the amount fed and repeat the cycle.

Veterinary Health Care Team Followup
Postoperatively. In most cases, food can be reintroduced within 24-36 hours. Feed small meals frequently and introduce gradually (see Consider How to Offer the Food: Postoperatively above).
  PERSISTENT VOMITING. Judicious use of antiemetics and/or metoclopramide in conjunction with continuous feeding may allow adequate nutrient intake. If tube gastrostomy was chosen as the method of permanent gastropexy, use this indwelling catheter for feeding (Appendix H). Also see Miscellaneous below.
Postrecovery. Rechecks should include assessment of body weight and BCS. The ultimate marker of success in GDV

patients is prevention of recurrent disease. Rarely, GD will develop in dogs that have had a gastropexy.

MISCELLANEOUS

Persistent vomiting in postoperative patients unresponsive to dietary/medical management (above) may indicate outflow obstruction arising from an improperly positioned gastropexy site. Functional obstruction may occur if the angle between the pyloric antrum and duodenum is too acute.
  See Chapters 17, 25 and 52-54, Small Animal Clinical Nutrition, 5th edition, for more information.

Authors
Condensed from Chapter 53, Small Animal Clinical Nutrition, 5th edition, authored by Deborah J. Davenport, Rebecca L. Remillard and Christine Jenkins.

References
See Chapter 53, Small Animal Clinical Nutrition, 5th edition, on the website www.markmorrisinstitute.org for references.

Endnote
a. Brake-Fast Dog Food Bowl. Brake-Fast LLC., Virginia Beach, VA, USA.

Gastric Motility and Emptying Disorders

Chapter 41

CLINICAL POINTS

- Gastric motility disorders arise from conditions that directly/indirectly disrupt 3 gastric functions: storing ingesta, mixing food particles and timely expulsion of gastric contents into the duodenum.
- **Table 1** outlines a number of primary and secondary causes of gastric motility disorders. Their importance in the pet population is unknown; primary gastric motility disorders are considered rare.
- The stomach should empty after an average meal in 6-8 hours in dogs and 4-6 hours in cats; longer emptying times are considered delayed.
- Delayed gastric emptying due to any cause may result in vomiting. Owners may report vomiting of undigested or partially

Abbreviations
AAFCO = Association of American Feed Control Officials
BCS = body condition score (Appendix A)
KNF = key nutritional factor

  digested food more than 12 hours after ingestion of food.
- Gastric distention and tympany may be evident. Patients with unrelenting vomiting may present with dehydration, depression and malaise.
- Weight loss and poor body condition are often present in chronic primary or secondary cases. Other signs may include intermittent gastric bloating, nausea, partial or complete inappetence and belching. Occasionally, patients will present with unrelenting or projectile vomiting; suspect complete gastric outflow obstruction in such cases.
- Clinical signs may develop gradually in acquired cases of chronic hypertrophic pyloric gastropathy or acutely with

Table 1. Potential causes of gastric emptying disorders in dogs and cats.

Functional obstruction (primary motility defects)
Gastric ulcers
Idiopathic asynchronous motility
Idiopathic hypomotility
Infectious gastroenteritis
Postoperative ileus
Functional obstruction (secondary motility defects)
Drug therapy
    Anticholinergics
    Beta-adrenergic agonists
    Narcotic analgesics
Electrolyte disturbances
    Hypercalcemia
    Hypocalcemia
    Hypokalemia
    Hypomagnesemia
Inflammation
    Acute pancreatitis
    Peritonitis
Metabolic disorders
    Diabetes mellitus
    Hepatic encephalopathy
    Hypothyroidism
Mechanical obstruction
Congenital or acquired antral pyloric hypertrophy
Extraluminal compression
Gastric or duodenal foreign bodies
Gastric or duodenal granulomatous lesions
Gastric or duodenal neoplasia or polyps

Table 2. Key nutritional factors for foods for dogs and cats with gastric motility and emptying disorders.*

Factors	Recommended levels
Energy density	4.0 to 4.5 kcal/g (16.7 to 18.8 kJ/g)
Potassium	0.8 to 1.1%
Chloride	0.5 to 1.3%
Sodium	0.3 to 0.5%
Fat	≤15% for dogs ≤25% for cats
Crude fiber	≤5% crude fiber; avoid foods with gel-forming fiber sources such as pectins and gums (e.g., gum arabic, guar gum, carrageenan, psyllium gum, xanthan gum, carob gum, gum ghatti and gum tragacanth)
Food form consistency	Moist is best; initially liquid or semi-liquid
Food temperature	70 to 100°F (21 to 38°C)

*Nutrients expressed on a dry matter basis.

foreign bodies. Clinical signs due to congenital pyloric stenosis may have been present since weaning.

- "Bilious vomiting syndrome" is chronic intermittent vomiting of only bile, associated with an empty stomach. It is most common in dogs, typically occurring late at night or early morning. Bile reflux (secondary to motility dysfunction, gastritis or duodenitis) causes gastric mucosal damage.
- Congenital pyloric stenosis (i.e., primary cause) most often occurs in brachycephalic dogs and Siamese cats. Chronic hypertrophic pyloric gastropathy usually affects small, purebred, middle-aged dogs (e.g., Lhasa apso, Maltese, Shih Tzu and Pekingese).

- Young animals are more at risk for gastric foreign bodies; older pets are more likely to have neoplastic lesions that obstruct gastric outflow.
- Hematologic and serum biochemistry values may reveal underlying disorders. Dehydration, electrolyte (hypokalemia, hypochloremia) and acid-base abnormalities may be associated with chronic, persistent vomiting. Prerenal azotemia is common. Hypochloremic metabolic alkalosis with paradoxical aciduria may occur in cases of complete pyloric outflow obstruction.
- Survey abdominal radiographs and GI contrast studies may confirm the diagnosis. However, endoscopy is preferred (presence of food in the stomach after a 12-18 hour fast is considered abnormal). Endoscopy may be curative in cases with antropyloric or proximal duodenal foreign bodies.
- Feeding plan strategies with appropriate KNFs that enhance gastric emptying are desirable for foods intended for patients with gastric motility/emptying disorders. The formulation and nutrient content of the food and meal size influence the rate of gastric emptying.
- Serum electrolyte concentrations abnormalities (e.g., potassium, sodium and chloride) are common with chronic vomiting and can adversely affect gastric motility/emptying. Initially correct these with appropriate parenteral fluid therapy. Foods should contain adequate potassium, chloride and sodium.
- Because patients are often underweight due to chronic ineffective nutrient intake, food nutrient density may need to be increased. However, the food should not have high fat levels. Increased dietary fat stimulates cholecystokinin release, which delays gastric emptying.
- Avoid foods containing gel-forming soluble fibers because they increase viscosity of ingesta and slow gastric emptying; these fibers include pectins and gums (e.g., gum arabic, guar gum, carrageenan, psyllium gum, xanthan gum, carob gum, gum ghatti and gum tragacanth). However, increased levels of insoluble fiber (e.g., powdered cellulose) in dry foods do not affect gastric emptying in cats.
- Moist foods, warm foods and warm water reduce gastric retention time.
- Larger meals are emptied more slowly than smaller meals in cats and probably dogs. Liquids are emptied more quickly than solids due to lower digesta osmolality.
- Prognosis varies with the underlying cause; mechanical obstructions managed surgically or endoscopically (e.g., foreign body retrieval) have an excellent prognosis. Occasionally, patients with longstanding gastric outflow obstruction with gastric distention may have residual gastric motility abnormalities.
- Feeding goals: through proper food and feeding methods, meet the patient's nutrient needs while supporting normalization of gastric motility and complementing appropriate endoscopic, surgical and medical therapies, when applicable.

Table 3. Key nutritional factors in selected moist commercial veterinary therapeutic foods compared to recommended levels for dogs with gastric motility and emptying disorders.* (Numbers in red match optimal KNFs.)

Factors	Energy density (kcal/g)	Potassium (%)	Chloride (%)	Sodium (%)	Fat (%)	Crude fiber (%)
Recommended levels	4.0-4.5	0.8-1.1	0.5-1.3	0.3-0.5	≤15	≤5
Hill's Prescription Diet i/d Canine	4.4	0.95	1.22	0.44	14.9	1.0
Iams Veterinary Formula Intestinal Low-Residue	4.6	0.84	0.84	0.53	13.2	3.9
Medi-Cal Gastro Formula	na	0.6	na	0.6	11.7	1.0
Purina Veterinary Diets EN GastroENteric	4.0	0.61	0.78	0.37	13.8	0.9
Royal Canin Veterinary Diet Digestive Low Fat LF	4.0	0.74	1.06	0.39	6.9	3.0
Royal Canin Veterinary Diet Intestinal HE	4.3	0.8	0.92	0.57	11.8	1.4

Key: na = information not available from manufacturer.
*From manufacturers' published information or calculated from manufacturers' published as-fed values; all values are on a dry matter basis unless otherwise stated. Moist foods, foods with liquid or semi-liquid consistency are preferred. Foods should be offered at temperatures between 70 to 100°F (21 to 38°C).

Table 4. Key nutritional factors in selected moist commercial veterinary therapeutic foods compared to recommended levels for cats with gastric motility and emptying disorders.* (Numbers in red match optimal KNFs.)

Factors	Energy density (kcal/g)	Potassium (%)	Chloride (%)	Sodium (%)	Fat (%)	Crude fiber (%)
Recommended levels	4.0-4.5	0.8-1.1	0.5-1.3	0.3-0.5	≤25	≤5
Hill's Prescription Diet i/d Feline	4.2	1.06	1.18	0.33	24.1	2.4
Iams Veterinary Formula Intestinal Low-Residue	4.0	0.93	0.69	0.40	11.7	3.7
Medi-Cal Hypoallergenic/Gastro	na	1.1	na	0.7	35.9	1.2
Medi-Cal Sensitivity CR	na	1.1	na	1.1	35.1	2.5

Key: na = information not available from manufacturer.
*From manufacturers' published information or calculated from manufacturers' published as-fed values; all values are on a dry matter basis unless otherwise stated. Moist foods, foods with liquid or semi-liquid consistency are preferred. Foods should be offered at temperatures between 70 to 100°F (21 to 38°C).

KEY NUTRITIONAL FACTORS

- Foods should provide recommended allowances of all required nutrients (nutritional adequacy), but should also contain specific levels of KNFs (certain nutrients and food features that may assist in managing gastric motility/emptying disorders).
- Table 2 lists KNF recommendations for foods for patients with gastric motility/emptying disorders. A detailed review of these recommendations can be found in Chapter 54, Small Animal Clinical Nutrition, 5th edition. In addition to KNFs in Table 2, other KNFs may be important depending on the patient's lifestage (e.g., growth; Chapters 5 and 11). Water is particularly important because dehydration is common.

FEEDING PLAN

Before a feeding plan is initiated, correct dehydration, electrolyte and acid-base abnormalities with appropriate parenteral fluid therapy; correct gastric outflow obstruction with surgical or endoscopic intervention.

Assess and Select the Food
Ensure the Food's Basic Nutritional Adequacy. AAFCO nutritional adequacy statements are usually found on a product's label. AAFCO approval does not ensure a food will effectively manage gastric motility/emptying disorders.
Compare the Food's KNF Content with the Recommended Levels. Tables 3 and 4 include the KNF content of selected commercial foods marketed for GI diseases (for dogs and cats, respectively) and compare them to the recommended levels for patients with gastric motility/emptying disorders. Select foods that most closely match KNF recommended levels.

PATIENTS WITH MILD DISEASE. Foods may not need to be changed for patients with mild clinical signs.

PATIENTS WITH COMPLETE PYLORIC OUTFLOW OBSTRUCTION. Depending on the patient's condition, assisted feeding that bypasses the obstruction may be advisable until the obstruction can be relieved (below). Use foods appropriate for the feeding route (Chapters 12 and 13).

Food Form. Liquids are emptied from the stomach more quickly than solids due to lower digesta osmolality. Consider gruels based on blenderized moist foods. Alternatively, liquid enteral products with appropriate KNF content may be used (Chapter 12).
Food Temperature. Cold meals and cold water slow gastric emptying; food and water temperature should be between room and body temperature (70 to 100°F [21 to 38°C]).

Assess and Determine the Feeding Method
Determine How Much Food to Feed. Estimate from feeding

guides on product labels or by calculation (Appendix C). These estimates are only starting points and will likely need to be adjusted, especially in chronic cases with associated weight loss (see Followup below).

Consider How to Offer the Food. For most patients, small-volume, frequent meals (≥3/day) are recommended.

PATIENTS WITH COMPLETE PYLORIC OUTFLOW OBSTRUCTION. Assisted feeding (Chapters 12 and 13) may be necessary to nutritionally rehabilitate patients before surgical alleviation of the obstruction. This is indicated when the patient's body condition is poor (BCS <2/5) and the patient is at increased risk for postsurgical complications. For enteral support, consider the jejunostomy tube approach to bypass the stomach.

PATIENTS WITH RESTORED GASTRIC FUNCTION. Use feeding methods similar to those used for normal pets (Chapters 1 and 7), if gastric function returns after endoscopy or surgery. Determine the most effective method for each patient by trial/error based on the degree of gastric function restored.

BILIOUS VOMITING SYNDROME. Late evening meals with or without prokinetic therapy (Appendix M) may help resolve clinical signs in affected dogs. Food may buffer irritating effects of refluxed bile and/or may enhance gastric motility.

FOLLOWUP

Owner Followup

Note any further episodes of vomiting. Obtain body weight (if possible) and/or grade body condition (BCS) monthly. The amount fed to underweight patients should be increased by 10% and the patient rechecked every 2 weeks for 1 month. At that point, if necessary, the amount fed should be increased again and the cycle repeated until normal body weight/BCS are achieved.

Veterinary Health Care Team Followup

Monitor changes in body weight and BCS. Assist owners with food dosages and adjust as indicated by the patient's body weight/BCS. Determine the extent of ongoing vomiting, if any, and if vomiting continues, alter the food or feeding pattern. Gradually attempt to normalize the feeding regimen if the patient is doing well. Feeding more solid foods and larger, less frequent meals are more convenient for pet owners.

Persistent Vomiting. Dividing the daily food intake into smaller meals may increase GI tolerance. Use prokinetic agents (Appendix M) if vomiting persists despite modifying the feeding plan.

MISCELLANEOUS

See Chapters 13, 17, 20, 24-26 and 54, Small Animal Clinical Nutrition, 5th edition, for more information.

Authors

Condensed from Chapter 54, Small Animal Clinical Nutrition, 5th edition, authored by Deborah J. Davenport, Rebecca L. Remillard and Christine Jenkins.

References

See Chapter 54, Small Animal Clinical Nutrition, 5th edition, on the website www.markmorrisinstitute.org for references.

CLINICAL POINTS

- This chapter addresses the management of patients with acute onset of diarrhea with or without vomiting.
- Acute gastroenteritis is one of the most common illnesses of dogs and cats. A number of infectious, toxic and dietary factors can trigger diarrhea with/without vomiting (Appendix N).
- Patients are usually presented for sudden onset of diarrhea, vomiting or both. Owners often report that the pet acts depressed and has a poor appetite.
- Large fluid stools are typical of small bowel disorders (Appendix N). Occasionally, patients may present with signs of small and large bowel involvement. Melenic/hemorrhagic stools may indicate a life-threatening disorder (Appendix N).
- Food-induced diarrhea is relatively common (e.g., a recent change to a moist high-fat or meat-based food; uncooked homemade meat-based foods) as is dietary indiscretion (e.g., table foods or access to garbage or carrion). Cats that ingest wild birds may be exposed to *Salmonella* spp. and dogs eating raw salmon are at risk for salmon poisoning.
- Young animals are more susceptible to a variety of infectious pathogens.
- A genetic influence has been recognized in some dog breeds (Appendix N). Chinese Shar-Peis, German shepherd dogs and beagles may have IgA deficiency, making them more susceptible to several GI conditions (Appendix N).
- Pets in unsanitary or overcrowded conditions are much more likely to develop infectious enteropathies.
- Review vaccination and anthelmintic treatment records.
- Because many potential causes of acute gastroenteritis and enteritis exist, a definitive diagnosis can be difficult to make and not always necessary for treatment. It is more important to determine if the condition is self-limiting or potentially life-threatening (Appendix N).
- Small-bowel disuse atrophy begins within days in the absence of luminal stimulation by food.
- Abdominal discomfort may be recognized on palpation. Always evaluate for septic shock.
- Evaluate seriously ill patients using hematology, serum biochemistry, urinalyses and fecal examinations (parasites and other infectious pathogens). Consider abdominal or GI contrast radiography to rule out obstruction.
- Diagnostics for apparent self-limiting cases are often limited to assessment of hydration status and thorough examination of feces for parasites and bacterial pathogens.
- Water is the most important nutrient for patients with acute gastroenteritis/enteritis because of the potential for life-threatening dehydration due to excessive fluid loss and inability of the patient to replace those losses.

Abbreviations

AAFCO = Association of American Feed Control Officials
BCS = body condition score (Appendix A)
DM = dry matter
KNF = key nutritional factor
NPO = nothing per os
SIBO = small intestinal bacterial overgrowth

- Mild hypokalemia, hypochloremia and either hypernatremia or hyponatremia are electrolyte abnormalities most commonly associated with acute vomiting and diarrhea. Foods should contain levels of potassium, chloride and sodium above minimum recommended allowances.
- Dietary fiber: predominant effects are on the large bowel but, depending on type and amount, fiber can also modify gastric, small intestinal and pancreatic function in ways that benefit patients with small bowel diarrhea.
- 2 approaches using types/levels of fiber are advocated for gastroenteritis/enteritis patients: 1) low-fiber foods (≤5% DM mixed fiber) that are highly digestible and 2) fiber-enhanced foods containing insoluble fiber at levels between 7-15% DM. Either strategy can be valuable for managing selected patients with acute gastroenteritis/enteritis.
- Mixed fibers include beet pulp, brans (rice, wheat or oat), pea, soy fibers, soy hulls and mixtures of soluble and insoluble fibers. Insoluble fibers include purified cellulose and peanut hulls. Soluble fiber sources include fruit pectins, guar gums and psyllium.
- Digestive capacity is often diminished in patients with gastroenteritis; therefore, consider food digestibility. The term "highly digestible" describes foods with protein digestibility ≥87% and fat and carbohydrate digestibility ≥90%.
- Fiber-enhanced foods typically have lower protein and fat digestibilities but the carbohydrate digestiblity should be about the same as for highly digestible foods. Digestibility recommendations for fiber-enhanced foods are ≥80% for protein and fat and ≥90% for carbohydrate.
- Smaller meals may promote gastric emptying and increase food digestibility.
- The prognosis for recovery in most cases of acute gastro-enteritis/enteritis is good.
- Dietary goal: provide a food that meets the patient's nutrient requirements, allows normalization of GI motility and function and helps control vomiting/diarrhea.

Table 1. Key nutritional factors for dogs and cats with acute gastroenteritis or enteritis.*

Factors	Recommended levels
Sodium	0.3 to 0.5%
Chloride	0.5 to 1.3%
Potassium	0.8 to 1.1%
Fat	12 to 15% for dogs (highly digestible foods)
	15 to 25% for cats (highly digestible foods)
	8 to 12% for dogs (increased-fiber foods)
	9 to 18% for cats (increased-fiber foods)
Energy density	4.0 to 4.5 kcal/g (16.7 to 18.8 kJ/g) (highly digestible foods)
	≥3.2 kcal/g (≥13.4 kJ/g) for dogs and ≥3.4 kcal/g (≥14.2 kJ/g) for cats (increased-fiber foods)
Fiber	≤5% in highly digestible foods (mixed fiber sources are best)
	7 to 15% in fiber-enhanced foods (insoluble fiber sources are best)
Digestibility	≥87% for protein and ≥90% for fat and carbohydrate (highly digestible foods)
	≥80% for protein and fat and ≥90% for carbohydrate (fiber-enhanced foods)

*Nutrient levels are on a dry matter basis.

Table 2. Selected commercial oral rehydration solutions available for use in dogs and cats.

Products (manufacturers)	Na	K	Cl	Mg	Ca	P	Citrate	ME (kcal/l)	Comments
Electramine (Life Science Products)	69.8	15.4	69.7	–	–	–	–	–	Contains glycine
Enfamil Enfalyte (Mead Johnson)	50	25	45	–	–	–	34	126	mOsm/l = 167
Pedialyte Solution unflavored (Abbott Nutrition)	45	20	35	–	–	–	30	100	mOsm/l = 250-270
Rebound OES (Virbac)	52.2-65.2	20.5-25.6	10-20	–	–	–	–	253	–

Key: mEq/l = milliequivalents per liter, Na = sodium, K = potassium, Cl = chloride, Mg = magnesium, Ca = calcium, P = phosphorus, ME = metabolizable energy.

KEY NUTRITIONAL FACTORS

- Foods should provide recommended allowances of all required nutrients (nutritional adequacy), but should also contain specific levels of KNFs (certain nutrients and food features that may assist in the management of gastroenteritis/enteritis).
- **Table 1** lists KNF recommendations for foods for patients with gastroenteritis/enteritis. Included are KNFs for highly digestible foods and fiber-enhanced foods. A detailed review of these recommendations can be found in Chapter 56, Small Animal Clinical Nutrition, 5th edition. Other KNFs may also be important depending on the patient's lifestage (e.g., growth; Chapters 5 and 11).

FEEDING PLAN

The first step in managing acute gastroenteritis/enteritis is to correct dehydration and electrolyte, glucose and acid-base imbalances, if present. Use appropriate IV fluid therapy for moderate/ severe dehydration; SQ or oral fluid therapy is reserved for non-vomiting patients with minor fluid deficits or to supply maintenance fluid requirements. **Table 2** lists oral rehydration solutions for dogs/cats; these fluids are most useful in secretory diarrheas, which are uncommon.

Assess and Select the Food

Ensure the Food's Basic Nutritional Adequacy. AAFCO nutritional adequacy statements are usually found on a product's label. AAFCO approval does not ensure a food will be effective for managing gastroenteritis/enteritis.

Compare the Food's KNF Content with the Recommended Levels. 3 different plausible dietary approaches are suggested and they may be attempted in any order.

ACUTE GASTROENTERITIS/ENTERITIS. The traditional approach is based on feeding highly digestible, low-residue foods formulated for GI disease that may contain small amounts of soluble/mixed fiber (**Tables 3** and **4**, for dogs and cats, respectively). An alternative approach is based on feeding fiber-enhanced foods that contain moderate amounts of fiber (**Tables 5** for dogs and **6** for cats). All aforementioned tables include KNF contents of selected commercial foods and compare them to recommended levels.

PROTRACTED SMALL BOWEL DISUSE. If there has been 3 days or more of low/no food intake, provide enteral nutrition

Table 3. Key nutritional factors in selected highly digestible commercial veterinary therapeutic foods marketed for dogs with acute gastroenteritis or acute enteritis.* (Numbers in red match optimal KNFs.)

Dry foods	Na (%)	Cl (%)	K (%)	Fat (%)	Energy density (kcal/g)	Fiber (%)**	Protein digestibility (%)	Fat digestibility (%)	Carbohydrate digestibility (%)	Ingredient comments
Recommended levels	0.3-0.5	0.5-1.3	0.8-1.1	12-15	4.0-4.5	≤5	≥87	≥90	≥90	–
Hill's Prescription Diet i/d Canine	0.45	1.04	0.92	14.1	4.2	2.7	92	93	94	–
Iams Veterinary Formula Intestinal Low-Residue	0.35	0.66	0.90	10.7	3.8	2.1	na	na	na	FOS, MOS prebiotics
Medi-Cal Gastro Formula	0.5	na	0.8	13.9	na	1.9	na	na	na	OS prebiotic, *Bacillus subtilis* dried fermentation extract
Purina Veterinary Diets EN GastroENteric Formula	0.6	0.85	0.66	12.6	4.2	1.5	84.5	91.4	94.4	MCT
Royal Canin Veterinary Diet Digestive Low Fat LF 20	0.49	1.10	0.88	6.6	3.7	2.3	na	na	na	FOS, MOS prebiotics
Royal Canin Veterinary Diet Intestinal HE 28	0.55	0.99	0.88	22.0	4.5	1.6	na	na	na	FOS, MOS prebiotics

Moist foods	Na (%)	Cl (%)	K (%)	Fat (%)	Energy density (kcal/g)	Fiber (%)**	Protein digestibility (%)	Fat digestibility (%)	Carbohydrate digestibility (%)	Ingredient comments
Recommended levels	0.3-0.5	0.5-1.3	0.8-1.1	12-15	4.0-4.5	≤5	≥87	≥90	≥90	–
Hill's Prescription Diet i/d Canine	0.44	1.22	0.95	14.9	4.4	1.0	88	94	93	–
Iams Veterinary Formula Intestinal Low-Residue	0.53	0.84	0.84	13.2	4.6	3.9	na	na	na	–
Medi-Cal Gastro Formula	0.6	na	0.6	11.7	na	1.0	na	na	na	FOS prebiotic
Purina Veterinary Diets EN GastroENteric Formula	0.37	0.78	0.61	13.8	4.0	0.9	85.1	95.6	92.2	MCT
Royal Canin Veterinary Diet Digestive Low Fat LF	0.39	1.06	0.74	6.9	4.0	3.0	na	na	na	–
Royal Canin Veterinary Diet Intestinal HE	0.57	0.92	0.80	11.8	4.3	1.4	na	na	na	Inulin prebiotic

Key: Na = sodium, Cl = chloride, K = potassium, fiber = crude fiber, na = information not available from manufacturer, FOS = fructooligosaccharide, MOS = mannanoligosaccharide, MCT = medium-chain triglyceride.
*Nutrients expressed on a dry matter basis. To convert kcal to kJ, multiply kcal by 4.184.
**Mixed fiber sources are best in highly digestible foods (see text).

continuously by nasoesophageal tube (see Feeding Through Vomiting/Diarrhea below) using a liquid food (Tables 4 and 5, Chapter 12).

Assess and Determine the Feeding Method

Determine How Much Food to Feed. Estimate from feeding guides on product labels or by calculation (Appendix C). These estimates are only starting points and will likely need to be adjusted (see Followup below).

Consider How to Offer the Food. 2 feeding methods have been described for patients with acute gastric disorders: NPO and feeding through vomiting/diarrhea.

NPO. Withhold food and water for 24-48 hours followed by small amounts of water/ice cubes every few hours. If water is tolerated, provide small amounts of GI food 6-8 times/day. If no vomiting/diarrhea occurs, increase the amount the fed gradually over 3-4 days until the patient is receiving its estimated daily food dose in 2-3 meals/day. If the patient begins to vomit or develops diarrhea during this period, withdraw food and offer it again in a few hours. Transition to the original food after the patient's condition has stabilized on GI food (see Manage Food Changes below).

FEEDING THROUGH VOMITING/DIARRHEA. This feeding method is suggested for patients with persistent vomiting/diarrhea and 3 days or more of low/no food intake. Refeed by constant infusion, if possible, via nasoesophageal tube. Effectiveness may be related to positive nutritional effects on the GI tissues themselves. Some patients may continue to vomit; however, most cases cease vomiting within 24 hours after liquid food administration is begun. Then, offer small frequent meals of a GI food (**Tables 3** and **4**) 24 hours after the last episode of vomiting/diarrhea.

METOCLOPRAMIDE. Persistent vomiting may complicate refeeding in some cases of parvoviral enteritis; some puppies may develop gastroparesis and require administration of prokinetic drugs. If so, metoclopramide or other antiemetic agents are

Table 4. Key nutritional factors in selected highly digestible commercial veterinary therapeutic foods marketed for cats with acute gastroenteritis or acute enteritis.* (Numbers in red match optimal KNFs.)

Dry foods	Na (%)	Cl (%)	K (%)	Fat (%)	Energy density (kcal/g)	Fiber (%)**	Protein digestibility (%)	Fat digestibility (%)	Carbohydrate digestibility (%)	Ingredient comments
Recommended levels	0.3-0.5	0.5-1.3	0.8-1.1	15-25	4.0-4.5	≤5	≥87	≥90	≥90	–
Hill's Prescription Diet i/d Feline	0.37	1.11	1.07	20.2	4.3	2.8	88	92	90	–
Iams Veterinary Formula Intestinal Low-Residue	0.25	0.63	0.66	13.7	3.9	1.8	na	na	na	FOS, MOS prebiotics
Medi-Cal HYPOallergenic/ Gastro	0.4	na	0.8	11.5	na	3.1	na	na	na	FOS prebiotic, *Bacillus subtilis* dried fermentation extract
Purina Veterinary Diets EN GastroENteric	0.64	0.58	0.99	18.4	4.4	1.3	94.0	93.1	79.7	–
Royal Canin Veterinary Diet Intestinal HE 30	0.65	0.97	0.97	23.7	4.4	5.8	na	na	na	FOS, MOS prebiotics

Moist foods	Na (%)	Cl (%)	K (%)	Fat (%)	Energy density (kcal/g)	Fiber (%)**	Protein digestibility (%)	Fat digestibility (%)	Carbohydrate digestibility (%)	Ingredient comments
Recommended levels	0.3-0.5	0.5-1.3	0.8-1.1	15-25	4.0-4.5	≤5	≥87	≥90	≥90	–
Hill's Prescription Diet i/d Feline	0.33	1.18	1.06	24.1	4.2	2.4	91	89	91	–
Iams Veterinary Formula Intestinal Low-Residue	0.40	0.69	0.93	11.7	4.0	3.7	na	na	na	FOS prebiotic
Medi-Cal HYPOallergenic/Gastro	0.7	na	1.1	35.9	na	1.2	na	na	na	FOS prebiotic
Medi-Cal Sensitivity CR	1.1	na	1.1	35.1	na	2.5	na	na	na	–

Key: Na = sodium, Cl = chloride, K = potassium, fiber = crude fiber, na = information not available from manufacturer, FOS = fructooligosaccharide, MOS = mannanoligosaccharide.
*Nutrients expressed on a dry matter basis. To convert kcal to kJ, multiply kcal by 4.184.
**Mixed fiber sources are best in highly digestible foods (see text).

recommended after GI obstruction has been ruled out (Appendix M). Rarely, some patients may require parenteral feeding (Chapter 13).

Manage Food Changes.

INITIATION OF GI FOOD. For transition feeding to GI food, see NPO, above.

RETURN TO REGULAR FOOD. Following recovery, gradually change back to the original food. Example: to change to the original food, replace 25% of the GI food with the original food on Day 1 and continue this incremental change daily until the change is complete on Day 4. Appendix E provides additional information.

Food and Water Receptacle Husbandry. Food and water bowls should be washed regularly with warm soapy water and rinsed well. Dishes used for gruels and moist foods need daily cleaning. Discard gruels, moist or moistened dry foods after 2-4 hours of room temperature exposure to avoid foodborne illnesses (Appendix F).

FOLLOWUP

Owner Followup

After the clinic visit for uncomplicated gastroenteritis, some owners, with guidance can manage dietary treatment at home (see NPO above). If possible, body weight should be recorded daily until recovery is complete.

Veterinary Health Care Team Followup

Nutritional reassessment of patients with gastroenteritis/enteritis includes monitoring changes in body weight and condition (BCS) and determining the extent of vomiting/diarrhea. Changes in body weight from day to day usually reflect changes in hydration status rather than loss or gain of body tissue. The daily food dose should be adjusted as indicated by changes in body weight, BCS and the patient's GI tolerance.

Persistent Severe Vomiting/Diarrhea. Acute worsening of clinical signs, especially when accompanied by abdominal pain in a young dog with gastroenteritis, may indicate intestinal intussusception. In such cases, abdominal radiography and/or ultrasonography are indicated.

Table 5. Key nutritional factors in selected fiber-enhanced commercial veterinary therapeutic foods marketed for dogs with acute gastroenteritis or acute enteritis.* (Numbers in red match optimal KNFs.)

Dry foods	Na (%)	Cl (%)	K (%)	Fat (%)	Energy density (kcal/g)	Fiber (%)**	Protein digestibility (%)	Fat digestibility (%)	Carbohydrate digestibility (%)	Primary sources of fiber**
Recommended levels	0.3-0.5	0.5-1.3	0.8-1.1	8-12	≥3.2	7-15	≥80	≥80	≥90	–
Hill's Prescription Diet w/d Canine	0.22	0.46	0.70	8.8	3.3	16.4	84	92	95	Cellulose, soybean mill run, beet pulp
Medi-Cal Fibre Formula	0.3	na	1.0	10.6	na	14.3	na	na	na	Tomato pomace, rice hulls, oat hulls, flax meal, apple pomace
Purina Veterinary Diets DCO Dual Fiber Control	0.34	0.82	0.70	12.4	3.7	7.6	79.9	80.4	90.6	Beet pulp, pea fiber
Purina Veterinary Diets OM Overweight Management Formula	0.31	0.97	0.83	7.2	2.9	10.3	81.9	78.9	72.3	Soybean hulls, pea fiber, cellulose
Royal Canin Veterinary Diet Calorie Control CC 26 High Fiber	0.33	0.77	0.90	10.4	3.1	17.6	na	na	na	Cellulose, pea fiber, rice hulls, beet pulp, psyllium husk
Royal Canin Veterinary Diet Diabetic HF 18	0.27	0.88	0.88	9.9	3.3	12.1	na	na	na	Cellulose, rice hulls, guar gum

Moist foods	Na (%)	Cl (%)	K (%)	Fat (%)	Energy density (kcal/g)	Fiber (%)**	Protein digestibility (%)	Fat digestibility (%)	Carbohydrate digestibility (%)	Primary sources of fiber**
Recommended levels	0.3-0.5	0.5-1.3	0.8-1.1	8-12	≥3.2	7-15	≥80	≥80	≥90	–
Hill's Prescription Diet w/d Canine	0.24	0.76	0.64	12.7	3.6	12.4	88	90	92	Cellulose
Medi-Cal Fibre Formula	0.5	na	0.7	9.1	na	15.0	na	na	na	Tomato pomace, guar gum, flax meal, carrageenan
Purina Veterinary Diets OM Overweight Management Formula	0.28	0.51	1.06	8.4	2.5	19.2	80.9	89.8	62.9	Pea fiber, beet pulp, carrageenan
Royal Canin Veterinary Diet Calorie Control CC 26 High Fiber	0.53	0.70	0.82	12.5	3.6	8.8	na	na	na	Tomato pomace, guar gum, flax meal, carrageenan

Key: Na = sodium, Cl = chloride, K = potassium, fiber = crude fiber, na = information not available from manufacturer.
*Nutrients expressed on a dry matter basis. To convert kcal to kJ, multiply kcal by 4.184.
**Insoluble fiber sources are best in fiber-enhanced foods (see text).

Multiple or Recurrent Small Bowel Diarrhea. Further diagnostic workup may be required and, most probably, a combination of dietary and medical therapies. Parasitic causes, however, should be ruled out and/or treated empirically before pursuing additional diagnostics.

MISCELLANEOUS

See Chapters 17, 24-26 and 56, Small Animal Clinical Nutrition, 5th edition, for more information.

Authors

Condensed from Chapter 56, Small Animal Clinical Nutrition, 5th edition, authored by Deborah J. Davenport and Rebecca L. Remillard.

References

See Chapter 56, Small Animal Clinical Nutrition, 5th edition, on the website www.markmorrisinstitute.org for references.

Table 6. Key nutritional factors in selected fiber-enhanced commercial veterinary therapeutic foods marketed for cats with acute gastroenteritis or acute enteritis.* (Numbers in red match optimal KNFs.)

Dry foods	Na (%)	Cl (%)	K (%)	Fat (%)	Energy density (kcal/g)	Fiber (%)**	Protein digestibility (%)	Fat digestibility (%)	Carbohydrate digestibility (%)	Primary sources of fiber**
Recommended levels	0.3-0.5	0.5-1.3	0.8-1.1	9-18	≥3.4	7-15	≥80	≥80	≥90	–
Hill's Prescription Diet w/d Feline	0.30	0.84	0.84	9.8	3.5	7.6	90	87	86	Cellulose
Hill's Prescription Diet w/d with Chicken Feline	0.35	0.82	0.80	9.9	3.5	7.6	91	85	94	Cellulose
Medi-Cal Fibre Formula	0.5	na	0.9	12.2	na	14.9	na	na	na	Pea fiber, beet pulp, flax meal
Purina Veterinary Diets OM Overweight Management	0.57	0.84	0.89	8.5	3.6	5.6	91.1	87.7	66.8	Oat fiber, cellulose
Royal Canin Veterinary Diet Calorie Control CC 29 High Fiber	0.51	0.92	0.88	10.2	3.3	14.0	na	na	na	Cellulose, pea fiber, rice hulls, beet pulp, psyllium

Moist foods	Na (%)	Cl (%)	K (%)	Fat (%)	Energy density (kcal/g)	Fiber (%)**	Protein digestibility (%)	Fat digestibility (%)	Carbohydrate digestibility (%)	Primary sources of fiber**
Recommended levels	0.3-0.5	0.5-1.3	0.8-1.1	9-18	≥3.4	7-15	≥80	≥80	≥90	–
Hill's Prescription Diet w/d with Chicken Feline	0.38	0.89	0.89	16.6	3.5	10.6	92	na	na	Cellulose, oat fiber, guar gum, locust bean gum, carrageenan
Medi-Cal Fibre Formula	0.4	na	0.8	17.1	na	16.7	na	na	na	Pea fiber, flax meal, guar gum
Purina Veterinary Diets OM Overweight Management	0.31	0.93	0.91	14.6	3.9	10.2	87.3	88.6	84	Pea fiber, oat fiber, guar gum
Royal Canin Veterinary Diet Calorie Control CC High Fiber	0.38	0.51	0.77	21.3	4.1	7.7	na	na	na	Cellulose, guar gum, flaxseed

Key: Na = sodium, Cl = chloride, K = potassium, fiber = crude fiber, na = information not available from manufacturer.
*Nutrients expressed on a dry matter basis. To convert kcal to kJ, multiply kcal by 4.184.
**Insoluble fiber sources are best in fiber-enhanced foods (see text).

CLINICAL POINTS

- IBD is a group of chronic, idiopathic GI disorders characterized by histopathologic lesions of mucosal inflammation. The lymphoplasmacytic form is probably the most common type.
- IBD is considered the most common cause of chronic diarrhea and vomiting.
- Genetic influences have been recognized in some dog breeds (Appendix N).
- Overcrowded, contaminated quarters are a risk for development of parasitic infections, viral and bacterial enteritis and SIBO, all of which may play a role in the pathogenesis of IBD.
- Apparently no age or gender predisposition exists.
- Severity varies from relatively mild clinical signs to life-threatening PLEs.
- In cats, the stomach and small bowel are affected most often. In dogs, IBD is common in both small and large intestines.
- Clinical signs may be mixed because multiple segments of bowel are often involved. The most common signs are chronic vomiting, diarrhea and weight loss. The predominant sign varies with the portion(s) of the GI tract affected. Occasionally, thickened loops of bowel may be detected by abdominal palpation (more easily detected in cats).
- Small intestinal involvement results in loose, fluid or steatorrheic stools. Diarrhea marked by tenesmus, mucus and small scanty stools is noted with colonic lesions (Appendix N).
- Signs may be intermittent or persistent and tend to increase in frequency and intensity as IBD progresses temporally. Some pets present with a history of depression, malaise and inappetence; others are alert and active.
- Multiple fecal examinations using concentration techniques are necessary to rule out parasitism in chronic cases.
- Hematologic findings vary and may indicate blood loss anemia, anemia of chronic disease and/or eosinophilia.
- Serum biochemistry alterations in patients with chronic diarrhea may include hypokalemia, hypoproteinemia and hypoalbuminemia (severe cases with PLE) and prerenal azotemia (dehydrated patients).
- IBD in cats may be associated with pancreatitis and hepatitis (triaditis). Neutrophilia, increased hepatic enzyme activities, hyperbilirubinemia and increased serum pancreatic lipase immunoreactivity may be noted. Hypereosinophilic syndrome may occur in cats with eosinophilic gastroenteritis.
- Radiographic findings are usually nonspecific and non-diagnostic. Endoscopic abnormalities include mucosal granularity, hyperemia, friability and inability to visualize colonic submucosal blood vessels. For definitive histopathologic diagnosis, collect and evaluate multiple biopsy specimens, even

Abbreviations
AAFCO = Association of American Feed Control Officials
BCS = body condition score (Appendix A)
EPI = exocrine pancreatic insufficiency
GALT = gut-associated lymphatic tissue
IBD = inflammatory bowel disease
KNF = key nutritional factor
PLE = protein-losing enteropathy
SIBO = small intestinal bacterial overgrowth

if the gross appearance is normal.
- IBD development involves hypersensitivity; 2 related theories have been proposed: 1) mucosal barrier defects and loss of mucosal integrity result in increased gut permeability and hypersensitivity responses to normally tolerated antigens and 2) GALT suppressor function defects may predispose to hypersensitivity to normally tolerated antigens. Both pathways culminate in release of inflammatory mediators, which further damage the mucosa and set up cycles of inflammation with barrier function loss.
- Mucosal inflammation results in malabsorption and osmotic diarrhea. Altered gut permeability can result in intraluminal leakage of fluid, protein and blood. Malabsorbed fats, carbohydrates and bile acids result in secretory diarrhea. Inflammatory mediators may directly trigger secretion and mucus production by goblet cells. Mucosal inflammatory infiltrates may alter motility patterns. Inflammation of the stomach and upper small bowel trigger vomiting.
- Justifications for nutritional management: 1) dietary factors may contribute to initiation/perpetuation of IBD and need to be managed, 2) malnutrition is commonly associated with IBD due to anorexia, malabsorption and increased nutrient losses.
- Dehydration occurs frequently with IBD. Reduced water consumption is often aggravated by fluid losses from vomiting and/or diarrhea.
- Foods for IBD patients should have adequate potassium because hypokalemia is particularly common.
- Smaller volumes of food minimize GI distention and secretions. However, energy/nutrient-dense foods are typically higher in fat, which may contribute to osmotic diarrhea and protein losses, further complicating IBD. Thus, moderate fat foods are recommended.
- Protein malnutrition may occur due to maldigestion/absorption and fecal losses. High biologic value, highly digestible (≥87%) protein sources should be used in foods for IBD. Because dietary antigens are suspected to play a role in the pathogenesis, "hypoallergenic" elimination foods are often recommended.
- Advantages of highly digestible foods: nutrients are more completely absorbed, osmotic diarrhea is reduced due to fat and carbohydrate malabsorption, production of intestinal gas is reduced due to carbohydrate malabsorption and antigen loads

Table 1. Key nutritional factors for dogs and cats with inflammatory bowel disease.*

Factors	Recommended levels
Potassium	0.8 to 1.1%
Energy density	4.0 to 4.5 kcal/g (16.7 to 18.8 kJ/g) for highly digestible foods for dogs and cats
	≥3.2 kcal/g (≥13.4 kJ/g) for fiber-enhanced foods for dogs and ≥3.4 kcal/g (≥14.2 kJ/g) for cats
Fat	12 to 15% for dogs and 15 to 25% for cats for highly digestible foods
	For fiber-enhanced foods:
	8 to 12% for dogs
	9 to 18% for cats
Protein	≥25% for dogs
	≥35% for cats
	If using a limited protein (elimination food) approach, restrict protein to one or two sources and use protein sources to which the patient has not been exposed previously or feed a protein hydrolysate (Chapter 19); also use lower protein levels (16 to 26% for dogs and 30 to 45% for cats)
Crude fiber	≤5% for highly digestible foods (mixed fiber) for dogs and cats
	7 to 15% for increased-fiber foods (insoluble fibers are best) for dogs and cats
Digestibility	≥87% for protein and ≥90% for fat and digestible carbohydrate for highly digestible foods
	≥80% for protein and fat and ≥90% for carbohydrate for fiber-enhanced foods

*Nutrients expressed on a dry matter basis.

Table 2. Key nutritional factors in selected highly digestible veterinary therapeutic foods marketed for dogs with inflammatory bowel disease compared to recommended levels.* (See Chapter 19 if foods with novel protein sources or protein hydrolysates are desired). (Numbers in red match optimal KNFs.)

Dry foods	K (%)	Energy density (kcal/g)	Fat (%)	Protein (%)	Fiber (%)	Protein digestibility (%)	Fat digestibility (%)	Carbohydrate digestibility (%)
Recommended levels	0.8-1.1	4.0-4.5	12-15	≥25	≤5	≥87	≥90	≥90
Hill's Prescription Diet i/d Canine	0.92	4.2	14.1	26.2	2.7	92	93	94
Iams Veterinary Formula Intestinal Low-Residue	0.90	3.8	10.7	24.6	2.1	na	na	na
Medi-Cal Gastro Formula	0.8	na	13.9	22.9	1.9	na	na	na
Medi-Cal Vegetarian Formula	0.8	na	10.5	20.9	3.2	na	na	na
Purina Veterinary Diets EN GastroENteric Formula	0.66	4.2	12.6	27.0	1.5	84.5	91.4	94.4
Royal Canin Veterinary Diet Digestive Low Fat LF 20	0.88	3.7	6.6	24.2	2.3	na	na	na
Royal Canin Veterinary Diets Intestinal HE 28	0.88	4.5	22.0	33.0	1.6	na	na	na

Moist foods	K (%)	Energy density (kcal/g)	Fat (%)	Protein (%)	Fiber (%)	Protein digestibility (%)	Fat digestibility (%)	Carbohydrate digestibility (%)
Recommended levels	0.8-1.1	4.0-4.5	12-15	≥25	≤5	≥87	≥90	≥90
Hill's Prescription Diet i/d Canine	0.95	4.4	14.9	25.0	1.0	88	94	93
Iams Veterinary Formula Intestinal Low-Residue	0.84	4.6	13.2	35.9	3.9	na	na	na
Medi-Cal Gastro Formula	0.6	na	11.7	22.1	1.0	na	na	na
Medi-Cal Vegetarian Formula	0.7	na	11.5	26.4	1.9	na	na	na
Purina Veterinary Diets EN GastroENteric Formula	0.61	4.0	13.8	30.5	0.9	85.1	95.6	92.2
Royal Canin Veterinary Diet Digestive Low Fat LF	0.74	4.0	6.9	31.9	3.0	na	na	na
Royal Canin Veterinary Diet Intestinal HE	0.80	4.3	11.8	23.1	1.4	na	na	na

Key: K = potassium, Fiber = crude fiber, na = information not available from manufacturer.
*Manufacturers' published values. Nutrients expressed on a dry matter basis. To convert kcal to kJ, multiply kcal by 4.184.

are decreased because smaller amounts of protein are absorbed intact.

- Fiber sources including beet pulp, soy fiber, inulin and fructooligosaccharides produce volatile fatty acids that may be beneficial in IBD.
- Moderate levels of insoluble fiber (e.g., cellulose) add nondigestible bulk, which buffers toxins, holds excess water and provides intraluminal stimuli to reestablish actions of hormones, neurons, smooth muscle, enzyme delivery, digestion and absorption.
- Some patients may only require dietary therapy; others require adjunctive pharmacologic agents: antibiotics (e.g., tylosin,

Table 3. Key nutritional factors in selected highly digestible veterinary therapeutic foods marketed for cats with inflammatory bowel disease compared to recommended levels.* (See Chapter 19 if foods with novel protein sources or protein hydrolysates are desired). (Numbers in red match optimal KNFs.)

Dry foods	K (%)	Energy density (kcal/g)	Fat (%)	Protein (%)	Fiber (%)	Protein digestibility (%)	Fat digestibility (%)	Carbohydrate digestibility (%)
Recommended levels	0.8-1.1	4.0-4.5	15-25	≥35	≤5	≥87	≥90	≥90
Hill's Prescription Diet i/d Feline	1.07	4.3	20.2	40.3	2.8	88	92	90
Iams Veterinary Formula Intestinal Low-Residue	0.66	3.9	13.7	35.8	1.8	na	na	na
Medi-Cal Hypoallergenic/Gastro	0.8	na	11.5	29.8	3.1	na	na	na
Purina Veterinary Diets EN GastroENteric Formula	0.99	4.4	18.4	56.2	1.3	94.0	93.1	79.7
Royal Canin Veterinary Diet Intestinal HE 30	0.97	4.4	23.7	34.4	5.8	na	na	na

Moist foods	K (%)	Energy density (kcal/g)	Fat (%)	Protein (%)	Fiber (%)	Protein digestibility (%)	Fat digestibility (%)	Carbohydrate digestibility (%)
Recommended levels	0.8-1.1	4.0-4.5	15-25	≥35	≤5	≥87	≥90	≥90
Hill's Prescription Diet i/d Feline	1.06	4.2	24.1	37.6	2.4	91	89	91
Iams Veterinary Formula Intestinal Low-Residue	0.93	4.0	11.7	38.4	3.7	na	na	na
Medi-Cal Hypoallergenic/Gastro	1.1	na	35.9	35.5	1.2	na	na	na
Medi-Cal Sensitivity CR	1.1	na	35.1	34.5	2.5	na	na	na

Key: K = potassium, Fiber = crude fiber, na = information not available from manufacturer.
*Manufacturers' published values. Nutrients expressed on a dry matter basis. To convert kcal to kJ, multiply kcal by 4.184.

tetracycline, enrofloxacin, metronidazole), anthelmintics (e.g., fenbendazole) and immunosuppressive agents (e.g., corticosteroids, budesonide, cyclosporine, azathioprine, cyclophosphamide) are often used for managing IBD.

- Prognosis is good to excellent in properly treated mild to moderate cases but varies more with increasing disease severity at initial presentation. Managing compliance and the specific underlying pathology also affect outcomes. Some forms are refractory to treatment and response may be poor in patients presented late in the disease or those with PLE.
- Feeding goals: control clinical signs while providing adequate nutrients to meet requirements and compensate for ongoing losses through the GI tract.

KEY NUTRITIONAL FACTORS

- Foods should provide recommended allowances of all required nutrients (nutritional adequacy), but should also contain specific levels of KNFs (certain nutrients and food features that may assist in the management of IBD).
- **Table 1** lists KNF recommendations for foods for patients with IBD. Included are KNFs for highly digestible foods, fiber-enhanced foods and elimination foods. A detailed review of these recommendations can be found in Chapter 57, Small Animal Clinical Nutrition, 5th edition. Other KNFs may also be important depending on the patient's lifestage (e.g., growth, Chapters 5 and 11).
- Water is the most important nutrient for patients with IBD because of the potential for life-threatening dehydration due to excessive fluid loss and inability of the patient to replace those

losses.

FEEDING PLAN

Assess and Select the Food

3 types of foods may be useful in managing IBD: 1) highly digestible GI foods, 2) fiber-enhanced foods and 3) elimination foods. Because physical exam findings, laboratory test results and historical facts will not indicate which food is best for a given patient, dietary "trial and error" is often needed.

Ensure the Food's Basic Nutritional Adequacy. AAFCO nutritional adequacy statements are usually found on a product's label. AAFCO approval does not ensure a food will be effective in the management of IBD.

Compare the Food's KNF Content with the Recommended Levels. The 3 different food approaches may be attempted in any order to see which is effective in a given patient. Comparison tables for highly digestible foods and fiber-enhanced foods include KNF contents of selected commercial foods and compare them to recommended levels for IBD (below). Compare KNF recommendations in **Table 1** to KNFs in Tables 3 and 4, Chapter 19, for elimination foods. Consider a food that most closely matches KNF recommendations.

HIGHLY DIGESTIBLE GI FOODS. May contain small amounts of soluble/mixed fiber (**Tables 2** and **3** for dogs and cats, respectively). This is the most common food strategy for IBD.

FIBER-ENHANCED FOODS. Contain moderate amounts of fiber (**Tables 4** for dogs and **5** for cats). Typically, these foods have lower energy density and IBD patients may have difficulty maintaining normal body weight and condition (BCS).

Table 4. Key nutritional factors in selected fiber-enhanced veterinary therapeutic foods marketed for dogs with inflammatory bowel disease compared to recommended levels.* (See Chapter 19 if foods with novel protein sources or protein hydrolysates are desired). (Numbers in red match optimal KNFs.)

Dry foods	K (%)	Energy density (kcal/g)	Fat (%)	Protein (%)	Fiber (%)	Protein digestibility (%)	Fat digestibility (%)	Carbohydrate digestibility (%)
Recommended levels	0.8-1.1	≥3.2	8-12	≥25	7-15	≥80	≥80	≥90
Hill's Prescription Diet w/d Canine	0.70	3.3	8.8	18.9	16.4	84	92	95
Medi-Cal Fibre Formula	1.0	na	10.6	26.2	14.3	na	na	na
Purina Veterinary Diets DCO Dual Fiber Control	0.7	3.7	12.4	25.3	7.6	79.9	80.4	90.6
Purina Veterinary Diets OM Overweight Management	0.83	2.9	7.2	31.1	10.3	81.9	78.9	72.3
Royal Canin Veterinary Diet Calorie Control CC 26 High Fiber	0.9	3.1	10.4	30.9	17.6	na	na	na
Moist foods	K (%)	Energy density (kcal/g)	Fat (%)	Protein (%)	Fiber (%)	Protein digestibility (%)	Fat digestibility (%)	Carbohydrate digestibility (%)
Recommended levels	0.8-1.1	≥3.2	8-12	≥25	7-15	≥80	≥80	≥90
Hill's Prescription Diet w/d Canine	0.64	3.5	12.7	17.9	12.4	88	90	92
Medi-Cal Fibre Formula	0.7	na	9.1	24.8	15.0	na	na	na
Purina Veterinary Diets OM Overweight Management	1.06	2.5	8.4	44.1	19.2	80.9	89.8	62.9
Royal Canin Veterinary Diet Calorie Control CC High Fiber	0.82	3.6	12.5	25.9	8.8	na	na	na

Key: K = potassium, Fiber = crude fiber, na = information not available from manufacturer.
*Manufacturers' published values. Nutrients expressed on a dry matter basis. To convert kcal to kJ, multiply kcal by 4.184.

Table 5. Key nutritional factors in selected fiber-enhanced veterinary therapeutic foods marketed for cats with inflammatory bowel disease compared to recommended levels.* (See Chapter 19 if foods with novel protein sources or protein hydrolysates are desired). (Numbers in red match optimal KNFs.)

Dry foods	K (%)	Energy density (kcal/g)	Fat (%)	Protein (%)	Fiber (%)	Protein digestibility (%)	Fat digestibility (%)	Carbohydrate digestibility (%)
Recommended levels	0.8-1.1	≥3.4	9-18	≥35	7-15	≥80	≥80	≥90
Hill's Prescription Diet w/d Feline	0.84	3.5	9.8	39.0	7.6	90	87	86
Hill's Prescription Diet w/d with Chicken Feline	0.80	3.5	9.9	39.9	7.6	91	85	94
Medi-Cal Fibre Formula	0.9	na	12.2	34.2	14.9	na	na	na
Purina Veterinary Diets OM Overweight Management	0.89	3.6	8.5	56.2	5.6	91.1	87.7	66.8
Royal Canin Veterinary Diet Calorie Control CC 29 High Fiber	0.88	3.3	10.2	33.5	14.0	na	na	na
Moist foods	K (%)	Energy density (kcal/g)	Fat (%)	Protein (%)	Fiber (%)	Protein digestibility (%)	Fat digestibility (%)	Carbohydrate digestibility (%)
Recommended levels	0.8-1.1	≥3.4	9-18	≥35	7-15	≥80	≥80	≥90
Hill's Prescription Diet w/d with Chicken Feline	0.89	3.5	16.6	39.6	10.6	92	na	na
Medi-Cal Fibre Formula	0.8	na	17.1	40.0	16.7	na	na	na
Purina Veterinary Diets OM Overweight Management	0.91	3.9	14.6	44.6	10.2	87.3	88.6	84.0
Royal Canin Veterinary Diet Calorie Control CC High Fiber	0.77	4.1	21.3	33.5	7.7	na	na	na

Key: K = potassium, Fiber = crude fiber, na = information not available from manufacturer.
*Manufacturers' published values. Nutrients expressed on a dry matter basis. To convert kcal to kJ, multiply kcal by 4.184.

ELIMINATION FOODS. Contain limited numbers of highly digestible, novel protein sources or protein hydrolysates to which a patient has not been previously exposed (Tables 3 for dogs and 4 for cats, Chapter 19). Eliminate all other possible dietary sources of protein and carbohydrate including treats, snacks, table foods, vitamin-mineral supplements and chewable/flavored medications.

OMEGA-3 (N-3) FATTY ACIDS. Many elimination foods contain increased levels to influence inflammatory mediators and provide other benefits (Tables 2 and 3, Chapter 21).
Manage Treats and Snacks. Recommend initially withholding treats/snacks until the patient' condition has stabilized. Consider commercial treats that match the food being fed. Most companies offer treats that correspond to their specific veterinary therapeutic

foods. An option is to use the opposite form of the food being fed; i.e., if a dry food is fed, offer small amounts of the same food in moist form as a snack and vice versa. Keep kibbles of dry food in a separate container away from the usual feeding area and use as treats. Treats/snacks should not be fed excessively (<10% of the total diet on a volume, weight or calorie basis).

Assess and Determine the Feeding Method

Determine How Much Food to Feed. Estimate from feeding guides on product labels or by calculation (Appendix C). These estimates are only starting points and will likely need to be adjusted (see Followup below).

Consider How to Offer the Food. Initially, recommend multiple (6-8) small meals/day as indicated by acceptance and GI tolerance for the prescribed food. Meal size can be increased and meal frequency can be reduced as tolerated by the patient after clinical signs have been successfully managed for several weeks.

Manage Food Changes.

INITIATION OF PRESCRIBED FOOD. For transition feeding, provide small amounts of the new food 6-8 times/day. If no vomiting/diarrhea develops, the amount fed can be increased gradually over several days until the patient receives the estimated daily food dose in 2-3 meals/day. If the patient begins to vomit/have diarrhea during this period, the owner should withdraw the food and offer it again in a few hours.

RETURN TO REGULAR FOOD. After recovery, the patient can continue to be fed the prescribed food; however, patients are rarely transitioned back to the original food.

Food and Water Receptacle Husbandry. Food and water bowls should be washed regularly with warm soapy water and rinsed well. Dishes used for gruels and moist foods need daily cleaning. Owners should discard gruels, moist or moistened dry foods after 2-4 hours of room temperature exposure to avoid foodborne illnesses (Appendix F).

FOLLOWUP

Owner Followup

Note GI signs daily. Weigh the patient (if possible) and/or grade its BCS monthly. If necessary, change the amount fed by 10% increments and recheck the patient every 2 weeks for 1 month. Then, if necessary, change the amount fed again and repeat the cycle until the patient reaches normal body weight/BCS.

Compliance. Work with the veterinary health care team to ensure compliance with home care orders for dietary and medical management. Do not feed unprescribed foods or treats. Deny access to other foods if the patient lives in a multi-pet household.

Veterinary Health Care Team Followup

Regaining/maintaining optimal body weight and BCS, normal activity and alertness and absence of clinical signs are measures of successful dietary and medical management. Often, medical therapy can be withdrawn after 3-6 months; thereafter, appropri-

ate foods should maintain the patient's remission. In some cases, however, medical therapy may be required for life.

Elimination Foods. Signs should abate within 3 weeks of initiating strict dietary management (i.e., feeding only the prescribed food/treats). After signs abate, owners may add individual specific ingredients previously fed to identify allergen(s); GI signs usually recur <12 hours after eating the offending ingredient. Many owners elect to skip this step and continue feeding the elimination food.

Poor Response to Treatment. The most common causes include owner noncompliance and inadequate dietary/medical management plans. Intercurrent illnesses (e.g., triaditis in cats, SIBO or EPI) or misdiagnosis of alimentary lymphosarcoma or progression of IBD to lymphosarcoma (dogs) can also be causes.

MISCELLANEOUS

See Chapters 17, 24, 31, 32 and 57, Small Animal Clinical Nutrition, 5th edition, for more information.

Vitamin Malnutrition

May occur in patients with IBD due to limited stores vs. increased losses and decreased intake resulting from diarrhea (impaired absorption) and increased fluid fluxes. Amounts in food are usually sufficient after signs abate.

Thiamin (B_1). Deficiency occurs commonly and can negatively affect appetite. Consider parenteral supplementation (see product label for dose).

Cobalamin (B_{12}). Deficiencies are observed for several reasons and can result in severe metabolic abnormalities. Consider laboratory tests to assess serum cobalamin levels for patients receiving parenteral cobalamin for hypocobalaminemia (<300 ng/l). Recommended SQ dose: 250 µg/week (cats) and 500 µg/week (dogs) until levels return to normal. Once/twice monthly therapy may be necessary for longer term maintenance.

Folate (B_{10} and B_{11}). Disease of the proximal small intestine can interfere with folate absorption. Consider laboratory tests to assess the necessity for, and adequacy of supplementation (see product label for dose).

Fat-Soluble Vitamins (A, D, E and K). Losses can be significant in patients with steatorrhea. Initially, parenteral administration (1 ml ADE,[a] divided into 2 IM sites) should be satisfactory for 3 months. Administer vitamin K_1 at a dose of 0.5-1.0 mg/kg SQ, if a vitamin K-responsive coagulopathy is suspected.

Zinc Malnutrition

Several potential mechanisms exist for zinc deficiency in IBD patients (Table 6). Consider supplemental oral zinc (zinc sulfate: 10 mg/kg/day; zinc methionine: 2 mg/kg/day) if poor coat quality or dermatitis occurs. Do not give with food.

Supplemental Omega-3 Fatty Acids

May modulate inflammatory mediators and provide other benefits. The dose is 50-300 mg omega-3 fatty acids/kg/day.

Table 6. Potential causes of zinc deficiency in patients with inflammatory bowel disease.

Decreased absorption
Intestinal inflammation
Supplemental iron and/or copper
Surgical resection of distal duodenum
Inadequate dietary intake
Anorexia
High fiber or phytate intake
Parenteral nutrition
Increased losses
Chronic blood loss
Increased metabolism
Increased requirements
Growth
Lactation
Pregnancy
Wound healing

Authors
Condensed from Chapter 57, Small Animal Clinical Nutrition, 5th edition, authored by Deborah J. Davenport, Albert E Jergens and Rebecca L. Remillard.

References
See Chapter 57, Small Animal Clinical Nutrition, 5th edition, on the website www.markmorrisinstitute.org for references.

Endnote
a. Vital E-A+D containing 100 IU of D and 300 IU of α-tocopherol/ml. Schering-Plough Animal Health Corp., Kenilworth, NJ, USA.

Chapter 44
Protein-Losing Enteropathies

CLINICAL POINTS

- PLE is a broad term encompassing intestinal disorders characterized by GI protein loss that causes hypoalbuminemia.
- Lymphangiectasia, one form of PLE, is characterized by abnormalities of the intestinal lymphatic system that cause lymphatic hypertension. Lymphangiectasia may occur as a primary lymphatic defect or as a consequence of severe intestinal infiltrative disease (e.g., IBD, alimentary lymphosarcoma, fungal enteritis).
- Lymphangiectasia is a common cause of PLE in dogs but is rare in cats.
- Dog breeds at risk include: Chinese Shar-Peis, Rottweilers and Lundehunds for PLE (it may occur in conjunction with protein-losing nephropathy in soft-coated wheaten terriers); Yorkshire terriers, poodles, golden retrievers and dachshunds for primary lymphatic defects; Basenjis and Lundehunds for lymphangiectasia secondary to IBD.
- Signs of PLE are insidious in onset and follow a waxing/waning course over several weeks to months before becoming overt. The clinical manifestations are generally attributable to the loss of lymph constituents (i.e., albumin, lymphocytes, fat and cholesterol) or to the underlying enteric disease.
- Many patients present with chronic intermittent diarrhea or vomiting; however, not all patients have GI signs. Weight

Abbreviations
AAFCO = Association of American Feed Control Officials
BCS = body condition score (Appendix A)
DM = dry matter
IBD = inflammatory bowel disease
KNF = key nutritional factor
LCT = long-chain triglyceride
MCT = medium-chain triglyceride
PLE = protein-losing enteropathy
RER = resting energy requirement (Appendix C)

loss, often with a good appetite, is a consistent finding in longstanding cases. Excessive protein loss from leaky intestinal lymphatics results in hypoalbuminemia and loss of colloidal oncotic pressure with associated signs.
- Typical lab results include hypoglobulinemia, hypoalbuminemia and hypocholesterolemia. Other findings may include anemia of chronic disease, a stress leukogram and hypocalcemia (caused by malabsorption of calcium and/or vitamin D).
- Fecal α-1-protease inhibitor protein is a sensitive and specific test for intestinal protein loss in dogs and cats.
- Endoscopy can be useful; mucosal granularity and glistening white patches, which indicate dilated lacteals may be noted. A definitive diagnosis is made through histopathology.
- Lymphatic defects are not limited to the GI tract in some patients (e.g., primary lymphangiectasia); abnormal lymph

flow may result in chylothorax, chylous abdominal effusion and subcutaneous chyle accumulation.

- Controlling dietary fat intake is important. LCT absorption increases lymph protein content and lymph flow 2-3 fold for several hours postprandially. Limiting fat intake minimizes lymph flow and protein loss. Generally, MCTs do not require micellarization for absorption; they are absorbed directly into the portal vasculature and do not affect lymph flow as much as LCTs. MCTs should be incorporated into the food.
- Foods for patients with PLE should contain enough high biologic value protein to support protein synthesis and replace depleted tissue proteins. Low-fat, elimination foods should be considered if severe IBD is the underlying cause.
- Highly digestible foods provide several advantages: 1) nutrients are more completely absorbed in the proximal gut, 2) reduced osmotic diarrhea related to fat and carbohydrate malabsorption, 3) reduced intestinal gas due to carbohydrate malabsorption and 4) decreased antigen loads because smaller amounts of protein are absorbed intact.
- Feeding goal: decrease enteric loss of plasma protein by dietary manipulation alone or with concurrent medical management.

KEY NUTRITIONAL FACTORS

- Foods should provide recommended allowances of all required nutrients (nutritional adequacy) and contain specific levels of KNFs (certain nutrients and food features that may assist in the management of PLE).
- **Table 1** lists KNF recommendations for foods for patients with PLE. A detailed review of these recommendations can be found in Chapter 58, Small Animal Clinical Nutrition, 5th edition. Inclusion of MCTs is desirable. Protein sources may be important if IBD is the underlying cause (Chapter 43).

FEEDING PLAN

Assess and Select the Food
Two types of foods may be useful for managing PLE: 1) highly digestible GI foods or 2) elimination foods.
Ensure the Food's Basic Nutritional Adequacy. AAFCO nutritional adequacy statements are usually found on a product's label. AAFCO approval does not ensure a food will be effective for managing PLE.
Compare the Food's KNF Content with the Recommended Levels. Comparison tables for highly digestible foods include the KNF contents of selected commercial foods and compare them to recommended KNF levels for PLE (below).
HIGHLY DIGESTIBLE GI FOODS. Tables 2 and **3** list selected veterinary therapeutic GI foods marketed for PLE in dogs and cats, respectively, and compare them to recommended levels. It is usually best to choose the food that most closely matches the KNF recommendations.

Table 1. Key nutritional factors for foods for patients with lymphangiectasia/protein-losing enteropathy.*

Factors	Recommended levels
Energy density	>3.5 kcal/g (>14.6 kJ/g)
Fat**	<15% for dogs and cats
Protein	≥25% for dogs
	≥35% for cats
Crude fiber	≤5%
Digestibility	≥87% for protein and ≥90% for fat and digestible carbohydrate

*Nutrients expressed on a dry matter basis.
**Inclusion of medium-chain triglycerides is desirable.

MCTs. If a patient cannot maintain normal body weight and condition (BCS) when fed an appropriate food, supplemental MCT oil may be used cautiously; introduce MCTs gradually and do not exceed 25% of the caloric requirement (<1 ml/lb [<0.5 ml/kg]/day).

SUPPLEMENTAL PROTEIN. Some patients may require additional protein. Dogs may be fed a low-fat (<10% DM fat) cat food that has a higher protein (>35% DM) content (**Table 3**) than a comparable dog food. Protein may also be added as cooked egg whites. Provide 1-2 cooked large egg whites/10 kg as needed to maintain serum albumin >2 g/dl.

ELIMINATION FOODS. Consider these foods for PLE patients with severe IBD as the underlying cause. Compare KNF recommendations in **Table 1** to the KNFs in Tables 3 and 4, Chapter 19. Consider a food that most closely matches KNF recommendations for IBD.

FOODS FOR ASSISTED FEEDING. For debilitated, anorectic patients, consider assisted feeding by nasoesophageal, pharyngostomy or esophagostomy tube using liquid foods (Tables 4 and 5, Chapter 12). Foods with lower fat content are preferred. Longstanding hospitalized patients in poor body condition should be fed parenterally. Calories can easily be administered via peripheral vein using an isosmolar 20% lipid solution piggybacked with standard fluid therapy sufficient to meet the patient's RER (Chapter 13).

Manage Treats and Snacks. Consider commercial treats that match the food being fed. Most companies offer treats that correspond to their specific veterinary therapeutic foods. An option is to use the opposite form of the food being fed; i.e., if a dry food is fed, the owners can offer small amounts of the same food in moist form as a snack and vice versa; keep dry food kibbles in a separate container away from the usual feeding area and use as treats. Treats/snacks should not be fed excessively (<10% of the total diet on a volume, weight or calorie basis).

Assess and Determine the Feeding Method
Determine How Much Food to Feed. Estimate from feeding guides on product labels or by calculation (Appendix C). These estimates are only starting points and will likely need to be adjusted (see Followup below).
Consider How to Offer the Food. Initially, feed multiple (6-8) small meals/day as indicated by acceptance and GI tolerance for the prescribed food. Meal size can be increased and meal frequency can be reduced as tolerated by the patient after clinical

Table 2. Key nutritional factors in selected veterinary therapeutic foods for dogs with lymphangiectasia/protein-losing enteropathy compared to recommended levels.* (See Chapter 19 if foods with novel protein sources or protein hydrolysates are desired). (Numbers in red match optimal KNFs.)

Dry foods	Energy density (kcal/g)	Fat (%)	Protein (%)	Fiber (%)	Protein digestibility (%)	Fat digestibility (%)	Carbohydrate digestibility (%)
Recommended levels	>3.5	<15	≥25	≤5	≥87	≥90	≥90
Hill's Prescription Diet i/d Canine	4.2	14.1	26.2	2.7	92	93	94
Iams Veterinary Formula Intestinal Low-Residue	3.8	10.7	24.6	2.1	na	na	na
Medi-Cal Low Fat LF 20	na	6.6	24.2	5.2	na	na	na
Purina Veterinary Diets EN GastroENteric Formula**	4.2	12.6	27.0	1.5	84.5	91.4	94.4
Royal Canin Veterinary Diet Digestive Low Fat LF 20	3.7	6.6	24.2	2.3	na	na	na

Moist foods	Energy density (kcal/g)	Fat (%)	Protein (%)	Fiber (%)	Protein digestibility (%)	Fat digestibility (%)	Carbohydrate digestibility (%)
Recommended levels	>3.5	<15	≥25	≤5	≥87	≥90	≥90
Hill's Prescription Diet i/d Canine	4.4	14.9	25.0	1.0	88	94	93
Iams Veterinary Formula Intestinal Low-Residue	4.6	13.2	35.9	3.9	na	na	na
Medi-Cal Low Fat LF	na	9.0	32.8	3.1	na	na	na
Purina Veterinary Diets EN GastroENteric Formula**	4.0	13.8	30.5	0.9	85.1	95.6	92.2
Royal Canin Veterinary Diet Digestive Low Fat LF	4.0	6.9	31.9	3.0	na	na	na

Key: Fiber = crude fiber, na = information not available from manufacturer.
*Manufacturers' published values. Nutrients expressed as % dry matter.
**Food contains medium-chain triglycerides.

Table 3. Key nutritional factors in selected veterinary therapeutic foods for cats with lymphangiectasia/protein-losing enteropathy compared to recommended levels.* (See Chapter 19 if foods with novel protein sources or protein hydrolysates are desired). (Numbers in red match optimal KNFs.)

Dry foods	Energy density (kcal/g)	Fat (%)	Protein (%)	Fiber (%)	Protein digestibility (%)	Fat digestibility (%)	Carbohydrate digestibility (%)
Recommended levels	>3.5	<15	≥35	≤5	≥87	≥90	≥90
Hill's Prescription Diet i/d Feline	4.3	20.2	40.3	2.8	88	92	90
Iams Veterinary Formula Intestinal Low-Residue	3.9	13.7	35.8	1.8	na	na	na
Medi-Cal Hypoallergenic/Gastro	na	11.5	29.8	3.1	na	na	na
Purina Veterinary Diets EN GastroENteric Formula	4.4	18.4	56.2	1.3	94.0	93.1	79.7
Royal Canin Veterinary Diet Intestinal HE	4.4	23.7	34.4	5.8	na	na	na

Moist foods	Energy density (kcal/g)	Fat (%)	Protein (%)	Fiber (%)	Protein digestibility (%)	Fat digestibility (%)	Carbohydrate digestibility (%)
Recommended levels	>3.5	<15	≥35	≤5	≥87	≥90	≥90
Hill's Prescription Diet i/d Feline	4.2	24.1	37.6	2.4	91	89	91
Iams Veterinary Formula Intestinal Low-Residue	4.0	11.7	38.4	3.7	na	na	na
Medi-Cal Hypoallergenic/Gastro	na	35.9	35.5	1.2	na	na	na
Medi-Cal Sensitivity CR	na	35.1	34.5	2.5	na	na	na

Key: Fiber = crude fiber, na = information not available from manufacturer.
*Manufacturers' published values. Nutrients expressed as % dry matter.

signs have been successfully managed for several weeks.

Manage Food Changes. For transition feeding, provide small amounts of the new food 6-8 times/day. If no untoward GI effects occur, the amount fed can be increased gradually over several days until the patient receives the estimated daily food dose in 2-3 meals/day.

Food and Water Receptacle Husbandry. Food and water bowls should be washed regularly with warm soapy water and rinsed well. Dishes used for moist foods need daily cleaning. Discard moist or moistened dry foods after 2-4 hours of room temperature exposure to avoid foodborne illnesses (Appendix F).

ADJUNCTIVE MEDICAL & SURGICAL MANAGEMENT

Immunosuppressive Therapy
Indicated when PLE occurs as a consequence of IBD. Drugs with reported efficacy include glucocorticoids and cyclosporine.

Colloid Therapy
Plasma, concentrated human albumin, dextran or hetastarch infusions may be necessary when hypoalbuminemia is severe to restore colloidal oncotic pressure. In general, aggressive nutritional support is more successful than plasma transfusions for restoring normoalbuminemia. Plasma transfusions may benefit patients with hypercoagulability resulting from panhypoproteinemia; plasma is a rich source of coagulation factors and antithrombin III.

FOLLOWUP

Owner Followup
Note clinical signs and food intake daily for review by the veterinary health care team.

Compliance. Adhere to homecare orders for dietary and medical management. Do not feed unprescribed foods or treats. Deny access to other foods if the patient lives in a multi-pet household.

Veterinary Health Care Team Followup
Initially, after discharge from the hospital, reassess the patient weekly including body weight and BCS. Adjust food intake as necessary and tolerance permits. Obtain serum albumin and calcium and a hemogram (lymphocyte count) every 2 weeks. Serial radiography helps assess resolution of abdominal or thoracic effusion. If the patient's condition improves, continue dietary therapy until the underlying enteropathy and associated clinical

signs have resolved. Otherwise, continue dietary therapy for life.

Inability to Maintain Normal Weight or Skin/Coat Quality. Attempt to increase dietary fat and essential fatty acid intake by prolonged (days to weeks), gradual transition to a higher fat food.

MISCELLANEOUS

See Chapters 25, 26, 31, 57 and 58, Small Animal Clinical Nutrition, 5th edition, for more information.

Fat-Soluble Vitamin Malnutrition
Fat-soluble vitamin supplementation is warranted in cases of long-term fat malabsorption. Administer 1 ml of a vitamin A, D and E solution,[a] divided into 2 IM sites. This therapy should supply fat-soluble vitamins for approximately 3 months. If vitamin K-responsive coagulopathy is suspected, consider administration of vitamin K_1, at a dose of 0.5-1 mg/kg, SQ.

Mineral Malnutrition
When fed foods containing higher levels of fat, patients with fat malabsorption may have increased divalent cation losses (i.e., calcium, magnesium, zinc or copper) because of intraluminal saponification.

Calcium. Supplementation is generally not needed because serum levels usually increase in conjunction with serum albumin concentrations. However, IV calcium should be administered if hypocalcemic tetany develops.

Magnesium. Hypomagnesemia has been reported to occur in Yorkshire terriers with lymphangiectasia. Anorexia and malabsorption complicated by the use of magnesium-free fluids are likely causes of the low serum magnesium levels. If necessary, magnesium repletion can be accomplished with appropriate IV fluids.

Authors
Condensed from Chapter 58, Small Animal Clinical Nutrition, 5th edition, authored by Deborah J. Davenport, Albert E. Jergens and Rebecca L. Remillard.

References
See Chapter 58, Small Animal Clinical Nutrition, 5th edition, on the website www.markmorrisinstitute.org for references.

Endnote
a. Vital E-A+D containing 100 IU of D and 300 IU of α-tocopherol/ml. Schering-Plough Animal Health Corp., Kenilworth, NJ, USA.

Chapter
45

Short Bowel Syndrome

CLINICAL POINTS

- SBS is an uncommon malassimilative condition that may develop after massive resection (≥50%) of the small intestine; mild malassimilation may occur even if 25% is removed (estimate percentage by subtracting the amount removed from the total length, which is approximately 4x the crown-rump distance).
- Conditions that may lead to resection include linear foreign bodies, intussusception, volvulus, infarction, neoplasia, entrapment, GI surgical site dehiscence and fungal infections.
- Puppies and young adult dogs are most likely to have GI conditions that require extensive small bowel resection. Young cats are at particular risk for linear foreign bodies.
- Large-breed dogs, especially German shepherd dogs, are more likely to have intussusception and mesenteric volvulus, which may require extensive resection.
- SBS is characterized by diarrhea, malnutrition and weight loss. The degree and nature of malassimilation depend on the length and portion of bowel resected.
- Dogs typically develop diarrhea (intermittent or persistent) 1 day after small bowel resection. Stools range from soft, cow-pie consistency to explosive, watery diarrhea. Longstanding cases may have weight loss with polyphagia.
- Initially, after resection, incomplete digestion/absorption of nutrients occurs, which leads to osmotic diarrhea. In addition, unabsorbed bile acids and fatty acids may result in secretory diarrhea of the large intestine.
- Eventually, the remaining small bowel undergoes morphologic and functional adaptation, which results from exposure to intraluminal nutrients.
- Adaptation is marked by enterocyte hyperplasia and an increase in bowel diameter, villous height, crypt depth and number of enterocytes per length of the villous/crypt unit. Mucosal changes begin to occur within 1-2 days and can result in a 4x increase of mucosal surface area within 2 weeks, if intraluminal nutrients are provided. Adaptation may take 1-2 months.
- Occasionally, patients present weeks to months after surgery with small intestinal diarrhea, flatulence and borborygmus. Delayed onset of signs often is associated with SIBO, which can develop as a sequela to resection of the ileocolic valve.
- Physical exam findings are usually unremarkable. The patient's body condition (BCS) may be poor if the predisposing condition was debilitating; most patients are alert and active with an increased appetite.
- Hematology and biochemical findings vary. Hypoproteinemia and hypoalbuminemia may be present in longstanding cases. Mild, normocytic, normochromic nonregenerative anemia may be a consequence of chronic disease. Patients with

Abbreviations
AAFCO = Association of American Feed Control Officials
BCS = body condition score (Appendix A)
EN = enteral nutrition
KNF = key nutritional factor
PN = parenteral nutrition
RER = resting energy requirement
SBS = short bowel syndrome
SIBO = small intestinal bacterial overgrowth
TNA = total nutrient admixture

ileal resection may have microcytic anemia consistent with cobalamin deficiency.
- After resection, diagnostic radiography is usually not helpful.
- Because this is a malassimilative condition, highly digestible foods (fat and digestible carbohydrate ≥90% and protein ≥87%) are indicated.
- Besides being a concentrated form of energy, dietary fat also stimulates small intestinal adaptation and slows gastric emptying, which may better match nutrient delivery to the compromised capabilities of the shortened small bowel.
- Various fiber sources help modulate GI motility and may stimulate adaptive processes by GI trophic factors; limited amounts have minimal effects on digestibility. Soluble or mixed fibers are recommended.
- Mixed fibers include beet pulp, brans (rice, wheat and oat), pea, soy fibers, soy hulls and mixtures of soluble and insoluble fibers. Insoluble fibers include purified cellulose and peanut hulls. Soluble fiber sources include fruit pectins, guar gums and psyllium.
- Dry foods are preferred because they increase gastric retention time; it takes longer to reduce osmolality for gastric emptying of dry foods vs. moist foods.
- Avoid lactose-containing ingredients because extensive small bowel resection results in the loss of brush border disaccharidases.
- Prognosis varies and cannot be based solely on the extent of resection. Preoperative condition, functional integrity of the remnant bowel, site of resection, degree of intestinal adaptation and owner commitment are also important.
- Feeding goals: provide adequate nutritional support during intestinal adaptation and stimulate adaptive changes that increase function in the remaining small bowel to control diarrhea. The feeding plan is often used in combination with medical therapy.

KEY NUTRITIONAL FACTORS

- Foods for oral feeding should provide recommended allowances of all required nutrients (nutritional adequacy) and contain specific levels of KNFs (certain nutrients and food features that may assist in the management of SBS).
- Table 1 lists KNF recommendations for foods for patients with SBS and malassimilative diseases. Dietary fiber can also be important. A detailed review of these recommendations can be found in Chapter 59, Small Animal Clinical Nutrition, 5th edition.
- Nutrients in liquid foods should contain glutamine (and if possible, soluble fiber) (Tables 4 and 5, Chapter 12).
- Nutrients included in TNAs for PN support are intended to meet basic needs (Chapter 13).

FEEDING PLAN

There are 3 broad categories of SBS patients: 1) patients with a good prognosis (<50% small bowel resected, ileocolic sphincter intact, remnant bowel healthy, normal BCS), 2) patients with a guarded prognosis (varies with combinations of % small bowel resected, ileocolic sphincter status, health of remnant bowel and BCS) and 3) patients with a poor prognosis (>50% small bowel resected, ileocolic sphincter not intact, remnant bowel compromised, poor BCS). Feeding methods and food selections are patient dependent and often require trial and error. Patients in categories 1 and 2 are often fed similarly but may have different outcomes.

Assess and Select the Food

Ensure the Food's Basic Nutritional Adequacy. AAFCO nutritional adequacy statements are usually found on a product's label. AAFCO approval does not ensure a food will be effective for managing SBS.

Compare the Food's KNF Content with the Recommended Levels.

PATIENTS WITH A GOOD/GUARDED PROGNOSIS. 2 types of foods are used: 1) highly digestible GI foods or 2) fiber-enhanced foods. Because physical exam findings, laboratory test results and historical facts will not predict which food is best for a given patient, dietary trial and error is often necessary. Tables 2 and 3 provide the KNF content of selected highly digestible foods marketed for malabsorptive-type diseases in dogs and cats, respectively and contain KNF recommendations for comparison. Tables 4 and 5, Chapter 43, provide the fiber content and type of selected fiber-enhanced foods. Foods containing mixed fiber sources are recommended.

FOOD FORM. Dry foods are less likely to overwhelm the remnant bowel compared to moist foods because they are emptied from the stomach more slowly.

Table 1. Key nutritional factors for foods for dogs and cats with short bowel syndrome.*

Factors	Recommended levels
Digestibility	≥87% for protein and ≥90% for fat and digestible carbohydrate
Fat	12 to 15% for dogs
	15 to 25% for cats
Fiber	≤5% (soluble or mixed fiber)
Carbohydrate	Lactose free
Food form	Dry foods are preferred due to slower gastric emptying vs. moist foods

*Nutrients expressed on a dry matter basis.

PATIENTS WITH A POOR PROGNOSIS.

BLENDERIZED HIGHLY DIGESTIBLE GI FOODS. Consider these for patients that will eat on their own. Mix blenderized food with prescribed dry food; gradually transition totally to dry food.

LIQUID FOODS/PN SOLUTIONS. Consider these for anorectic patients. Use assisted EN alone or in combination with PN. Recommend liquid foods with added glutamine (Tables 4 and 5, Chapter 12) and soluble fiber (obtain from product label information). Use TNA solutions for PN support (Chapter 13). Augment PN with ≥30% EN (calorie basis) to stimulate adaptation. If PN/EN feeding is used, transition to assisted EN as soon as tolerated and to self-feeding as soon as the patient's appetite returns.

Assess and Determine the Feeding Method

As with food selection, feeding methods are often based on trial and error.

Determine How Much to Feed.

PATIENTS WITH A GOOD/GUARDED PROGNOSIS. Estimate from feeding guides on product labels or by calculation (Appendix C). These estimates are only starting points and will likely need to be adjusted (see Followup below), depending primarily on the patient's GI tolerance.

PATIENTS WITH A POOR PROGNOSIS. Initially feed to meet the patient's RER (EN and PN). Gradually increase EN feeding based on the patient's GI tolerance and BCS. Chapters 12 and 13 provide guidelines.

Consider How to Offer the Food.

PATIENTS WITH A GOOD/GUARDED PROGNOSIS. Multiple (6-8) small meals/day are recommended during the intestinal adaptation period. Eventually, the daily number of meals can be decreased as the remnant bowel adapts.

PATIENTS WITH A POOR PROGNOSIS. See EN/PN feeding guidelines in Chapters 12 and 13. If the patient responds and its prognosis improves, feed accordingly (above).

Manage Food Changes. Replace 25% of the previous food with the GI food on Day 1 and continue this incremental change daily until the change is complete on Day 4 or 5. Appendix E provides additional information.

Food and Water Receptacle Husbandry. Food and water bowls should be washed regularly with warm soapy water and rinsed well. Clean dishes used for gruels and moist foods daily. Discard moist or moistened foods after 2-4 hours of room temperature exposure to avoid foodborne illnesses (Appendix F).

Table 2. Key nutritional factors in selected commercial veterinary therapeutic foods for dogs with short bowel syndrome compared to recommended levels.* (Numbers in red match optimal KNFs.)

Dry foods	Protein digestibility (%)	Fat digestibility (%)	Carbohydrate digestibility (%)	Fat (%)	Fiber (%)**	Primary sources of fiber**	Lactose free (Yes/No)
Recommended levels	≥87	≥90	≥90	12-15	≤5	–	Yes
Hill's Prescription Diet i/d Canine	92	93	94	14.1	2.7	Cellulose, beet pulp	Yes
Iams Veterinary Formula Intestinal Low-Residue	na	na	na	10.7	2.1	Beet pulp	Yes
Medi-Cal Gastro Formula	na	na	na	13.9	1.9	Flax meal, pea fiber	Yes
Medi-Cal Low Fat Formula	na	na	na	6.6	5.2	Beet pulp, cellulose	Yes
Purina Veterinary Diets EN GastroENteric Formula	84.5	91.4	94.4	12.6	1.5	–	Yes
Royal Canin Veterinary Diet Digestive Low Fat LF 20	na	na	na	6.6	2.3	Beet pulp, cellulose	Yes
Royal Canin Veterinary Diet Intestinal HE 28	na	na	na	22.0	1.6	Beet pulp, psyllium husks	Yes

Moist foods	Protein digestibility (%)	Fat digestibility (%)	Carbohydrate digestibility (%)	Fat (%)	Fiber (%)**	Primary sources of fiber**	Lactose free (Yes/No)
Recommended levels	≥87	≥90	≥90	12-15	≤5	–	Yes
Hill's Prescription Diet i/d Canine	88	94	93	14.9	1.0	Soy fiber	Yes
Iams Veterinary Formula Intestinal Low-Residue	na	na	na	13.2	3.9	Beet pulp	Yes
Medi-Cal Gastro Formula	na	na	na	11.7	1.0	Oat bran, guar gum, flax meal	No
Medi-Cal Low Fat Formula	na	na	na	9.0	3.1	Cellulose, beet pulp, guar gum, carrageenan	Yes
Purina Veterinary Diets EN GastroENteric Formula	85.1	95.6	92.2	13.8	0.9	Gum arabic	Yes
Royal Canin Veterinary Diet Digestive Low Fat LF	na	na	na	6.9	3.0	Cellulose, guar gum	Yes
Royal Canin Veterinary Diet Intestinal HE	na	na	na	11.8	1.4	Oat bran, guar gum, carrageenan, flaxseed	No

Key: Fiber = crude fiber, na = information not available from manufacturer.
*Manufacturers' published values; nutrients expressed as % dry matter; dry foods are preferred because they have slower gastric emptying compared to moist foods.
**Foods with soluble or mixed fiber sources are best (see text).

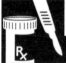

ADJUNCTIVE MEDICAL & SURGICAL MANAGEMENT

Commonly used drugs include opiate antidiarrheal agents (e.g., loperamide, diphenoxylate), antibiotics (e.g., tetracycline, tylosin) and bile salt binding agents (e.g., cholestyramine, ursodeoxycholic acid).

FOLLOWUP

Owner Followup

Evaluate stools daily and body weight, if possible, and body condition (BCS) weekly. As stools improve, the number of meals/day may be decreased. If a trend of increasing or decreasing body weight or condition is noted, change the amount fed by 10% increments and recheck the patient every 2 weeks for 1 month. At that point change the amount fed and repeat the cycle if necessary. Work closely with the veterinary health care team to ensure optimal dietary and medical management.

Veterinary Health Care Team Followup

Adaptation may be underway in 1-2 weeks but usually occurs within 1-2 months; diarrhea may resolve in that time. In some cases, adaptation continues for years; stool quality may improve over a similar time frame. Stools may never appear normal. *Persistent Diarrhea.* Consider adjunctive medical management (above) if dietary therapy alone does not sufficiently improve stool quality and maintain body weight. Evaluate well-compensated patients immediately if a decline in body condition is noted. This development suggests concurrent GI disease or the onset of SIBO in dogs without an ileocolic sphincter. If large bowel diarrhea develops, consider bile acid overload and manage medically.

MISCELLANEOUS

See Chapters 25, 26 and 59, Small Animal Clinical Nutrition, 5th edition, for more information.

Fat-Soluble Vitamin Malnutrition

Fat-soluble vitamin supplementation is warranted in cases of long-term fat malabsorption. Administer 1 ml of a vitamin A,

Table 3. Key nutritional factors in selected commercial veterinary therapeutic foods for cats with short bowel syndrome compared to recommended levels.* (Numbers in red match optimal KNFs.)

Dry foods	Protein digestibility (%)	Fat digestibility (%)	Carbohydrate digestibility (%)	Fat (%)	Fiber (%)**	Primary sources of fiber**	Lactose free (Yes/No)
Recommended levels	≥87	≥90	≥90	15-25	≤5	–	Yes
Hill's Prescription Diet i/d Feline	88	92	90	20.2	2.8	Cellulose, beet pulp	Yes
Iams Veterinary Formula Intestinal Low-Residue	na	na	na	13.7	1.8	Beet pulp	Yes
Medi-Cal Hypoallergenic/Gastro	na	na	na	11.5	3.1	Beet pulp, rice bran	Yes
Purina Veterinary Diets EN GastroENteric Formula	94.0	93.1	79.7	18.4	1.3	Cellulose	Yes
Royal Canin Veterinary Diet Intestinal HE 30	na	na	na	23.7	5.8	Cellulose, beet pulp	Yes

Moist foods	Protein digestibility (%)	Fat digestibility (%)	Carbohydrate digestibility (%)	Fat (%)	Fiber (%)**	Primary sources of fiber**	Lactose free (Yes/No)
Recommended levels	≥87	≥90	≥90	15-25	≤5	–	Yes
Hill's Prescription Diet i/d Feline	91	89	91	24.1	2.4	Beet pulp, cellulose, guar gum	Yes
Iams Veterinary Formula Intestinal Low-Residue	na	na	na	11.7	3.7	Beet pulp	Yes
Medi-Cal Hypoallergenic/Gastro	na	na	na	35.9	1.2	Cellulose, carrageenan, guar gum, flax meal	Yes
Medi-Cal Sensitivity CR	na	na	na	35.1	2.5	Cellulose, guar gum, carrageenan, carob gum	Yes

Key: Fiber = crude fiber, na = information not available from manufacturer.
*Manufacturers' published values; nutrients expressed as % dry matter; dry foods are preferred because they have slower gastric emptying compared to moist foods.
**Foods with soluble or mixed fiber sources are best (see text).

D and E solution,[a] divided into 2 IM sites. This should supply fat-soluble vitamins for approximately 3 months. Vitamin K_1 at a dose of 0.5-1 mg/kg SQ is recommended if vitamin K-responsive coagulopathy is suspected.

Cobalamin Malnutrition

B_{12} deficiency occurs with distal ileum resection; this portion of the bowel is responsible for B_{12} absorption. For dogs, administer ~600 mg cobalamin IM weekly for 6 weeks followed by injections every other week for 6 weeks then monthly until serum B_{12} normalizes. For cats, 250 mg/week IM for 4-6 weeks is recommended. Bacterial uptake of B_{12} may exacerbate deficiency if complicated by SIBO.

Authors
Condensed from Chapter 59, Small Animal Clinical Nutrition, 5th edition, authored by Deborah J. Davenport, Chris L. Ludlow and Rebecca L. Remillard.

References
See Chapter 59, Small Animal Clinical Nutrition, 5th edition, on the website www.markmorrisinstitute.org for references.

Endnote
a. Vital E-A+D containing 100 IU of D and 300 IU of α-tocopherol/ml. Schering-Plough Animal Health Corp., Kenilworth, NJ, USA.

Chapter
46 Small Intestinal Bacterial Overgrowth

CLINICAL POINTS

- SIBO (also known as antibiotic-responsive diarrhea) is a diarrheic disorder characterized by excessive numbers of bacteria in the small intestine.
- The incidence of SIBO is unknown and debated; some clinicians speculate that it is present in as many as 50% of dogs with chronic small bowel diarrhea whereas others say that it rarely occurs.
- Affected dogs usually present with a history of weight loss and intermittent small bowel diarrhea; borborygmus and flatulence are also common complaints.
- German shepherd dogs appear to be predisposed, possibly because of IgA deficiency. EPI is also a predisposing factor.
- Kennel-housed dogs may be at increased risk: reasons include environment (i.e., cleanliness), coprophagia and breed-specific characteristics (e.g., IgA deficiency).
- SIBO can develop any time normal host defenses are impaired including losses of gastric acid secretion, normal intestinal peristalsis, interdigestive ("housekeeper") motility, ileocolic valve function or local IgA production.
- Physical exam findings are often unremarkable. Poor body condition may be present in longstanding cases.
- Serum cobalamin levels may be low but are not pathognomonic for SIBO.
- The gold standard for diagnosing SIBO is quantitative aerobic and anaerobic cultures of undiluted duodenal juice; however, quantitative microbiology is difficult and not readily available. Other diagnostic tests are available but have various shortcomings. Response to antibiotic therapy may be indicative but is not specific.
- Highly digestible foods (fat and digestible carbohydrate ≥90% and protein ≥87%) provide several advantages: 1) nutrients are more completely absorbed in the proximal gut, 2) reduced osmotic diarrhea caused by fat and carbohydrate malabsorption and 3) reduced production of intestinal gas resulting from carbohydrate malabsorption.
- Moderate fat levels are best. High-fat foods may contribute to osmotic diarrhea and GI protein losses, which complicate SIBO.

Table 1. Key nutritional factors for foods for dogs and cats with small intestinal bacterial overgrowth.*

Factors	Recommended levels
Digestibility	≥87% for protein and ≥90% for fat and digestible carbohydrate
Fat	12 to 15% for dogs 15 to 25% for cats

*Nutrients expressed on a dry matter basis.

- Because SIBO results in loss of brush border disaccharidases, lactose-free foods avoid the complication of lactose intolerance.
- Prognosis: in general, SIBO can be managed effectively with a combination of proper dietary and medical therapies.
- Feeding plan goals: control/resolve clinical signs through the use of proper foods and feeding methods that augment medical management.

KEY NUTRITIONAL FACTORS

- Foods should provide recommended allowances of all required nutrients (nutritional adequacy), but should also contain specific levels of KNFs (certain nutrients and food features that may assist in the management of SIBO).
- Table 1 lists KNF recommendations for foods for patients with SIBO. A detailed review of these recommendations can be found in Chapter 60, Small Animal Clinical Nutrition, 5th edition.

FEEDING PLAN

Assess and Select the Food
Ensure the Food's Basic Nutritional Adequacy. AAFCO nutritional adequacy statements are usually found on a product's label. AAFCO approval does not ensure a food will be effective for managing SIBO.
Compare the Food's KNF Content with the Recommended Levels. Tables 2 and 3 include the KNF content of selected veterinary therapeutic GI foods for dogs and cats, respectively, and compare them to the recommended levels. Select foods that most closely match KNF recommendations for SIBO. For puppies and kittens, foods should also provide KNFs for growth (Chapters 5 and 11).
Manage Treats and Snacks. Consider commercial treats that match the food being fed. Most companies offer treats that correspond to their specific veterinary therapeutic foods. An option is to use the opposite form of the food being fed; e.g., if a dry food is fed, offer small amounts of the same food in moist form as a snack and vice versa; keep dry food kibbles in a separate

Table 2. Key nutritional factors in selected highly digestible commercial veterinary therapeutic foods marketed for dogs with small intestinal bacterial overgrowth compared to recommended levels.* (Numbers in red match optimal KNFs.)

Dry foods	Fat (%)	Protein digestibility (%)	Fat digestibility (%)	Carbohydrate digestibility (%)	Ingredient comments
Recommended levels	12-15	≥87	≥90	≥90	–
Hill's Prescription Diet i/d Canine	14.1	92	93	94	–
Iams Veterinary Formula Intestinal Low-Residue	10.7	na	na	na	FOS, MOS prebiotics
Medi-Cal Gastro Formula	13.9	na	na	na	FOS prebiotic, *Bacillus subtilis* dried fermentation extract
Medi-Cal Low Fat LF 20	6.6	na	na	na	MCT
Purina Veterinary Diets EN GastroENteric Formula	12.6	84.5	91.4	94.4	Sodium silico aluminate, FOS, MOS prebiotics
Royal Canin Veterinary Diet Digestive Low Fat LF 20	6.6	na	na	na	FOS, MOS prebiotics

Moist foods	Fat (%)	Protein digestibility (%)	Fat digestibility (%)	Carbohydrate digestibility (%)	Ingredient comments
Recommended levels	12-15	≥87	≥90	≥90	–
Hill's Prescription Diet i/d Canine	14.9	88	94	93	–
Iams Veterinary Formula Intestinal Low-Residue	13.2	na	na	na	–
Medi-Cal Gastro Formula	11.7	na	na	na	FOS prebiotic
Medi-Cal Low Fat LF	9.0	na	na	na	–
Purina Veterinary Diets EN GastroENteric Formula	13.8	85.1	95.6	92.2	MCT
Royal Canin Veterinary Diet Digestive Low Fat	6.9	na	na	na	Inulin prebiotic

Key: na = information not available from manufacturer, FOS = fructooligosaccharide, MOS = mannanoligosaccharide, MCT = medium-chain triglyceride.
*Manufacturers' published values. Nutrients expressed as % dry matter.

Table 3. Key nutritional factors in selected highly digestible commercial veterinary therapeutic foods marketed for cats with small intestinal bacterial overgrowth compared to recommended levels.* (Numbers in red match optimal KNFs.)

Dry foods	Fat (%)	Protein digestibility (%)	Fat digestibility (%)	Carbohydrate digestibility (%)	Ingredient comments
Recommended levels	15-25	≥87	≥90	≥90	–
Hill's Prescription Diet i/d Feline	20.2	88	92	90	–
Iams Veterinary Formula Intestinal Low-Residue	13.7	na	na	na	FOS, MOS prebiotics
Medi-Cal Hypoallergenic/Gastro	11.5	na	na	na	FOS prebiotic, *Bacillus subtilis* dried fermentation extract
Purina Veterinary Diets EN GastroENteric Formula	18.4	94.0	93.1	79.7	–
Royal Canin Veterinary Diet Intestinal HE	23.7	na	na	na	FOS, MOS prebiotics, sodium silico aluminate

Moist foods	Fat (%)	Protein digestibility (%)	Fat digestibility (%)	Carbohydrate digestibility (%)	Ingredient comments
Recommended levels	15-25	≥87	≥90	≥90	–
Hill's Prescription Diet i/d Feline	24.1	91	89	91	–
Iams Veterinary Formula Intestinal Low-Residue	11.7	na	na	na	FOS prebiotic
Medi-Cal Hypoallergenic/Gastro	35.9	na	na	na	FOS prebiotic
Medi-Cal Sensitivity CR	35.1	na	na	na	–

Key: na = information not available from manufacturer, FOS = fructooligosaccharide, MOS = mannanoligosaccharide.
*Manufacturers' published values. Nutrients expressed as % dry matter.

container away from the usual feeding area and use as treats. Treats/snacks should not be fed excessively (<10% of the total diet on a volume, weight or calorie basis).

Assess and Determine the Feeding Method

Determine How Much Food to Feed. Estimate either from feeding guides on product labels or by calculation (Appendix C). Feeding guidelines and calculations are based on population averages and may need to be adjusted for individual patients (see Followup below).

Consider How to Offer the Food. Initially, feed multiple (6-8) small meals/day as indicated by acceptance and GI tolerance for the prescribed food. Meal size can be increased and meal frequency can be reduced as tolerated by the patient after clinical signs have been successfully managed for several weeks.

Manage Food Changes. Replace 25% of the previous food with the GI food on Day 1 and continue this incremental change daily until the change is complete on Day 4 or 5. Appendix E provides additional information.

Food and Water Receptacle Husbandry. Food and water bowls should be washed regularly with warm soapy water and rinsed well. Dishes used for gruels and moist foods need daily cleaning. Discard moist or moistened foods after 2-4 hours of room temperature exposure to avoid foodborne illnesses (Appendix F).

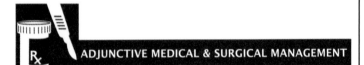

ADJUNCTIVE MEDICAL & SURGICAL MANAGEMENT

Antibiotic Therapy

Antibiotics are often used in conjunction with dietary management. Base antibiotic selection on culture and sensitivity testing of specific pathogens identified in duodenal aspirates. Consider using tetracycline or tylosin if no pathogen is isolated. Consult medical texts for specific information.

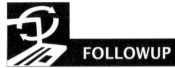

FOLLOWUP

Owner Followup

Note the frequency and character of diarrhea daily along with borborygmi and flatus. Record body weight (if possible) and condition (BCS) every 2 weeks to assess resolution of malabsorption and to facilitate adjustments in food dose.

Veterinary Health Care Team Followup

Conduct reassessments as necessary based on consultations with the owner regarding response to initial dietary and medical management. Consider obtaining serum folate and cobalamin levels in 1-2 months as another indicator of recovery.

MISCELLANEOUS

See Chapters 17, 24 and 60, Small Animal Clinical Nutrition, 5th edition, for more information.

Cobalamin (B_{12}) Deficiency

Low serum cobalamin levels may result from microbial uptake, preventing absorption. Consider laboratory tests to assess serum cobalamin levels for patients receiving parenteral cobalamin (hypocobalaminemia = <300 ng/l). The recommended SQ dose: 250 µg/week (cats) and 500 µg/week (dogs) until levels return to normal. Once/twice monthly therapy may be necessary for longer term maintenance.

Authors

Condensed from Chapter 60, Small Animal Clinical Nutrition, 5th edition, authored by Deborah J. Davenport, Chris L. Ludlow, Karen L. Johnston and Rebecca L. Remillard.

References

See Chapter 60, Small Animal Clinical Nutrition, 5th edition, on the website www.markmorrisinstitiute.org for references.

CLINICAL POINTS

- Colitis occurs commonly in dogs and cats and can be acute or chronic. Several infectious, toxic, inflammatory and dietary factors can trigger an episode of large bowel diarrhea (Appendix N).
- Lymphoplasmacytic colitis is thought to be the most common cause of chronic large bowel diarrhea.
- Certain breeds appear to be at risk for specific colonic disorders (Appendix N).
- Puppies and kittens are more susceptible to infectious causes.
- Hospitalization and administration of chemotherapeutic drugs are associated with nosocomial infections. Immunocompromised pets are at risk for viral and bacterial enteritides.
- Pets in insanitary/overcrowded conditions are more likely to have large bowel infections. Records of anthelmintic treatments may be helpful.
- Dietary history is important. Food-induced diarrhea is common and can include a recent change to a moist high-fat or meat-based food or dietary indiscretions including feeding table foods or access to garbage, carrion or abrasive materials, such as bones.
- Systemic signs are variable. Most patients are alert and active but some present with depression, malaise and anorexia.
- A common clinical sign for either acute or chronic colitis is diarrhea characterized by tenesmus, dyschezia, urgency and passage of mucus and blood (Appendix N). Hemorrhagic stools indicate a potentially life-threatening disorder. Signs may be intermittent or persistent and tend to increase in frequency and intensity as colitis progresses.
- Patients with acute colitis may be dehydrated and exhibit pain on abdominal palpation. Evaluate for septic shock and treat patients that have accompanying fever and congested mucous membranes more aggressively.
- Because there are many potential and obscure causes of acute colitis, obtaining a definitive diagnosis can be difficult and it is more important to determine if the condition is self-limiting or potentially life-threatening (Appendix N). More aggressive diagnostics are warranted in more serious cases. Diagnostics in self-limiting cases are often limited to assessment of hydration status and fecal examinations.
- Physical exam findings vary with chronic colitis; many patients appear normal but rarely may present with weight loss (suspect serious infiltrative disorders or concurrent small intestinal disease). Occasionally, thickened loops of bowel may be palpable, especially in cats. This finding is consistent with eosinophilic gastroenterocolitis (cats) and granulomatous enteritis (dogs). Also distinguish from intussusceptions, foreign

bodies, histoplasmosis and neoplastic lesions.
- Lab results in chronic colitis are often nonspecific. Hematologic findings are variable and may include blood loss anemia, anemia of chronic disease, eosinophilia and lymphopenia. Serum biochemistry profiles and urinalyses help assess systemic effects and rule out concurrent diseases. Fecal exams are very important.
- Endoscopic findings in chronic colitis may include mucosal granularity, hyperemia, increased friability and inability to visualize colonic submucosal blood vessels. Definitive diagnosis of IBD is based on histopathologic interpretation of biopsy specimens.
- Water is the most important nutrient in acute colitis patients because of the potential for life-threatening dehydration resulting from excessive fluid losses and inability of the patient to replace those losses.
- Hypokalemia may be profound if losses are not matched by sufficient dietary potassium intake. Foods for patients with colitis should contain potassium, sodium and chloride at levels above minimum allowances.
- Dietary protein should be sufficient for the patient's lifestage. Presence of PLE may require increased protein intake. With chronic colitis, limited protein source elimination-type foods may be effective because of the suspected role of dietary antigens.
- The action of bacterial flora on unabsorbed fats in the colon may result in hydroxyl fatty acid production, which can be an important cause of large bowel diarrhea. Avoid high-fat foods in colitis patients.
- 3 different dietary approaches may prove useful: 1) highly digestible foods, 2) fiber-enhanced foods or 3) elimination foods for suspected cases of antigen-induced inflammation.
- Highly digestible (fat and digestible [soluble] carbohydrate ≥90% and protein ≥87%) foods provide advantages for colitis patients: 1) less osmotic diarrhea due to reduced colonic fat/carbohydrate, 2) reduced production of intestinal gas due to reduced digestible carbohydrate in the colon and 3) less antigenic because fewer protein are absorbed intact.
- Dietary fiber predominately affects the large bowel; benefits include: 1) normalize colonic motility, 2) buffer bile acids and bacterial enterotoxins, 3) bind/hold excess water, 4) support normal microflora and 5) provide fuel for colonocytes. Fiber-enhanced foods may have lower digestibility values.
- Omega-3 (n-3) fatty acids may help decrease inflammatory mediators.

Table 1. Key nutritional factors for dogs and cats with colitis.*

Factors	Recommended levels
Protein	Adult dogs: 15 to 30% Growing puppies: 22 to 32% Adult cats: 30 to 45% Growing kittens: 35 to 50% Option: consider elimination foods or protein hydrolysates (Tables 3 for dogs and 4 for cats, Chapter 19)
Fat	Dogs: 8 to 15% Cats: 9 to 25%
Digestibility	Highly digestible foods: ≥87% for protein and ≥90% for fat and digestible carbohydrate Fiber-enhanced foods: ≥80% for protein and fat and ≥90% for digestible carbohydrate
Fiber	Highly digestible foods: ≤5% Fiber-enhanced foods: ≥7%
Electrolytes	Sodium: 0.3 to 0.5% Chloride: 0.5 to 1.3% Potassium: 0.8 to 1.1%

*All values expressed on a dry matter basis.

- Prognosis for recovery in most cases of acute colitis is good, whereas chronic colitis patients may have to be managed for the rest of their lives, depending on underlying causes.
- Feeding plan goals: for acute colitis, provide a food that meets the patient's nutrient requirements and allows normalization of colonic motility and function and fecal water balance. In addition, for chronic colitis patients, compensate for ongoing nutrient losses through the GI tract and, if inflammatory/immune-mediated, remove offending food antigen(s).

KEY NUTRITIONAL FACTORS

- Foods should provide recommended allowances of all required nutrients (nutritional adequacy), but should also contain specific levels of KNFs (certain nutrients and food features that may assist in the management of acute and chronic colitis).
- **Table 1** lists KNF recommendations for foods for patients with colitis. Included are KNFs for highly-digestible foods, fiber-enhanced foods and elimination foods. A detailed review of these recommendations can be found in Chapter 62, Small Animal Clinical Nutrition, 5th edition. Protein and other KNF levels should be sufficient for the patient's lifestage (e.g., growth; Chapters 5 and 11), unless PLE is present (Chapter 44).

FEEDING PLAN

The first step in managing acute colitis is to correct dehydration and electrolyte, glucose and acid-base imbalances, if present. Correct moderate to severe disturbances with parenteral rather than oral fluid therapy.

Assess and Select the Food
Ensure the Food's Basic Nutritional Adequacy. AAFCO nutritional adequacy statements are usually found on a product's label. AAFCO approval does not ensure a food will be effective in the management of acute/chronic colitis.
Compare the Food's KNF Content with the Recommended Levels. There are 3 different plausible dietary approaches.

ACUTE COLITIS. A popular approach is use of fiber-enhanced foods that contain moderate amounts of fiber (**Tables 2** for dogs, **3** for cats).

FIBER SUPPLEMENTATION. Alternatively, fiber supplementation (Appendix N) can be used in conjunction with the patient's original food. The optimal fiber level is determined by trial and error.

HIGHLY DIGESTIBLE GI FOOD APPROACH. An alternative approach is highly digestible GI foods that may contain small amounts of soluble/mixed fiber (**Tables 4** and **5**; dogs and cats, respectively). Dietary trials are often needed to determine which food type works best for a given patient. Foods for extended feeding of puppies/kittens with colitis should also meet KNF recommendations for growth (Chapters 5 and 11). All aforementioned tables include KNF contents of selected commercial foods and compare them to recommended levels.

CHRONIC COLITIS. In addition to the 2 types of food suggested for acute colitis (above), elimination foods (Tables 3 and 4 for dogs and cats, respectively, Chapter 19) are a consideration for mild to moderate lymphoplasmacytic and eosinophilic colitis. In some of these cases, elimination foods successfully control signs without medical intervention.
Manage Treats and Snacks.

ACUTE COLITIS. Recommend initially withholding treats/snacks until the patient has stabilized.

CHRONIC COLITIS. Consider commercial treats that match the KNFs in the food being fed. Most companies offer treats that correspond to their specific veterinary therapeutic foods. An option is to use the opposite form of the food being fed; i.e., if a dry food is fed, offer small amounts of the same food in moist form as a snack and vice versa; keep kibbles of dry food in a separate container away from the usual feeding area and use as treats. Treats/snacks should not be fed excessively (<10% of the total diet on a volume, weight or calorie basis).

Assess and Determine the Feeding Method
Determine How Much Food to Feed. Estimate from feeding guides on product labels or by calculation (Appendix C). These estimates are only starting points and will likely need to be adjusted (see Followup below).
Consider How to Offer the Food.

ACUTE COLITIS. Initially withhold all food for 1-2 days while providing fluid/electrolyte support by parenteral administration. Then offer small amounts of the prescribed food 6-8 times/day. If the patient tolerates food without recurrence of diarrhea, the amount fed can be increased over 3-4 days until it is receiving its estimated daily energy requirement in 2-3 meals per day. After feeding the prescribed food for another 3-4 days, the pet's regular food may be reintroduced over another 3-day period. In some cases, initial fasting alone reduces/resolves diarrhea by

Table 2. Key nutritional factors in selected fiber-enhanced veterinary therapeutic foods marketed for dogs with acute or chronic colitis compared to recommended levels.* (See Table 3, Chapter 19, if foods with novel protein sources or protein hydrolysates are desired.) (Numbers in red match optimal KNFs.)

Dry foods	Protein (%)	Fat (%)	Protein digestibility (%)	Fat digestibility (%)	Carbohydrate digestibility (%)	Fiber (%)	Na (%)	Cl (%)	K (%)
Recommended levels	15-30	8-15	≥80	≥80	≥90	≥7	0.3-0.5	0.5-1.3	0.8-1.1
Hill's Prescription Diet w/d Canine	18.9	8.8	84	92	95	16.4	0.22	0.46	0.70
Medi-Cal Fibre Formula	26.2	10.6	na	na	na	14.3	0.3	na	1.0
Purina Veterinary Diets DCO Dual Fiber Control	25.3	12.4	79.9	80.4	90.6	7.6	0.34	0.82	0.70
Purina Veterinary Diets OM Overweight Management Formula	31.1	7.2	81.9	78.9	72.3	10.3	0.31	0.97	0.83
Royal Canin Veterinary Diet Calorie Control CC 26 High Fiber	30.9	10.4	na	na	na	17.6	0.33	0.77	0.90
Royal Canin Veterinary Diet Diabetic HF 18	22	9.9	na	na	na	12.1	0.27	0.88	0.88

Moist foods	Protein (%)	Fat (%)	Protein digestibility (%)	Fat digestibility (%)	Carbohydrate digestibility (%)	Fiber (%)	Na (%)	Cl (%)	K (%)
Recommended levels	15-30	8-15	≥80	≥80	≥90	≥7	0.3-0.5	0.5-1.3	0.8-1.1
Hill's Prescription Diet w/d Canine	17.9	12.7	88	90	92	12.4	0.24	0.76	0.64
Medi-Cal Fibre Formula	24.8	9.1	na	na	na	15.0	0.5	na	0.70
Purina Veterinary Diets OM Overweight Management Formula	44.1	8.4	80.9	89.8	62.9	19.2	0.28	0.51	1.06

Key: Fiber = crude fiber, Na = sodium, Cl = chloride, K = potassium, na = information not available from manufacturer.
*Nutrients expressed on a dry matter basis.

Table 3. Key nutritional factors in selected fiber-enhanced veterinary therapeutic foods marketed for cats with acute or chronic colitis compared to recommended levels.* (See Table 4, Chapter 19, if foods with novel protein sources or protein hydrolysates are desired.) (Numbers in red match optimal KNFs.)

Dry foods	Protein (%)	Fat (%)	Protein digestibility (%)	Fat digestibility (%)	Carbohydrate digestibility (%)	Fiber (%)	Na (%)	Cl (%)	K (%)
Recommended levels	30-45	9-25	≥80	≥80	≥90	≥7	0.3-0.5	0.5-1.3	0.8-1.1
Hill's Prescription Diet w/d Feline	39.0	9.8	90	87	86	7.6	0.30	0.84	0.84
Hill's Prescription Diet w/d Feline with Chicken	39.9	9.9	91	85	94	7.6	0.35	0.82	0.80
Medi-Cal Fibre Formula	34.2	12.2	na	na	na	14.9	0.5	na	0.90
Purina Veterinary Diets OM Overweight Management Formula	56.2	8.5	91.1	87.7	66.8	5.6	0.57	0.84	0.89
Royal Canin Veterinary Diets Calorie Control CC 29 High Fiber	33.5	10.2	na	na	na	14.0	0.51	0.92	0.88

Moist foods	Protein (%)	Fat (%)	Protein digestibility (%)	Fat digestibility (%)	Carbohydrate digestibility (%)	Fiber (%)	Na (%)	Cl (%)	K (%)
Recommended levels	30-45	9-25	≥80	≥80	≥90	≥7	0.3-0.5	0.5-1.3	0.8-1.1
Hill's Prescription Diet w/d Feline with Chicken	39.6	16.6	92	na	na	10.6	0.38	0.89	0.89
Medi-Cal Fibre Formula	40.0	17.1	na	na	na	16.7	0.4	na	0.80
Purina Veterinary Diets OM Overweight Management Formula	44.6	14.6	87.3	88.6	84.0	10.2	0.31	0.93	0.91
Royal Canin Veterinary Diets Calorie Control CC High Fiber	33.5	21.3	na	na	na	7.7	0.38	0.51	0.77

Key: Fiber = crude fiber, Na = sodium, Cl = chloride, K = potassium, na = information not available from manufacturer.
*Nutrients expressed on a dry matter basis.

Table 4. Key nutritional factors in selected highly digestible veterinary therapeutic foods marketed for dogs with acute or chronic colitis compared to recommended levels.* (See Table 3, Chapter 19, if foods with novel protein sources or protein hydrolysates are desired.) (Numbers in red match optimal KNFs.)

Dry foods	Protein (%)	Fat (%)	Protein digestibility (%)	Fat digestibility (%)	Carbohydrate digestibility (%)	Fiber (%)	Na (%)	Cl (%)	K (%)
Recommended levels	15-30**	8-15	≥87	≥90	≥90	≤5	0.3-0.5	0.5-1.3	0.8-1.1
Hill's Prescription Diet i/d Canine	26.2	14.1	92	93	94	2.7	0.45	1.04	0.92
Iams Veterinary Formula Intestinal Low-Residue	24.6	10.7	na	na	na	2.1	0.35	0.66	0.90
Medi-Cal Gastro Formula	22.9	13.9	na	na	na	1.9	0.5	na	0.8
Purina Veterinary Diets EN GastroENteric Formula	27.0	12.6	84.5	91.4	94.4	1.5	0.60	0.85	0.66
Royal Canin Veterinary Diet Intestinal HE 28	33.0	22.0	na	na	na	1.6	0.55	0.99	0.88

Moist foods	Protein (%)	Fat (%)	Protein digestibility (%)	Fat digestibility (%)	Carbohydrate digestibility (%)	Fiber (%)	Na (%)	Cl (%)	K (%)
Recommended levels	15-30**	8-15	≥87	≥90	≥90	≤5	0.3-0.5	0.5-1.3	0.8-1.1
Hill's Prescription Diet i/d Canine	25.0	14.9	88	94	93	1.0	0.44	1.22	0.95
Iams Veterinary Formula Intestinal Low-Residue	35.9	13.2	na	na	na	3.9	0.53	0.84	0.84
Medi-Cal Gastro Formula	22.1	11.7	na	na	na	1.0	0.6	na	0.6
Purina Veterinary Diets EN GastroENteric Formula	30.5	13.8	85.1	95.6	92.2	0.9	0.37	0.78	0.61
Royal Canin Veterinary Diet Intestinal HE	23.1	11.8	na	na	na	1.4	0.57	0.92	0.80

Key: Fiber = crude fiber, Na = sodium, Cl = chloride, K = potassium, na = information not available from manufacturer.
*Nutrients expressed on a dry matter basis.
**22 to 32% are recommended levels for growing puppies.

Table 5. Key nutritional factors in selected highly digestible veterinary therapeutic foods marketed for cats with acute or chronic colitis compared to recommended levels.* (See Table 4, Chapter 19, if foods with novel protein sources or protein hydrolysates are desired.) (Numbers in red match optimal KNFs.)

Dry foods	Protein (%)	Fat (%)	Protein digestibility (%)	Fat digestibility (%)	Carbohydrate digestibility (%)	Fiber (%)	Na (%)	Cl (%)	K (%)
Recommended levels	30-45**	9-25	≥87	≥90	≥90	≤5	0.3-0.5	0.5-1.3	0.8-1.1
Hill's Prescription Diet i/d Feline	40.3	20.2	88	92	90	2.8	0.37	1.11	1.07
Iams Veterinary Formula Intestinal Low-Residue	35.8	13.7	na	na	na	1.8	0.25	0.63	0.66
Medi-Cal Hypoallergenic/Gastro	29.8	11.5	na	na	na	3.1	0.4	na	0.8
Purina Veterinary Diets EN GastroENteric Formula	56.2	18.4	94.0	93.1	79.7	1.3	0.64	0.58	0.99
Royal Canin Veterinary Diets Intestinal HE 30	34.4	23.7	na	na	na	5.8	0.65	0.97	0.97

Moist foods	Protein (%)	Fat (%)	Protein digestibility (%)	Fat digestibility (%)	Carbohydrate digestibility (%)	Fiber (%)	Na (%)	Cl (%)	K (%)
Recommended levels	30-45**	9-25	≥87	≥90	≥90	≤5	0.3-0.5	0.5-1.3	0.8-1.1
Hill's Prescription Diet i/d Feline	37.6	24.1	91	89	91	2.4	0.33	1.18	1.06
Iams Veterinary Formula Intestinal Low-Residue	38.4	11.7	na	na	na	3.7	0.40	0.69	0.93
Medi-Cal Hypoallergenic/Gastro	35.5	35.9	na	na	na	1.2	0.7	na	1.1
Medi-Cal Sensitivity CR	34.5	35.1	na	na	na	2.5	1.1	na	1.1

Key: Fiber = crude fiber, Na = sodium, Cl = chloride, K = potassium, na = information not available from manufacturer.
*Nutrients expressed on a dry matter basis.
**35 to 50% are recommended levels for growing kittens.

removing the effects of unabsorbed food and offending agents from the colon and the patient's previous food can be gradually reintroduced.

CHRONIC COLITIS. Initially feed multiple small meals per day as indicated by acceptance and tolerance of the food. After successful management of clinical signs for several weeks, increase meal size and decrease meal frequency as tolerated by the patient. *Manage Food Changes.*

INITIATION OF PRESCRIBED FOOD. For transition feeding to the prescribed food, see Consider How to Offer the Food, above.

RETURN TO REGULAR FOOD. After recovery from acute colitis, gradually change back to the original food. Example: to change to the original food, replace 25% of the prescribed food with the original food on Day 1 and continue this incremental change daily until the change is complete on Day 4. Appendix E provides additional information.

Food and Water Receptacle Husbandry. Food and water bowls should be washed regularly with warm soapy water and rinsed well. Dishes used for gruels and moist foods need daily cleaning. Discard gruels, moist or moistened dry foods after 2-4 hours of room temperature exposure to avoid foodborne illnesses (Appendix F).

ADJUNCTIVE MEDICAL & SURGICAL MANAGEMENT

Concurrent Medical Therapy
May include antibiotics (e.g., metronidazole, tylosin, fluoroquinolones [for histiocytic colitis]), anthelmintics, motility modifying agents (e.g., loperamide) and immunosuppressant agents (e.g., corticosteroids and azathioprine). Local-acting antiinflammatory drugs such as sulfasalazine and olsalazine/mesalamine may also be used. Lifelong dietary therapy may be required to control clinical signs in longstanding colitis cases.

FOLLOWUP

Owner Followup
Acute Colitis. Note body weight (if possible) and GI signs daily for consulting with the veterinary health care team.

Chronic Colitis. Initially, note body weight (if possible) and/or grade the patient's body condition (BCS) weekly. After stabilization, if necessary, the amount fed should be changed by 10% increments and the patient rechecked every 2 weeks for 1 month. Then, the amount fed can be changed again and the cycle repeated until the patient reaches a normal body weight/BCS.

COMPLIANCE-ELIMINATION FOODS. All unprescribed foods (multi-pet households), treats, snacks, table foods, vitamin-mineral supplements and chewable/flavored medications should be discontinued.

Veterinary Health Care Team Followup
Acute Colitis. Often resolves within 2-4 days with conservative medical and nutritional management. Body weight should be recorded daily until recovery is complete. Changes in body weight from day to day usually reflect changes in hydration status rather than loss or gain of lean or adipose tissue.

PERSISTENT DIARRHEA/OTHER GI SIGNS. Further diagnostics are warranted if persistent diarrhea or if clinical signs indicative of concurrent small bowel disease become apparent (vomiting, hypoalbuminemia and melena).

Chronic Colitis. At clinic visits, review the owner's records for body weight, BCS and stool evaluations. Regaining or maintaining optimal body weight and BCS, normal level of activity and alertness and absence of clinical signs indicate successful dietary and medical management. Advise the owner to change the amount fed as needed to maintain body weight and condition. Consider adjunctive medical therapies (above) if dietary therapy alone fails to improve stool quality and maintain body weight.

PERSISTENT DIARRHEA. Patients presenting with multiple or recurrent episodes of diarrhea require further diagnostic workup and, most probably, a combination of dietary and medical therapies; however, rule out parasitic causes or treat empirically before pursuing further diagnostics.

MISCELLANEOUS

See Chapters 17, 24, 31, 57 and 58, Small Animal Clinical Nutrition, 5th edition, for more information.

Vitamins
Folate (B_{10} & B_{11}) Malnutrition. Folic acid supplementation is recommended for patients receiving long-term sulfasalazine therapy. Supplement with 0.5-1 mg folate per os, q24h, until sulfasalazine therapy is discontinued and/or folate levels return to normal.

Authors
Condensed from Chapter 62, Small Animal Clinical Nutrition, 5th edition, authored by Deborah J. Davenport, Rebecca L. Remillard and Maureen Carroll.

References
See Chapter 62, Small Animal Clinical Nutrition, 5th edition, on the website www.markmorrisinstitute.org for references.

CLINICAL POINTS

- IBS is a poorly defined functional disorder believed to be caused by GI dysmotility. In people, it is characterized by recurrent abdominal pain associated with altered bowel movements (constipation and diarrhea). No associated histopathology has been identified.
- IBS has been reported to account for 5-17% of large bowel disorders in dogs but is uncommon in cats.
- IBS is most common in large working breeds and small, nervous breeds. Dogs with behavioral disorders such as separation anxiety may be predisposed.
- Clinical signs include chronic, intermittent bouts of predominantly large bowel diarrhea (Appendix N). Diarrhea is often accompanied by nausea, vomiting, dyschezia, tenesmus and bloating. Borborygmus, belching and flatus are frequent complaints. Occasionally, explosive bouts of diarrhea and flatus occur, often in association with abdominal pain. Rarely, hematochezia may be seen.
- Affected dogs may exhibit discomfort during abdominal palpation if examined during an acute episode. Sometimes abdominal pain is relieved by eating, eructation or defecation. Typically, signs are variable and may change from bout to bout.
- In some cases, GI signs can be linked to identifiable stressors such as showing, work, boarding or changes in environment (e.g., owner anxiety or new spouse, child, pet, house or apartment).
- Generally, dogs with IBS are in good physical condition and do not exhibit weight loss as is often associated with organic GI disorders.
- In IBS, colonic dysfunction exists in the absence of structural, biochemical or microbiologic lesions and therefore is a diagnosis of exclusion following an appropriate diagnostic workup. Laboratory tests are usually within normal limits; radiography and colonoscopy are rarely useful other than as tools to rule out organic disorders.

Table 1. Key nutritional factors for foods for dogs with idiopathic bowel syndrome.*

Factors	Recommended levels
Soluble fiber**	1 to 5%
Mixed fiber**	5 to 10%
Insoluble fiber**	10 to 15%
Crude fiber***	≥8%

*All values are on a dry matter basis.
**Any one of the three types of fiber listed at the recommended levels can be effective, depending on patient response. See Chapter 5, Small Animal Clinical Nutrition, 5th edition, for more information about dietary fiber types and associated ingredient sources.
***Crude fiber is the only fiber value readily available for pet foods.

Abbreviations
AAFCO = Association of American Feed Control Officials
BCS = body condition score (Appendix A)
IBS = idiopathic (irritable) bowel syndrome
KNF = key nutritional factor

- The etiology of IBS is undefined. The postulated pathogenesis includes abnormalities of GI motility, visceral sensations, the brain and gut complex, personality and postepisodic infections in the colonic mucosa.
- Reports note clinical improvement with increased dietary fiber intake.
- Increasing dietary fiber may provide these effects: altered fecal water content, colonic motility, intestinal transit time and gut microbial populations and increased production of butyrate (soluble fiber), all of which may benefit patients with IBS. Positive responses may occur with foods containing small amounts of soluble fiber or moderate amounts of insoluble fiber or mixed fibers.
- Insoluble fiber sources include cellulose and peanut hulls. Soluble fiber sources include citrus and apple pectins, psyllium and gums. Rice bran, oat bran, wheat bran, soy fibers, soy hulls, pea fiber and beet pulp are sources of mixed fibers.
- Most IBS patients respond favorably to dietary management and can be managed successfully long-term with appropriate food and intermittent medical management. If possible, reduce/eliminate stressful events that trigger diarrheic episodes.
- Feeding goals: reduce frequency and severity of clinical signs, either alone or in combination with medical treatment.

KEY NUTRITIONAL FACTORS

Foods for IBS should provide recommended allowances of all required nutrients (nutritional adequacy) but should also contain the level and type of the single KNF (i.e, dietary fiber) that may assist in the management of IBS. A detailed review of this recommendation can be found in Chapter 63, Small Animal Clinical Nutrition, 5th edition.

FEEDING PLAN

Assess and Select the Food
Ensure the Food's Basic Nutritional Adequacy. Table 1 lists KNF recommendations for foods for patients with IBS. AAFCO nutritional adequacy statements are usually found on a

Table 2. Key nutritional factors in selected veterinary therapeutic foods for dogs with idiopathic bowel syndrome.* (Numbers in red match optimal KNFs.)

Dry foods Recommended levels	Crude fiber (%) ≥8	Primary sources of fiber –
Hill's Prescription Diet w/d Canine	16.4	Cellulose, soybean mill run, beet pulp
Hill's Prescription Diet w/d with Chicken Canine	17.1	Cellulose, soybean mill run, beet pulp
Medi-Cal Fibre	14.3	Tomato pomace, rice hulls, oat hulls, flax meal, apple pomace
Purina Veterinary Diets DCO Dual Fiber Control	7.6	Soybean hulls, pea fiber, cellulose
Purina Veterinary Diets OM Overweight Management	10.3	Soybean hulls, pea fiber, cellulose
Royal Canin Veterinary Diet Calorie Control CC 26 High Fiber	17.6	Cellulose, pea fiber, rice hulls, beet pulp, psyllium husk
Royal Canin Veterinary Diet Diabetic HF 18	12.1	Cellulose, rice hulls, guar gum
Moist foods Recommended levels	**Crude fiber (%) ≥8**	**Primary sources of fiber –**
Hill's Prescription Diet w/d Canine	12.4	Cellulose
Iams Veterinary Formula Intestinal Low-Residue	3.9	Beet pulp
Medi-Cal Fibre Formula	15.0	Tomato pomace, guar gum, flax meal, carrageenan
Purina Veterinary Diets OM Overweight Management Formula	19.2	Pea fiber, beet pulp, carrageenan
Royal Canin Veterinary Diet Calorie Control CC High Fiber	8.8	Tomato pomace, guar gum, flax meal, carrageenan

*All values expressed on a dry matter basis.

product's label. AAFCO approval does not ensure a food will be effective in the management of IBS.

Compare the Food's KNF Content with the Recommended Levels. Table 2 compares fiber levels/sources in selected fiber-enhanced veterinary therapeutic dog foods to recommended KNF levels/types. Consider changing to one of these foods if the current food's fiber level is low and/or the type of fiber it contains is unknown. If the fiber content of the current food is within the recommended ranges, changing to a new food should still be considered. The most effective combination of fiber type and level cannot be predicted and should be determined systematically by trial and error.

DETERMINING EFFECTIVE FIBER AMOUNT/TYPE. One approach is to begin with a food containing mixed-fiber types. If response is inadequate after 2-3 weeks, try other foods with either soluble or insoluble fibers (**Table 2**).

FIBER SUPPLEMENTATION. If an owner insists on feeding the current food or the current food is necessary for managing concurrent conditions, fiber can be added (Appendix N). In some cases, supplemental fiber may increase the severity of clinical signs; if so, discontinue immediately because clinical signs are unlikely to improve with time. Consider another fiber supplement or a fiber-enhanced food option.

Manage Treats and Snacks. Consider commercial treats that match the KNFs in the food being fed. Most companies offer treats that correspond to their specific veterinary therapeutic foods. An option is to use the opposite form of the food being fed; i.e., if a dry food is fed, offer small amounts of the same food in moist form as a snack and vice versa; keep kibbles of dry food in a separate container away from the usual feeding area and use as treats. Treats/snacks should not be fed excessively (<10% of the total diet on a volume, weight or calorie basis).

Assess and Determine the Feeding Method

Determine How Much Food to Feed. Estimate from feeding guides on product labels or by calculation (Appendix C). These estimates are only starting points and will likely need to be adjusted (see Followup below).

Consider How to Offer the Food. Both free-choice and restricted-feeding methods are acceptable. If restricted feeding is used, consider offering the food multiple times/day to reduce the amount of digesta passing into the large bowel at any one time.

Manage Food Changes. Replace 25% of the original food with the prescribed food on Day 1 and continue this incremental change daily until the change is complete on Day 4. Appendix E provides additional information.

Food and Water Receptacle Husbandry. Wash food and water bowls regularly with warm soapy water and rinse well. Dishes used for moist or moistened dry foods need daily cleaning. Discard moist or moistened dry foods after 2-4 hours of room temperature exposure to avoid foodborne illnesses (Appendix F).

ADJUNCTIVE MEDICAL & SURGICAL MANAGEMENT

Medical treatment with psychotropic and/or GI antispasmodic drugs may be beneficial (Appendix N).

FOLLOWUP

Owner Followup

Keep records of bouts of IBS and initially note body weight (if possible) and/or grade condition (BCS) every 2 weeks. If a trend of increasing or decreasing body weight or BCS is noticed, the amount fed should be changed by 10% increments and the patient rechecked every 2 weeks for 1 month. At that point, if necessary, the amount fed should be changed again and the cycle repeated until the desired body weight/BCS is attained.

Compliance. Foods other than those determined to control clinical signs should be strictly avoided for dogs in which recurring bouts are initiated by food changes, access to garbage or feeding table foods or unprescribed treats or snacks.

Veterinary Health Care Team Followup

Maintenance of body weight and BCS, normal activity level and behavior and absence of clinical signs indicate successful dietary management. Well-compensated patients should be evaluated immediately if a decline in condition is noted.

Persistent Signs. Consider adjunctive medical therapy (above) if dietary management alone is insufficient to improve clinical signs. Reevaluate the patient's home life to identify/alleviate possible inciting stressors. Be available for client support/guidance when they are dealing with pets afflicted by unpredictable signs of IBS (essential to successful management).

MISCELLANEOUS

See Chapter 63, Small Animal Clinical Nutrition, 5th edition, for more information.

Authors

Condensed from Chapter 63, Small Animal Clinical Nutrition, 5th edition, authored by Deborah J. Davenport, Maureen Carroll and Rebecca L. Remillard.

References

See Chapter 63, Small Animal Clinical Nutrition, 5th edition, on the website www.markmorrisinstitute.org for references.

Chapter

49 Constipation/Obstipation/Megacolon

CLINICAL POINTS

- The term constipation is applied to patients that pass stools infrequently or exhibit tenesmus when defecating. Obstipation is severe constipation that requires dietary and medical management for relief.
- Constipation in cats occurs most commonly in young adult males of domestic shorthair breeding; less common but still overrepresented are domestic longhairs and Siamese.
- A number of commonly used drugs are associated with constipation (**Table 1**).
- Dietary indiscretion (e.g., eating bones, rocks or clay) frequently causes constipation in dogs. Constipation and obstipation have been reported in dogs consuming bones and raw food diets. Cats may become constipated as a result of trichobezoar formation.
- Dehydration and electrolyte imbalances may induce constipation by altered colonic muscular activity (e.g., cats with chronic kidney disease).
- Mechanical obstructions from a variety of causes may result in constipation. Additionally, cauda equina syndrome, dysautonomia and diabetic or hypothyroid polyneuropathy may result in reduced colonic motility.
- Normal colonic motility is both propulsive and non-propulsive. Digesta and associated somatic activity stimulate propulsive contractions, which move contents distally. Non-propulsive motility mixes colonic contents and promotes water absorption. Destruction/damage to the parasympathetic nervous system or

Abbreviations
AAFCO = Association of American Feed Control Officials
BCS = body condition score (Appendix A)
DM = dry matter
IBD = inflammatory bowel disease
KNF = key nutritional factor
PLE = protein losing enteropathy

intrinsic myenteric and submucosal plexuses reduces colonic motility and potentiates constipation.
- Feline idiopathic megacolon is a frustrating, chronic, recurring form of obstipation that often results in euthanasia. A similar condition occurs in dogs but is relatively rare.
- Constipated dogs and cats typically exhibit tenesmus, dyschezia and abdominal pain. Chronically affected patients may present with systemic signs of illness including weight loss, inappetence, vomiting and depression.
- Constipated cats are usually presented for reduced, absent or painful defecation for a period ranging from days to weeks or months. Some make multiple, unproductive attempts to defecate; others may sit in the litter box for prolonged periods without assuming a defecation posture.
- Cats with megacolon usually present for repeated constipation or obstipation. Many cats that present for constipation are obese; chronically obstipated cats often exhibit weight loss and poor body condition.
- Abdominal palpation and digital rectal examination often reveal colonic distention and the presence of dry hard feces.
- History and physical exam findings are usually diagnostic. However, all obstipated/chronically constipated pets should have

a workup that includes a complete blood count, biochemistry profile, urinalysis, thyroxine analysis and abdominal radiography. Further diagnostic evaluation may require abdominal ultrasound, GI contrast studies and/or colonoscopy.

- Maintaining hydration is important for managing patients with chronic constipation or obstipation. Ensuring adequate water intake is often overlooked. Moist foods are recommended for both constipation and obstipation.
- Dietary fiber is important but should be altered in opposite directions: increase to manage constipation and decrease for obstipation.
- Many constipated patients improve when fed fiber-enhanced foods. Fiber can increase fecal water content, colonic motility and intestinal transit rate. Insoluble, mixed and soluble fibers are all recommended. However, limit soluble fibers (fruit pectins, guar gum, psyllium) to ≤5% (DM) because of the increased potential for flatulence, diarrhea and abdominal cramping.
- Motility patterns of obstipated patients are severely impaired (e.g., severe endstage megacolon in cats). Fiber may be ineffective in stimulating colonic motility; worse, it can contribute to obstipation. Foods for patients with megacolon should have ≤5% DM crude fiber.
- Feed patients with chronic obstipation and megacolon (where colonic motility is completely lost) highly digestible foods with increased nutrient density to reduce fecal mass. This practice may markedly reduce home management (i.e., administering stool softeners and enemas) and owners can often remove feces by means of cleansing enemas only 1-2 times/week.
- Prognosis is good for constipation/intermittent obstipation and can usually be managed with food alone. Chronic obstipation has a guarded prognosis and megacolon patients have a poor prognosis unless they receive a subtotal colectomy.
- Feeding plan goals: control constipation/intermittent obstipation by using proper foods and feeding methods (and complementary medical management if needed). Facilitate management of megacolon patients with appropriate dietary management.

KEY NUTRITIONAL FACTORS

- Foods should provide recommended allowances of all required nutrients (nutritional adequacy), but should also contain specific levels of KNFs (certain nutrients and food features that may assist in the management of constipation, obstipation and feline megacolon).
- KNFs for constipation/intermittent obstipation differ from KNFs for chronic obstipation/feline megacolon; **Table 2** summarizes KNFs for both.

Table 1. Drugs associated with constipation.

Antacids	Bismuth subsalicylate
Anticholinergics	Diuretics
Anticonvulsants (phenytoin)	Hematinics
Antidepressants	Opiates
Barium sulfate	Sucralfate

Table 2. Key nutritional factors and their recommended levels for foods for patients with chronic constipation or obstipation.*

Factors	Recommended levels
Water	>75% for cats and dogs with constipation or obstipation (moist foods)
Fiber	≥7% crude fiber (insoluble or mixed is best) for cats and dogs with chronic constipation and intermittent obstipation
	≤5% for cats with chronic obstipation (megacolon)
Digestibility	High digestibility for cats with chronic obstipation (megacolon) (fat and digestible carbohydrate ≥90% and protein ≥87%)
Energy density	≥4 kcal/g for cats with chronic obstipation (megacolon)

*All values are on a dry matter basis except water; to convert kcal to kJ, multiply kcal by 4.184.

FEEDING PLAN

Initial management of chronic constipation includes owner education, encouraging increased water intake, appropriate dietary changes and judicious use of laxatives and enemas. Consider a weight-reduction program if the patient is overweight (Chapter 14). Obstipation often requires multiple cleansing enemas with or without mechanical removal of impacted feces before dietary changes are instituted.

Assess and Select the Food

Ensure the Food's Basic Nutritional Adequacy. AAFCO nutritional adequacy statements are usually found on a product's label. AAFCO approval does not ensure a food will be effective for managing constipation/obstipation and feline megacolon.
Compare the Food's KNF Content with the Recommended Levels.

Constipation/Intermittent Obstipation Patients. Tables 3 and 4 list selected commercial veterinary therapeutic foods for chronic constipated dogs and cats and compare the KNF content of these foods to recommended levels. Consider prescribing a food that most closely matches the KNF recommendations.

Food Form. Feed moist foods (>75% water) to increase water intake (see Water below).

Water. A variety of methods can be used to increase water intake including providing multiple bowls of water in prominent locations in the pet's environment, adding small amounts of flavoring substances (e.g., bouillon or broth) to water sources,

Table 3. Key nutritional factors in selected veterinary therapeutic foods for dogs with constipation and intermittent obstipation compared to recommended levels.* (Numbers in red match optimal KNFs.)

Moist foods	Crude fiber (%)	Primary sources of fiber**
Recommended levels	≥7	–
Hill's Prescription Diet w/d Canine	12.4	Cellulose
Iams Veterinary Formula Intestinal Low-Residue	3.9	Beet pulp
Medi-Cal Fibre Formula	15.0	Tomato pomace, guar gum, flax meal, carrageenan
Purina Veterinary Diets OM Overweight Management Formula	19.2	Pea fiber, beet pulp, carrageenan
Royal Canin Veterinary Diet Calorie Control CC High Fiber	8.8	Tomato pomace, guar gum, flax meal, carrageenan

Dry foods	Crude fiber (%)	Primary sources of fiber**
Recommended levels	≥7	–
Hill's Prescription Diet w/d Canine	16.4	Cellulose, soybean mill run, beet pulp
Iams Veterinary Formula Intestinal Low-Residue	2.1	Beet pulp
Medi-Cal Fibre Formula	14.3	Tomato pomace, rice hulls, oat hulls, flax meal, apple pomace
Purina Veterinary Diets DCO Dual Fiber Control	7.6	Beet pulp, pea fiber
Purina Veterinary Diets OM Overweight Management	10.3	Soybean hulls, pea fiber, cellulose
Royal Canin Veterinary Diet Calorie Control CC 26 High Fiber	17.6	Cellulose, pea fiber, rice hulls, beet pulp, psyllium husk
Royal Canin Veterinary Diet Diabetic HF 18	12.1	Cellulose, rice hulls, guar gum

*Moist foods are best. Manufacturers' published values. Values expressed on a dry matter basis.
**Fiber sources should be insoluble or mixed. Increased levels of soluble fiber are not recommended (see text).

Table 4. Key nutritional factors in selected veterinary therapeutic foods for cats with constipation and intermittent obstipation compared to recommended levels.* (Numbers in red match optimal KNFs.)

Moist foods	Crude fiber (%)	Primary sources of fiber**
Recommended levels	≥7	–
Hill's Prescription Diet w/d with Chicken Feline	10.6	Cellulose, oat fiber, guar gum, locust bean gum, carrageenan
Iams Veterinary Formula Intestinal Low-Residue	3.7	Beet pulp
Medi-Cal Fibre Formula	16.7	Pea fiber, flax meal, guar gum
Purina Veterinary Diets OM Overweight Management	10.2	Pea fiber, oat fiber, guar gum
Royal Canin Veterinary Diet Calorie Control CC High Fiber	7.7	Cellulose, guar gum, flaxseed

Dry foods	Crude fiber (%)	Primary sources of fiber**
Recommended levels	≥7	–
Hill's Prescription Diet w/d Feline	7.6	Cellulose
Hill's Prescription Diet w/d Feline with Chicken	7.6	Cellulose
Iams Veterinary Formula Intestinal Low-Residue	1.8	Beet pulp
Medi-Cal Fibre Formula	14.9	Pea fiber, beet pulp, flax meal
Purina Veterinary Diets OM Overweight Management	5.6	Oat fiber, cellulose
Royal Canin Veterinary Diet Calorie Control CC High Fiber	14.0	Cellulose, pea fiber, rice hulls, beet pulp, psyllium

*Moist foods are best. Manufacturers' published values. Values expressed on a dry matter basis.
**Fiber sources should be insoluble or mixed. Increased levels of soluble fiber are not recommended (see text).

Table 5. Key nutritional factors in selected veterinary therapeutic foods for cats with chronic obstipation (megacolon) compared to recommended levels.* (Numbers in red match optimal KNFs.)

Moist foods	Crude fiber (%)	Protein digestibility (%)	Fat digestibility (%)	Carbohydrate digestibility (%)	Energy density (kcal/g)**
Recommended levels	≤5	≥87	≥90	≥90	≥4
Hill's Prescription Diet a/d Canine/Feline	1.3	90	89	96	4.8
Hill's Prescription Diet i/d Feline	2.4	91	89	91	4.2
Iams Veterinary Formula Intestinal Low-Residue	3.7	na	na	na	4
Iams Veterinary Formula Stress/Weight Gain Formula Maximum-Calorie	2.7	na	na	na	5.8
Medi-Cal Hypoallergenic/Gastro	1.2	na	na	na	na
Medi-Cal Recovery Formula	3.4	na	na	na	na
Medi-Cal Sensitivity CR	2.5	na	na	na	na
Royal Canin Veterinary Diet Recovery RS	3.4	na	na	na	4.4

Dry foods	Crude fiber (%)	Protein digestibility (%)	Fat digestibility (%)	Carbohydrate digestibility (%)	Energy density (kcal/g)**
Recommended levels	≤5	≥87	≥90	≥90	≥4
Hill's Prescription Diet i/d Feline	2.8	88	92	90	4.3
Iams Veterinary Formula Intestinal Low-Residue	1.8	na	na	na	3.9
Medi-Cal Hypoallergenic/Gastro	3.1	na	na	na	na
Purina Veterinary Diets EN GastroENteric Formula	1.3	94.0	93.1	79.7	4.4
Royal Canin Veterinary Diet Intestinal HE 30	5.8	na	na	na	4.4

Key: na = information not available from manufacturer.
*Moist foods are best. Manufacturers' published values. All values expressed on a dry matter basis.
**To convert to kJ, multiply kcal by 4.184.

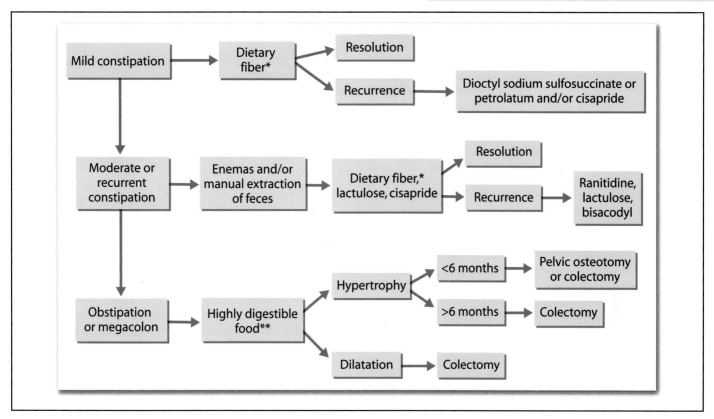

Figure 1. An algorithm for combined dietary and medical management for constipation and obstipation.
*Tables **3** and **4**.
Table **5.

offering ice cubes as treats and adding canned pumpkin and/or sweet potato (~90% water) to the food. Appendix L provides tips for increasing water intake in cats.

FIBER SUPPLEMENTATION. Fiber intake can be increased by adding an enhanced-fiber food to the current food or adding fiber supplements (Appendix N), but it is generally better to switch to a fiber-enhanced food. It is prudent to increase the fiber concentration gradually over several weeks until clinical signs improve or resolve; some patients may experience worsened constipation if transitioned too quickly to high-fiber foods. Soluble fiber content should not exceed 5% (DM) because of potential side effects.

FELINE MEGACOLON PATIENTS. Prescribe foods that are highly digestible and have increased nutrient density. **Table 5** lists KNF contents for foods for such cats and compares them to recommended levels. Patients with severe megacolon may need foods for enteral-assisted feeding (**Table 6**, Chapter 12).

Manage Treats and Snacks.

CONSTIPATION/INTERMITTENT OBSTIPATION PATIENTS. Suggest commercial treats that match the KNFs in the food being fed. Most companies offer treats that correspond to their specific veterinary therapeutic foods. An option is to use the opposite form of the food being fed; i.e., if a dry food is fed, offer small amounts of the same food in moist form as a snack and vice versa; keep kibbles of dry food in a separate container away from the usual feeding area and use as treats. Treats/snacks should not be fed excessively (<10% of the total diet on a volume, weight or calorie basis).

Assess and Determine the Feeding Method

Determine How Much Food to Feed. Estimate from feeding guides on product labels or by calculation (Appendix C). These estimates are only starting points and will likely need to be adjusted (see Followup below).

Consider How to Offer the Food. Smaller, more frequent meals may aid colonic motility patterns and reduce the amount of digesta entering the colon at any one time. Ask owners to walk dogs immediately after feeding; mild exercise and the gastrocolic reflex will often result in defecation during the postprandial period.

Manage Food Changes. Gradually transition to the prescribed food. Example: replace 25% of the original food with the prescribed food on Day 1 and continue this incremental change daily until the change is complete on Day 4. Appendix E provides additional information.

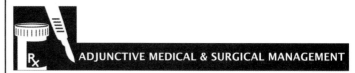
ADJUNCTIVE MEDICAL & SURGICAL MANAGEMENT

The specific medical/surgical plan depends on the severity of constipation/obstipation, recurrence and the underlying cause (**Figure 1**).

Patients with Mild/Moderate Constipation

Consider enemas, stool softeners, laxatives (**Table 6**) and colonic motility modifiers (e.g., cisapride,[a] 0.25 mg/kg body weight, t.i.d. to q.i.d.).

Table 6. Non-dietary medical therapies.

Emollient/lubricant laxatives/stool softeners
Dioctyl sodium succinate (Colace, Regulax SS, Surfak)
Dioctyl calcium sulfosuccinate (Sufax)
Mineral oil (Fleet mineral oil)
Hyperosmolar laxatives
Glycerin
Lactulose (Cephulac, Chronulac, Duphalac)
Polyethylene glycol (Miralax)
Polyethylene glycol with electrolytes (Colyte, GoLYTELY, NuLYTELY)
Sugar alcohols
    Sorbitol (potentially toxic to small dogs and cats)
    Mannitol
Saline laxatives
Magnesium citrate (Evac-Q-Mag)
Magnesium hydroxide (Phillip's Milk of Magnesia)
Magnesium sulfate
Sodium phosphate (Fleet enema, Fleet Phospho-Soda, Visicol)
Stimulant laxatives
Aloe
Anthraquinones
    Cascara sagrada (Colamin, Sagrada-lax)
    Senna (Senokot, Ex-Lax)
    Castor oil (Purge, Neoloid, Emulsoil)
Diphenylmethanes
    Phenolphthalein
    Bisacodyl (Dulcolax, Correctol)
    Sodium picosulfate (Lubrilax, Sur-Lax)
GI prokinetic therapy
Cisapride
Prucalopride (Resolor) (not approved in the U.S.)
New applications of existing drug classifications
Acetylcholinesterase inhibitors (ranitidine, nizatidine, neostigmine)
Erythromycin
Metoclopramide
Prostaglandin E_1 analogues (misoprostol)

Feline Megacolon Patients
Usually respond inadequately to dietary/medical therapy. Subtotal colectomy is often necessary for a positive outcome.

FOLLOWUP

Owner Followup
Note bowel movements (quality and frequency) daily and body weight (if possible) and condition (BCS) every 2 weeks. Well-compensated patients should be evaluated immediately if a change or decline in condition is noted. If a trend of increasing or decreasing body weight or BCS is noted, change the amount fed by 10% increments and recheck every 2 weeks for 1 month. Then, if necessary, change the amount fed and repeat the cycle.

Veterinary Health Care Team Followup
Regaining/maintaining normal body weight and BCS, normal activity level, normal behavior and absence of clinical signs indicate successful dietary management. The first episodes are often transient and resolve without medical therapy.
Persistent Constipation. Consider adjunctive medical management (above) if dietary management fails to improve stool quality and maintain body weight. Although case specific, many patients can eventually be managed with diet alone after medical therapies are gradually discontinued. Manage possible predisposing factors (e.g., pelvic osteotomy to relieve pelvic stricture). Figure 1 summarizes management recommendations if problems recur.

MISCELLANEOUS

See Chapters 25, 27 and 64, Small Animal Clinical Nutrition, 5th edition, for more information.

Authors
Condensed from Chapter 64, Small Animal Clinical Nutrition, 5th edition, authored by Deborah J. Davenport, Rebecca L. Remillard and Maureen Carroll.

References
See Chapter 64, Small Animal Clinical Nutrition, 5th edition, on the website www.markmorrisinstitute.org for references.

Endnote
a. Available from compounding pharmacies.

CLINICAL POINTS

- Flatulence is the presence of excessive gases in GI tract. Flatus is gas expelled through the anus. Belching is the noisy voiding of gas from the stomach through the mouth. Borborygmus is a rumbling noise caused by the movement of gas through the intestines.
- Excessive flatulence is usually associated with noticeable flatus, belching, borborygmus, abdominal distention or a combination of these signs. Excessive flatus is a chronic objectionable problem that occurs often in dogs and less commonly in cats.
- Gas in the GI tract is normal and may be derived from 3 sources: air swallowing, intraluminal gas production and diffusion of gas from the blood to the GI tract.
- Excessive aerophagia is a risk factor for flatulence and is seen with brachycephalic, working and sporting dogs and pets with aggressive and/or competitive eating behaviors.
- Dietary indiscretion and ingestion of certain food ingredients may be risks for certain individuals.
- Large amounts of gas may be formed from colonic microbial fermentation of poorly digestible carbohydrates and certain fibers. Odorless gases (i.e., N_2, O_2, CO_2, H_2 and CH_4) compose up to 99% of flatus. The rest is composed of odoriferous gases that contribute the objectionable odors.
- Flatus, belching and borborygmus occur in normal pets but when excessive, may be associated with small intestinal or colonic disorders. Maldigestive or malabsorptive diseases are often associated with excessive flatus because malassimilated substrates are delivered to the colon and fermented.
- Obtaining a thorough dietary history is important in evaluating patients with excessive flatulence. Knowledge of specific foods, major food ingredients, treats, supplements and opportunities for dietary indiscretion facilitates management.
- Foods such as onions, nuts, spices, cruciferous vegetables and high protein ingredients can increase production of odoriferous sulfur-containing gases.
- Foods that contain large amounts of nonabsorbable oligo-saccharides (e.g., soybeans, beans, peas) may produce large amounts of intestinal gas. Dogs/cats lack the specific enzymes needed to digest these sugars into absorbable monosaccharides and colonic microbes ferment them to CO_2 and H_2. Flatus may be present in pets with lactose intolerance.
- Dietary protein sources and amount may affect flatus odor. NH_3 and volatile amines containing sulfur are odoriferous and may result from microbial fermentation of food protein, mucus or bile acid residues reaching the large intestine. Soybean meal is commonly used in pet foods as a protein source.
- In most cases, physical exam findings are unremarkable although abdominal distention is sometimes noted in cats.

Abbreviations
AAFCO = Association of American Feed Control Officials
BCS = body condition score (Appendix A)
KNF = key nutritional factor

- Laboratory testing is usually not indicated. However, further evaluation is in order if concomitant GI signs are present.
- The focus of dietary management of flatulence is to decrease intestinal gas production attributable to bacterial fermentation of undigested food.
- Digestibility, especially of carbohydrate ingredients, is an important food factor for patients with excessive flatus. Feeding highly digestible foods reduces residues available for colonic fermentation. Foods with high digestibility (fat and digestible [soluble] carbohydrate ≥90% and protein ≥87%) are recommended for patients with objectionable flatus.
- Studies in dogs indicate that foods with rice as the major carbohydrate source result in less intestinal gas formation than foods containing wheat or corn.
- Soluble fibers (e.g., fruit pectins, guar gum, carrageenan) are readily fermentable by gut microbes and may result in gas production, contributing to excessive flatus in some patients. Even some mixed fibers (brans, soy fiber, soy hulls, pea fiber and beet pulp) can be a source of flatus and may contain non-fiber ingredients that worsen objectionable flatus (e.g., soy hulls and pea fiber).
- A series of dietary elimination trials may be required to determine which food(s) are most efficacious in reduction of excessive flatus.
- Feeding two or more times/day may result in fewer episodes of flatus than feeding once/day.
- Prognosis is good in most cases.
- Feeding plan goals: reduce excessive flatulence through the use of appropriate foods and feeding methods.

KEY NUTRITIONAL FACTORS

- Foods should provide recommended allowances of all required nutrients (nutritional adequacy), but should also contain specific levels of KNFs (certain nutrients proven to assist in the management of excessive flatulence).
- **Table 1** lists KNF recommendations (including ingredients to avoid) for foods for dogs and cats with excessive flatulence. A detailed review of these recommendations can be found in Chapter 65, Small Animal Clinical Nutrition, 5th edition. In the case of puppies/kittens with excessive flatulence, protein and other KNF levels should be sufficient for growth (Chapters 5 and 11).

Table 1. Key nutritional factors for foods, treats and snacks for dogs and cats with excessive flatulence.*

Factors	Recommendations
Digestibility	Increased digestibility
	Fat and carbohydrate digestibility ≥90%
	Protein digestibility ≥87%
Carbohydrate	Change source: rice is preferred
Protein	Avoid high-protein foods
	Adult dogs: limit to ≤30% or less
	Adult cats: limit to ≤40% or less
	Avoid legumes (see below)
Fiber	Dogs and cats: limit to ≤5% fiber (most important aspect regarding fiber)
	Avoid high-fiber foods, especially soluble/fermentable and mixed fibers (soy fiber, soybean hulls, pea fiber, psyllium, pectin, carrageenan, guar gum, bran and beet pulp)
Legumes	Avoid all beans (including soybeans), peas, lentils, peanuts
Lactose sources	Avoid milk, ice cream, cheese, yogurt
Sulfur-containing vegetables	Avoid broccoli, cauliflower, Brussels sprouts, cabbage
Onions	Avoid
Nuts	Avoid
Spices	Avoid
Fructose	Avoid fruits and high-fructose corn syrup
Vitamin-mineral supplements	Avoid; unnecessary with most commercial foods

*Nutrient values are on a dry matter basis.

FEEDING PLAN

Assess and Select the Food

Ensure the Food's Basic Nutritional Adequacy. AAFCO nutritional adequacy statements are usually found on a product's label. AAFCO approval does not ensure a food will be effective for managing excessive flatulence.

Compare the Food's KNF Content with the Recommended Levels. **Tables 2** and **3** list commercially available highly digestible foods marketed for managing GI diseases in dogs and cats (respectively) and compare KNF content of these foods with recommended levels for managing excessive flatulence. Contact manufacturers for information for foods not in the tables (manufacturer contact information is listed on product labels). Select a food that best approximates the recommended KNF levels. Dietary trials may be necessary to select a food that reduces flatulence.

    INGREDIENTS. Evaluate foods and treats/snacks for specific ingredients that might contribute to excessive flatulence by comparing product label ingredient lists to ingredients recommended to avoid/limit, provided in **Table 1**. If a product's major ingredients are a concern, change to one that has a KNF profile and ingredient list that more closely compares to the recommendations in **Table 1**.

Manage Treats and Snacks. Suggest commercial treats that match the KNFs of the prescribed food. Most companies offer treats that correspond to their specific veterinary therapeutic foods. An option is to use the opposite form of the food being fed; i.e., if a dry food is fed, offer small amounts of the same food in moist form as a snack and vice versa; keep kibbles of dry food in a separate container away from the usual feeding area and use as treats. Treats/snacks should not be fed excessively (<10% of the total diet on a volume, weight or calorie basis). **Table 1** lists human foods to avoid as treats/snacks.

Assess and Determine the Feeding Method

Determine How Much Food to Feed. Estimate from feeding guides on product labels or by calculation (Appendix C). Estimates are only starting points and will likely need to be adjusted (see Followup below).

Consider How to Offer the Food. Reducing aerophagia is important, especially in brachycephalic dog breeds. Feeding several small meals/day may reduce rapid eating and gulping of air and improve digestibility thereby reducing food residues available for colonic fermentation. Feeding in a quiet, isolated location will eliminate competitive eating and reduce aerophagia. Walking dogs outdoors within 30 minutes of eating encourages defecation, which may help eliminate a source of intestinal gas.

Manage Food Changes. Most dogs and cats adapt well to new foods but a transition period to avoid GI upsets is good practice. Gradually transition the patient to the prescribed food. Example: replace 25% of the original food with the prescribed food on Day 1 and continue this incremental change daily until the change is complete on Day 4. Appendix E provides additional information.

Food and Water Receptacle Husbandry. Food and water bowls should be washed regularly with warm soapy water and rinsed well. Dishes used for moist foods need daily cleaning. Discard moist or moistened dry foods after 2-4 hours of room temperature exposure to avoid foodborne illnesses (Appendix F).

Table 2. Key nutritional factors in selected commercial veterinary therapeutic foods for dogs with excessive flatulence compared to recommended levels.* (Numbers in red match optimal KNFs.)

Dry foods	Protein digestibility (%)	Fat digestibility (%)	Carbohydrate digestibility (%)	Protein (%)	Crude fiber (%)
Recommended levels	≥87	≥90	≥90	≤30	≤5
Hill's Prescription Diet i/d Canine	92	93	94	26.2	2.7
Iams Veterinary Formula Intestinal Low-Residue	na	na	na	24.6	2.1
Medi-Cal Gastro Formula	na	na	na	22.9	1.9
Purina Veterinary Diets EN GastroENteric Formula	84.5	91.4	94.4	27.0	1.5
Royal Canin Veterinary Diet Digestive Low Fat LF 20	na	na	na	24.2	2.3
Royal Canin Veterinary Diet Intestinal HE 28	na	na	na	33.0	1.6

Moist foods	Protein digestibility (%)	Fat digestibility (%)	Carbohydrate digestibility (%)	Protein (%)	Crude fiber (%)
Recommended levels	≥87	≥90	≥90	≤30	≤5
Hill's Prescription Diet i/d Canine	88	94	93	25.0	1.0
Iams Veterinary Formula Intestinal Low-Residue	na	na	na	35.9	3.9
Medi-Cal Gastro Formula	na	na	na	22.1	1.0
Purina Veterinary Diets EN GastroENteric Formula	85.1	95.6	92.2	30.5	0.9
Royal Canin Veterinary Diet Digestive Low Fat LF	na	na	na	31.9	3.0
Royal Canin Veterinary Diet Intestinal HE	na	na	na	23.1	1.4

Key: na = information not available from manufacturer; see **Table 1** for specific ingredients to avoid.
*Protein and crude fiber levels are on a dry matter basis.

Table 3. Key nutritional factors in selected commercial veterinary therapeutic foods for cats with excessive flatulence compared to recommended levels* (Numbers in red match optimal KNFs.)

Dry foods	Protein digestibility (%)	Fat digestibility (%)	Carbohydrate digestibility (%)	Protein (%)	Crude fiber (%)
Recommended levels	≥87	≥90	≥90	≤40	≤5
Hill's Prescription Diet i/d Feline	88	92	90	40.3	2.8
Iams Veterinary Formula Intestinal Low-Residue	na	na	na	35.8	1.8
Medi-Cal Hypoallergenic/Gastro	na	na	na	29.8	3.1
Purina Veterinary Diets EN GastroENteric Formula	94.0	93.1	79.7	56.2	1.3
Royal Canin Veterinary Diet Intestinal HE 30	na	na	na	34.4	5.8

Moist foods	Protein digestibility (%)	Fat digestibility (%)	Carbohydrate digestibility (%)	Protein (%)	Crude fiber (%)
Recommended levels	≥87	≥90	≥90	≤40	≤5
Hill's Prescription Diet i/d Feline	91	89	91	37.6	2.4
Iams Veterinary Formula Intestinal Low-Residue	na	na	na	38.4	3.7
Medi-Cal Hypoallergenic/Gastro	na	na	na	35.5	1.2
Medi-Cal Sensitivity CR	na	na	na	34.5	2.5

Key: na = information not available from manufacturer; see **Table 1** for specific ingredients to avoid.
*Protein and crude fiber levels are on a dry matter basis.

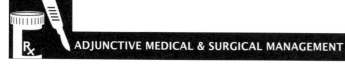

ADJUNCTIVE MEDICAL & SURGICAL MANAGEMENT

Carminatives

Consider using these if feeding plan changes do not result in significant improvement to help reduce excessive flatulence. The best evidence exists for short-term use of bismuth subsalicylate, zinc acetate and nonabsorbable antibiotics. Less evidence exists for use of activated charcoal, simethicone, digestive enzyme preparations, *Yucca* extract, grape seed extract and probiotics. For more information, see Box 65-1, Small Animal Clinical Nutrition, 5th edition.

FOLLOWUP

Owner Followup

Initially, owners should note body weight (if possible) and condition (BCS) every 2 weeks to determine if the feeding amount/method needs to be adjusted. If a trend of increasing or decreasing body weight or BCS is noted, change the amount fed by 10% increments and recheck every 2 weeks for 1 month. At that point, change the amount fed and repeat the cycle if necessary.

Veterinary Health Care Team Followup

Manage owner expectations; inform owners about normal intestinal gas production and to not expect complete cessation of flatulence.

Persistent Flatulence. Relapses in pets that have been controlled indicate dietary indiscretion. However, if there is good compliance then evaluate for malassimilation. If the feeding plan changes (i.e., lack of significant improvement), consider the use of carminatives (above).

OTHER FOOD OPTIONS. Changing to foods with different sources of protein/carbohydrate may benefit some pets. Consider elimination foods (Tables 3 [dogs] and 4 [cats], Chapter 19) and compare them to KNF recommendations in **Table 1.** Vegetarian-based foods often include potentially odoriferous sulfur-containing vegetables/legumes. Lactose-containing ingredients (e.g., cheese, ice cream, milk) in foods and treats may be factors for adult pets, especially those with lactase deficiency or underlying GI disease. Dietary trials may be necessary to find a food that lessens flatulence in individual pets.

MISCELLANEOUS

See Chapters 17, 24, 31 and 67, Small Animal Clinical Nutrition, 5th edition, for more information. Also see Current Veterinary Therapy XIV.

Authors
Condensed from Chapter 65, Small Animal Clinical Nutrition, 5th edition, authored by Philip Roudebush, Deborah J. Davenport and Rebecca L. Remillard.

References
See Chapter 65, Small Animal Clinical Nutrition, 5th edition, on the website www.markmorrisinstitute.org for references.

Chapter
51
Exocrine Pancreatic Insufficiency

CLINICAL POINTS

- Malassimilation results from failure of nutrients to pass across the intestinal barrier at a rate necessary to maintain body condition or weight; both maldigestive and malabsorptive diseases may be causes.
- Defects in intraluminal digestion may occur from gastric, pancreatic or biliary dysfunction and result in maldigestion; EPI is the most common cause of maldigestion in dogs.
- Potential causes of EPI include congenital acinar atrophy and chronic/acute pancreatitis.
- EPI attributable to acinar atrophy occurs most commonly in younger large-breed dogs. German shepherd dogs, Eurasians and rough-coated collies appear to have a genetic predisposition. However, any breed can be affected.
- Congenital EPI may be subclinical or clinical due to partial or complete loss of pancreatic enzymes; clinical signs develop when 85-90% of exocrine function is lost. Congenital EPI usually occurs at 6-18 months of age.
- Acquired EPI can result from chronic inflammation and fibrosis; diabetes mellitus may develop concurrently.
- EPI is rare in cats; however, juvenile and acquired forms have been recognized.

Abbreviations
AAFCO = Association of American Feed Control Officials
BCS = body condition score (Appendix A)
DM = dry matter
EPI = exocrine pancreatic insufficiency
KNF = key nutritional factor
PN = parenteral nutrition
RER = resting energy requirement (Appendix C)
SIBO = small intestinal bacterial overgrowth
TLI = trypsin-like immunoreactivity

- Tentative diagnosis is based on history and clinical findings; definitive diagnosis is based on low fasting TLI values (<2.5 µg/l) in both dogs and cats; serum amylase, isoamylase and lipase are of little value.
- History of chronic small bowel diarrhea (usually characterized as osmotic), failure to thrive and weight loss are common.
- Typically, stools are frequent (6-10/day), voluminous, steatorrheic and pale.
- Clinical signs commonly include polyphagia, borborygmus, flatulence, pica and coprophagia; vomiting and polydipsia occur less commonly.
- Poor coat quality may also be noted due to maldigestion of nutrients; cats may have soiled hair in the perineal region.
- Congenital pancreatic atrophy usually results in stunted animals compared to breed standards.

- Because chronic pancreatitis may result in acquired EPI, risk factors are the same as those for pancreatitis (Chapter 52).
- Several different causes of inadequate digestion exist in EPI including lack of exocrine pancreatic enzymes and pancreatic secretory components (e.g., bicarbonate, trophic factors, antibacterial factors).
- Dogs with EPI often have SIBO, which exacerbates the condition by damaging mucosal surfaces.
- Food digestibility is the most important nutritional factor; carbohydrate and protein digestibilities should be ≥90 and ≥87%, respectively; fiber content should be ≤5% (DM).
- Fat should be kept between 10-15% DM for dogs and 15-25% DM for cats; highly digestible fats are preferred.
- In addition to dietary management, oral administration of pancreatic enzymes is essential (see below).
- Fat digestion will not return to normal even with pancreatic enzyme therapy; a finding probably attributable to inactivation of lipase by gastric acid.
- Prognosis: congenital cases may do well if there is good owner compliance. If owner compliance is poor or EPI is acquired, prognosis can be grave, especially for indoor pets.
- Feeding goals: regaining/maintaining optimal body weight and condition (BCS), normal activity level and absence/reduction of clinical signs.

KEY NUTRITIONAL FACTORS

- Foods should provide recommended allowances of all required nutrients (nutritional adequacy), but should also contain specific levels of KNFs appropriate for EPI.
- Table 1 lists KNFs for foods for EPI patients and recommended amounts to feed; these KNFs and feeding amounts are discussed in more detail in Chapter 66, Small Animal Clinical Nutrition, 5th edition.

Concurrent Diabetes Mellitus

These patients often require a modified KNF profile: foods containing 10-15% DM fat, 50-55% DM digestible carbohydrate and 5-10% fiber may be used (Chapter 16).

FEEDING PLAN

If the patient presents with a low BCS due to underlying chronic pancreatitis (Chapter 52), PN support (Chapter 13) may be required during the initial treatment period.

Assess and Select the Food
Ensure the Food's Basic Nutritional Adequacy. AAFCO nutritional adequacy statements are usually found on a product's label. AAFCO approval does not ensure a food will be effective for nutritional management of EPI.

Table 1. Key nutritional factors for foods for patients with exocrine pancreatic insufficiency.*

Factors	Recommended levels
Digestibility	≥87% for protein and ≥90% for fat and digestible carbohydrate
Fat	10 to 15% for dogs 15 to 25% for cats
Fiber	≤5%**

*Nutrients expressed on a dry matter basis.
**Lower is better.

Compare the Food's KNF Content with the Recommended Levels. Several commercial foods are marketed for management of EPI in dogs and cats (**Tables 2** and **3**, respectively). Feeding highly digestible foods may reduce the amount of supplemental oral pancreatic enzymes required to control signs. Foods used for EPI in puppies and kittens should also meet the KNF requirements for growth (Chapters 5 and 11). Choose a food that most closely fits recommended levels.

Manage Treats and Snacks. Suggest commercial treats that match the food being fed. Most companies offer treats that correspond to their specific veterinary therapeutic foods. An option is to use the opposite form of the food being fed; i.e., if a dry food is fed, offer small amounts of the same food in moist form as a snack and vice versa; keep kibbles of dry food in a separate container away from the usual feeding area and use as treats. Treats/snacks should not be fed excessively (<10% of the total diet on a volume, weight or calorie basis). Offer concurrently with the pancreatic enzyme supplemented food. See Appendix B for other treats/snacks information.

Assess and Determine the Feeding Method
Determine How Much to Food to Feed. Estimate from feeding guides on product labels or by calculation (Appendix C). Estimates are only starting points and will likely need to be adjusted (see Followup below). If body weight and condition (BCS) are not ideal, adjust food dosage estimates appropriately. Increase the amount fed for underweight patients above that for normal weight patients (e.g., 2x RER for their estimated ideal weight) until ideal body weight and BCS of 2.5-3.5/5 are attained. It may be necessary to offer an above average amount of food to offset persistent maldigestion, even after achieving ideal weight/BCS.

Consider How to Offer the Food. Multiple small meals/day are recommended to improve digestibility and help prevent dietary overload and subsequent osmotic diarrhea.

Manage Food Changes. A transition period to avoid GI upsets and facilitate acceptance of a new food is good practice. Gradually, transition to the prescribed food. Example: replace 25% of the original food with the prescribed food on Day 1 and continue this incremental change daily until the change is complete on Day 4. If GI problems occur while increasing the amount of prescribed food, reduce the amount fed to the previous level for several days then initiate a more gradual transition to full feeding of the prescribed food. Appendix E provides additional information about managing food changes.

Table 2. Key nutritional factors in selected commercial veterinary therapeutic foods for dogs with exocrine pancreatic insufficiency compared to recommended levels.* (Numbers in red match optimal KNFs.)

Dry foods	Protein digestibility (%)	Fat digestibility (%)	Carbohydrate digestibility (%)	Fat (%)	Crude fiber (%)
Recommended levels	≥87	≥90	≥90	10-15	≤5**
Hill's Prescription Diet i/d Canine	92	93	94	14.1	2.7
Iams Veterinary Formula Intestinal Low-Residue	na	na	na	10.7	2.1
Medi-Cal Gastro Formula	na	na	na	13.9	1.9
Purina Veterinary Diets EN GastroENteric Formula***	84.5	91.4	94.4	12.6	1.5
Purina Veterinary Diets HA Hypoallergenic Formula***	90.7	93.1	95.7	10.54	1.58
Royal Canin Veterinary Diet Low Fat LF 20	na	na	na	6.6	2.3
Royal Canin Veterinary Diet Hypoallergenic HP 19	na	na	na	20.9	2.3

Moist foods	Protein digestibility (%)	Fat digestibility (%)	Carbohydrate digestibility (%)	Fat (%)	Crude fiber (%)
Recommended levels	≥87	≥90	≥90	10-15	≤5**
Hill's Prescription Diet i/d Canine	88	94	93	14.9	1.0
Iams Veterinary Formula Intestinal Low-Residue	na	na	na	13.2	3.9
Medi-Cal Gastro Formula	na	na	na	11.7	1.0
Purina Veterinary Diets EN GastroENteric Formula***	85.1	95.6	92.2	13.8	0.9
Royal Canin Veterinary Diet Low Fat LF	na	na	na	6.9	3.0

Key: na = information not available from manufacturer.
*All values are on a dry matter basis; values obtained from manufacturer.
**Lower is better.
***Contains medium-chain triglycerides; see text.

Table 3. Key nutritional factors in selected commercial veterinary therapeutic foods for cats with exocrine pancreatic insufficiency compared to recommended levels.* (Numbers in red match optimal KNFs.)

Dry foods	Protein digestibility (%)	Fat digestibility (%)	Carbohydrate digestibility (%)	Fat (%)	Crude fiber (%)
Recommended levels	≥87	≥90	≥90	15-25	≤5**
Hill's Prescription Diet i/d Feline	88	92	90	20.2	2.8
Iams Veterinary Formula Intestinal Low-Residue	na	na	na	13.7	1.8
Medi-Cal Hypoallergenic/Gastro	na	na	na	11.5	3.1
Purina Veterinary Diets EN GastroENteric Formula	94.0	93.1	79.7	18.4	1.3
Royal Canin Veterinary Diets Hypoallergenic HP 23	na	na	na	21.5	4.8

Moist foods	Protein digestibility (%)	Fat digestibility (%)	Carbohydrate digestibility (%)	Fat (%)	Crude fiber (%)
Recommended levels	≥87	≥90	≥90	15-25	≤5**
Hill's Prescription Diet i/d Feline	91	89	91	24.1	2.4
Iams Veterinary Formula Intestinal Low-Residue	na	na	na	11.7	3.7
Medi-Cal Hypoallergenic/Gastro	na	na	na	35.9	1.2

Key: na = information not available from manufacturer.
*All values are on a dry matter basis; values obtained from manufacturer.
**Lower is better.

Food and Water Receptacle Husbandry. Food and water bowls should be washed regularly with warm soapy water and rinsed well. Dishes used for moist foods need daily cleaning. Discard moist or moistened dry foods after 2-4 hours of room temperature exposure to avoid foodborne illnesses (Appendix F).

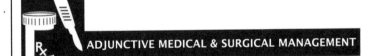

ADJUNCTIVE MEDICAL & SURGICAL MANAGEMENT

Pancreatic Enzyme Therapy

Dried pancreatic enzyme supplementation is necessary (Table 4) for successful management of EPI. For dogs, initiate at a dose of 1 tsp of powdered extract/10 kg/meal. The starting dose for cats is 1 tsp/meal. Mix enzymes with food immediately before the meal is fed. The dose may be reduced based on individual response. Most dogs require ≥1 tsp of enzyme product/

Table 4. Enzyme preparations used in patients with exocrine pancreatic insufficiency.*

Products (manufacturers)	Lipase	Protease	Amylase	Formulation
Viokase-V Powder (Fort Dodge)	71,400	388,000	460,000	Powder
Viokase-V Tablets (Fort Dodge)	9,000	57,000	64,000	Tablets
Viokase Powder (Axcan Scandipharm)	16,800	70,000	70,000	Powder
Pancrezyme Powder (Daniels Pharmaceuticals)	71,400	388,000	460,000	Powder
Pancrezyme Tablets (Daniels Pharmaceuticals)	9,000	57,000	64,000	Tablets
Pancrease MT16 Capsules (McNeil)	18,000	18,000	48,000	Enteric-coated microtablets
Pancrease MT20 Capsules (McNeil)	20,000	44,000	56,000	Enteric-coated microtablets
Pancreatic Plus Powder (Butler)	71,400	388,000	460,000	Powder
Pancreatic Plus Tablets (Butler)	9,000	57,000	64,000	Tablets
Pancrelipase Capsules (Mutual)	18,000	18,000	48,000	Enteric-coated pellets
Lypex Pancreatic Enzyme Capsules (Vio-Vet)	30,000	18,750	1,200	Capsules

*Enzymatic contents (IU) per capsule, tablet or tsp of powder (2.8 g).

meal. If available, raw bovine, porcine or ovine pancreas may be an option (can keep frozen for several months). Dogs should receive 30-90 g (1-3 oz.) and cats 30 g (1 oz.) of freshly thawed, chopped pancreas/meal.

Side Effects. Pancreatic enzyme extract may cause oral mucosal irritation/hemorrhage and reluctance to eat. Decreasing the dose and mixing well with food may mitigate the problem. If not, consider feeding raw pancreas.

Antacid/H₂ Blockers. Some EPI cases may respond better if gastric acid secretion is decreased, which reduces destruction of added enzymes.

Oral Antibiotics. Antibiotics may help resolve clinical signs in dogs and cats with concurrent SIBO. Tetracycline (20 mg/kg per os, t.i.d., for 21 days) or tylosin (25 mg/kg per os, b.i.d., for 6 weeks) are recommended; however, metronidazole (10-20 mg/kg per os, every 24 hours for 7-14 days) may be more effective if anaerobic bacteria are suspected.

Insulin. May be required in patients with concurrent diabetes mellitus (Chapter 16).

FOLLOWUP

Owner Followup

Record daily food intake, stool quantity and stool character; note BCS and body weight (if practical) every 2 weeks. If necessary, the amount fed should be changed by 10% increments and rechecked every 2 weeks for 1 month. At that point, the amount fed can be changed again and the cycle repeated until the patient reaches a normal body weight/BCS.

Compliance. Work with the veterinary health care team to ensure compliance with home-care orders for dietary and medical management. Do not feed unprescribed foods or treats. If the patient comes from a multi-pet household, deny access to other pets' foods.

Veterinary Health Care Team Followup

Improvement in the patient's attitude, appetite and activity and resolution/reduction in severity of clinical signs are good indicators of success.

Use of Owner Data. If owners record food intake and stool character daily and BCS/body weight every 2 weeks, occasionally correlate these findings with measures taken by a member of the veterinary health care team. If owner data correlate, some rechecks/food adjustments can be done by phone and alternated with in-clinic exams. In addition, owner records of vomiting, diarrhea and other complications may help assess progress.

Recurrence of Clinical Signs. If the patient is well managed and suddenly decompensates, rule out SIBO.

MISCELLANEOUS

See Chapters 17, 24, 26, 29, 57 and 66, Small Animal Clinical Nutrition, 5th edition, for more information.

Vitamin Malnutrition

Fat-soluble vitamins, folate and cobalamin may need to be supplemented in patients with EPI.

Fat-Soluble Vitamins (A,D,E &K). Fat-soluble vitamin supplementation is warranted in cases of long-term fat malabsorption. Administer 1 ml of a vitamin A, D and E solution,[a] divided into 2 IM sites. This should supply fat-soluble vitamins for approximately 3 months. Vitamin K_1 at a dose of 0.5-1 mg/kg, SQ, is recommended if vitamin K-responsive coagulopathy is suspected.

Cobalamin (B₁₂). Consider laboratory tests to assess serum cobalamin levels (<300 ng/l indicates hypocobalaminemia). Recommended SQ dose: 250 μg/week (cats) and 500 μg/week (dogs) until levels return to normal. Once/twice monthly therapy may be necessary for longer term maintenance. If complicated by SIBO, bacterial uptake of B_{12} may exacerbate deficiency.

Folate (B₁₀ & B₁₁). Serum folate levels may be elevated in EPI with concurrent SIBO due to microbial synthesis. However, it may be decreased in dogs with EPI and concurrent enteropathies involving the ileum. Folate deficiency inhibits pancreatic exocrine function in rats. Supplement with 0.5-1 mg folate per os, once/day until ileal pathology is resolved.

Authors
Condensed from Chapter 66, Small Animal Clinical Nutrition, 5th edition, authored by Deborah J. Davenport, Rebecca L. Remillard and Kenny W. Simpson.

References
See Chapter 66, Small Animal Clinical Nutrition, 5th edition, on the website www.markmorrisinstitute.org for references.

Endnote
a. Vital E-A+D containing 100 IU of D and 300 IU of α-tocopherol/ml. Schering-Plough Animal Health Corp., Kenilworth, NJ, USA.

Chapter
52 Acute and Chronic Pancreatitis

CLINICAL POINTS

- Pancreatitis, an inflammatory disease of the pancreas, can be either acute or chronic. Acute pancreatitis, if treated early and properly, is often reversible. Chronic pancreatitis denotes longstanding inflammatory disease and is often associated with irreversible morphologic changes.
- Pancreatitis is more common in dogs than cats. Pancreatitis may be an inciting cause of EPI.

Table 1. Risk factors for pancreatitis in dogs and cats.

Breed
Boxer
Briard
Cavalier King Charles spaniel
Cocker spaniel
Collie
Miniature schnauzer
Sheltie
Yorkshire terrier
Himalayan cat
Dietary factors
High-fat, low-protein foods
Ingestion of garbage or table scraps
Drug administration
Azathioprine
Corticosteroids
L-asparaginase
Organophosphate insecticides (cats)
Fasting hyperlipidemia
Gender
Castrated males
Spayed females
Hepatobiliary disease
Feline suppurative cholangiohepatitis
Triaditis (IBD, cholangiohepatitis, pancreatitis)
Hypercalcemia
Hyperparathyroidism
Intravenous calcium infusion
Increasing age
Intervertebral disk disease
Ischemia or reperfusion
Postgastric dilatation-volvulus
Obesity

Abbreviations
AAFCO = Association of American Feed Control Officials
BCS = body condition score (Appendix A)
EN = enteral nutrition
EPI = exocrine pancreatic insufficiency
IBD = inflammatory bowel disease
KNF = key nutritional factor
NPO = nothing by mouth
PLI = pancreatic lipase immunoreactivity
PN = parenteral nutrition
TNA = total nutrient admixture

- Pancreatitis occurs as a consequence of intracellular pancreatic acinar enzymatic activation and the resultant autodigestion of the pancreas. After damage has incurred, inflammatory mediators perpetuate the cycle of damage and pancreatitis becomes self-propagating and can cause untoward systemic consequences.
- Several factors are associated with increased risk (**Table 1**); the most common are hypertriglyceridemia, obesity and certain drugs.
- In dogs, dietary indiscretion, high-fat foods (including struvite litholytic foods) and corticosteroids may be associated with onset of disease.
- In some cats, pancreatitis can present concurrently with other diseases such as diabetes mellitus and triaditis (hepatic lipidosis, cholangiohepatitis or IBD).
- Dogs with acute pancreatitis usually present with vomiting and abdominal pain; other clinical signs include depression, anorexia, fever and occasionally large bowel diarrhea or icterus.
- Cats have highly variable signs. Some mimic typical canine presentations; others follow a more indolent course that results in a mild chronic illness. The most common signs in cats include anorexia, lethargy, dehydration and weight loss.
- Acute hemorrhagic or necrotizing pancreatitis is a medical emergency.
- Chronic pancreatitis is subtle and variable in clinical presentation; weight loss and low BCS often are the only signs noted.

- Abdominal radiograpic (dogs and cats) and ultrasonograpic (dogs) diagnostic imaging can be useful.
- An inflammatory leukogram is typical for acute pancreatitis. Also, a CBC, serum biochemistry profile and urinalysis help rule out other potential causes of clinical signs and may aid in the diagnosis of concurrent conditions (e.g., diabetes mellitus, hepatic lipidosis, interstitial nephritis and cholangiohepatitis).
- Species specific PLI is an important tool for the diagnosis of pancreatitis in dogs and cats and is not falsely elevated in renal disease or by corticosteroid administration.
- Foods providing excess dietary protein may contribute to further episodes of acute pancreatitis and should be avoided; free amino acids in the duodenum are potent stimuli for pancreatic secretion via cholecystokinin.
- Dietary fat also causes release of cholecystokinin. Low-fat foods are indicated for obese/overweight and hypertriglyceridemic patients recovering from pancreatitis. Other pancreatitis patients can tolerate moderate dietary fat levels.
- Prognosis for acute edematous pancreatitis is good but guarded/poor for acute necrotizing pancreatitis. Chronic pancreatitis, by its very nature, has a guarded prognosis.
- Feeding goals include: decreasing stimuli for pancreatic exocrine secretion while providing adequate nutrition via appropriate foods and feeding methods to support tissue repair and recovery.

KEY NUTRITIONAL FACTORS

- Foods used to facilitate recovery and prevent recurrence should provide recommended allowances of all required nutrients (nutritional adequacy), but should also contain specific levels of KNFs appropriate for dietary management of pancreatitis, depending on body weight/BCS.
- **Table 2** lists KNFs for foods (normal weight patients) intended for pancreatitis, which are discussed in more detail in Chapter 67, Small Animal Clinical Nutrition, 5th edition. **Tables 3** and **4** cover recommendations for dogs and cats that are of normal weight, respectively. **Tables 5** and **6** cover recommendations for dogs and cats that are obese prone/hypertriglyceridemic; Chapter 67, Small Animal Clinical Nutrition, 5th edition, covers these KNFs in more detail.
- As much as possible, these KNFs should be considered for liquid foods (Chapter 12) if used for EN support during the immediate recovery period (below).
- Water and electrolytes are the most important nutrients for initial acute pancreatitis because of potential ongoing vomiting and resultant dehydration and electrolyte/acid-base imbalances.

FEEDING PLAN

Initially, NPO is recommended for ≤3 days (including days of anorexia pre-presentation) to control vomiting. At the same

Table 2. Key nutritional factors for foods for canine and feline patients with pancreatitis.*

Factors	Recommended levels
Fat	≤15% for non-obese and non-hypertriglyceridemic dogs
	≤ 25% for non-obese and non-hypertriglyceridemic cats
	≤10% for obese and/or hypertriglyceridemic dogs
	≤15% for obese and/or hypertriglyceridemic cats
Protein	15 to 30% for dogs
	30 to 40% for cats

*Nutrients expressed on a dry matter basis.

time, begin parenteral fluid therapy to correct dehydration and electrolyte and acid-base disturbances and consider concurrent medical therapy (below). The rest of the feeding plan is patient-dependent.

Patients with Intractable Vomiting
If the patient continues to vomit beyond the prescribed NPO period, institute continuous feeding by tube (Chapter 12, Appendix H) in combination with antiemetic therapy (below). Another option is PN support (Chapter 13) concurrent with fluid and medical therapy until the patient has stabilized and can be fed orally.

Debilitated or Triaditis Patients
Recommend early EN support (liquid foods) (Chapter 12) with concurrent medical therapy until the patient has stabilized and can be fed orally.

Stabilized Patients
Initially offer small amounts of water, ice cubes and/or oral rehydration solutions. Monomeric liquid human foods can also be given to canine patients (these foods minimally stimulate pancreatic secretion) (Chapter 12). If these offerings are tolerated, select a food that facilitates recovery and prevents recurrence.

Assess and Select the Food
Ensure the Food's Basic Nutritional Adequacy. AAFCO nutritional adequacy statements are usually found on a product's label. AAFCO approval does not ensure a food will be effective for managing pancreatitis. Nutritional adequacy is important for recovery/prevention-type foods because once successfully initiated, they are usually fed for life.
Compare the Food's KNF Content with the Recommended Levels.
  PN SOLUTIONS. For PN-assisted feeding, premixed TNA solutions are easiest to use and may be administered by peripheral vein, depending on osmolarity (Chapter 13).
  HUMAN MONOMERIC LIQUID FOODS. Table 4, Chapter 12, lists available foods. These foods are for canine patients (not nutritionally complete for cats) during the very early recovery period and are usually fed short-term.
  LIQUID FOODS FOR EN-ASSISTED FEEDING. Foods for EN support for canine and feline patients are listed in Tables 4 and 5 (Chapter 12), respectively. These tables include glutamine;

Table 3. Key nutritional factors in selected commercial veterinary therapeutic foods for dogs with pancreatitis compared to recommended levels.* (See **Table 5** if the patient is obese or hypertriglyceridemic). (Numbers in red match optimal KNFs.)

Moist foods	Fat (%)	Protein (%)
Recommended levels	≤15	15-30
Hill's Prescription Diet i/d Canine	14.9	25.0
Iams Veterinary Formula Intestinal Low-Residue	13.2	35.9
Medi-Cal Gastro Formula	11.7	22.1
Purina Veterinary Diets EN GastroENteric Formula	13.8	30.5
Royal Canin Veterinary Diet Digestive Low Fat LF	6.9	31.9
Royal Canin Veterinary Diet Intestinal HE	11.8	23.1
Dry foods	**Fat (%)**	**Protein (%)**
Recommended levels	≤15	15-30
Hill's Prescription Diet i/d Canine	14.1	26.2
Iams Veterinary Formula Intestinal Low-Residue	10.7	24.6
Medi-Cal Gastro Formula	13.9	22.9
Purina Veterinary Diets EN GastroENteric Formula	12.6	27.0
Royal Canin Veterinary Diet Digestive Low Fat LF 20	6.6	24.2
Royal Canin Veterinary Diet Intestinal HE 28	22.0	33.0

*Manufacturers' published values. Nutrients expressed as % dry matter.

Table 4. Key nutritional factors in selected commercial veterinary therapeutic foods for cats with pancreatitis compared to recommended levels.* (See **Table 6** if the patient is obese or hypertriglyceridemic). (Numbers in red match optimal KNFs.)

Moist foods	Fat (%)	Protein (%)
Recommended levels	≤25	30-40
Hill's Prescription Diet i/d Feline	24.1	37.6
Iams Veterinary Formula Intestinal Low-Residue	11.7	38.4
Medi-Cal HYPOallergenic/Gastro	35.9	35.5
Medi-Cal Sensitivity CR	35.1	34.5
Dry foods	**Fat (%)**	**Protein (%)**
Recommended levels	≤25	30-40
Hill's Prescription Diet i/d Feline	20.2	40.3
Iams Veterinary Formula Intestinal Low-Residue	13.7	35.8
Medi-Cal HYPOallergenic/Gastro	11.5	29.8
Purina Veterinary Diets EN GastroENteric	18.4	56.2
Royal Canin Veterinary Diet Intestinal HE 30	23.7	34.4

*Manufacturers' published values. Nutrients expressed as % dry matter.

glutamine may facilitate reestablishment of GI tract integrity/function following NPO/prolonged inadequate food intake. The KNF contents of these foods can be compared to the KNF recommendations in **Table 2** to help with food selection.
Foods for Recovery/Prevention of Recurrence. Several commercial foods are marketed for management of pancreatitis. **Tables 3** (dogs) and **4** (cats) list foods marketed for patients of normal body weight/BCS and compare their KNF contents to KNF recommendations. **Tables 5** and **6** (dogs and cats, respectively) provide KNF contents of foods for obese and/or hypertriglyceridemic pancreatitis patients and compare them to recommended levels. Prescribe a food that most closely fits recommended KNF levels.

Assess and Determine the Feeding Method
Careful introduction of the prescribed food for recovery/prevention of recurrence is necessary to avoid relapse. Chapters 12 and 13 provide feeding method information for EN/PN support.
Determine Much Food to Feed. The amount to feed can be obtained from product labels (or other supporting materials or Appendix C). If body weight and BCS are not ideal, adjust food

dosage estimates appropriately over time (see Followup below).
Manage Food Changes. After the patient's condition has stabilized, gradually reintroduce the prescribed food to avoid relapse and facilitate acceptance. Care must be taken: initially feed ≤10% of the estimated dose of the prescribed food on Day 1 and continue this incremental increase daily until the total food dose estimate is achieved in 7-10 days. If problems occur, delay the increase or cut back to the previous day's level for a few days before continuing reintroduction of food. Appendix E provides additional information.
Consider How to Offer the Food. Initially, divide the amount being fed into multiple small offerings/day to help minimize pancreatic stimulation and potential for relapse. The patient's regular feeding methods can be reintroduced following several days without clinical signs, unless dietary indiscretion or inappropriate foods or feeding methods contributed to the original problem.
Manage Treats and Snacks. After the successful transition to the prescribed food, if the owner desires to feed treats/snacks, commercial treats that match the nutritional profile recommended for pancreatitis are best. Most companies offer treats

Table 5. Key nutritional factors in selected commercial veterinary therapeutic foods for obese or hypertriglyceridemic dogs with pancreatitis compared to recommended levels.* (Numbers in red match optimal KNFs.)

Moist foods	Fat (%)	Protein (%)
Recommended levels	≤10	15-30
Hill's Prescription Diet w/d Canine	12.7	17.9
Medi-Cal Fibre Formula	9.1	24.8
Purina Veterinary Diets OM Overweight Management Formula	8.4	44.1
Dry foods	Fat (%)	Protein (%)
Recommended levels	≤10	15-30
Hill's Prescription Diet w/d Canine	9.0	18.9
Medi-Cal Fibre Formula	10.6	26.2
Purina Veterinary Diets DCO Dual Fiber Control	12.4	25.3
Purina Veterinary Diets OM Overweight Management Formula	7.2	31.1
Royal Canin Veterinary Diet Calorie Control CC 26 High Fiber	10.4	30.9
Royal Canin Veterinary Diet Diabetic HF 18	9.9	22

*Manufacturers' published values. Nutrients expressed as % dry matter.

Table 6. Key nutritional factors in selected commercial veterinary therapeutic foods for obese or hypertriglyceridemic cats with pancreatitis compared to recommended levels.* (Numbers in red match optimal KNFs.)

Moist foods	Fat (%)	Protein (%)
Recommended levels	≤15	30-40
Hill's Prescription Diet w/d Feline with Chicken	16.6	39.6
Medi-Cal Fibre Formula	17.1	40.0
Purina Veterinary Diets OM Overweight Management Formula	14.6	44.6
Royal Canin Veterinary Diets Calorie Control CC High Fiber	21.3	33.5
Dry foods	Fat (%)	Protein (%)
Recommended levels	≤15	30-40
Hill's Prescription Diet w/d Feline	9.8	39.0
Hill's Prescription Diet w/d Feline with Chicken	9.9	39.9
Medi-Cal Fibre Formula	12.2	34.2
Purina Veterinary Diets OM Overweight Management Formula	8.5	56.2
Royal Canin Veterinary Diets Calorie Control CC 29 High Fiber	10.2	33.5

*Manufacturers' published values. Nutrients expressed as % dry matter.

that correspond to their specific veterinary therapeutic foods. Treats/snacks should not be fed excessively (<10% of the total diet on a volume, weight or calorie basis). For more information see Appendix B.

Food and Water Receptacle Husbandry. Food and water bowls should be washed regularly with warm soapy water and rinsed well. Dishes used for moist foods need daily cleaning. Discard moist or moistened dry foods after 2-4 hours of room temperature exposure to avoid foodborne illnesses (Appendix F).

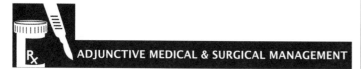

ADJUNCTIVE MEDICAL & SURGICAL MANAGEMENT

Antiemetics
Maropitant, dolasetron and ondansetron are potent injectable antiemetics and are recommended to encourage food intake during initial reintroduction of foods or for intractable vomiting. They can also be used with continuous EN feeding by tube to allow for early initiation of nutritional support.

Analgesics
Aggressive pain control with single agents or combination therapy with opioids, lidocaine, ketamine or epidurals is recommended.

Gastric Acidity Modifiers
Consider H_2-receptor blockers or proton pump inhibitors to control gastric acidity.

Antibiotics
Indicated if signs of sepsis are present.

Surgery
Exploration of the abdomen may be necessary for extirpation/drainage of pancreatic abscesses or pseudocysts; if so, consider inserting a jejunostomy tube at the time of surgery for assisted feeding to facilitate recovery.

FOLLOWUP

Owner Followup

After the patient returns home, the owner should observe for recurrence of signs indicative of a relapse; if signs recur, immediately notify the veterinarian. Record daily food intake and BCS (and body weight if practical) every 2 weeks. If necessary, change the amount fed by 10% increments and recheck the patient every 2 weeks for 1 month. At that point, the amount fed can be changed again and the cycle repeated until the patient reaches a normal body weight/BCS.

Compliance. Work with the veterinary health care team to ensure compliance with home care orders for dietary and medical management. Do not feed unprescribed foods or treats. Deny access to other foods, if the house has multiple pets.

Veterinary Health Care Team Followup

Assess hospitalized patients frequently. Resolution of abdominal pain, improvement in attitude, appetite and activity level and resolution of GI signs are important indicators of progress. Monitor leukograms and serum for lipemia, amylase, lipase, PLI and bilirubin.

Recurrence of Clinical Signs. Reevaluate for pancreatic pseudocysts, necrosis or abscesses, which can be sequelae to acute pancreatitis. Consider possible home care compliance issues.

MISCELLANEOUS

See Chapters 7, 25, 26, 43, 67 and 68, Small Animal Clinical Nutrition, 5th edition, for more information.

Cobalamin

Assessment of serum cobalamin is recommended in cats with pancreatitis complicated by IBD or triaditis. If levels are depleted, parenteral supplementation is recommended (weekly SQ cobalamin therapy [250 μg/cat] for 4-6 weeks or until serum levels return to the normal range. Once/twice monthly therapy may be required for longer-term maintenance.

Antioxidants

In people with chronic pancreatitis, supplemental selenium, vitamin C, vitamin E, β-carotene and methionine, resulted in a 50% reduction in painful days/month. Similar trials have not been performed in chronic or acute pancreatitis in veterinary patients. Chapter 7, Small Animal Clinical Nutrition, 5th edition, provides more information about antioxidants.

Authors

Condensed from Chapter 67, Small Animal Clinical Nutrition, 5th edition, authored by Deborah J. Davenport, Rebecca L. Remillard and Kenny W. Simpson.

References

See Chapter 67, Small Animal Clinical Nutrition, 5th edition, on the website www.markmorrisinstitute.org for references.

CLINICAL POINTS

- See Chapter 54 for feeding plans and general information about feline hepatic lipidosis and feline cholangitis patients.
- Hepatobiliary diseases can have numerous etiologies, all of which have the potential to disrupt the broad-spectrum of liver functions including: drug metabolism, removal of noxious substances, synthesis of important substances (e.g., albumin, clotting factors) and food digestion/nutrient metabolism.
- An estimated 2-3% of all patients presented at one veterinary teaching hospital had some form of hepatobiliary disease; **Table 1** provides a frequency distribution of liver diseases.
- Reactive hepatopathies result from the liver being damaged secondarily by other diseases.
- Chronic hepatitis can result from many different causes including copper accumulation, infectious diseases, drugs, breed-associated hepatitis and possibly autoimmune disease. Cirrhosis results from fibrosis and impairs blood and bile flow and nutrient exchange, perpetuating hepatocellular injury.
- Neoplasia may be localized or diffuse; the most common types are metastases, lymphoma, hemangiosarcoma, hepatocellular carcinoma and cholangiocarcinoma. Due to the tremendous regenerative capacity of the liver, tumors may go undetected for long periods.
- There are various types of congenital PSS and, depending on the type, they occur most frequently in certain dog breeds and mixed-breed cats. Acquired PSS can be due to cirrhosis, tumors or portal vein thrombosis.
- Bedlington terriers often develop copper storage disease. The role of copper in liver diseases in other breeds is less clear. Breeds thought to have primary copper-associated hepatopathies include West Highland white terriers, Skye terriers, Doberman pinschers, Dalmatian dogs and Labrador retrievers. The disease seen in these dogs is different than in Bedlington terriers; hepatic copper levels are lower and do not increase with age.
- Hepatic copper content is also increased in patients with cholestatic liver disease. Copper plays a minimal role, if any, in feline liver diseases.
- HE is a neurologic syndrome that may arise due to liver dysfunction or PSS. Chronic HE results from disturbances in various neurotransmitter systems caused by a variety of gut-derived toxins and compounds; acute HE is uncommon.
- Irrespective of the primary liver disease, the hepatic reaction pattern is similar; thus, most liver disorders (if severe/longstanding) lead to syndromes with potentially serious consequences (e.g., cholestasis, icterus, portal hypertension, ascites and HE).
- Malnutrition may be a problem with longstanding liver disease

Abbreviations
AAFCO = Association of American Feed Control Officials
BCS = body condition score (Appendix A)
CKD = chronic kidney disease
DM = dry matter
HE = hepatic encephalopathy
KNF = key nutritional factor
PSS = portosystemic shunt

and is often associated with anorexia, nausea and vomiting; however, it can also occur in the face of normal food intake due to impaired nutrient digestion, absorption and metabolism.
- Understanding the specific etiology of a patient's liver disease is important for formulating an effective treatment plan; additional laboratory, imaging and/or histopathology may be required because clinical signs are often nondefinitive. **Table 2** lists the most important clinical signs of liver diseases and the frequencies with which they occur.
- Liver disease is often discovered by hematologic, serum biochemistry and urine tests performed either as part of a routine wellness screen or diagnostic evaluation of a sick patient. It is beyond the scope of this chapter to review in detail the laboratory tests and imaging techniques recommended for diagnosis of the various hepatobiliary diseases.
- Hepatic tissue has a high capacity for repair and regeneration with appropriate nutritional and medical support.
- Provision of proper energy/nutrient intake is the cornerstone of successful dietary management of patients with chronic hepatitis, cirrhosis, PSS and copper-associated hepatotoxicosis.
- Adequate dietary protein, arginine and taurine are important for patients with chronic hepatitis, cirrhosis and portal hypertension and dogs with copper-associated hepatotoxicosis. However, protein restriction may be necessary for patients with endstage cirrhosis, hyperammonemia and HE. The goal is to provide adequate protein to support hepatic regeneration while avoiding excesses that might contribute to HE.
- Dogs with chronic liver disease and HE may develop hypokalemia due to inadequate potassium intake, vomiting and other contributing factors. Hypokalemia, especially in combination with alkalosis, is problematic because it may prolong anorexia and exacerbate HE. Foods for liver-disease patients should provide adequate potassium; supplementation may be required in certain cases.
- Liver-disease patients with ascites, portal hypertension and/or significant hypoalbuminemia should not be fed foods that provide excess sodium and chloride.
- Trace minerals such as copper and iron should be minimized to avoid toxic accumulation in patients susceptible to sequestering these minerals in their livers. Controlling copper intake before serious injury occurs is important for dogs susceptible to copper-associated hepatotoxicosis.

Table 1. Frequency distribution of liver diseases in dogs and cats.

Dogs*	Frequency (%)
Reactive hepatitis	25
Chronic hepatitis/cirrhosis	17
Portosystemic shunts	16
Liver tumors (primary, metastases)	14
Malignant lymphoma	14
Other conditions	12
Extrahepatic cholestasis	2
Cats**	
Lipidosis (idiopathic and secondary)	26
Cholangitis	25
Neoplasia (malignant and benign)	20
Reactive hepatopathies	16
Other conditions	8
Vascular anomalies	5

*Adapted from Rothuizen J, Meyer HP. History, physical examination, and signs of liver disease. In: Ettinger SJ, Feldman EC, eds. Textbook of Veterinary Internal Medicine: Diseases of the Dog and Cat, 5th ed. Philadelphia, PA: WB Saunders Co, 2000; 1272-1277.
**Twedt DC. 175 consecutive liver biopsies in cats: Unpublished data. College of Veterinary Medicine and Biomedical Sciences, Colorado State University, Fort Collins, Colorado.

Table 2. Clinical signs that most often accompany primary liver disease in dogs.*

Signs	Frequency of occurrence (%)
Apathy and listlessness	60
Reduced appetite	59
Vomiting	58
Weight loss	50
Polydipsia/polyuria	45
Diarrhea	27
Reduced endurance	27
Ascites	25
Neurologic signs	12
Icterus	12
Acholic feces	7

*Adapted from Rothuizen J, Meyer HP. History, physical examination, and signs of liver disease. In: Ettinger SJ, Feldman EC, eds. Textbook of Veterinary Internal Medicine: Diseases of the Dog and Cat, 5th ed. Philadelphia, PA: WB Saunders Co, 2000; 1272-1277.

Table 3. Key nutritional factors for dogs and cats with hepatobiliary disease.*

Factors	Dogs	Cats
Energy density (kcal/g)	≥4.0	≥4.2
Energy density (kJ/g)	≥16.7	≥17.6
Protein (%)	15-20**	30-35**
Arginine (%)	–	1.5 to 2.0
Taurine (%)	≥0.1	≥0.3
Sodium (%)	0.08 to 0.25	0.07 to 0.3
Copper (mg/kg)	≤5	–
Zinc (mg/kg)	>200	>200
Iron (mg/kg)	80 to 140	80 to 140
Vitamin E (IU/kg)	≥400	≥500
Vitamin C (mg/kg)	≥100	100 to 200

*Nutrients expressed on a dry matter basis.
**For liver disease patients with signs of hepatic encephalopathy, dry matter dietary protein levels should be limited to 10 to 15% for dogs and 25 to 30% for cats until signs resolve.

- In addition to the direct hepatoprotective effects of zinc (e.g., antioxidant/antifibrotic activities), it also blocks intestinal absorption of copper in dogs with copper-associated hepatotoxicosis. Besides containing appropriate copper levels, foods for these patients should provide adequate zinc and/or be supplemented with zinc.
- Lipid peroxidation may be involved in the pathogenesis of some forms of acute liver injury and chronic hepatitis; increased levels of antioxidant vitamins E and C in foods for liver disease patients may be beneficial.
- For hepatobiliary-disease patients, multiple small meals/day may help improve digestibility, improve nitrogen balance and may be better accepted by nauseated patients. Also, multiple meals may decrease the amount of digesta entering the colon at any one time, which reduces the potential for excessive toxin production.
- Prognoses vary by specific disease: Predicting individual response to dietary/medical/surgical management of PSS is difficult.
- Feeding goals: The goals of nutritional management for hepatobiliary diseases include: 1) correcting fluid/electrolyte disturbances, 2) supporting the liver's normal metabolic processes and homeostatic functions, 3) providing nutrients that support hepatocellular repair and regeneration, 4) mitigating further oxidative damage to liver tissue and 5) preventing/managing HE.

KEY NUTRITIONAL FACTORS

- Foods should provide recommended allowances of all required nutrients (nutritional adequacy), but should also contain specific levels of KNFs appropriate for dietary management of liver diseases.
- KNFs for managing hepatobiliary diseases cover profiles that will benefit most liver-disease patients in the following categories: 1) patients with general hepatobiliary diseases and 2) patients with liver disease with HE. However, due to the wide ranges of liver diseases within a category and their differing severity, the recommended KNF category profiles might not always be ideal for a given patient. KNFs for foods for dogs and cats with hepatobiliary disease and recommended amounts are listed in **Table 3**. KNF recommendations for liver disease patients with HE are also included in **Table 3** (footnote). All KNFs are discussed in more detail in Chapter 68, Small Animal Clinical Nutrition, 5th edition.
- Copper restriction (≤mg DM copper/kg food) is a KNF for foods for dogs with inherited copper-related hepatotoxicosis and cholestatic disease (note: this level of restriction is almost twice the minimum recommended allowance).

Table 4. Levels of key nutritional factors in selected commercial veterinary therapeutic foods marketed for dogs with hepatobiliary disease compared to recommended levels.* (Numbers in red match optimal KNFs.)

Dry foods	Energy density (kcal/cup)**	Energy density (kcal ME/g)	Protein (%)***	Taurine (%)	Sodium (%)	Copper (mg/kg)	Zinc (mg/kg)	Iron (mg/kg)	Vit. E (IU/kg)	Vit. C (mg/kg)
Recommended levels	–	≥4.0	15-20	≥0.1	0.08-0.25	≤5	>200	80-140	≥400	≥100
Hill's Prescription Diet										
l/d Canine	399	4.4	18.1	0.08	0.22	4.9	301	170	385	116
Medi-Cal Hepatic LS 14	342	na	17.6	na	0.2	na	300	na	na	na
Medi-Cal Vegetarian Formula	317	na	20.9	na	0.4	na	na	na	na	na
Purina Veterinary Diets										
EN GastroENteric	397	4.2	27.0	na	0.60	na	na	na	577	na
Royal Canin Veterinary										
Diet Hepatic LS 14	333	4.4	17.6	0.22	0.21	4.4	253	187	725	na

Moist foods	Energy density (kcal/can)**	Energy density (kcal ME/g)	Protein (%)***	Taurine (%)	Sodium (%)	Copper (mg/kg)	Zinc (mg/kg)	Iron (mg/kg)	Vit. E (IU/kg)	Vit. C (mg/kg)
Recommended levels	–	≥4.0	15-20	≥0.1	0.08-0.25	≤5	>200	80-140	≥400	≥100
Hill's Prescription Diet										
l/d Canine	472/13 oz.	4.5	17.6	0.10	0.20	4.2	258	118	693	190
Iams Veterinary Formula										
Stress/Weight Gain	333/6 oz.	5.8	41.8	0.33	0.24	na	na	na	na	na
Formula Maximum-Calorie										
Medi-Cal Vegetarian										
Formula	319/396 g	na	26.4	na	0.5	na	na	na	na	na
Purina Veterinary Diets										
EN GastroENteric	423/12.5 oz.	4.0	30.5	na	0.37	na	260	na	505	139

Key: ME = metabolizable energy, Vit. E = vitamin E, Vit. C = vitamin C, na = information not available from manufacturer.
*From manufacturers' published information or calculated from manufacturers' published as-fed values; all values are on a dry matter basis unless otherwise stated.
**Energy density values are listed on an as fed basis and are useful for determining the amount to feed; cup = 8-oz. measuring cup. To convert to kJ, multiply kcal by 4.184.
***For liver disease patients with signs of hepatic encephalopathy (HE), dietary protein levels should be limited to 10 to 15% dry matter until signs resolve. In these cases, several commercial veterinary therapeutic foods designed for patients with kidney disease that provide less protein than the foods intended for liver disease may be appropriate (Table 3, Chapter 26). If these foods are used, the patient should be transitioned to the selected food specifically formulated for liver disease after signs of HE have subsided.

FEEDING PLAN

For best success, dietary therapy for liver disease is performed in conjunction with appropriate medical/surgical management (see Adjunctive Medical & Surgical Management below). In acute hepatic failure, correction of fluid/electrolyte imbalances and treatment of other complications take precedence over initiation of nutritional support.

Assess and Select the Food

Ensure the Food's Basic Nutritional Adequacy. AAFCO nutritional adequacy statements are usually found on a product's label. AAFCO approval does not ensure a food will be effective for management of hepatobiliary diseases.

Compare the Food's KNF Content with the Recommended Levels. Several commercial foods are marketed for management of hepatobiliary diseases (**Tables 4** [dogs] and **5** [cats]). Choose a food that most closely fits recommended levels.

PATIENTS WITH HE. Limit dietary protein levels to 10-15% (DM) for dogs and 25-30% (DM) for cats until signs resolve. Consider foods designed for CKD patients (Tables 3 and 4, Chapter 26, for dogs and cats, respectively). These foods typically provide less protein. After signs of HE have resolved, transition patients to the food prescribed for liver disease.

COPPER-ASSOCIATED HEPATOTOXICOSIS PATIENTS. Foods with moderate copper restriction (≤5mg copper/kg food [DM]) are recommended. However, for Bedlington terriers with clinical/subclinical liver disease, adjunctive treatment with copper chelating agents may be indicated (see Adjunctive Medical & Surgical Management below).

POSTOPERATIVE PSS PATIENTS. After recovery from surgery, patients can often be fed their regular foods.

Manage Treats and Snacks. After a patient has stabilized and is readily consuming a prescribed food, if the owner desires to feed treats/snacks, suggest commercial treats that match the KNFs in the food being fed. Most companies offer treats that correspond to their specific veterinary therapeutic foods. An option is to use the opposite form of the food being fed; i.e., if a dry food is fed, offer small amounts of the same food in moist form as a snack and vice versa; keep kibbles of dry food in a separate container away from the usual feeding area and use as treats. Treats/snacks should not be fed excessively (<10% of the total diet on a volume, weight or calorie basis).

COPPER-ASSOCIATED HEPATOTOXICOSIS PATIENTS. Avoid using commercial treats (unless the copper content is appropriate [<5 mg copper/kg food DM]) or human foods with increased copper content as treats/snacks. Liver and shellfish are

Table 5. Levels of key nutritional factors in selected commercial veterinary therapeutic foods marketed for cats with hepatobiliary disease, compared to recommended levels.* (Numbers in red match optimal KNFs.)

Dry foods	Energy density (kcal/cup)**	Energy density (kcal ME/g)	Protein (%)***	Arginine (%)	Taurine (%)	Sodium (%)	Zinc (mg/kg)	Iron (mg/kg)	Vit. E (IU/kg)	Vit. C (mg/kg)
Recommended levels	–	≥4.2	30-35	1.5-2.0	≥0.3	0.07-0.30	>200	80-140	≥500	100-200
Hill's Prescription Diet										
l/d Feline	505	**4.5**	**31.8**	**1.98**	**0.53**	**0.27**	**305**	173	267	**109**
Medi-Cal Mature Formula	355	na	29.2	na	**0.4**	0.4	na	na	na	na
Medi-Cal Reduced Protein	440	na	28.1	na	**0.4**	**0.3**	na	na	na	na
Medi-Cal Renal LP 21	409	na	24.7	na	0.2	**0.2**	na	na	na	na
Purina Veterinary Diets EN										
GastroENteric	572	**4.4**	56.2	na	**0.32**	0.64	na	na	232	na
Royal Canin Veterinary Diet										
Modified Formula	432	**4.7**	27.1	**1.51**	0.23	**0.23**	**320**	241	380	na

Moist foods	Energy density (kcal/can)**	Energy density (kcal ME/g)	Protein (%)***	Arginine (%)	Taurine (%)	Sodium (%)	Zinc (mg/kg)	Iron (mg/kg)	Vit. E (IU/kg)	Vit. C (mg/kg)
Recommended levels	–	≥4.2	30-35	1.5-2.0	≥0.3	0.07-0.30	>200	80-140	≥500	100-200
Hill's Prescription Diet										
l/d Feline	183/5.5 oz.	**4.7**	**31.6**	**2.00**	**0.52**	**0.20**	**336**	212	**836**	**124**
Medi-Cal Mature Formula	205/170 g	na	41.5	na	**0.3**	**0.3**	na	na	na	na
Medi-Cal Reduced										
Protein	265/170 g	na	**33.9**	na	**0.3**	**0.2**	na	na	na	na
Medi-Cal Renal LP	125/85 g pouch	na	29.3	na	**0.8**	0.6	na	na	na	na
Royal Canin Veterinary	256/170 g									
Diet Modified Formula	596/396 g	**6.1**	**34.7**	2.07	0.28	**0.28**	**208**	545	178	na

Key: ME = metabolizable energy, Vit. E = vitamin E, Vit. C = vitamin C, na = information not available from manufacturer.
*From manufacturers' published information or calculated from manufacturers' published as-fed values; all values are on a dry matter basis unless otherwise stated.
**Energy density values are listed on an as fed basis and are useful for determining the amount to feed; cup = 8-oz. measuring cup. To convert to kJ, multiply kcal by 4.184.
***For liver disease patients with signs of hepatic encephalopathy (HE), dietary protein levels should be limited to 25 to 30% dry matter until signs resolve. In these cases, several commercial veterinary therapeutic foods designed for patients with kidney disease that provide less protein than the foods intended for liver disease may be appropriate (Table 4, Chapter 26). If these foods are used, the patient should be transitioned to the selected food specifically formulated for liver disease after signs of HE have subsided.

high in copper; cheese, cottage cheese, rice and tofu are low in copper.

Assess and Determine the Feeding Method

Determine How Much Food to Feed. The amount to feed can be obtained from product labels (or other supporting material) or calculated (Appendix C). After the patient has transitioned to the prescribed food, food dosages will likely need to be modified to achieve/maintain optimal body weight/BCS (see Followup below). Feeding amounts for patients with HE are determined similarly.

Consider How to Offer the Food. The predetermined food dose (above) should be divided into multiple small meals fed throughout the day.

Manage Food Changes. A transition period to avoid GI upsets and facilitate acceptance of the prescribed food is good practice. Replace 25% of the original food with the prescribed food on Day 1 and continue this incremental change daily until the change is complete on Day 4. If problems occur, delay the increase or cut back to the previous level of transition for several more days before continuing the food change. Appendix E provides additional information.

Food and Water Receptacle Husbandry. Food and water bowls should be washed regularly with warm soapy water and rinsed well. Dishes used for moist foods need daily cleaning. Discard moist or moistened dry foods after 2-4 hours of room temperature exposure to avoid foodborne illnesses (Appendix F).

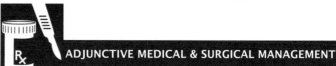

ADJUNCTIVE MEDICAL & SURGICAL MANAGEMENT

Table 6 summarizes general therapy for patients with hepatobiliary diseases including medical/surgical recommendations. Other surgical interventions that may be necessary include partial/total ligation of congenital PSS and removal of focal liver masses.

Copper Chelators

In addition to copper-restricted foods, adjunctive treatment with copper chelators may be necessary, particularly for Bedlington terriers with clinical/subclinical copper-associated hepatotoxicosis. Chelator treatment is also used for dogs with copper-associated chronic hepatitis and cirrhosis that have been documented by histopathology and/or elevated hepatic copper levels (generally >1,000-2,000 ppm dry weight). Copper chelating agents include D-penicillamine and trientine.

Zinc

Zinc is also used to reduce dietary copper absorption. If foods do

Table 6. General therapy for patients with hepatobiliary disease.*

Fluid therapy	
Maintain hydration	Give appropriate parenteral fluid therapy
Prevent hypokalemia	Add KCl to maintenance fluids
Maintain acid-base balance	Use potassium-replete food or potassium supplement
Prevent or control hypoglycemia	Avoid alkalosis in patients with hepatic encephalopathy
	Add dextrose to parenteral fluids as needed
Nutritional support	
Maintain caloric intake	Ensure that daily energy requirement is being met; if not, begin assisted feeding
Provide adequate vitamins and minerals	Add B vitamins to fluids or give as injection
Modify feeding plan to control complications	Use complete and balanced food
	See specific complications below
Control hepatic encephalopathy	
Modify food and prevent formation and absorption of enteric toxins	Avoid excess dietary protein
	Use retention enemas q6h containing lactulose or povidone iodine solution
	Give lactulose orally
Control GI hemorrhage	Treat GI parasites, treat gastric ulcers, avoid drugs that exacerbate GI hemorrhage (e.g., aspirin, glucocorticoids)
Correct metabolic imbalances	See fluid therapy above
Avoid drugs or therapies that exacerbate hepatic encephalopathy	Do not administer sedatives, analgesics, anesthetics, diuretics, stored blood or methionine-containing products
Control seizures	Use appropriate anticonvulsant drugs (e.g., potassium bromide)
Control infection	Give systemic antimicrobials (see below)
Control ascites and edema	Avoid excess dietary sodium chloride
	Administer diuretics (e.g., furosemide, spironolactone)
Control coagulation defects and anemia	Give vitamin K_1 parenterally
	Give fresh plasma or blood transfusion as needed
Control GI ulceration	Give H_2 blockers (e.g., ranitidine) or cytoprotective agents (e.g., sucralfate)
Control infection and endotoxemia	Give systemic antibiotics (e.g., penicillin, ampicillin, cephalosporins, aminoglycosides, metronidazole)
	Give intestinal antibiotics (e.g., neomycin)
Manage cholestasis	Give bile "altering" or choleretic drugs (e.g., ursodiol)
	Correct extrahepatic bile duct obstruction

*Adapted from Johnson SE, Sherding RG. Diseases of the liver and biliary tract. In: Birchard SJ, Sherding RG, eds. Manual of Small Animal Practice. Philadelphia, PA: WB Saunders Co, 1994; 730.

not contain >200 mg/kg zinc (DM) consider oral supplemental zinc in the form of zinc acetate (50-100 mg zinc/day b.i.d. [between meals]), zinc gluconate (3 mg/kg/day) or zinc sulfate (2 mg/kg/day) divided into 3 doses.

Antioxidant Vitamins E and C

Besides ensuring increased amounts in foods, consider supplemental amounts for dogs with inflammatory liver disease; oral doses are 50-400 IU vitamin E/day and 500-1,000 mg vitamin C/day.

Lactulose

Considered one of the treatments of choice for HE. Beneficial effects are probably due to: 1) increased intraluminal colonic nitrogen retention, 2) increased intestinal transit rate and 3) decreased ammonia generation. Dosage varies: 2.5-25 ml, t.i.d. for dogs and 1-3 ml, t.i.d. for cats. Titrate to produce a "porridge-like" stool. Reduce dose if stool becomes watery.

S-adenosylmethionine (SAMe)

SAMe acts in part like an antioxidant by replenishing hepatic glutathione stores, either by increasing glutathione (cats) or by preventing depletion (dogs). Glutathione depletion can increase hepatocyte oxidative stress.

Silymarin

A flavonolignan from "milk thistle" that has antioxidant properties and several other purported benefits for liver disease. Has been shown to be hepatocytoprotective against certain toxins. Unfortunately, purity of various products and ideal therapeutic doses are unknown, which limit its use.

 FOLLOWUP

Owner Followup

After the patient returns home, if possible, record daily food intake and frequency/severity of vomiting, diarrhea, icterus and neurobehavioral signs. Note BCS (and body weight if practical) every 2 weeks. If necessary, change the amount of food being fed by 10% increments and recheck the patient every 2 weeks for 1 month. At that point, the amount fed can be changed again and the cycle repeated until the patient reaches a normal body weight/BCS.

Veterinary Health Care Team Followup

In-clinic reassessment includes review of owner data (above). Improvement of attitude, activity, appetite and resolution of GI signs (vomiting and diarrhea) are good indicators of success. Serial laboratory evaluations (every few days-weeks) of serum liver enzyme activity, bile acids and potassium and blood ammonia are useful. Serial hepatic biopsy specimens can be evaluated every 4-6 months for copper content and presence/absence of inflammatory hepatopathies. Many patients can be returned to their regular foods after hepatobiliary disease has resolved.

Patients With Ascites. Monitor body weight and abdominal configuration; ultrasonography is useful.

Patients With Persistent Vomiting. Be sure small frequent meals are fed. Continuous tube feeding and antiemetics may be helpful. For HE patients, more aggressive medical treatment (e.g., lactulose) may be necessary.

MISCELLANEOUS

See Chapters 25, 37 and 68, Small Animal Clinical Nutrition, 5th edition, for more information.

Appetite Stimulants

Anabolic steroids and benzodiazepines are not recommended. If used, do so advisedly due to the potential for hepatotoxicity; also, benzodiazepines may be involved in the pathogenesis of HE.

Authors

Condensed from Chapter 68, Small Animal Clinical Nutrition, 5th edition, authored by Hein P. Meyer, David C. Twedt, Philip Roudebush and Elizabeth Dill-Macky.

References

See Chapter 68, Small Animal Clinical Nutrition, 5th edition, on the website www.markmorrisinstitute.org for references.

Chapter
54 Feline Hepatic Lipidosis and Cholangitis

CLINICAL POINTS

- Feline hepatic lipidosis and cholangitis are distinct liver diseases; however, they have similar feeding plans and, therefore, are included together in this chapter. They are the 2 most common liver diseases in cats.
- Feline hepatic lipidosis is characterized by accumulation of excess fat in hepatocytes with resulting cholestasis and hepatic dysfunction.
- Hepatic lipidosis usually results from prolonged inadequate food intake but may be secondary to diabetes mellitus, diseases resulting in anorexia and weight loss (e.g., pancreatitis, IBD) or as an idiopathic disorder of unknown etiology. Obese patients experiencing rapid weight loss are at increased risk.
- Clinical signs of hepatic lipidosis may include anorexia, weight loss, jaundice, GI signs (vomiting, diarrhea or constipation), weakness/inactivity, HE, ptyalism (especially with HE) and abnormalities associated with underlying disease, if present.
- Laboratory findings associated with hepatic lipidosis include anemia (variable), hyperbilirubinemia and increased AP, ALT and GGT (mildly elevated) values; the leukogram may reflect

Abbreviations
AAFCO = Association of American Feed Control Officials
ALT = alanine aminotransferase
AP = alkaline phosphatase
BCS = body condition score (Appendix A)
CKD = chronic kidney disease
DM = dry matter
EN = enteral nutrition
GGT = gamma glutamyltransferase
HE = hepatic encephalopathy
IBD = inflammatory bowel disease
KNF = key nutritional factor
PE = parenteral nutrition

an underlying disorder.
- Imaging results for hepatic lipidosis: survey abdominal radiographs may indicate hepatomegaly; ultrasonography may show hyperechogenicity.
- Cytology and histopathology should be used to evaluate liver biopsy specimens obtained from suspected hepatic lipidosis patients (pretreat with vitamin K_1).
- Cholangitis is inflammation of the biliary ducts (especially intrahepatic ducts and surrounding liver tissue). It is the

most common feline inflammatory liver disease and is usually caused by enteric bacteria (leukocytic form) or immunologic mechanisms (lymphocytic form). Cholangitis is often associated with concurrent cholecystitis, pancreatitis and IBD. Chronic cholangitis may progress to biliary cirrhosis.

- Many cats with cholangitis develop significant cholestasis and may have sludged/inspissated bile causing partial/complete biliary obstruction.
- The leukocytic form is more common in middle-aged/older cats; whereas the lymphocytic form is more common in younger cats.
- Clinical signs of cholangitis are form dependent: leukocytic-cholangitis patients present with anorexia, pyrexia, jaundice and abdominal pain; lymphocytic-cholangitis patients often present with jaundice and/or progressive ascites; they may/may not appear ill. Polyphagia may be present in lymphocytic-form patients with/without weight loss and hepatomegaly may be the most prominent physical exam finding. HE may develop in the latter stages if extensive cirrhosis and portal hypertension have occurred.
- Laboratory findings include leukocytosis with neutrophilia and a left shift in the leukocytic form and lymphopenia for the lymphocytic form. Increased AP, ALT, GGT and bilirubin occur in both forms (may be higher in lymphocytic form). If concurrent IBD or pancreatitis is present laboratory findings may also reflect abnormalities associated with these diseases (Chapters 43 and 52).
- Imaging results for cholangitis: survey abdominal radiographs may indicate hepatomegaly with lymphocytic forms; ultrasonography may reveal a hyperechoic liver in both forms with signs of biliary stasis in the leukocytic form.
- Liver biopsy specimens from cholangitis patients should be submitted for bacterial culture in addition to histopathology.
- Provision of adequate energy intake is the cornerstone of successful dietary management of cats with hepatic lipidosis but is also important for patients with cholangitis.
- Adequate dietary protein, arginine and taurine are important for cats with hepatic lipidosis. However, protein restriction may be necessary for patients with HE. The goal is to provide adequate protein to support hepatic regeneration/recovery while avoiding excesses that might contribute to HE.
- Cats with hepatic lipidosis with/without HE may develop hypokalemia due to inadequate potassium intake, vomiting and/or various other contributing factors. Hypokalemia, especially in combination with alkalosis, is problematic because it may prolong anorexia and exacerbate HE. Foods for hepatic lipidosis or cholangitis patients should provide adequate potassium; supplementation may be required in certain cases.
- Lipid peroxidation may be involved in the pathogenesis of some forms of liver tissue injury; increased food amounts containing antioxidant vitamins E and C may be beneficial.
- Dietary L-carnitine-supplemented foods appear to prevent obese cats undergoing rapid weight loss from accumulating excessive lipid in their hepatocytes. Adequate dietary L-carnitine intake may also benefit cats being treated for hepatic lipidosis.
- Feed multiple small meals/day to help minimize release of free fatty acids from adipose tissue, improve digestibility, improve nitrogen balance and increase acceptance in nauseated patients. Also, multiple meals may reduce the amount of digesta entering the colon at any one time, which reduces the potential for excessive toxin production and HE.
- Prognoses: hepatic lipidosis is reversible but resolution depends on the underlying disorder and appropriate nutritional support. Leukocytic cholangitis may be cured; long-term remission is possible for the chronic lymphocytic form.
- Manage underlying medical conditions if present; cats with cholangitis often develop significant cholestasis causing partial/complete biliary obstruction. Concurrent cholecystitis, pancreatitis and IBD are common in feline cholangitis patients and may warrant specific medical therapy.
- Feeding goals include providing nutritional support for: 1) hepatocellular repair and regeneration, 2) normal metabolic processes and homeostatic mechanisms performed by the liver, 3) mitigating further oxidative damage to liver tissue and 4) preventing HE or managing it if present.

KEY NUTRITIONAL FACTORS

- Foods should provide recommended allowances of all required nutrients (nutritional adequacy), but should also contain specific levels of KNFs appropriate for dietary management of hepatic lipidosis or cholangitis.
- Table 1 lists KNFs for the initial management of cats with hepatic lipidosis or cholangitis. After patients are eating on their own, refer to KNFs in Table 2 for foods for general liver disease patients. KNF recommendations for foods for patients with HE are included in Table 2. All KNFs are discussed in more detail in Chapter 68, Small Animal Clinical Nutrition, 5th edition.

FEEDING PLAN

In acute hepatic failure, correction of fluid/electrolyte imbalances and treatment of other complications take precedence over initiation of nutritional support. If patients are not eating on their own, initially provide assisted EN or PN feeding. For best success, dietary therapy is performed in conjunction with appropriate medical management (see Adjunctive Medical & Surgical Management below).

Assess and Select the Food
Ensure the Food's Basic Nutritional Adequacy. AAFCO nutritional adequacy statements are usually found on a product's label. AAFCO approval does not ensure a food will be effective for management of hepatic lipidosis or cholangitis.
Compare the Food's KNF Content with the Recommended Levels.

ANORECTIC PATIENTS. The patients require EN or PN

Table 1. Key nutritional factors for foods for assisted feeding of cats with hepatic lipidosis or cholangitis.	
Factors	**Recommended levels**
Osmolarity (mOsm/l)	250-400*
Energy density (kcal/ml)**	1 to 2
Energy density (kJ/ml)	4.184 to 8.37
Protein (g/100 kcal)	6.8 to 10.2
Arginine (mg/100 kcal)	340 to 450
Taurine (mg/100 kcal)	≥68
Potassium (mg/100 kcal)	180 to 230
L-carnitine (mg/100 kcal)	≥4.5

*250 is optimal.
**Energy density on an as fed basis.

Table 2. Key nutritional factors for cats with hepatobiliary disease.*	
Factors	**Recommended levels**
Energy density (kcal/g)	≥4.2
Energy density (kJ/g)	≥17.6
Protein (%)	30-35**
Arginine (%)	1.5 to 2.0
Taurine (%)	≥0.3
Sodium (%)	0.07 to 0.3
Zinc (mg/kg)	>200
Iron (mg/kg)	80 to 140
Vitamin E (IU/kg)	≥500
Vitamin C (mg/kg)	100 to 200

*Nutrients expressed on a dry matter basis.
**For liver disease patients with signs of hepatic encephalopathy, dry matter dietary protein levels should be limited to 25 to 30% until signs resolve.

support (Chapters 12 and 13). If necessary, be sure fluid/electrolyte abnormalities are corrected before initiation of assisted feeding. **Table 3** provides KNF information for foods for assisted EN feeding and compares them to KNF recommendations. Patients may develop learned aversions to foods if GI disturbances accompany liver disease; therefore, it is better to initially institute tube feeding rather than offer several different foods and possibly have the patient develop aversions. After signs of liver disease have completely resolved, transition patients to a food for liver disease or to maintenance foods.

Patients Eating on Their Own. Several commercial foods are marketed and (**Table 4**) suitable for cats with hepatic lipidosis or cholangitis. Choose a food that most closely fits recommended KNF levels.

Patients with HE. Limit dietary protein levels to 25-30% (DM) until signs resolve. Consider foods designed for CKD patients (Table 4, Chapter 26); they typically provide less protein. Again, after signs of HE have resolved, transition patients to the selected food for liver disease (**Table 4**).

Manage Treats and Snacks. After a patient has stabilized and is readily consuming a prescribed food, if the owner desires to feed treats/snacks, suggest commercial treats that match the KNFs in the food being fed. Most companies offer treats that correspond to their specific veterinary therapeutic foods. An option is to use the opposite form of the food being fed; i.e., if a dry food is fed, offer small amounts of the same food in moist form as a snack

and vice versa; keep kibbles of dry food in a separate container away from the usual feeding area and use as treats. Treats/snacks should not be fed excessively (<10% of the total diet on a volume, weight or calorie basis).

Assess and Determine the Feeding Method
Determine How Much Food to Feed.
Anorectic Patients. Refer to guidelines for EN or PN support, Chapters 12 and 13.
Patients Eating on Their Own. The amount to feed can be obtained from product labels (or other supporting material) or calculated (Appendix C). After the patient has transitioned to the prescribed food, food dosages will likely need to be modified to achieve/maintain optimal body weight/BCS (see Followup below). Amount to feed HE patients is determined similarly.
Consider How to Offer the Food.
Anorectic Patients. Methods for providing assisted EN or PN support for cats are described in Chapters 12 and 13.
Patients Eating on Their Own. The predetermined food dose (above) should be divided into multiple small meals fed throughout the day. This is particularly important for HE patients.
Manage Food Changes.
Anorectic Patients. Methods for transitioning patients on to/off of assisted EN or PN support are described in Chapters 12 and 13, respectively. To avoid refeeding syndrome in malnourished hepatic lipidosis patients, transition gradually: provide approximately 25% of the patient's estimated daily feeding amount on Day 1 and increase to the full amount over 6-7 days. If electrolyte abnormalities occur (refeeding syndrome), reduce amount being fed by 50% and initiate corrective fluid/electrolyte therapy. Following stabilization, continue the gradual transition. Chapter 12 also provides information about refeeding syndrome.
Patients Eating on Their Own. A transition period to avoid GI upsets and facilitate acceptance of the prescribed food is good practice. Replace 25% of the original food with the prescribed food on Day 1 and continue this incremental change daily until the change is complete on Day 4. If problems occur, delay the increase or cut back to the previous level of transition for several more days before continuing the food change. Appendix E provides additional information.
Food and Water Receptacle Husbandry. Food and water bowls should be washed regularly with warm soapy water and rinsed well. Dishes used for moist foods need daily cleaning. Discard moist or moistened dry foods after 2-4 hours of room temperature exposure to avoid foodborne illnesses (Appendix F).

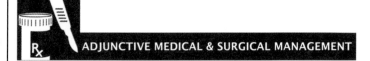

ADJUNCTIVE MEDICAL & SURGICAL MANAGEMENT

Antibiotic Therapy
This is a priority for cholangitis patients with the leukocytic form. Consider long-term potentiated broad-spectrum penicillin, cephalosporin or fluoroquinolone combined with metronidazole.

Table 3. Key nutritional factor content of selected commercial veterinary liquid foods used for enteral-assisted feeding of critically ill cats compared to recommended levels.* (Numbers in red match optimal KNFs.)

Factors	Osmolarity (mOsm/l)	Energy density (kcal/ml)**	Protein (g)	Arginine (mg)	Taurine (mg)	Potassium (mg)	L-carnitine (mg)
Recommended levels	250-400***	1-2	6.8-10.2	340-450	≥68	180-230	≥4.5
Abbott CliniCare Canine/Feline Liquid Diet	315	1.0	8.2	350	68	160	0.04
Abbott CliniCare RF Liquid Diet	235	1.0	6.3	350	64	125	0.06
PetAg Formula V Enteral Care HLP	312	1.2	8.5	413	48	92	na
PetAg Formula V Enteral Care MLP	256	1.1	7.5	393	48	66	na

Key: na = information not available from manufacturer.
*Liquid veterinary foods in this table are formulated to meet minimum requirements of the Association of American Feed Control Officials; all nutrient values = units/100 kcal, unless otherwise stated; to convert to kJ, multiply kcal by 4.184.
**Energy density values are listed on an as fed basis.
***250 is optimal.

Table 4. Levels of key nutritional factors in selected commercial veterinary therapeutic foods marketed for cats with hepatobiliary disease compared to recommended levels.* (Numbers in red match optimal KNFs.)

Dry foods	Energy density (kcal/cup)**	Energy density (kcal ME/g)	Protein (%)***	Arginine (%)	Taurine (%)	Sodium (%)	Zinc (mg/kg)	Iron (mg/kg)	Vit. E (IU/kg)	Vit. C (mg/kg)
Recommended levels	–	≥4.2	30-35	1.5-2.0	≥0.3	0.07-0.30	>200	80-140	≥500	100-200
Hill's Prescription Diet l/d Feline	505	4.5	31.8	1.98	0.53	0.27	305	173	267	109
Medi-Cal Mature Formula	355	na	29.2	na	0.4	0.4	na	na	na	na
Medi-Cal Reduced Protein	440	na	28.1	na	0.4	0.3	na	na	na	na
Medi-Cal Renal LP 21	409	na	24.7	na	0.2	0.2	na	na	na	na
Purina Veterinary Diets EN GastroENteric	572	4.4	56.2	na	0.32	0.64	na	na	232	na
Royal Canin Veterinary Diet Modified Formula	432	4.7	27.1	1.51	0.23	0.23	320	241	380	na

Moist foods	Energy density (kcal/can)**	Energy density (kcal ME/g)	Protein (%)***	Arginine (%)	Taurine (%)	Sodium (%)	Zinc (mg/kg)	Iron (mg/kg)	Vit. E (IU/kg)	Vit. C (mg/kg)
Recommended levels	–	≥4.2	30-35	1.5-2.0	≥0.3	0.07-0.30	>200	80-140	≥500	100-200
Hill's Prescription Diet l/d Feline	183/5.5 oz.	4.7	31.6	2.00	0.52	0.20	336	212	836	124
Medi-Cal Mature Formula	205/170 g	na	41.5	na	0.3	0.3	na	na	na	na
Medi-Cal Reduced Protein	265/170 g	na	33.9	na	0.3	0.2	na	na	na	na
Medi-Cal Renal LP	125/85 g pouch	na	29.3	na	0.8	0.6	na	na	na	na
Royal Canin Veterinary Diet Modified Formula	256/170 g 596/396 g	6.1	34.7	2.07	0.28	0.28	208	545	178	na

Key: ME = metabolizable energy, Vit. E = vitamin E, Vit. C = vitamin C, na = information not available from manufacturer.
*From manufacturers' published information or calculated from manufacturers' published as-fed values; all values are on a dry matter basis unless otherwise stated.
**Energy density values are listed on an as fed basis and are useful for determining the amount to feed; cup = 8-oz. measuring cup. To convert to kJ, multiply kcal by 4.184.
***For liver disease patients with signs of hepatic encephalopathy (HE), dietary protein levels should be limited to 25 to 30% dry matter until signs resolve. In these cases, several commercial veterinary therapeutic foods designed for patients with kidney disease that provide less protein than the foods intended for liver disease may be appropriate (Table 4, Chapter 26). If these foods are used, the patient should be transitioned to the selected food specifically formulated for liver disease after signs of HE have subsided.

Lactulose

Considered one of the treatments of choice for HE. Dosage varies: 1-3 ml per os, t.i.d. (cats). Titrate to produce a "porridge-like" stool. Reduce the dose if the stool becomes watery.

FOLLOWUP

Owner Followup

After the patient returns home, if possible, record daily food intake and frequency/severity of vomiting, diarrhea, icterus and neurobehavioral signs. Note BCS (and body weight if practical) every 2 weeks. If necessary, change the amount of food being fed by 10% increments and recheck the patient every 2 weeks for 1 month. At that point, the amount fed can be changed again and the cycle repeated until the patient reaches a normal body weight/BCS.

Veterinary Health Care Team Followup

Anorectic Patients. Feeding tubes can often be removed after a cat has shown clinical improvement and is eating 66-75% of its estimated normal food dose, of the prescribed food, on its own. This may take weeks-months for hepatic lipidosis patients. Subsequently, if no signs of hepatobiliary disease exist, many patients can be fed their regular maintenance foods.

Patients with Persistent Vomiting. Be sure small, frequent meals are fed. Continuous rate infusion tube feeding (Chapter 12) and antiemetics may be helpful. More aggressive medical treatment (e.g., lactulose) may be necessary for patients with HE.

Patients with Refeeding Syndrome. Severely malnourished patients can suffer from metabolic electrolyte disturbances within 12-72 hours after initiating EN support, which can lead to neurologic, pulmonary, cardiac, neuromuscular and hematologic complications. Initial gradual transition to EN support is important (above) to avoid refeeding syndrome.

Patients Eating on Their Own. In-clinic reassessment includes review of owner data (above). Improvement in attitude, activity, appetite and resolution of signs (vomiting and diarrhea) are good indicators of success. Serial laboratory evaluations (every few days-weeks) of serum liver enzyme activity, bile acids and potassium and blood ammonia are useful. Serial hepatic biopsies every 4-6 months can be evaluated for presence/absence of inflammatory hepatopathies. Many patients can be fed their regular maintenance foods after hepatobiliary disease has resolved.

MISCELLANEOUS

For more information about feline lipidosis and cholangitis, see Chapters 25, 26, 37, 57, 67 and 68, Small Animal Clinical Nutrition, 5th edition.

Appetite Stimulants

Anabolic steroids and benzodiazepines are not recommended. If used, do so advisably because of the potential for hepatotoxicity; also, benzodiazepines may be involved in the pathogenesis of HE.

Authors

Condensed from Chapter 68, Small Animal Clinical Nutrition, 5th edition, authored by Hein P. Meyer, David C. Twedt, Philip Roudebush and Elizabeth Dill-Macky.

References

See Chapter 68, Small Animal Clinical Nutrition, 5th edition, on the website www.markmorrisinstitute.org for references.

Appendices

Appendix A. Body Condition Scoring Guidelines.

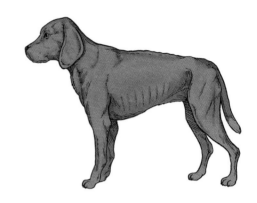

BCS 1. Very thin ▶

The ribs are easily palpable with no fat cover. The tailbase has a prominent raised bony structure with no tissue between the skin and bone. The bony prominences are easily felt with no overlying fat. Dogs over six months of age have a severe abdominal tuck when viewed from the side and an accentuated hourglass shape when viewed from above.

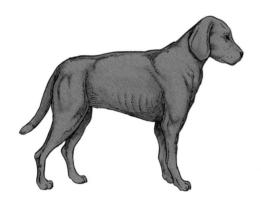

◀ BCS 2. Underweight

The ribs are easily palpable with minimal fat cover. The tailbase has a raised bony structure with little tissue between the skin and bone. The bony prominences are easily felt with minimal overlying fat. Dogs over six months of age have an abdominal tuck when viewed from the side and a marked hourglass shape when viewed from above.

BCS 3. Ideal ▶

The ribs are palpable with a slight fat cover. The tailbase has a smooth contour or some thickening. The bony structures are palpable under a thin layer of fat between the skin and bone. The bony prominences are easily felt under minimal amounts of overlying fat. Dogs over six months of age have a slight abdominal tuck when viewed from the side and a well-proportioned lumbar waist when viewed from above.

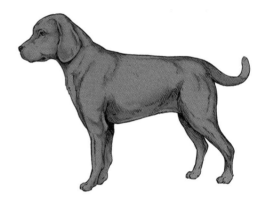

◀ BCS 4. Overweight

The ribs are difficult to feel with moderate fat cover. The tailbase has some thickening with moderate amounts of tissue between the skin and bone. The bony structures can still be palpated. The bony prominences are covered by a moderate layer of fat. Dogs over six months of age have little or no abdominal tuck or waist when viewed from the side. The back is slightly broadened when viewed from above.

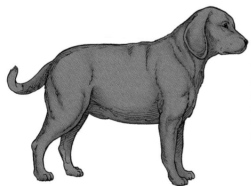

BCS 5. Obese ▶

The ribs are very difficult to feel under a thick fat cover. The tailbase appears thickened and is difficult to feel under a prominent layer of fat. The bony prominences are covered by a moderate to thick layer of fat. Dogs over six months of age have a pendulous ventral bulge and no waist when viewed from the side due to extensive fat deposits. The back is markedly broadened when viewed from above. A trough may form when epaxial areas bulge dorsally.

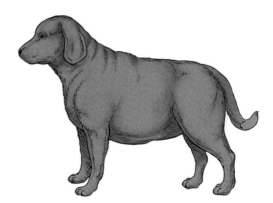

Figure 1. Body condition score (BCS) descriptors for dogs in a five-point system.

BCS 1. Very thin ▶
The ribs are easily palpable with no fat cover. The bony prominences are easily felt with no overlying fat. Cats over six months of age have a severe abdominal tuck when viewed from the side and an accentuated hourglass shape when viewed from above.

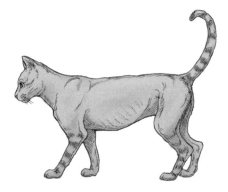

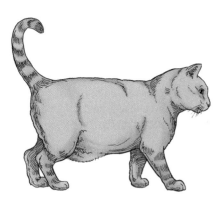

◀ **BCS 2. Underweight**
The ribs are easily palpable with minimal fat cover. The bony prominences are easily felt with minimal overlying fat. Cats over six months of age have an abdominal tuck when viewed from the side and a marked hourglass shape when viewed from above.

BCS 3. Ideal ▶
The ribs are palpable with a slight fat cover. The bony prominences are easily felt under a slight amount of overlying fat. Cats over six months of age have an abdominal tuck when viewed from the side and a well-proportioned lumbar waist when viewed from above.

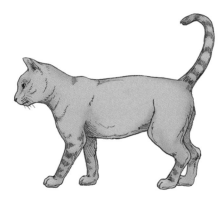

◀ **BCS 4. Overweight**
The ribs are difficult to feel with moderate fat cover. The bony structures can still be palpated. The bony prominences are covered by a moderate layer of fat. Cats over six months of age have little or no abdominal tuck or waist when viewed from the side. The back is slightly broadened when viewed from above. A moderate abdominal fat pad is present.

BCS 5. Obese ▶
The ribs are very difficult to feel under a thick fat cover. The bony prominences are covered by a moderate to thick layer of fat. Cats over six months of age have a pendulous ventral bulge and no waist when viewed from the side due to extensive fat deposits. The back is markedly broadened when viewed from above. A marked abdominal fat pad is present. Fat deposits may be found on the limbs and face.

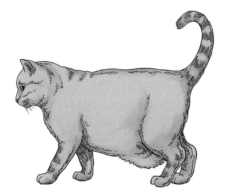

Figure 2. Body condition score (BCS) descriptors for cats in a five-point system.

Appendix B. Treats, Snacks and Table Foods.

BOX 1. IMPACT OF TREATS ON DAILY INTAKE IN DOGS.

From 60 to 86% of owners regularly give their dogs commercial treats. If table foods are considered, 90% or more of dogs receive treats, snacks and biscuits as a supplement to their regular food. People like to give treats and snacks for emotional reasons, to change their pet's behavior or to improve and maintain oral health. Because several daily treats will have a marked effect on a dog's cumulative nutritional intake, specific questions about treats should be asked when taking the dietary history. Specific recommendations about treats should be provided when prescribing a food regimen for diseased or healthy dogs. This information is critical when managing specific problems such as developmental orthopedic disease in growing large- and giant-breed dogs, adverse reactions to food, obesity, urolithiasis, diabetes mellitus, heart failure and renal disease.

The impact of snacks on a dog's daily nutrient intake depends on two factors: 1) the nutrient profile of the treat and 2) the number of treats provided daily. It is best to recommend a treat that matches the nutritional profile preferred for a given lifestage or disease. Snacks provide energy; a handful of dog snacks, for example, can easily be equivalent to 40% of a small dog's daily energy requirement (DER) or 10% of a large-breed dog's DER. Therefore, the owner must compensate for the additional energy by feeding less of the dog's usual food. This recommendation is especially important for dogs in which

a small snack can have a marked impact (i.e., toy- and small-breed dogs). The following two examples illustrate the impact of treats.

A six-year-old, neutered male miniature pinscher weighing 4.5 kg is fed two commercial biscuit treats per day, in addition to its regular food. Each biscuit provides 15 kcal (62.8 kJ), so the dog receives a total of 30 kcal (125.5 kJ) per day from the treats. The dog's DER is about 330 kcal (1,381 kJ). Therefore, the treats provide almost 10% of the dog's DER. If the dog's DER is being met with the regular food, then the treats may contribute to long-term excess energy intake and obesity.

A five-month-old, 20-kg, female German shepherd dog is given a commercial treat marketed as a snack with "real marrow bone." Calcium is not declared on the guaranteed or typical analysis of the treat label. The owner gives the dog 10 treats daily as part of a training program. This number of treats is within the feeding guidelines on the label. However, analysis shows that each treat contains 426 mg of calcium. Consuming 10 treats daily increases the dog's daily calcium intake by more than 80% compared with feeding a commercial food formulated for large-breed puppies. This feeding practice increases the risk of developmental orthopedic disease (Chapter 22). To facilitate learning, dogs do not need to receive edible reinforcement every time and the pieces can be very small. If praise is paired with treats, praise alone will rapidly become sufficient reinforcement for the desired behavior.

Appendix B. Treats, Snacks and Table Foods, continued.

BOX 2. COMMERCIAL TREATS AND TABLE FOODS FOR CATS.

An estimated 41 to 60% of cats are regularly fed table foods and 34% of cats are fed commercial treats.[a] Feeding treats and table food allows more social interaction with the owner, increases diet variety and provides additional caloric intake. Some commercial treats claim dental benefits either by mechanical cleansing or through use of an active ingredient (Chapter 36). When fed in excess, treats and table foods may negatively affect a well-balanced food. Because most commercial cat foods contain vitamins and minerals well above the nutritional needs of cats, table foods and treats fed at less than 10% of the total daily intake should be safe. Providing high-calorie treats or table foods can also contribute to obesity and must be considered in the calculation of total calories for a cat.

MILK

One of the most common human foods offered to cats is milk. Milk is highly palatable and small quantities are well tolerated by most healthy cats. However, after weaning, intestinal lactase activity declines unless milk is a regular part of the diet. Undigested lactose is subject to bacterial fermentation and promotes osmotic diarrhea. Feeding milk to cats unaccustomed to receiving it may overwhelm digestive capacity resulting in diarrhea, flatulence or gastrointestinal distress. Lactase supplements may alleviate signs of lactose

intolerance, lactose avoidance is more prudent for affected cats.

NUTRITIONAL SUPPLEMENTS

Although many supplements are legitimate sources of essential nutrients, others represent food fads that reflect current trends in human nutrition. Poor-quality foods are rarely "fixed" by adding a supplement. Changing to a higher quality food is a more appropriate recommendation and often less expensive.

Calcium

Breeders sometimes provide supplemental calcium during pregnancy, lactation or growth. Additional calcium is rarely necessary, except for cats fed a homemade food or queens with eclampsia, and may lead to nutritional excess or nutrient imbalances in cats fed complete and balanced commercial cat foods.

Chromium

Chromium has been called a "glucose tolerance factor" for its role in normal glucose homeostasis and insulin action in experimental animals. Chromium supplementation promotes lean tissue accretion in growing livestock. Thus, health food stores now stock chromium as an "anti-diabetic" nutrient and "fat-burner" for people. Little information exists about the effect of chromium supplementation in cats. Some caution may be warranted given excess chromium has been associated with chromosomal damage.

Brewer's Yeast/Thiamin

Brewer's yeast and thiamin have been promoted as coat condition-

Appendix B. Treats, Snacks and Table Foods, continued.

ers and flea preventives for dogs and cats. Although brewer's yeast is a good source of B vitamins, particularly thiamin, research has not proven its efficacy as a flea repellent.

RAW MEATS

Breeders and owners commonly feed raw meats to cats. Raw muscle and organ meats are highly palatable, digestible and generally nutritious when supplemented with appropriate vitamins and minerals. Cooking destroys some nutrients and increases the availability of others. A benefit to feeding raw meat to cats has not been documented, and the disadvantages far outweigh any advantages. Raw meat, even when "flash frozen," may contain harmful bacteria (e.g., *Salmonella* spp. and *Escherichia coli*) and parasites (e.g., *Toxoplasma gondii*, *Cryptosporidium parvum*) (Chapter 11, Small Animal Clinical Nutrition, 5th edition). Some of these microbes can also be a health risk for people. Unless supplemented with vitamins and minerals, raw meat is nutritionally incomplete and can lead to nutritional secondary hyperparathyroidism, iodine deficiency or both. Meat mixes composed of large percentages of organ meats may provide excessive levels of vitamin A. Finally, cats fed raw meat diets sometimes develop fixed-food preferences, making subsequent food changes difficult.

FEEDING BONES

Bones are a concentrated source of calcium, phosphorus and magnesium. Steamed bone meal is a very good choice for supplying calcium in homemade or all-meat diets. However, feeding whole bones to cats should be discouraged. Bones with jagged or sharp points are often to blame for oral trauma and can become esophageal foreign bodies. Bone feeding is also associated with colitis and constipation in small animals. Commercial foods approved by the Association of American Feed Control Officials (AAFCO) are replete in calcium, phosphorus and magnesium and should not be supplemented.

VEGETARIAN AND VEGAN DIETS

Although the nutritional needs of cats are best met by a carnivorous diet, vegetarian diets can be designed to provide adequate nutrition. Vegetarian formulas are commercially available and several commercial supplements are available to provide nutrients normally missing, inadequate or poorly available in plant-based diets. The commonly reported pitfalls of commercially available feline vegan diets include taurine, arachidonic acid and vitamin A deficiencies. Several nutrients (below) require special attention in vegetarian formulations.

Protein

Plants are typically low in protein relative to the dietary needs of cats. Additionally, the quality of protein, in many cases, is much lower than protein from animal sources. Concentrated sources of plant protein available to supplement feline foods include isolated soybean protein and corn gluten meal. Care must be taken to feed sufficient protein both to meet the overall nitrogen needs and the minimum requirements of available individual amino acids.

Amino Acids

Taurine is not present in plant ingredients. Therefore, cats fed plant-based foods require taurine supplementation. Chemically synthesized sources of taurine are available from pharmacies and health food stores. Similarly, only animal tissues synthesize carnitine, a vitamin-like amino acid. Although healthy cats do not require dietary carnitine, a dietary source may be conditionally essential during growth or under disease conditions. Synthetic supplements are available. The common limiting amino acids in plants are methionine, lysine and tryptophan. Diets must be closely evaluated to ensure the availability of sufficient quantities of these amino acids. Plant proteins contain large amounts of glutamate. Cats may poorly tolerate high-glutamate foods.

Vitamins

Because cats cannot use β-carotene, pre-formed vitamin A must be supplied in the food. Also, many vitamin A supplements contain vitamin D. All sources of vitamin D should be considered to avoid excess. Vegetarian diets also require supplementation with vitamin B_{12}, which is not supplied by plant ingredients. Vitamin B_{12}-enriched yeast and synthetic supplements are commercially available. Finally, the niacin content of vegetarian diets should be closely evaluated. Although niacin is present in high amounts in many plant ingredients, the availability is often poor and additional supplementation may be required.

Minerals

Providing adequate calcium is a concern in any homemade food. A variety of calcium supplements are available from health food stores and pharmacies. Many plant ingredients contain components (e.g., fibers or phytates) that severely compromise the availability of certain trace elements. The availability of iron, zinc and copper is of particular concern in high-phytate and high-fiber foods (Chapter 5, Small Animal Clinical Nutrition, 5th edition). These minerals should be provided as a highly available source.

Fat

Of the nutrients required by cats, arachidonic acid is the one not commercially available. To provide arachidonate directly, cats must be given animal fat or tissue as a nutritional source. However, cats can convert γ-linolenic acid (18:3n6) to arachidonic acid (20:4n6) via delta 5-desaturase. γ-linolenic acid is available from plant oils (e.g., borage and evening primrose oils). Prolonged feeding and reproductive trials using γ-linolenic acid have not been reported; thus, the suitability of these oils as long-term arachidonic acid supplements is unknown. Because cats fed foods high in polyunsaturated fatty acids may develop steatitis, cats fed vegetarian foods with large quantities of plant oils should be protected with added vitamin E.

DOG FOOD

Most dog foods are not nutritionally adequate for the maintenance, growth and reproduction of cats. Nutrients most likely to be deficient are protein, taurine, niacin, vitamin B_6, methionine and choline. Clinical signs of deficiency depend on which nutrients are deficient and to what degree.

FOOD TOXINS

Food toxicities are relatively infrequent in cats. Most notable is hemolytic anemia caused by onion toxicity. Certain disulfides found ▶

Appendix D. Feeding Methods: Pros and Cons.

The amount fed is usually offered in one of three ways: 1) free-choice feeding (dogs and cats), 2) food-restricted meal feeding (dogs and cats) and 3) time-restricted meal feeding (dogs). The number of feedings per day must be considered when the last two methods are used.

Free-choice feeding (also referred to as ad libitum or self feeding) is a method in which more food than the dog or cat will consume is always available; therefore, the animal can eat as much as it wants, whenever it chooses. The major advantage of free-choice feeding is that it is quick and easy. All that is necessary is to ensure that reasonably fresh food is always available. Free-choice feeding is the method of choice during lactation. Free-choice feeding also has a quieting effect in a kennel and timid dogs have a better chance of getting their share if dogs are fed in a group.

Disadvantages include: 1) anorectic animals may not be noticed for several days, especially if two or more animals are fed together, 2) if food is always available, some dogs and cats will continuously overeat and may become obese (such animals should be meal fed) and 3) moist foods and moistened dry foods left at room temperature for prolonged periods can spoil and are inappropriate for free-choice feeding (Appendix F).

When changing a dog from meal feeding to free-choice feeding, first feed it the amount of the food it is used to receiving at a meal. After this food has been consumed and the dog's appetite has been somewhat satisfied, set out the food to be fed free choice. This transitioning method helps prevent engorgement by dogs unaccustomed to free-choice feeding. Engorgement is generally not a problem when transitioning cats to free-choice feeding. Although dogs and cats unaccustomed to free-choice feeding may overeat initially, they generally stop doing so within a few days, after they learn that food is always available. Avoid taking the food away at any time during this transition period. Each time food is taken away increases the difficulty in changing the animals to a free-choice feeding regimen.

With food-restricted meal feeding, the dog or cat is given a specific, but lesser, amount of food than it would eat if the amount offered were not restricted (i.e., free choice). Time-restricted meal feeding is a method in which the animal is given more food than it will consume within a specified period of time, generally five to 15 minutes. Time-restricted meal feeding is of limited usefulness with dogs and has little if any practical application in cats. Many dogs can eat an entire meal in less than two minutes. Both types of meal feeding are repeated at a specific frequency such as one or more times a day. Some people combine feeding methods, such as free-choice feeding a dry or semi-moist food and meal feeding a moist food or other foods such as meat or table scraps.

Food consumption resulting from frequent meal and free-choice feeding has several advantages. Small meals fed frequently throughout the day result in a greater loss of energy due to an increase in daily meal-induced heat production. Also, providing frequent small meals generally result in greater total food intake than does less frequent feeding. Frequent feeding of small meals benefits animals with dysfunctional ingestion, digestion, absorption or use of nutrients.

Frequent feeding is also desirable in normal animals that require a high food intake. Puppies and kittens less than six months old, some dogs engaged in heavy work (high levels of physical activity), dogs and cats experiencing ambient temperature extremes, bitches and queens during the last month of gestation and during lactation should be fed at least three times per day to ensure that their nutritional needs are met. These animals may require one and one-half to four times as much food per unit of body weight than most normal adult dogs and cats. A reduced frequency might limit total food intake in these situations. Also, more frequent feeding during periods of variable appetite suppression, such as occurs with psychologic stress or high ambient temperatures, helps ensure adequate food intake.

Most clinically normal adult dogs that are not lactating, working or experiencing stress will have a sufficient appetite and physical capacity to consume all of the food required daily in a single 10-minute period (assuming food of typical nutrient density [about 3.5 kcal/g or 14.64 kJ/g dry matter]). Cats are less likely to eat their entire meal in one 10-minute sitting, but once-a-day feeding is adequate for most healthy adults. Although many dogs and cats are fed once daily without noticeable detrimental effects, at least twice daily feeding is generally recommended.

In summary, how the food is provided and how often it is fed depend on the animal's condition and in some cases the lifestyle of the owner. Each animal's situation will dictate which feeding method is most desirable (free choice, time-restricted meal feeding or food-restricted meal feeding). For many physiologic and disease conditions this consideration will not be important. For others it will be very important. Recommendations for the best method of providing the food and the number of times per day the food is offered are included in each individual chapter.

Appendix E. Changing Foods.

Changing foods for most healthy dogs and cats is of minor consequence. Some owners switch their pets from one food to another daily. Most dogs and cats tolerate these changes. However, vomiting, diarrhea, belching, flatulence or a combination of signs may occur with sudden, rapid switching of foods, probably because of ingredient differences. It is prudent, therefore, to recommend that owners change their pet's food over the course of at least three days. A seven-day period is even better, as owners increase the proportion of new food and decrease the proportion of old food (**Table 1**).

Nearly all pets readily tolerate a seven-day transition period. A much longer transitional period is recommended in cases in which the food change is known to be significant, the pet has demonstrated a poor tolerance to such changes in the past or food refusal is expected (**Table 1**). For example, a long transition schedule is likely to be needed for an old cat recently diagnosed with kidney disease when the food must be switched from a highly palatable grocery "gourmet" food to an appropriate veterinary therapeutic food.

Table 1. Recommended short- and long-term food transition schedules for dogs and cats.

Short schedule*	Long schedule**		Food percentages	
Dogs and cats (days)	Dogs (days)	Cats (weeks)	Previous food	New food
1,2	1-3	1	75	25
3,4	4-6	2	50	50
5,6	7-9	3	25	75
7	10	4	0	100

*Recommended for most healthy dogs and cats.
**Recommended for situations in which the food change is known to be significant, the dog or cat has demonstrated low tolerance to such changes in the past or food refusal is anticipated.

Appendix F. Prevention of Foodborne Illness in Animals.

COMMERCIAL PET FOODS (MOIST OR DRY KIBBLES)
Discard foods from bulging or leaking cans and damaged bags.
Discard all foods with an abnormal color, foreign materials, odor or moldy appearance.
Discard dry foods 30 minutes after adding water.
Avoid frozen raw diets.

HOMEMADE DIETS
Use raw ingredients appropriate for human consumption.
Cook ground meat thoroughly to the center.
Sear the surface of whole meat cuts, which may lower risks.
Cook all eggs: whole, yolks, whites and shells if used as calcium supplement.
Wash all raw fruits and vegetables.

CONTROL FOOD CONTAMINATION
Use stainless steel utensils, feeding bowls, etc. whenever possible.
Keep food preparation areas, cooking utensils and food bowls spotlessly clean. Wash and disinfect bowls and utensils daily.
Store dry, commercial foods in a cool, dry environment, free from insects and rodents.

Empty the feeding bowl of moist or moistened foods not consumed within two to four hours if the ambient temperature is above 10°C (50°F).
Clean, wash and disinfect food utensils and food bowls after each feeding.
If feeding free choice, check food daily for mold and spoilage.

CONTROL MICROORGANISMS IN FOOD USING PHYSICAL MEANS
Cook all home-prepared foods at 82°C (180°F) for a minimum of 10 minutes.
Verify cooking temperatures with a cooking thermometer and internal meat temperatures with a meat thermometer.
Validate thermometer accuracy periodically with boiling water.
Cover all perishable foods and opened cans of pet food and store in the refrigerator at 4°C (40°F) when not being prepared, cooked or consumed.

CONTROL THE PET'S ACCESS TO UNINTENTIONAL FOODS
Minimize roaming on trash pick up days.
Monitor closely when off leash.

Appendix G. Alternative Eating Behaviors.

BOX 1. ALTERNATIVE CANINE EATING BEHAVIORS.

RESPONSE TO FOOD VARIETY

Dogs may display preferences for specific types of foods according to taste and texture. However, the notion that dogs require a variety of flavors or taste in their meals is incorrect and may be detrimental in some instances. Dogs prefer novel foods or flavors to familiar foods; therefore, feeding a variety of novel foods free choice may lead to overeating and obesity. Dogs may correct for excessive energy intake by decreasing or refusing food intake the next day(s). Reduction of food intake to maintain weight following engorgement may erroneously be interpreted as a dislike of the current food instead of an auto-regulatory mechanism to achieve the previous set-point weight.

GARBAGE EATING

Garbage eating is probably normal behavior. Many dogs prefer food in an advanced stage of decomposition. However, garbage eating is oftentimes unhealthy. Ingestion of garbage may cause brief, mild gastroenteritis or more serious intoxication (Chapter 11, Small Animal Clinical Nutrition, 5th edition). Because the etiology is complex and may involve bacterial toxins, mycotoxins and by-products from putrefaction or decomposition, the clinical signs vary widely from vomiting, diarrhea, abdominal pain, weakness, incoordination and dyspnea, to shock, coma and death. Scavenging dogs may eat less of their regular meal; therefore, garbage eating may be mistaken for anorexia at home.

Spraying garbage bags with a dog repellent usually will not stop the problem. Preventing access to garbage is the obvious best solution.

GRASS EATING

Owners often ask why dogs eat grass. Plant and grass eating is normal behavior. Herbivores are the natural prey for wolves and most other canids. The viscera of prey are often eaten first and contain partially digested vegetable material. Because dogs' ancestors and close relatives in the wild regularly ingest plant material, some investigators have suggested that domestic dogs must also eat grass. Probably the better explanation is that, to date, no one knows for sure why dogs eat plants or grass, but they may simply like the way plants taste or prefer the texture. Plant chlorophyll can bind mycotoxins, such as those found in moldy grains, decreasing their absorption.

BEGGING FOR FOOD

Begging for food may be fun when dogs sit up or perform other tricks; however, the behavior can become annoying when whining, barking, persistent nudging and scratching take over. Begging for food was one of the most common complaints addressed in a study involving more than 1,400 owners and was perceived as a problem in one-third of the dogs. Additionally, begging may encourage owners to feed more of the dog's regular food. Begging tends to increase with age and may indicate that most owners don't realize that they reinforce begging by continuing to offer tidbits to their begging pet. Treats reinforce begging. Also, the fact that begging for food is directly proportional to the number of people in the family may be related to an increase in the number of tidbits fed.

Treatment consists of ignoring behaviors such as begging, barking and whining. Owners should be prepared for a prolonged period of such behaviors before begging subsides completely. Intermittent reinforcement of begging when these behaviors become problematic can be more powerful than continuous rewarding, even though the owner may have refused to provide snacks in the interim. It may also help to keep the dog out of the kitchen and dining areas when preparing and eating food and to feed the dog before or after the family has eaten.

PICA

Pica is defined as perverted appetite with craving for and ingestion of non-food items. The etiology of true pica is unknown. Suggested causes include mineral deficiencies, permanent anxiety and psychological disturbances. A few cases of pica have been noted in relation to zinc intoxication and hepatic encephalopathy. Pica is common in dogs with exocrine pancreatic insufficiency, probably as a manifestation of polyphagia, and perhaps as a consequence of some specific nutritional deficiency. Sometimes, coprophagy and garbage eating are mistakenly considered forms of pica.

Pica can be treated with aversion therapy by offering a counter attraction at the moment the dog begins to eat foreign material and by punishment if there is no response. Outdoors, the dog should be kept on a leash or even muzzled. Most treatments for pica are unrewarding, therefore physical prevention is sometimes the only solution.

COPROPHAGY

Coprophagy is defined as eating feces and may involve consumption of the animal's own stools or the feces of other animals. Coprophagy is probably widespread among pet dogs and is probably more disturbing to owners than it is harmful to dogs. Bitches normally eat the feces of their puppies during the first three weeks of lactation. Feral dogs and dogs in rural areas have access to and consume large-animal feces, which is considered normal behavior. In many cases, however, coprophagy is a behavioral problem and the etiology is unknown. Coprophagy can also be related to certain diseases.

Table 1 lists behavioral and metabolic disorders that may be associated with coprophagy. The risk of transmitting parasitic diseases is probably the most important health reason for managing coprophagy; however, the associated halitosis is of primary concern to owners. The dog's motivation must be reduced to correct coprophagy. Several measures have been proposed.

Punishment may deter the dog's behavior, but may violate the confidence between owner and pet. Punishment may also aggravate the coprophagic behavior. Walking the dog on a leash and keeping it away from feces after the dog defecates is helpful.

Repulsive substances can be used to create aversion for feces. Many products have been recommended including spices (e.g., pepper, sambal, hot pepper sauce), quinine, strong perfumes and products such as cythioate, meat tenderizers and For-Bid.[a] Adding repulsive substances to feces can be time-consuming and has questionable efficacy.

Food changes to deter coprophagy have been recommended; however, most of these recommendations lack substantiation. Using foods with increased fiber levels has been reported to help. Free-choice feeding ▶

Appendix G. Alternative Eating Behaviors, continued.

has also been recommended, whereas a strict schedule of two meals per day and avoiding all tidbits or table foods has worked for others.

Table 1. Factors associated with coprophagy.

Behavior
Confinement in a kennel leading to stress or competitive behavior
Confinement leading to boredom with exploratory effort focused on feces
Reaction to punishment during housetraining
Strong dominance or extreme submissive attitude towards the owner
To attract the owner's attention
Young animals with a natural interest in feces

ENDNOTE
a. Alpar Laboratories Inc., La Grange, IL, USA.

Gastrointestinal disorders
Malassimilation
Parasitic infections
Polyphagia due to diabetes mellitus or Cushing's syndrome

Food
Overfeeding
Poorly digestible food

Appendix G. Alternative Eating Behaviors, continued.

BOX 2. ALTERNATIVE FELINE EATING BEHAVIORS.

Although there are such things as aberrant eating behaviors, many of the behaviors observed are normal behaviors that owners happen to find objectionable.

COPROPHAGIA

Coprophagia, or consumption of excreta, is normal behavior for queens with kittens less than 30 days of age. The queen stimulates the kittens' elimination reflexes by grooming the kittens' perineal areas and then consumes the products of elimination. This process is important as an aid to elimination in young kittens. In addition, coprophagia maintains sanitation and reduces odors in the nest area. Thus, coprophagia has important survival value in wild or feral cats by reducing factors that could attract predators to the nest site. It is very uncommon for cats to continue coprophagia after the kittens are weaned.

CANNIBALISM/INFANTICIDE

Cannibalism or infanticide is often normal behavior in male and female cats. Queens typically cannibalize aborted, dead and weak kittens. This behavior may serve to reduce the spread of disease to healthy kittens, conserve maternal resources and optimize survival of the fittest kittens and help keep the nest box clean. In addition, the queen derives nutritional benefits from consuming dead kittens. Occasionally, queens will kill an apparently healthy litter. Environmental factors that cause kittens to mimic early signs of illness (e.g., inactivity, hyperthermia or hypothermia) may trigger infanticide and cannibalism. Maternal stress, malnourishment and hormonal insufficiency may contribute to unexplained cannibalism as well. Maternal experience or parity does not appear to play a role.

Tomcats may indiscriminately kill unrelated kittens. This behavior usually occurs when a strange male enters a new territory and encounters a lactating queen and kittens. A queen rapidly returns to estrus after the loss of its kittens. Thus, infanticide optimizes a male's genetic potential because it now has an opportunity to sire subsequent litters. Infanticide is an uncommon behavior by resident male cats.

The health status, dietary management and husbandry practices should be reviewed in queens or catteries experiencing persistent problems with cannibalism. Males should not have access to young kittens to reduce the chance of infanticide. Although resident male cats rarely pose a problem, it is prudent to err on the side of safety. Factors contributing to maternal stress should be evaluated and, if possible, reduced.

PLANT AND GRASS EATING

Plant and grass eating is a natural behavior of both cats and dogs. A variety of explanations have been advanced for grass eating. Because grass is not digested within the cat's gastrointestinal (GI) tract, it acts as a local irritant and sometimes stimulates vomiting. Thus, grass eating may serve as a purgative to eliminate hair or other indigestible material. However, many cats readily seek out grass to eat, appear to enjoy eating it and do not vomit. Other explanations for the behavior include a response to nutritional deficiencies, boredom or a taste preference. In contrast to eating grass, eating other plants, including many indoor ornamental plants, carries risk of toxicity (e.g., lily toxicity).

RESPONSE TO CATNIP

The smell or ingestion of catnip (*Nepeta cataria*) can invoke unusual behavioral changes for five to 15 minutes after exposure. The active ingredient, cis-trans-nepetalactone, is thought to act as a hallucinogen although stimulation of neurologic centers associated with estrous behaviors has also been suggested. Cats may respond to catnip by head rubbing and shaking, salivating, gazing, skin twitching, rolling and animated leaping. Only 50 to 70% of cats exhibit a behavioral response, which may have a genetic basis. Prolonged exposure may lead to a chronic state of partial unawareness. Cats may become refractory for an hour or more after cessation of the initial response.

WOOL SUCKING

A commonly reported behavioral abnormality in cats is wool sucking. The behavior first appears near puberty when cats begin to lick, suck, chew or eat wool or other clothing articles. Although the cause is poorly understood, nutritional deficiencies are unlikely. Affected cats may be seeking the odor of lanolin or human sweat or the behavior may be a manifestation of prolonged nursing. Siamese, Siamese-cross and Burmese cats are primarily affected, suggesting a genetic link. ▶

Appendix G. Alternative Eating Behaviors, continued.

Wool sucking is managed by limiting access to attractive items and through behavior modification. Feeding a high-fiber food or providing a continuous supply of dry food may reduce the behavior.

PROLONGED NURSING

Prolonged nursing may occur in kittens that strive to satisfy a desire for non-nutritional sucking. Non-nutritional sucking normally subsides near weaning. Kittens may develop nursing vices when nursing fails to take place because they were orphaned, prematurely weaned or required bottle feeding. Within the litter, kittens will often nurse tails, ears, skin folds and/or the genitalia of their littermates. After a kitten is separated from its litter, it may transfer sucking vices to people, stuffed toys, clothing or other pets.

ANOREXIA

Although a few days of inappetence is not particularly detrimental to an otherwise healthy cat, prolonged inadequate calorie intake results in malnutrition, reduced immune function and increased risk for hepatic lipidosis. Anorexia may be caused by stress, unacceptable foods or concurrent disease. Most commonly, cats presented to veterinarians for anorexia have a concurrent disease. Cats may endure prolonged starvation rather than eat an unpalatable food. Therefore, advising owners that a cat will "eat when it gets hungry enough" can have deadly results. Anorexia of more than three days duration, even in an otherwise healthy-appearing cat, warrants investigation.

A thorough history is useful for differentiating potential causes of anorexia. To determine if inadequate food acceptance is the cause, offer a small selection of highly palatable foods along with the typical food. Because improperly stored foods may develop off flavors, bacterial contamination or fungal growth, confirm that the product is fresh and wholesome. Environmental or emotional factors reported to result in stress-mediated anorexia include hospitalization, boarding, travel, introduction of new people or pets to the household, loss of a companion, overcrowding, high temperatures and excessive handling. Stress-mediated anorexia is usually diagnosed from the history and by ruling out other diseases. Providing a quiet secluded area will often allow a cat to relax sufficiently enough to begin eating. Often, increasing the food's palatability will improve food intake. Warming food, changing the food form, adding water or choosing foods high in animal protein and fat can enhance food palatability. If cats are highly stressed or appropriate feeding sites are unavailable, mild tranquilizers or appetite stimulants (e.g., mirtazapine, oxazepam or cyproheptadine) may be beneficial (Chapter 25, Small Animal Clinical Nutrition, 5th edition). Force feeding may be accepted by some cats but others find the process so stressful that any benefit is far outweighed by the additional stress.

FIXED-FOOD PREFERENCES

The food type fed by the owner during a kitten's first six months influences the pattern of food preferences throughout life. Although uncommon, kittens exposed to a very limited number of foods may develop a food fixation, refusing to eat anything but a single food. Adult cats fed highly palatable, single-item foods have been reported to develop fixed-food preferences as well.

Cats with food fixations can be particularly troublesome if dietary modifications are necessary. Cats with strong food preferences should be transitioned to the new food over a prolonged period. Convert to the desired food by replacing 10 to 20% of the old food with an equal amount of the new food on Day 1, then gradually increase the ratio of new to old over the next 14 days. A more gradual transition may be required if food intake drops below 70% of maintenance levels. Cats should be monitored to ensure they are not selecting the preferred food from the food dish and that food intake remains adequate. Feeding kittens and cats a variety of foods (both different forms of food and different brands) and not feeding single-item foods can prevent food fixations. This approach is strongly recommended because disease management later in life often requires a dietary change.

LEARNED TASTE AVERSIONS

Cats may develop learned aversions to certain foods when feeding is paired with a negative GI experience. The negative experience can be physical, emotional or physiologic. Typically, aversions occur when cats consume a food immediately before an episode of nausea or vomiting. Foods that were readily consumed before the negative incident will be avoided subsequently. Clinically, aversions may develop when GI upset is induced by various diseases, drugs or treatment protocols. Foods with high salience (i.e., strong odors or high protein levels) are more likely to become aversive and should not be fed within 24 hours of anticipated GI upsets. Aversions have been documented to last up to 40 days in cats. Learned aversions are considered an adaptive response. By avoiding foods that previously caused gastric distress, cats will avoid eating foods likely to be spoiled or tainted. From a clinical perspective, consideration of food aversions often equates to delaying introduction of a therapeutic food, such as a diet for chronic kidney disease, until the cat's GI signs have been controlled with other medical management.

POLYPHAGIA

Various diseases, drugs and psychological stresses can mediate excessive food consumption. Rarely, polyphagia (hyperphagia) may occur with diseases involving the central nervous system, particularly with lesions of the ventromedial hypothalamus. Presence of weight loss or gain is of key diagnostic importance. Polyphagia with weight loss is almost always associated with an underlying disease process or simple underfeeding. Caloric intake should always be calculated because underfeeding can result in a ravenous appetite that may be misinterpreted as abnormal. Nutritional management of polyphagia requires an accurate diagnosis because treatment is aimed at the primary disease.

Appendix H. Assisted-Feeding Techniques.

SYRINGE FEEDING

Patients are often fed a liquid or moist homogenized product by syringe on a short-term basis. For dogs, the syringe tip is placed between the molar teeth and cheek with the head held in a normal or lowered position (**Figure 1**). For cats, the syringe tip is placed between the four canine teeth (**Figure 2**). The patient may choose to swallow the liquid or allow it to flow down the mouth into the esophagus by gravity. Some patients refuse to swallow the liquid or food; therefore, force feeding may increase the risk of aspiration. Syringe feeding should be discontinued if the patient does not swallow food voluntarily.

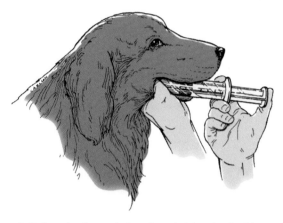

Figure 1. Syringe-feeding technique for administering liquid or moist homogenized foods to dogs.

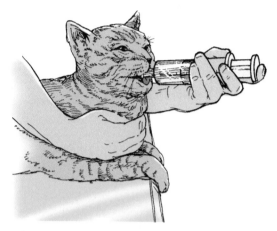

Figure 2. Syringe-feeding technique for administering liquid or moist homogenized foods to cats.

NASOESOPHAGEAL TUBE PLACEMENT

Nasoesophageal tubes are generally used for three to seven days, but are occasionally used longer (weeks if moved to the opposite side every seven days). Polyurethane tubes (6 to 8 Fr., 90 to 100 cm) with or without a weighted tip and silicone feeding tubes (3.5 to 10 Fr., 20 to 105 cm) may be placed in the caudal esophagus or stomach. The preferred placement of all tubes originating cranial to the stomach is in the caudal esophagus to minimize gastric reflux and subsequent esophagitis. An 8-Fr. tube will pass through the nasal cavity of most dogs; a 5- Fr. tube is more comfortable for cats.

The length of tube to be inserted is determined by measuring from the nasal planum along the side of the animal to the caudal margin of the last rib (**Figure 1**) and marking the tube at a point that is approximately three-fourths of the total measured length with a piece of adhesive tape or an indelible marker. This mark is how far the tube should be inserted. Tape will also provide a tab to secure the tube. The animal's nose is desensitized by placing a few drops of topical anesthetic (2% lidocaine or 0.5% proparacaine) into a nostril and tilting the head upward for a few seconds. The tip of the tube is lubricated with a water-soluble lubricant or 2 to 5% lidocaine ointment/jelly before passage.

To pass the tube, direct the tip in a caudoventral, medial direction into the ventrolateral aspect of the external nares. The head is generally held in a normal static position. As soon as the tip of the catheter reaches the medial septum at the floor of the nasal cavity in dogs, the external nares are pushed dorsally, which opens the ventral meatus, ensuring passage of the tube into the oropharynx (**Figure 2**). To aid passage, the proximal end of the tube is lifted as

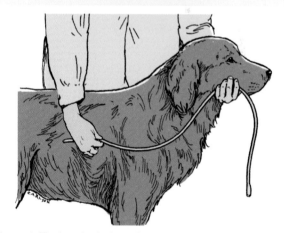

Figure 1. The length of tube to insert is determined by measuring from the nose to the last rib. Marking the tube at three-quarters of the distance between the last rib and the nose will place the end of the tube in the caudal esophagus. This location is marked with an indelible marker or a piece of adhesive tape. Tape can also serve as a suture tab to secure the tube.

▶

Appendix H. Assisted-Feeding Techniques, continued.

the nose is pushed upward (**Figure 2**). In cats, because of the lack of a well-developed alar fold, the tube can be inserted initially in a ventromedial direction and continued directly into the oropharynx. The tube is inserted until the adhesive tape tab or indelible mark is reached (**Figure 3**).

To evaluate proper tube placement, 3 to 15 ml of sterile water or saline solution may be injected through the tube and the animal evaluated for coughing (**Figure 4**). A lateral radiograph may be taken of the neck to confirm the tube is placed in the caudal esophagus (i.e., over the larynx). After confirmation of position, the tube is secured with either sutures or glue. The first tape tab is secured to the skin just lateral to the external nares. A second tape tab is secured to the skin on the dorsal nasal midline, just rostral to the level of the eyes. An Elizabethan collar is used in most animals to prevent inadvertent removal of the tube (**Figure 5**).

Complications of nasoesophageal intubation include epistaxis, lack of tolerance of the procedure and inadvertent removal of the tube by the animal. Incidence of tube removal by the animal has been reported to be as high as 50% even with use of collars. Nasoesophageal tubes should not be used in vomiting patients or those with respiratory disease.

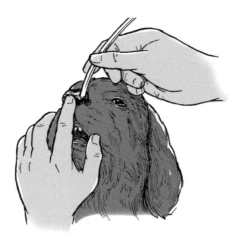

Figure 2. The external nares are pushed dorsally and the proximal end of the tube is lifted to facilitate passage of the tube into the ventral nasal meatus.

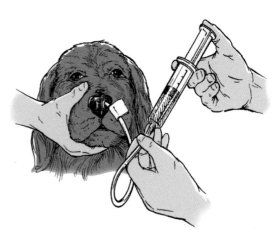

Figure 4. A test injection of sterile water or saline solution is made to ensure proper tube placement.

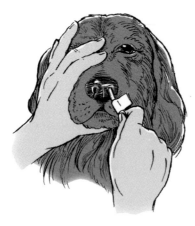

Figure 3. The tube is inserted until the indelible mark or adhesive tape tab is reached. Sutures or glue are used to secure the tape tab to the skin.

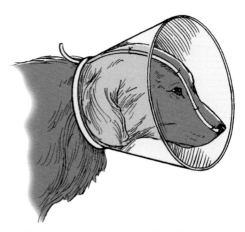

Figure 5. Securing the tube at several locations by suturing or gluing tape tabs to the skin and applying collars will help decrease inadvertent removal of the tube by the animal.

Appendix H. Assisted-Feeding Techniques, continued.

PHARYNGOSTOMY TUBE PLACEMENT

in some instances, a pharyngostomy tube is used to bypass the nose and mouth of an animal requiring nutritional support (e.g., in cases of facial trauma) or when nasoesophageal tubes are not tolerated. Pharyngostomy tubes have been largely replaced by esophagostomy tubes or gastrostomy tubes placed percutaneously.

The patient is anesthetized, intubated and positioned in lateral recumbency. The area caudal to the mandible on either side is prepared for aseptic surgery. A 14- to 18-Fr. polyvinylchloride tube is premeasured as described in **Figure 1, Nasoesophageal Tube Placement**, except that the tube exit site will be caudal to the mandible.

With the mouth held open with a speculum, palpate the hyoid apparatus with one finger. The tube exit site must be carefully planned to avoid interfering with laryngeal opening and epiglottic movement. The tube should exit as far caudally and dorsally along the lateral pharyngeal wall as possible. The finger inside the mouth locates the hyoid apparatus and protrudes from the pharyngeal wall laterally at the selected exit site (**Figure 1**). Alternatively, forceps can be used to bulge the pharyngeal wall laterally. The finger locates the pulsating carotid artery, ensuring that it will be avoided, while providing a target for the tunneling forceps. A 1-cm skin incision is made over the bulging pharyngeal wall. Long, curved forceps are used to bluntly tunnel caudally through the tissues from outside to inside. Blunt dissection prevents injury to nearby nerves, carotid artery and jugular vein. Forceps are used to grasp one end of the feeding tube so it exits through the dissection site while the other end is advanced down the esophagus (**Figure 2**). The tube is then secured to the skin with tape and sutures.

Complications include airway obstruction, tube displacement, damage to cervical nerves and blood vessels and infection at the exit site. Placing the tube exit site caudal to the hyoid apparatus or use of very large diameter tubes is much more likely to result in airway obstruction or aspiration (**Figure 3**). The animal should be observed frequently for signs of respiratory embarrassment as it recovers from anesthesia. Frequent inspection and cleansing of the tube entrance/exit site help prevent skin infection. These tubes should not be used in vomiting patients or those with respiratory disease.

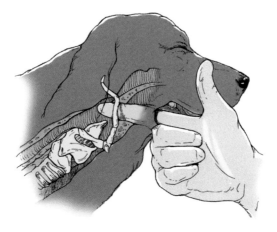

Figure 1. A finger is used to find the optimal exit site for the pharyngostomy tube. The tube should exit the pharyngeal wall as far caudally and dorsally as possible.

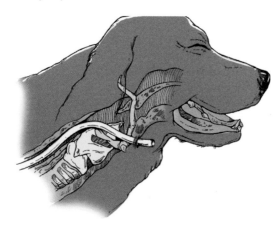

Figure 2. Proper placement of a pharyngostomy tube with the tube exiting dorsal and caudal to the larynx.

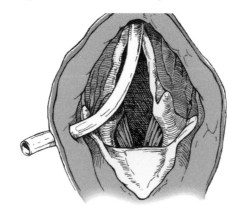

Figure 3. Inappropriate positioning of a pharyngostomy tube, as depicted here, causes the tube to course over the laryngeal opening and to interfere with movement of the epiglottis. This placement can lead to serious airway obstruction. The tube should exit the pharyngeal wall as far caudally and dorsally as possible.

Appendix H. Assisted-Feeding Techniques, continued.

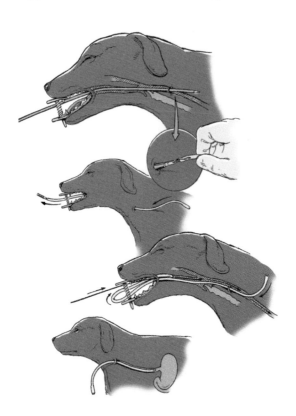

ESOPHAGOSTOMY TUBE PLACEMENT

Several techniques have been described for mid-cervical placement of esophagostomy tubes in dogs and cats. The animal receives light general anesthesia for esophagostomy tube placement. The entire lateral cervical region from the ventral midline to near the dorsal midline is clipped and aseptically prepared for surgery.

In one technique, appropriately sized, curved Kelly, Carmalt or similar forceps are inserted into the pharynx and then into the proximal cervical esophagus. The tip of the forceps is turned laterally and pressure is applied in an outward direction, thereby tenting up the cervical tissue so that the instrument tip can be seen and palpated externally. A small skin incision, just large enough to accommodate the feeding tube, is made over the tip of the forceps. In small dogs and cats, the tip of the forceps is forced bluntly through the esophagus. In larger dogs, a deeper incision is made to allow passage of the tip of the forceps through the esophagus. Tube sizes 12- to 19-Fr. are generally used. The tube is premeasured as described in **Figure 1, Nasoesophageal Tube Placement**, so that the distal tip resides in the mid to caudal esophagus. The distal tip of the tube is grasped with forceps, pulled into the esophagus and out through the mouth, turned around and redirected into the esophagus. The tube is then secured with tape and sutures. A light circumferential bandage containing antibiotic-impregnated gauze is then placed at the exit site.

Another technique uses a percutaneous feeding tube applicator (ELD Gastrostomy Tube Applicator) (**Figure 1**).

Reported complications of tube esophagostomy for nutritional support include tube displacement due to vomiting or scratching by the animal and skin infection around the exit site.

Figure 1. Insertion of a percutaneous feeding tube applicator into the mid-cervical esophagus. The distal tip is palpated and an incision is made through the skin and subcutaneous tissue over the tip of the applicator. The trocar is advanced through the esophageal wall and directed through the incision. The distal end of the feeding tube is secured to the eyelet of the trocar with suture material. The applicator and attached feeding tube are retracted into the esophagus and out the mouth. The feeding tube is redirected into the esophagus for final placement. A wire stylet can be inserted into the feeding tube if necessary to ease placement in the esophagus.

Appendix H. Assisted-Feeding Techniques, continued.

SURGICAL PLACEMENT OF GASTROSTOMY TUBES

A limited left flank celiotomy for gastrostomy tube placement provides an alternative when endoscopic or blind gastrostomy techniques are not performed. A gastrostomy tube may also be inserted when a celiotomy is performed for other reasons. General anesthesia is administered and the left flank is aseptically prepared for surgery. The prepared left paracostal area is draped and a 2- to 3-cm incision is made through the skin and subcutaneous tissue. The incision is made just caudal and parallel to the last rib, with its dorsal limit just below the ventral edge of the paravertebral epaxial musculature. The incision should be extended ventrally so that the intraperitoneal rather than the retroperitoneal space is accessed. The incision should be long enough to permit insertion of one or two fingers and a tissue forceps.

The greater curvature of the stomach is located and an Allis or Babcock tissue forceps is used to grasp and exteriorize the stomach through the incision. A stomach tube may be passed by an assistant and the stomach dilated with 10 to 15 ml of air/kg body weight if difficulty is encountered locating the stomach. Exteriorizing the stomach through a small flank incision can be difficult, especially in larger, deep-chested canine breeds. The left lateral aspect of the gastric body or the caudal aspect of the fundus is selected for the ostomy site. Two pursestring sutures are placed around the selected ostomy site (**Figure 1**). A stab incision is made through the ostomy site, the tube is inserted into the stomach and the pursestring sutures are tied snugly. Tube sizes 14 to 28 Fr. can be inserted.

The tube may exit the body wall through a separate stab wound or the original incision. The stomach is then fixed to the abdominal wall where the tube enters the peritoneum using a continuous suture pattern circling the gastrostomy tube placement (**Figure 2**). After the gastropexy sutures are placed, gentle traction is applied to the external end of the tube to ensure the stomach is adjacent to the abdominal wall (**Figure 3**). A rubber flange, which is slid down the tube to rest lightly against the skin, is sutured to the skin to secure the tube in place.

Potential risks with this procedure are the same as with any celiotomy and include wound infection, peritonitis and dehiscence. Pressure necrosis of the stomach may also occur if excessive tension is placed on the pursestring sutures. Wrapping the intraperitoneal tube with the omentum should contain leakage to a localized site. A layer of greater omentum can also be placed over the ostomy site before the stab incision is made into the stomach.

Percutaneous gastrostomy tube placement with gastropexy using a large-bore stiff plastic stomach tube has also been described. This technique is less invasive than the technique described here and may be more convenient for some veterinary practitioners.

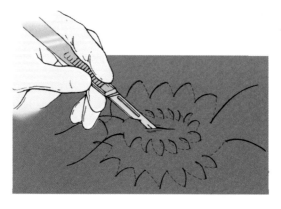

Figure 1. Two full-thickness pursestring sutures are placed concentrically around the selected gastrostomy site to help invert the stomach around the tube. A stab incision is made in the center of the suture pattern for tube placement.

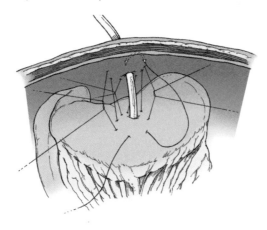

Figure 2. The stomach is sutured to the abdominal wall with four preplaced mattress sutures (or a simple continuous pattern). These sutures should include the strong abdominal fascia and the gastric submucosa. Tightening the loops brings the gastric serosa and omentum snugly in contact with the peritoneum.

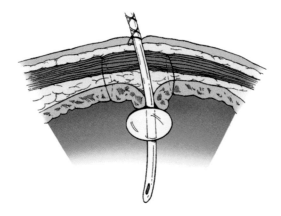

Figure 3. A mushroom-tip Pezzer catheter or one with an inflatable bulb is placed in the stomach. After the gastropexy sutures are placed, gentle traction is applied on the external end of the tube to ensure this area of the stomach is adjacent to the abdominal wall.

Appendix H. Assisted-Feeding Techniques, continued.

PERCUTANEOUS ENDOSCOPIC GASTROSTOMY TUBES

Percutaneous endoscopic gastrostomy (PEG) tubes are inserted with the aid of general anesthesia. The patient is placed in right lateral recumbency and an area of the left flank extending 4 to 6 inches caudal to the last rib is surgically prepared. **Figures 1** to **7** describe tube placement technique in detail. Landmarks for feeding tube placement are usually 1 to 2 cm caudal to the last rib and one-third the distance from the ventral border of the epaxial musculature to the ventral midline. Commercial PEG catheter assembly kits, ranging in size from 16 to 28 Fr., are available for small animal patients and provide cost-effective, convenient materials for PEG tube placement (**Figure 4**).

Following insertion, the tube is usually incorporated into a light bandage, with the free end brought to a convenient position for feeding. PEG tubes should be left in place for a minimum of five to seven days. Firm adhesions between the gastric serosa and the peritoneum have been reported to form within 36 to 48 hours of PEG tube placement in healthy dogs but do not reliably form in healthy cats. Adhesion formation may also be variable in undernourished animals.

The stomach should be empty when the tube is removed. Sedation or anesthesia is not generally required for tube extraction. Tubes are removed by exerting firm traction on the tube, while simultaneously applying counter-pressure around the exit site (**Figure 8**). An alternative method of removal, suitable for dogs weighing more than 10 kg, is to cut the catheter off flush with the skin, leaving the catheter tip to be passed in the feces. The resulting gastrocutaneous fistula usually heals rapidly.

Complications of PEG tube placement include vomiting, peristomal skin infection, cellulitis and pressure necrosis at the tube exit site.

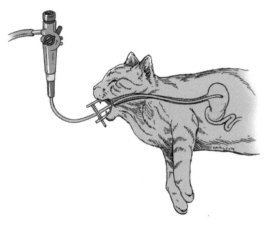

Figure 1. The animal is positioned in right lateral recumbency and an endoscope is introduced. The stomach is insufflated with air so that the gastric wall comes in contact with the body wall and the spleen is displaced caudally.

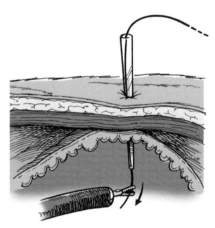

Figure 3. Nylon suture is advanced through the needle or catheter until it can be grasped with endoscopic retrieval forceps. The suture material is pulled out through the mouth as the endoscope is withdrawn.

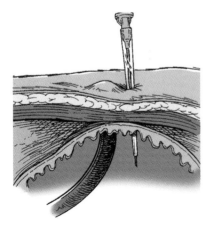

Figure 2. The lighted tip of the endoscope will be seen pressing outward against the abdominal wall. A large-bore needle or over-the-needle intravenous catheter is inserted into the stomach adjacent to the endoscope tip.

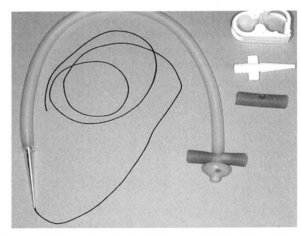

Figure 4. Commercial PEG catheter assembly kits provide the most convenient materials for PEG tube placement. The catheter guide is already secured to the free end of the feeding tube in commercial kits.

Appendix H. Assisted-Feeding Techniques, continued.

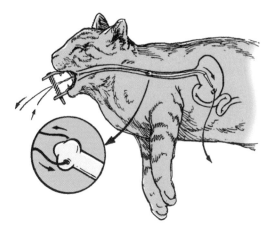

Figure 5. The lubricated catheter is drawn down the esophagus as the suture exiting the body wall is pulled. A second "safety" suture is placed through the openings in the mushroom-tip feeding tube (insert) and exits the mouth. This safety suture is used to retrieve the feeding tube from the stomach if problems occur during the placement procedure.

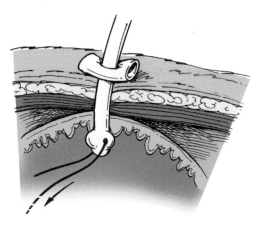

Figure 7. Gentle traction is used to bring the stomach and abdominal wall into loose contact. A rubber flange is fitted down the tube and a piece of tape attached to prevent tube slippage. The tube is not usually sutured or glued to the skin. The safety suture is removed via the mouth (arrow) after the feeding tube is secured.

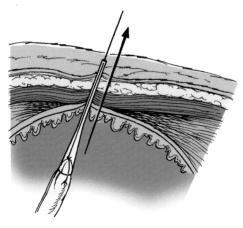

Figure 6. Resistance will be encountered when the catheter tip guide contacts the body wall. Steady traction and firm application of counter-pressure to the body wall will allow the guide tip to emerge through the skin (arrow). A small skin incision (2 to 3 mm) at the point of exit may help.

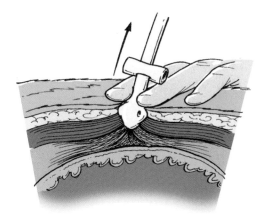

Figure 8. PEG tubes are usually removed by traction. The mushroom tip will usually collapse as it pulls through the abdominal wall. The resulting gastrocutaneous fistula usually heals rapidly.

Appendix I. Sodium Content of Human Foods/Taurine Concentrations of Natural Food Sources.

Table 1. Sodium content of selected human foods.*

Food	Amount	Sodium (mg)
Bread, cereals and potatoes		
Recommended		
Macaroni	1 cup	1-10
Potato	1 (medium)	<5
Puffed wheat	1 oz.	1-10
Rice (polished)	1/2 cup	1-10
Spaghetti	1 cup	1-10
Not recommended		
Bread	1 slice	200
Corn chips	1 oz.	230
Potato chips	1 oz.	300
Pretzel	1	275
Margarine and oil		
Recommended		
Unsalted margarine	1 tsp	0-1
Vegetable shortening	1 tbs	0-1
Not recommended		
Mayonnaise	1 tbs	60-90
Dairy products		
Not recommended		
American cheese	1 oz.	200-300
Butter	1 tsp	50
Cottage cheese	3 oz.	200-300
Cream cheese	1 1/2 oz.	100-120
Milk (regular and skim)	1 cup	122
Meats, poultry, fish		
Recommended		
Beef (fresh)	3 1/2 oz.	50
Chicken (no skin)		
Light meat	3 1/2 oz.	64
Dark meat	3 1/2 oz.	86
Lamb (fresh)	3 1/2 oz.	84
Pork (fresh)	3 1/2 oz.	62
Turkey (no skin)		
Light meat	3 1/2 oz.	82
Dark meat	3 1/2 oz.	98

Food	Amount	Sodium (mg)
Meats, poultry, fish (continued)		
Not recommended		
Bacon	2 slices	385
Egg	1	70
Frankfurter	1	560
Ham (processed)	3 oz.	940
Tuna (canned)	1 can	320
Vegetables (fresh or dietetic canned)		
Recommended		
Corn	1/2 cup	<5
Cucumber	1/2 cup	<5
Green beans	1/2 cup	<5
Green pepper	1/4 cup	<5
Lettuce	1/4 cup	<5
Peas	1/2 cup	<5
Tomato	1	<5
Not recommended		
Most canned vegetables	1/2 cup	190-450
Fruits		
Most fresh and canned fruits are low in sodium and are permitted		
Other food items		
Not recommended		
Macaroni with cheese	1 cup	1,000
Peanut butter	1 tbs	81
Pizza (cheese)	1 slice	650
Desserts		
Recommended		
Sherbet	1/2 cup	15-25
Not recommended		
Cookies	1	35-100
Gelatins	1/2 cup	60-85
Ice cream	1/2 cup	60-85
Puddings	1/2 cup	100-200

*Sodium amounts are on an as fed basis; adapted from Morris ML Jr, Ettinger SJ. In: Ettinger SJ, Feldman EC, eds. Textbook of Veterinary Internal Medicine, 4th ed. Philadelphia, PA: WB Saunders Co, 1995; 237.

Table 2. Taurine concentrations (mg/kg dry matter) in selected natural food sources.

Source	Concentration
Beef muscle, uncooked	1,200
Chicken muscle, uncooked	1,100
Cod fish, uncooked	1,000
Lamb muscle, uncooked	1,600
Mouse carcass	7,000
Pork muscle, uncooked	1,600
Tuna, canned	2,500

Appendix J. Inherited Diseases/IRIS Staging System/Feeding Tips for CKD Patients.

Table 1. Kidney diseases suspected or confirmed to be inherited in dogs and cats.

Kidney disease	Canine breeds	Feline breeds
Amyloidosis	Beagle, collie, foxhound, Chinese Shar-Pei, Walker hound	Abyssinian, Siamese, Oriental
Atrophic glomerulopathy	Rottweiler	–
Fanconi syndrome	Basenji, border terrier, miniature schnauzer, Norwegian elkhound, Shetland sheepdog	–
Glomerulonephropathy	Beagle, Bernese mountain dog, bull mastiff, Dalmatian, Doberman pinscher, soft-coated wheaten terrier	–
Glomerulosclerosis	Newfoundland	–
Hereditary nephritis	Bull terrier, English cocker spaniel, Samoyed	–
Medullary cystic disease	Miniature schnauzer	–
Polycystic kidney disease	Beagle, cairn terrier, collie, foxhound, miniature poodle	Domestic longhair cat, Himalayan, Persian
Primary renal glucosuria	Norwegian elkhound, Scottish terrier	–
Renal cystadenocarcinoma	German shepherd dog	–
Renal dysplasia	Alaskan malamute, beagle, boxer, bulldog, cavalier King Charles spaniel, chow chow, cocker spaniel, Dutch kookier, Great Dane, Great Pyrenees, golden retriever, Irish wolfhound, keeshond, Lhasa apso, Samoyed, Shih Tzu, soft-coated wheaten terrier, standard poodle, Yorkshire terrier	Persian
Renal telangiectasia	Pembroke Welsh corgi	–
Tubulointerstitial nephropathy	Norwegian elkhound	–
Unilateral renal agenesis	Beagle, Doberman pinscher	Domestic shorthair cat, Himalayan

Table 2. International Renal Interest Society (IRIS) Staging System for Chronic Kidney Disease in Dogs and Cats.

Stage	Serum creatinine (dogs)	Serum creatinine (cats)	Substage based on proteinuria and hypertension	Comments
1	<1.4 mg/dl (<125 µmol/l)	<1.6 mg/dl (<140 µmol/l)	Proteinuria: NP/BP/P* Hypertension: N/L/M/H/nc/c/RND**	Non-azotemic CKD Clinical signs (other than PU/PD) usually absent
2	1.4-2.0 mg/dl (125-179 µmol/l)	1.6-2.8 mg/dl (140-249 µmol/l)	Proteinuria: NP/BP/P* Hypertension: N/L/M/H/nc/c/RND**	Mild renal azotemia (overlaps with reference range) Clinical signs (other than PU/PD) usually mild or absent
3	2.1-5.0 mg/dl (180-439 µmol/l)	2.9-5.0 mg/dl (250-439 µmol/l)	Proteinuria: NP/BP/P* Hypertension: N/L/M/H/nc/c/RND**	Moderate renal azotemia Extrarenal clinical signs usually begin in this stage
4	>5.0 mg/dl (>440 µmol/l)	>5.0 mg/dl (>440 µmol/l)	Proteinuria: NP/BP/P* Hypertension: N/L/M/H/nc/c/RND**	Severe renal azotemia Many extrarenal clinical signs usually present

Key: PU/PD = polyuria/polydipsia, UPC = urine protein-creatinine ratio, BP = blood pressure.
*NP = non-proteinuric (UPC <0.2), BP = borderline proteinuric (UPC = 0.2 to 0.4 in cats and 0.2 to 0.5 in dogs), P = proteinuric (UPC >0.4 in cats and >0.5 in dogs).
**N = minimal risk of complications (systolic BP <150 mm Hg), L = low risk of complications (systolic BP 150 to 159 mm Hg),
M = moderate risk of complications (systolic BP 160 to 179 mm Hg), H = high risk of complications (systolic BP >180 mm Hg),
nc = no evidence of hypertensive complications, c = hypertensive complications present, RND = risk not determined (blood pressure not measured).
Adapted from www.iris-kidney.com.

Appendix J. Inherited Diseases/IRIS Staging System/Feeding Tips for CKD Patients, continued.

BOX 1. TIPS FOR ENCOURAGING ACCEPTANCE OF VETERINARY THERAPEUTIC RENAL FOODS IN PATIENTS WITH CHRONIC KIDNEY DISEASE.

Educate pet owners about the effectiveness of nutritional management for prolonging survival time and improving quality of life in patients with kidney disease. For treatment to succeed, owners must commit their time and money, which is more likely to occur if they understand the benefits of their efforts.

Begin nutritional management sooner rather than later. Current evidence supports feeding a veterinary therapeutic renal food when serum creatinine is ≥2 mg/dl. Waiting until later (e.g., when there are signs of uremia) is not advised because patients with more advanced disease may be less likely to accept a change in treatment and therefore will not receive optimal benefits of a renal therapeutic food.

Probably the single most important thing you can do to increase patient acceptance of a veterinary therapeutic renal food is gradually transition to the new food. The transition period should be a minimum of seven days; however, some patients (especially cats) need a transition of three to four weeks or longer. It is critical to discuss the need for this transition with pet owners, otherwise, they are likely to buy a new food, go home and switch from the old food to the new food at the next meal. In this scenario, many patients will refuse to eat the new food, which results in an unhappy owner and a patient that will likely not receive the benefits of nutritional management.

One option for transitioning to a renal food is to mix the old and new food, gradually adding more of the new food over time. Another approach is to provide both foods (old and new) in side-by-side food dishes. This technique assists with gradual transition and also allows cats to express their preferences. For more information, visit www.vet.osu.edu/indoorcat for The Indoor Cat Initiative.

If transitioning cats from dry to moist food, use a flat food dish (e.g., saucer) instead of a bowl. This avoids rubbing the cat's whiskers on the food dish, which could affect acceptance of new food.

Avoid offering veterinary therapeutic renal foods in stressful environments (e.g., sick and/or hospitalization, during force-feeding); a food aversion may develop causing decreased acceptance of the food when the patient is feeling better. Stated another way, while patients are hospitalized, do not feed them (especially cats) the food you want them to eat for the rest of their lives. In this situation, one option would be to feed a maintenance food that avoids excessive protein, phosphorus and sodium until the patient is feeling better and then gradually transition to a therapeutic renal food.

Use fresh food at room temperature. Some patients may eat refrigerated food that is warmed, but others will only eat food from a newly opened container. Some patients may eat food that has been refrigerated and stored in a plastic container vs. food stored in the original can.

Offer foods with different textures (e.g., minced formulas) or form (dry vs. moist). Some pets may prefer dry or moist food all their lives and when they develop kidney disease, their preferences may switch (e.g., a cat that has eaten dry food all its life may eat moist food after kidney disease occurs and vice versa).

Add flavor enhancers (low-sodium chicken broth or tuna juice) or a small amount of maintenance food to encourage the patient to eat all the veterinary therapeutic food. Excessive use of other foods will likely decrease the beneficial effects of the veterinary therapeutic renal food; therefore, the smallest amount possible should be used.

If you have followed the steps above and there is still reluctance to eat a veterinary therapeutic renal food, switch to a different brand. Although commercially available renal foods have general features in common, they are not the same. In addition, individual pets may express a preference for one brand over another. Avoid giving the owner samples of several different brands of foods at once; this could result in a food aversion to all veterinary therapeutic renal foods, especially if owners offer each sample at successive meals or on consecutive days.

Appendix K. Canine Urolithiasis.

Table 1. Mineral composition of 350,803 canine uroliths evaluated at the Minnesota Urolith Center by quantitative methods: 1981 to 2007.

Predominant mineral type	Proportion of predominant mineral (%)	Number	Percent
Magnesium ammonium phosphate•6H$_2$O	-	**149,199**	**42.53**
	100	(66,481)	-
	70-99*	(82,718)	-
Magnesium hydrogen phosphate•3H$_2$O	-	**52**	**0.01**
	100	(19)	-
	70-99*	(33)	-
Magnesium phosphate hydrate	70-100	**4**	**<0.01**
Calcium oxalate	-	**133,338**	**38.01**
Calcium oxalate monohydrate	100	(69,863)	-
	70-99*	(31,677)	-
Calcium oxalate dihydrate	100	(8,341)	-
	70-99*	(13,896)	-
Calcium oxalate monohydrate and dihydrate	100	(8,004)	-
	70-99*	(1,557)	-
Calcium phosphate	-	**1,801**	**0.51**
Calcium phosphate	100	(413)	-
	70-99*	(694)	-
Calcium hydrogen phosphate•2H$_2$O	100	(233)	-
	70-99*	(460)	-
Tricalcium phosphate	70-99*	(1)	-
Purines	-	**22,412**	**6.39**
Ammonium urate	100	(15,607)	-
	70-99*	(2,820)	-
Sodium urate	100	(1,577)	-
	70-99*	(118)	-
Sodium calcium urate (salts of uric acid)	100	(1,153)	-
	70-99*	(117)	-
Ammonium calcium urate	70-99*	(1)	-
Uric acid	100	(464)	-
	70-99*	(32)	-
Xanthine	100	(197)	-
	70-99*	(72)	-
Uric acid monohydrate (formerly unidentified uric acid)	100	(251)	-
	70-99*	(3)	-
Cystine	-	**3,402**	**0.97**
	100	(3,275)	-
	70-99*	(127)	-
Silica	-	**1,414**	**0.4**
	100	(982)	-
	70-99*	(432)	-
Other	-	**24**	**0.01**
Calcium carbonate	70-100	**6**	**<0.01**
Dolomite	100	**1**	**<0.01**
Mixed**	-	**8,146**	**2.32**
Compound***	-	**30,832**	**8.79**
Matrix	-	**153**	**0.04**
Drug metabolite	-	**19**	**0.01**

*Urolith composed of 70 to 99% of mineral type listed; no nucleus and shell detected.
**Uroliths did not contain at least 70% of mineral type listed; no nucleus or shell detected.
***Uroliths contained an identifiable nucleus and one or more surrounding layers of a different mineral type.

Appendix K. Canine Urolithiasis, continued.

Table 2. Clinical signs of uroliths that may be associated with urinary system dysfunction.

Urethroliths
Asymptomatic
Dysuria, pollakiuria, urge incontinence and/or periuria
Gross hematuria
Palpable urethral uroliths
Spontaneous voiding of small uroliths
Partial or complete urine outflow obstruction
    Overflow incontinence
    Anuria
    Palpation of an overdistended and painful urinary bladder
    Urinary bladder rupture, abdominal distention and
        abdominal pain
    Signs of postrenal azotemia (anorexia, depression, vomiting
        and diarrhea)
    Signs associated with concurrent urocystoliths, ureteroliths
        and/or renoliths

Urocystoliths
Asymptomatic
Dysuria, pollakiuria and urge incontinence
Gross hematuria
Palpable bladder uroliths
Palpably thickened urinary bladder wall
Partial or complete urine outflow obstruction of bladder neck
    (See Urethroliths.)
Other signs associated with concurrent urethroliths, ureteroliths
    and/or nephroliths

Ureteroliths
Asymptomatic
Gross hematuria
Constant abdominal pain
Unilateral or bilateral urine outflow obstruction
    Palpably enlarged kidney(s)
    Signs of postrenal azotemia (See Urethroliths.)
May have other signs associated with concurrent urethroliths,
    urocystoliths and/or nephroliths

Nephroliths
Asymptomatic
Gross hematuria
Constant abdominal pain
Signs of systemic illness if generalized renal infection is present
    (anorexia, depression, fever and polyuria)
Palpably enlarged kidney(s)
Signs of postrenal azotemia (See Urethroliths.)
Other signs associated with concurrent urethroliths, urocystoliths
    and/or ureteroliths

Table 3. Common characteristics of selected urine crystals.

Crystal types	Appearances	Urinary pH at which crystals commonly form		
		Acidic	Neutral	Alkaline
Ammonium urate	Yellow-brown spherulites, thorn apples	+	+	+
Amorphous urates	Amorphous or spheroidal yellow-brown structures	+	±	-
Bilirubin	Reddish-brown needles or granules	+	-	-
Calcium carbonate	Large yellow-brown spheroids with radial striations, or small crystals with spheroidal or dumbbell shapes	-	±	+
Calcium oxalate dihydrate	Small colorless envelopes (octahedral form)	+	+	±
Calcium oxalate monohydrate	Small spindles "hempseed" or dumbbells	+	+	±
Calcium phosphate	Amorphous or long thin prisms	±	+	+
Cholesterol	Flat colorless plates with corner notch	+	+	-
Cystine	Flat colorless hexagonal plates	+	+	±
Hippuric acid	Four- to six-sided colorless elongated plates or prisms with rounded corners	+	+	±
Leucine	Yellow-brown spheroids with radial and concentric laminations	+	+	-
Magnesium ammonium phosphate	Three- to six-sided colorless prisms	±	+	+
Sodium urate	Colorless or yellow-brown needles or slender prisms, sometimes in clusters or sheaves	+	±	-
Sulfa metabolites	Sheaves of needles with central or eccentric binding, sometimes fan-shaped clusters	+	±	-
Tyrosine	Fine colorless or yellow needles arranged in sheaves or rosettes	+	-	-
Uric acid	Diamond or rhombic rosettes, or oval plates, structures with pointed ends, occasionally six-sided plates	+	-	-
Xanthine	Yellow-brown amorphous, spheroidal or ovoid structures	+	±	-

Key: + = crystals commonly occur at this pH, ± = crystals may occur at this pH, but are more common at the other pH, - = crystals are uncommon at this pH.

Appendix K. Canine Urolithiasis, continued.

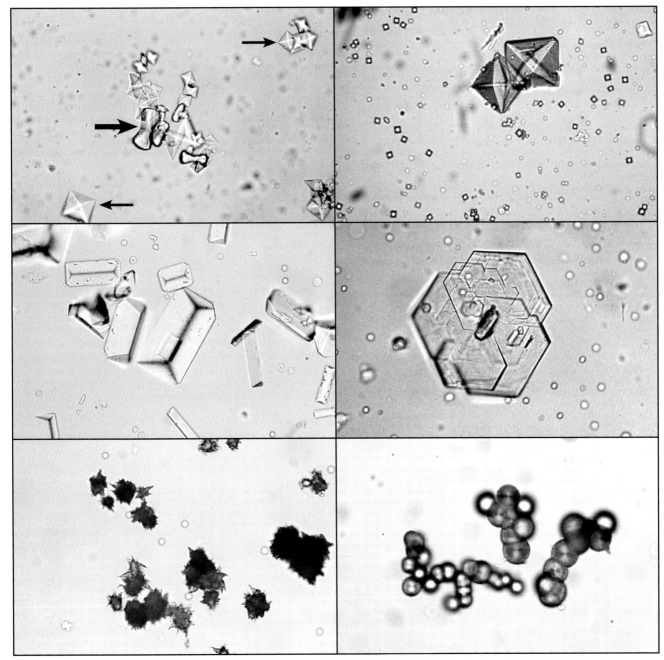

Figure 1. Photomicrographs of common crystals found in urine sediment. Calcium oxalate monohydrate (dumbbell form, large arrow) and calcium oxalate dihydrate (octahedral form, small arrows) (Top, Left). Calcium oxalate dihydrate; octahedral form (Top, Right). Magnesium ammonium phosphate (struvite); prisms (Middle, Left). Cystine; flat, colorless hexagonal plates (Middle, Right). Ammonium urate; thorn apple form (Bottom, Left). Amorphous xanthine; spheroids (Bottom, Right).

Appendix K. Canine Urolithiasis, continued.

Table 4. Voiding urohydropropulsion: A nonsurgical technique for removing small urocystoliths.

1. Perform appropriate diagnostic studies, including complete urinalysis, quantitative urine culture and diagnostic radiography. Determine the location, size, surface contour and number of urocystoliths.
2. Anesthetize the patient, if needed.
3. If the urinary bladder is not distended with urine, moderately distend it with a physiologic solution (e.g., saline, Ringer's, etc.) injected through a transurethral catheter. To prevent overdistention, palpate the bladder per abdomen during infusion. Remove the catheter.
4. Position the patient such that the vertebral spine is approximately vertical.
5. Gently agitate the urinary bladder, with the objective of promoting gravitational movement of urocystoliths into the bladder neck.
6. Induce voiding by manually expressing the urinary bladder. Use steady digital pressure rather than an intermittent squeezing motion.
7. Collect urine and uroliths in a cup. Compare urolith number and size to those detected by radiography and submit them for quantitative analysis.
8. If needed, repeat Steps 3 through 7 until the number of uroliths detected by radiography are removed or until uroliths are no longer voided.
9. Perform double-contrast cystography to ensure that no uroliths remain in the urinary bladder. Repeat voiding urohydropropulsion if small urocystoliths remain.
10. Administer prophylactic antimicrobials for three to five days, or longer if needed.
11. Monitor the patient for adverse complications (i.e., hematuria, dysuria, bacterial urinary tract infection and urethral obstruction with uroliths).
12. Formulate appropriate recommendations to minimize urolith recurrence or to manage uroliths remaining in the urinary tract on the basis of quantitative mineral analysis of voided urocystoliths.

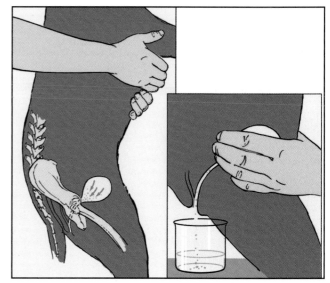

Figure 2. To remove urocystoliths by voiding urohydropropulsion, position the patient so that its vertebral column is approximately vertical (Left). The urinary bladder is then gently agitated to promote gravitational movement of urocystoliths into the bladder neck. To expel urocystoliths (Right), voiding is induced by applying steady digital pressure to the urinary bladder. (Adapted from Lulich JP, Osborne CA, Carlson M, et al. Nonsurgical removal of uroliths from dogs and cats by voiding urohydropropulsion. Journal of the American Veterinary Medical Association 1993; 203: 660-663.)

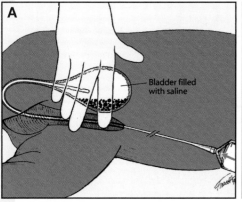
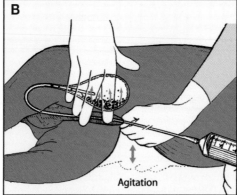
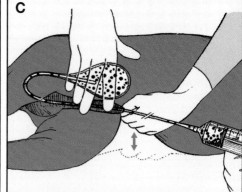

Figure 3. Illustration of catheter-assisted retrieval of urocystoliths. With the patient in lateral recumbency, uroliths have gravitated to the dependent portion of the urinary bladder (A). The bladder lumen has been distended by injection of 0.9% saline solution. Vigorous movement of the abdomen in an up-and-down motion disperses uroliths throughout fluid in the bladder lumen (B). Aspiration of fluid from the urinary bladder during movement of the abdominal wall (C) may result in movement of one or more small uroliths into the catheter and syringe. (Adapted from Lulich JP, Osborne CA. Catheter assisted retrieval of canine and feline urocystoliths. Journal of the American Veterinary Medical Association 1992; 201: 111-113.)

Appendix K. Canine Urolithiasis, continued.

Table 5. Contact information for urolith analysis laboratories.

Antech Diagnostics – East
111 Marcus Ave.
Lake Success, NY 11042
800.872.1001

Antech Diagnostics – West
17672 Cowan Ave.
Irvine, CA 92614
800.745.4725

Canadian Veterinary Urolith Centre
Laboratory Services Division
University of Guelph
95 Stone Road West
P.O. Box 3650
Guelph, ON N1H8J7

Gerald V. Ling Urinary Stone Analysis Laboratory
Department of Medicine
Room 3106 MSI-A
School of Veterinary Medicine
Davis, CA 95616
Phone: 530.752.3228
Fax: 530.752.0414
www.vetmed.ucdavis.edu/vme/labs.htm

Laboratory for Stone Research
81 Wyman Street
P.O. Box 129
Newton, MA 02168

Louis C. Herring and Company
1111 South Orange Ave.
Orlando, FL 32806-1236
P.O. Box 2191
Orlando, FL 32802
Phone: 407.841.770
Fax: 407.422.8896
www.herringlab.com

Minnesota Urolith Center
University of Minnesota
1352 Boyd Ave.
St. Paul, MN 55108
Phone: 612.625.4221
Fax: 612.624.0751
www.cvm.umn.edu/depts/minnesotaurolithcenter

Urolithiasis Laboratory
P.O. Box 25375
Houston, TX 77265-5375
800.235.4846
www.urolithiasis-lab.com

BOX 1. RECIPES FOR SUPPLEMENTING LOW-PROTEIN FOODS FOR URATE UROLITHIASIS.

Providing a safe and effective urate litholytic food for immature dogs presents a challenge. Growing dogs usually consume greater quantities of protein and, thus, purines than adult dogs. The safety and efficacy of low-protein litholytic foods in young dogs with urate uroliths are unknown. Adding non-purine-containing protein to the litholytic food may be effective; however, no studies have yet been performed to confirm this hypothesis. Also, the metabolism of allopurinol in puppies has not been evaluated. Therefore, surgical removal of large uroliths remains the option with the most predictable short-term outcome.

The dry formulation of a low-protein veterinary therapeutic food[a] often recommended for dogs with urate urolithiasis can be modified for growing dogs (**Table 1**). However, the long-term safety and efficacy of this modified food in young dogs with urate or other uroliths are unknown. Therefore, growing dogs should be appropriately monitored for protein-calorie malnutrition if fed foods based on these recipes.

Table 1. Modified recipes for growing dogs based on the dry formulation of a low-protein, low-purine veterinary therapeutic food.

Recipe A	Recipe B
1 cup Prescription Diet u/d Canine	1 cup Prescription Diet u/d Canine
1 tsp dicalcium phosphate	3/4 tsp dicalcium phosphate
1 cup cottage cheese	2 cooked eggs
Multivitamin-mineral supplement for dogs	Multivitamin-mineral supplement for dogs

Nutrient levels (% dry matter)		Nutrient levels (% dry matter)	
Protein	30.5	Protein	17.6
Fat	19.5	Fat	27.1
Calcium	1.0	Calcium	1.1
Phosphorus	1.0	Phosphorus	1.0
Magnesium	0.02	Magnesium	0.02
Sodium	0.6	Sodium	0.4
Potassium	0.5	Potassium	0.6

ENDNOTE
a. Hill's Prescription Diet u/d Canine dry. Hill's Pet Nutrition, Inc., Topeka, KS, USA.

Appendix K. Canine Urolithiasis, continued.

Table 6. Predicting mineral composition of common canine uroliths.

Mineral types	Urinary pH	Crystal appearance	Urine culture	Predictors — Radiographic density	Radiographic contour	Serum abnormalities	Breed predisposition	Gender predisposition (>80%)	Common ages
Magnesium ammonium phosphate	Neutral to alkaline	Three- to eight-sided colorless prisms	Urease-producing bacteria (staphylococci, Proteus spp., Ureaplasma spp.)	1+ to 4+ (sometimes laminated)	Smooth, round or faceted May assume shape of renal pelvis, ureter, bladder or urethra	None	Miniature schnauzer, miniature poodle, Bichon Frise, cocker spaniel	Females (>80%)	2 to 9 years
Calcium oxalate	Acidic to neutral	Colorless envelope or octahedral shape (dihydrate salt) Spindles or dumbbell shape (monohydrate salt)	Negative	2+ to 4+	Rough or speculated (dihydrate salt) Small, smooth, round (monohydrate salt) Sometimes jackstone	Usually normocalcemic, occasionally hypercalcemic	Miniature schnauzer, standard schnauzer, Lhasa apso, Yorkshire terrier, miniature poodle, Shih Tzu, Bichon Frise	Males (>70%)	5 to 12 years
Urate	Acidic to neutral	Yellow-brown amorphous shapes (ammonium urate)	Negative	0 to 2+	Smooth (occasionally irregular) round or oval	Low serum urea nitrogen and albumin values in dogs with hepatic portosystemic shunts	Dalmatian, English bulldog, miniature schnauzer, Yorkshire terrier, Shih Tzu	Males (>90%)	1 to 5 years
Calcium phosphate	Alkaline to neutral (brushite forms in acidic urine)	Amorphous or long thin prisms	Negative	2+ to 4+	Smooth or irregular, round or faceted	Occasionally hypercalcemic	Yorkshire terrier, miniature schnauzer, Shih Tzu	Males (>55%)	<1 year, 6 to 10 years
Cystine	Acidic to neutral	Flat colorless hexagonal plates	Negative	1+ to 2+	Smooth (occasionally irregular) round or oval	None	English bulldog, dachshund, basset hound, Newfoundland	Males (>98%)	1 to 7 years
Silica	Acidic to neutral	None observed	Negative	2+ to 3+	Round center with radial spoke-like projections (jackstone)	None	German shepherd, golden retriever, Labrador retriever, miniature schnauzer, cavalier King Charles spaniel	Males (95%)	3 to 10 years

Appendix K. Canine Urolithiasis, continued.

BOX 2. COMPOUND UROLITHIASIS.

Compound uroliths (nucleus composed of one mineral type and shells of a different mineral type) occurred in approximately 7% of the canine uroliths analyzed at the University of Minnesota (**Table 1**). Examples include: 1) a nucleus of 100% calcium oxalate monohydrate surrounded by a shell of 80% magnesium ammonium phosphate and 20% calcium phosphate, 2) a nucleus composed of 95% magnesium ammonium phosphate and 5% calcium phosphate surrounded by a shell of 95% ammonium acid urate and 5% magnesium ammonium phosphate and 3) a nucleus composed of 95% silica and 5% calcium oxalate monohydrate surrounded by a shell of 100% calcium oxalate monohydrate.

Voiding urohydropropulsion may be used to remove small compound urocystoliths (**Figure 2** and **Table 4**). Lithotripsy may be considered to remove uroliths lodged in the urethra. For most practitioners, surgery remains the most reliable method to remove large compound urocystoliths.

Because risk factors that predispose patients to precipitation (nucleation) of different minerals vary, the occurrence of compound uroliths poses a unique challenge in terms of preventing recurrence. In the absence of clinical evidence to the contrary, it seems logical to recommend management protocols designed primarily to minimize recurrence of minerals composing the nucleus (rather than those in shells) of compound uroliths. (See specific chapters for recommendations [Chapters 39 through 44, Small Animal Clinical Nutrition, 5th edition]). Followup studies designed to evaluate efficacy of preventive protocols should include complete urinalyses, radiography or ultrasonography and if available, evaluation of the urine concentration of lithogenic metabolites.

Appendix L. Feline Lower Urinary Tract Diseases.

BOX 1. ANCILLARY MANAGEMENT FOR PATIENTS WITH FELINE IDIOPATHIC CYSTITIS: ENVIRONMENTAL ENRICHMENT.

In addition to nutritional management, currently recommended treatment for patients with feline idiopathic cystitis (FIC) includes environmental enrichment, stress reduction and appropriate litter box maintenance. Recently, a prospective, uncontrolled study evaluated the effects of multimodal environmental modification in 46 client-owned cats with FIC. Significant reductions in lower urinary tract signs, fearfulness and nervousness were seen after treatment for 10 months, compared with the signs noted before using environmental enrichment.

Environmental enrichment includes providing opportunities for play/resting (e.g., horizontal and vertical surfaces for scratching, hiding places and climbing platforms). Food and water bowls should be clean and kept in safe places (e.g., not next to noisy appliances). Litter boxes should be clean and kept in locations that do not increase stress. An adequate number of litter boxes (generally defined as one more than the number of cats in the home) should be available. Most cats prefer clumping, unscented litter but individual preferences may differ for some cats and different strategies can be used to determine a cat's particular preference. More detailed and helpful information about environmental enrichment and litter box management is available elsewhere.

BEHAVIORAL MANAGEMENT

Even after successful implementation of strategies described above, some patients with FIC (or other lower urinary tract disorders) may continue to urinate in inappropriate locations. This undesirable behavioral pattern may be maintained for several reasons. Classic conditioning may play a role in persistent periuria. The litter box is associated with pain and discomfort that occurred when the cat urinated in the box previously; therefore, the cat might associate this experience with the litter box and avoid using it in the future. In this situation, it may help to change the location or physical characteristics of the litter box. It also is possible for cats to develop a litter box aversion secondary to lack of cleanliness, because the litter box may be used more frequently during episodes of FIC. If this happens, it may help to provide additional litter boxes and/or increase frequency of cleaning the litter box or changing litter. If a cat develops a litter box aversion secondary to FIC or experiences an urgency that causes elimination elsewhere, the possibility exists for development of a secondary location or substrate preference. In this situation, the litter box is not necessarily the problem; however, the cat may discover a better toileting option (e.g., a substrate that is softer, more absorbent, more accessible or cleaned more readily). To resolve this problem, the preferred inappropriate site should be made less attractive or unavailable while the litter box is improved to meet the preferences of the cat. Finally, the pain associated with an episode of FIC may result in increased irritability and subsequent social strife between previously friendly cats in the household. When signs of FIC resolve, cats may not return to their previously friendly relationship. In serious cases, full segregation and gradual reintroduction using desensitization and counter-conditioning may be necessary. Cats with persistent periuria can be very frustrating to manage and may be relinquished to a shelter if not handled appropriately. Therefore, consulting with a veterinary behaviorist (sooner rather than later) should be considered to increase chances of improving quality of life for the cat and the owner. **Boxes 2** and **3** provide more information about behavioral management of cats with inappropriate urination.

PAIN MANAGEMENT

Analgesics are indicated to manage patient discomfort during acute episodes of FIC. Drugs that have been used include buprenorphine[a] (0.03 mg/kg body weight administered topically via buccal mucosa every six to eight hours), butorphanol[b] (0.5 to 1 mg/kg body weight orally every six to eight hours) and meloxicam[c] (0.1 mg/kg body weight orally once daily for three to four days). Although other anal-

Appendix L. Feline Lower Urinary Tract Diseases, continued.

gesics and nonsteroidal antiinflammatory agents may be appropriate, selection is often based on clinician preference or experience and whether the patient has concomitant conditions (e.g., kidney disease) that might preclude their use. No clinical studies have evaluated opioid analgesics (e.g., butorphanol, buprenorphine) or nonsteroidal antiinflammatory agents in patients with FIC.

FELINE FACIAL PHEROMONE

Synthetic feline facial pheromone therapy has been recommended to decrease signs of stress in patients with FIC. In a double-blind, placebo-controlled clinical study of 20 hospitalized cats (13 with lower urinary tract disease and seven apparently healthy), exposure to feline facial pheromone[d] was associated with significant increases in grooming, interest in food and food intake; these results suggested an anxiolytic effect in some cats. Another study evaluated effects of feline facial pheromone in 12 patients with FIC. Although no significant difference was seen between treatment of the environment with placebo and feline facial pheromone for two months, a trend was identified for cats exposed to facial pheromone. Exposed cats had fewer days with clinical signs of cystitis, a reduced number of episodes and reduced negative behavioral traits (e.g., less aggression and fear). Further study is needed; however, it seems reasonable to consider treatment with facial pheromones in cats with signs of stress or when clinical signs persist after implementing environmental enrichment and methods to increase water intake.

GLYCOSAMINOGLYCANS

Glycosaminoglycan (GAG) replacers such as pentosan polysulfate have been used in people with interstitial cystitis and have been recommended for patients with FIC. Anecdotally, these agents have been mentioned as useful. However, only one GAG has been critically evaluated. In a randomized, double-blinded, controlled clinical study, administration of glucosamine hydrochloride[e] (125 mg orally once daily) was not associated with any difference in clinical signs compared with cats that received placebo. If signs of FIC persist despite other treatments, GAGs (such as pentosan polysulfate[f] [8 mg/kg body weight orally q12h] or a combination of glucosamine

and chondroitin sulfate[g] [250 mg/200 mg orally q24h]) may be attempted.

AMITRIPTYLINE

Amitriptyline[h] is a tricyclic antidepressant with anticholinergic, antihistaminic, sympatholytic, analgesic and antiinflammatory properties that has been used in treating people with interstitial cystitis and cats with FIC. In an uncontrolled study of cats with severe, recurrent FIC that failed to respond to other treatments, administration of amitriptyline for 12 months was associated with decreased clinical signs in nine (60%) of 15 cats during the last six months of treatment. A randomized, controlled clinical trial of amitriptyline treatment for seven days revealed no significant difference in rate of recovery from pollakiuria or hematuria; overall, clinical signs recurred significantly faster and more frequently in cats that had been treated with amitriptyline compared with control cats. In a similar study, amitriptyline combined with amoxicillin was no more effective than placebo and amoxicillin when given to cats with FIC for seven days. Based on current information, amitriptyline does not appear to be beneficial for short-term management of cats with FIC. It is possible that longer use (i.e., several months) may be helpful; however, this has not yet been demonstrated in a controlled, long-term clinical study.

ENDNOTES

a. Buprenex. Reckitt Benckiser Pharmaceuticals, Inc., Richmond, VA, USA.
b. Torbutrol and Torbugesic. Fort Dodge Animal Health, Fort Dodge, IA, USA.
c. Metacam. Boehringer Ingelheim Vetmedica, Inc., Saint Joseph, MO, USA.
d. Feliway. Veterinary Product Laboratories, Phoenix, AZ, USA.
e. Cystease. Ceva Animal Health, Chesam, United Kingdom.
f. Elmiron. Ortho McNeil Pharmaceutical, Inc., Raritan, NJ, USA.
g. Cosequin for Cats. Nutramax Laboratories, Inc., Edgewood, MO, USA.
h. Elavil. Astra-Zenaca, Wilmington, DE, USA.

Appendix L. Feline Lower Urinary Tract Diseases, continued.

BOX 2. BEHAVIORAL SCREEN FOR CATS WITH INAPPROPRIATE URINATION.*

All cats that urinate outside the litter box or in inappropriate places should receive a medical evaluation to identify and address underlying medical disease(s). In some cases, a primary medical reason for inappropriate urination will be identified, treatment implemented and the problem resolved. However, in other cases there will be no primary medical problem identified or even after resolution/control of an identified medical issue, inappropriate urination continues. In the latter case, the medical problem may have been the initiating cause but behavioral issues maintain inappropriate urination, despite successful control/resolution of primary medical problems. For cats with continued inappropriate urination despite diagnosis and management of all primary medical issues, the following questions should be considered:

Question**	Answer
1. Does your cat urinate on vertical surfaces outside the litter box?	☐ YES ☐ NO
2. Does your cat urinate on horizontal surfaces outside the litter box?	☐ YES ☐ NO
3. Does your cat seek out certain targets for urination?	☐ YES ☐ NO
4. Do these targets have a common quality (e.g. all soft, absorbent materials, certain room, always slick surfaces)?	☐ YES ☐ NO
5. Is the quantity of urine deposited very small?	☐ YES ☐ NO
6. Does your cat defecate outside the litter box?	☐ YES ☐ NO
7. Does your cat ever use the litter box?	☐ YES ☐ NO
8. Does your cat dig in its litter when it uses the litter box?	☐ YES ☐ NO
9. Is there more than one cat in the household?	☐ YES ☐ NO
10. Does your cat ever fight or appear frightened of other pets or people in the household?	☐ YES ☐ NO
11. Are the litter boxes all in the same site/room/area/floor of the home?	☐ YES ☐ NO

Total number of litter boxes in the house .... _____

Indicate number of boxes with each characteristic:

Box style:
Covered ___
Uncovered ___
Large ___
Medium ___
Small ___
With plastic liner ___

Litter type:
Unscented ___
Scented ___
Clumping (sand-like) ___
Recycled paper (pellets) ___
Crystal (silica) ___
Non-clumping clay ___
Wheat clumping ___
Corn clumping ___
Pine ___
Other ___

Cleaning schedule for litter boxes — Check rate
Scooping:
Multiple times per day ☐
Once per day ☐
Once every other day ☐
Twice a week ☐
Once a week or less often ☐

Complete box change (wash, new litter):
Daily ☐
Weekly ☐
Every two weeks ☐
Monthly ☐
Every 2-3 months ☐
Every 3-6 months ☐
Every year or more ☐
Never ☐

*Adapted from Neilson JC. FLUTD: When should you call the behaviorist? In: Proceedings. Hill's Symposium on Feline Lower Urinary Tract Disease, 2007: 20-28 (www.hillsvet.com/conferenceproceedings).
**"YES" answers for Questions 1 and 5 may indicate urine marking.

Appendix L. Feline Lower Urinary Tract Diseases, continued.

BOX 3. BEHAVIORAL MANAGEMENT FOR CATS WITH INAPPROPRIATE URINATION.*

Cats that urinate and/or defecate outside the litter box can do so for a variety of reasons including disease, communication (e.g., marking) and toileting preferences/aversions. Sometimes the medical problem can be an initiating factor for toileting problems. For example, medically triggered urgency to urinate causes the cat to select a convenient location like the bed; but even with resolution of the medical problem, the new behavior persists. These cats develop a new preference for toileting. (e.g., the bed is convenient, nicely absorbent and is cleaned readily) or have such negative associations with the litter box (e.g., painful urination when they were ill) that they persist in using a new, alternative, inappropriate site. Issues that should be addressed in cases of inappropriate elimination are listed below.

Resources	Recommendations	Explanations/consequences
Number of litter boxes	Number of litter boxes = number of cats +1	Too few litter boxes may result in problems that cause a cat to seek alternative toileting sites. These problems may include: volume of excrement in the litter box; box occupied by another cat; box being guarded by another cat.
Location of litter boxes	Should be spread throughout environment in easily accessible locations	Clustering litter boxes in one location may create access problems. These problems may include: guarding by another cat and physical challenges (e.g., stairs/distance) with getting to the litter box location.
Litter box style	Large	Boxes that are too small may be uncomfortable for cats to use, causing them to seek out other sites.
	Uncovered	Boxes that are covered may trap odors, creating an unpleasant environment and causing the cat to seek other toileting sites.
Litter	Clumping (sand-like) Unscented	Although individual preferences exist, the majority of cats prefer unscented clumping (finely particulate matter–similar to sand) litter.
Litter box hygiene	Daily litter box scooping Complete litter box cleaning/ change every 1 to 4 weeks	Cats tend to be fastidious and prefer clean toileting locations. Frequency of full box cleaning (wash/new litter) will depend on litter type; clumping type litters that allow owners to remove urine may require less frequent changes.
Scratching posts/pads	Multiple, sturdy, tall, prominently located	Scratching is a form of marking behavior. Encouraging scratch marking on appropriate targets may reduce the likelihood of other forms of marking and prevent destruction of household items.
Resting perches	Multiple, single cat sized, elevated, upholstered surfaces	Creative use of vertical space in the home can reduce inter-cat tension/ aggression. Cats tend to prefer upholstered surfaces over slick surfaces but individual preferences may exist.
Feeding/water stations	Number of stations = number of cats	Providing adequate resources spread throughout the environment allows cats to self-segregate; this may help to reduce social tension in multi-cat households.
Play/social interaction	At least 2 to 3 daily short sessions (5 to 10 minutes)	Cat age and personality may affect type and duration of interaction but it is important to recognize that domesticated cats are social and will often benefit from play/interaction. Indoor-only cats can especially benefit from owner-initiated activity such as playing with toys for overall stress reduction and exercise. Play activity also enhances the family-pet bond and is useful for overweight cats.

*Adapted from Neilson JC. FLUTD: When should you call the behaviorist? In: Proceedings. Hill's Symposium on Feline Lower Urinary Tract Disease, 2007: 20-28 (www.hillsvet.com/conferenceproceedings).

Appendix L. Feline Lower Urinary Tract Diseases, continued.

Table 1. Clinical presentations of cats with various lower urinary tract diseases.*

Presentation	Nonobstructive periuria	Obstructive dysuria	Behavioral periuria**	Urinary incontinence
Probable diagnoses	FIC Uroliths Infection Neoplasia	Urethral plugs Urethroliths Urethral strictures Functional obstruction Blood clots Foreign material	Toileting preferences/ aversions and/or marking with or without medical causes of lower urinary tract disease (e.g., FIC, uroliths, UTI, others)	Neurologic incontinence Anatomic abnormalities Partial obstruction
Initial tests	Urinalysis Diagnostic imaging	Abdominal radiographs Urinalysis	Urinalysis Diagnostic imaging	Neurologic examination Urinalysis Diagnostic imaging
Ancillary tests	Urine culture Abdominal ultrasound Contrast urethrocystography	Serum biochemistry profile Urine culture Contrast urethrocystography Complete blood count	Urine culture Abdominal ultrasound Contrast urethrocystography Coagulation profile Complete blood count	Urine culture Abdominal ultrasound Contrast urethrocystography Intravenous urography Cystoscopy

Key: FIC = feline idiopathic cystitis, UTI = urinary tract infection.
*Adapted from Lulich JP. FLUTD: Are you missing the correct diagnosis? In: Proceedings. Hill's Symposium on Feline Lower Urinary Tract Disease, 2007: 12-19 (www.hillsvet.com/conferenceproceedings).
**May occur with or without hematuria and signs of urinary tract inflammation.

Table 2. Clinical and diagnostic findings associated with the most common feline uroliths.*

Parameters	Struvite	Calcium oxalate	Purine (urate)
Breed predisposition	Chartreux Domestic longhair Domestic shorthair Foreign shorthair Himalayan Manx Oriental shorthair Ragdoll Siamese	Burmese British shorthair Exotic shorthair Foreign shorthair Havana brown Himalayan Persian Ragdoll Scottish fold Domestic shorthair	Siamese
Gender predisposition	Female >male Neutered >intact	Male >female	Neutered >intact
Common age (years)	Younger (<7 years)	Middle-aged to older (>7 years)	Young (if associated with portosystemic shunt)
Serum biochemistries	Normal	Hypercalcemia Acidemia (decreased TCO_2)	Normal (idiopathic) Evidence of hepatic disease (low urea nitrogen, increased ammonia)
Urinary pH**	Slightly acidic (>6.5) or alkaline	Acidic to neutral	Acidic to neutral
Bacteria	Usually sterile Occasionally associated with urease-producing bacteria	Usually sterile May be present in cats with infection secondary to uroliths	Usually sterile May be present in cats with infection secondary to uroliths
Typical crystals	Colorless, coffin-lid prisms, sometimes shaped like squares	Monohydrate–oval, dumbbell shaped Dihydrate-squares with diagonal lines	Spherical, tan in color May be green/brown Thorn apple appearance
Radiopacity	1+ to 4+	3+ to 4+	0 to 2+
Radiographic appearance	Rough or smooth, round or faceted, sometimes disk-shaped	Rough or smooth, usually small, occasionally jackstone shaped	Smooth, occasionally irregular

*Adapted from Osborne CA, Kruger JM, Lulich JP, et al. Disorders of the feline lower urinary tract. In: Osborne CA, Finco DR, eds. Canine and Feline Nephrology and Urology. Baltimore, MD: Williams & Wilkins 1995; 651.
**Concomitant infection with urease-producing bacteria may cause alkaline urine in cats with uroliths.

Appendix L. Feline Lower Urinary Tract Diseases, continued.

Table 3. Reported risk factors for selected feline lower urinary tract diseases.*

Parameters	Feline idiopathic cystitis	Struvite uroliths	Calcium oxalate uroliths
Patient characteristics	Four to 10 years old Breeds (purebred, longhaired, Persian) Neutered Overweight Lazy/little exercise	Younger cats (<7 years) Breeds (**Table 2**) Female Neutered Urinary tract infection (urease positive)	Older cats (>7 years) Breeds (**Table 2**) Male Neutered
Environmental conditions	Multi-cat household Less freedom to leave house Provided with litter box Living in conflict with another cat Moving within last three months High number of rainfall days in month before signs		Indoor environment
Nutritional factors	Fed dry cat food Decreased water intake	Alkalinizing foods (urinary pH >6.5) Magnesium content 0.14 to 0.56% (0.36 to 1.4 mg/kcal) Phosphorus content 1.27 to 1.88% (3.17 to 4.70 mg/kcal) Sodium content 0.57 to 1.48% (1.43 to 3.7 mg of Na/kcal) Fiber content ≥2.7 (≥0.71 g/100 kcal)	Dry foods 7 to 7.9% moisture Excessively acidifying foods (urinary pH = 5.8 to 6.29) Feeding single brand Sodium content 0.2 to 0.3% (0.48 to 0.77 mg/kcal) Potassium content 0.04 to 0.06% (0.95 to 1.6 mg/kcal) Protein content 21 to 32% (5.15 to 7.98 g/100 kcal) Magnesium content 0.04 to 0.07% (0.09 to 0.18 mg/kcal) or 0.14 to 0.56% (0.36 to 1.4 mg/kcal) Phosphorus content 0.34 to 0.70% (0.85 to 1.76 mg/kcal) or 1.27 to 1.88% (3.17 to 4.70 mg/kcal) Calcium content 0.39 to 0.82% (0.97 to 2.05 mg/kcal) or 1.5 to 2.0% (3.76 to 5.06 mg/kcal)

*Nutrient values expressed on a percent dry matter basis and assume a food energy density of 4 kcal metabolizable energy/g (17.6 kJ/g); however, dry matter nutrient content of foods with energy densities substatially higher or lower than 4 kcal/g will be under- or overrepresented, respectively. Thus, the energy basis nutrient values in this table (parenthetical values) are more accurate.

Table 4. Tips for increasing water consumption in cats.

Food
Feed moist food
Add small amount of water to moist food
Add warm water to dry food
Divide daily food amount into several smaller meals
Add flavor enhancers to food
    Low-sodium chicken or beef broth
    Clam juice
    Tuna juice (low sodium)
Water
Use fresh, clean water at all times (change at least once daily)
Try water from different sources
    Tap water   Filtered water
    Bottled water   Distilled water
Place ice cubes in water or provide cold water
Offer frozen cubes of water mixed with low-sodium tuna juice, etc.
Containers
Use non-reflective bowls for food and water
Use wide bowl so whiskers do not touch sides
Ensure ideal location of water and food bowls
    Quiet, draft-free environment (avoid noisy appliances and vents)
    In areas where cats can escape if needed
    Not in same area as litter boxes
    On different levels of multi-floor house
Provide access to other sources of water
    Water fountains with circulating water
    Dripping faucet

Appendix L. Feline Lower Urinary Tract Diseases, continued.

BOX 4. OTHER UROLITHS.

Pathogenesis of less commonly diagnosed urolith types is not well understood, although several factors may be involved in formation of uroliths composed of purine (e.g., ammonium acid urate, uric acid) or calcium phosphate (**Table 1** below). An underlying metabolic disorder is likely in these patients; however, often one is not identified. Detection of certain crystals (i.e., ammonium urate, cystine and xanthine), even in patients without clinical signs, suggests an important underlying metabolic defect, but not all cats with these crystals will develop uroliths. UTI may be associated with uncommon urolith types, but there is little evidence to support that UTI is the cause of these uroliths. Xanthine uroliths have been reported to occur in seven cats that had not received allopurinol; an underlying cause was not obvious. Cystinuria, presumably due to a defect in renal tubular transport of certain amino acids including cystine, has been identified in a small number of cats with cystine uroliths. **Table 2** summarizes key nutrtional factors for cats with less common urolith types.

Table 2. Key nutritional factors for preventing uncommon feline uroliths.

Factors	Dietary recommendations
Purine uroliths (urate, uric acid)	
Water	Promote water intake by using a moist food or other measures
Protein	Avoid excess dietary protein
	Recommend foods with 28 to 30% DM protein
	Recommend foods with low purine content
	Avoid proteins with high purine content such as liver, sardines and anchovies
Urinary pH	Use foods that maintain less acidic urine (6.6 to 6.8)
Calcium phosphate uroliths	
Water	Promote water intake by using a moist food or other measures
Calcium	Avoid excess dietary calcium
	Recommend foods with 0.6 to 0.8% DM calcium
Phosphorus	Avoid excess dietary phosphorus
	Recommend foods with <0.8% DM phosphorus
Sodium	Avoid excess dietary sodium
	Recommend foods with <0.30% DM sodium
Vitamin D	Avoid excess dietary vitamin D
	Recommend foods with <2,000 IU of vitamin D/kg DM

Key: DM = dry matter.

Table 1. Potential factors associated with formation of uncommon feline uroliths.

Factors	Causes	Pathogenesis
Urate		
Hyperuricosuria	Portosystemic shunt or severe hepatic disease	Decreased hepatic conversion of uric acid to allantoin, which is more soluble in urine
	Excessive purine intake	Promotes hyperuricemia with subsequent hyperuricosuria
Hyperammonuria	Excessive protein intake	Additional urea and glutamine available for conversion to ammonium (NH_4)
	Metabolic acidosis	Promotes metabolism of glutamine to NH_4
	Acidic urine	Ammonia (NH_3) is converted to NH_4, which is excreted in urine
	Hypokalemia	Results in intracellular acidosis (potassium exchanged for hydrogen) and subsequent excretion of NH_4
	Urinary tract infection with urease-producing organism	Converts urea in urine to NH_3 and NH_4
Aciduria	Acidic urine	Decreased solubility of uric acid in urine
Decreased urine volume	Decreased water intake	Increased urine concentration and saturation with uric acid
		Decreased urination causes retention of crystals and uroliths
Calcium phosphate		
Hypercalciuria	Hypercalcemia	Increased urinary calcium excretion
	Excessive vitamin D	Increased intestinal calcium absorption and suppressed parathyroid hormone secretion, which promote calcium excretion
	Hypophosphatemia	Stimulates vitamin D production, which augments intestinal absorption of calcium
	Acidosis	Promotes skeletal release of calcium and inhibits renal tubular reabsorption of calcium
	Excessive calcium intake	Increases urinary calcium excretion
	Excessive sodium intake	Increases urinary calcium excretion
Hyperphosphaturia	Excessive phosphorus intake	Increased urinary phosphorus excretion
	Alkaline urine	Increases urine concentration and saturation of phosphate
Alkaline urine	Alkaline urine	Reduces solubility of calcium phosphates, especially brushite
Decreased urine volume	Decreased water intake	Increased urine concentration and saturation with calcium phosphate
		Decreased urination causes retention of crystals and uroliths

Appendix M. Esophageal/Gastric Disorders and Pharmacologic Agents for Gastric Disorders.

BOX 1. REGURGITATION VS. VOMITING.

Differentiating regurgitation from vomiting is important in distinguishing esophageal from gastric disease. Characteristics of vomiting include expulsion of digested and bile-stained food and retching with involuntary abdominal contractions. Gastric contents are often highly acidic, which may be reflected in the pH of the vomitus. However, vomiting often involves reflux of bicarbonate-rich fluid into the stomach from the duodenum, which buffers gastric acid. The vomited material may then have a neutral or near-neutral pH.

Regurgitation involves less forceful casting up of tubular, bile-free, undigested food. Mucoid secretions mixed with the undigested food will usually have a pH of 6.5 to 7.0. Copious salivation may also be a confusing sign; it may be a primary sign of esophageal diseases (e.g., foreign body) or it may be part of the nausea that often accompanies vomiting.

Table 1. Breed-associated gastric disorders.

Disorders	Breeds
Atrophic gastritis	Lundehund
Chronic hypertrophic gastritis	Basenji
	Drentse patrijshond
Chronic hypertrophic pyloric gastropathy	Lhaso apso
	Maltese dog
	Pekingese
	Shih Tzu
Gastric dilatation-volvulus	Basset hound
	Doberman pinscher
	Gordon setter
	Great Dane
	Irish setter
	Saint Bernard
	Weimaraner
Gastric neoplasia	Beagle
	Belgian shepherd
	Rough collie
	Staffordshire bull terrier
Hemorrhagic gastroenteritis	Dachshund
	Miniature schnauzer
	Toy poodle
Pyloric stenosis	Boston terrier
	Boxer
	Siamese cat

Table 2. Pharmacologic agents useful in managing gastritis, gastroduodenal ulceration and gastric motility/emptying disorders.

Antacids
Mylanta (Al + Mg)
Amphojel (AlOH)
Tums (CaCO₃)   1 to 2 tabs or 5 to 10 ml PO every four to six hours

Antiemetic agents
Chlorpromazine   0.2 to 0.5 mg/kg body weight, PO, SQ, IM every six to eight hours
Prochlorpromazine   0.5 mg/kg body weight, PO, SQ, IM every six to eight hours
Odansetron   0.1 to 0.2 mg/kg body weight, SQ every eight hours or
    0.5 mg/kg body weight, IV (loading dose) followed by 0.5 mg/kg body weight as a constant IV infusion
        or 0.5 to 1.0 mg/kg body weight, PO every six to eight hours
Metoclopramide   0.2 to 0.4 mg/kg body weight, IM, SQ every eight hours or
    1.0 mg/kg body weight/day as a constant IV infusion
Butorphanol   0.4 mg/kg body weight, IM or 0.1 mg/kg body weight/hour as a constant IV infusion

Antihistamines
Diphenhydramine   2 to 4 mg/kg body weight, PO
Dimenhydrinate   25 to 50 mg PO per dog or 12.5 mg PO per cat

Anti-prostaglandin agent
Misoprostol   1 to 3 µg/kg body weight, PO every eight to 12 hours (dogs)

H₂-receptor blockers
Cimetidine   5 to 10 mg/kg body weight, PO, SQ every six to eight hours
Ranitidine   1 to 4 mg/kg body weight, PO, SQ, IV every eight to 12 hours
Famotidine   0.5 to 1.0 mg/kg body weight, PO, IV every 12 to 24 hours
Nizatidine   2.5 to 5.0 mg/kg body weight, PO every 24 hours

Prokinetic agents
Metoclopramide   0.2 to 0.4 mg/kg body weight, IM, SQ every eight hours or
    1.0 mg/kg body weight/day as a constant IV infusion
Cisapride   0.25 to 0.5 mg/kg body weight, PO every eight hours*
Erythromycin   0.5 to 1.0 mg/kg body weight, PO every eight hours (dogs)

Proton pump inhibitors
Omeprazole   0.2 to 0.7 mg/kg body weight, PO every 24 hours (dogs)

Mucosal protectants
Sucralfate   1 g/25 kg body weight, PO every six to eight hours
Colloidal bismuth

Key: PO = per os, SQ = subcutaneously, IM = intramuscularly, IV = intravenously.
*Available from compounding pharmacies.

Appendix M. Esophageal/Gastric Disorders and Pharmacologic Agents for Gastric Disorders, continued.

BOX 2. HAIRBALLS.

Hairballs occur commonly in cats because of their normal grooming behavior and sharp barbs on the tongue that enhance hair ingestion. Cats with longer, thicker coats and those with fastidious grooming behavior usually have more problems with hairballs. Swallowed hair initially accumulates as loose aggregates or more compacted, soft aggregates mixed with mucus. Hairballs are regurgitated periodically from the oropharynx or esophagus or vomited from the stomach, or they pass into the intestinal tract, where they are voided in the feces. Owners observe periodic gagging, retching and regurgitation or vomiting of hair and mucus (usually not containing food or bile). Hairballs are often tubular.

Trichobezoars are harder concretions within the stomach or intestines formed of hair, mucus and other material. Trichobezoars probably begin as simple aggregates of hair, but progress to larger and harder concretions. They are less common in cats than typical hairballs, but are more likely to cause severe clinical signs. Trichobezoars are a common cause of anorexia in pet rabbits (Chapter 70, Small Animal Clinical Nutrition, 5th edition). Large trichobezoars may obstruct pyloric outflow or the intestines and must be removed by surgery or endoscopy.

How cats eliminate aggregates of hair is probably similar to how they eliminate the pelts of small mammals that are ingested as part of a natural diet. Cats that hunt frequently may be seen vomiting the pelts of voles, mice, small rabbits and other mammals. This may be a protective mechanism for eliminating less digestible portions of prey.

Although hairballs do not usually cause significant clinical disease, their associated clinical signs are considered to be a nuisance by many cat owners. Hairballs generally can be controlled. Various laxatives, lubricants, treats and foods are available for routine management of these problems. Several commercial foods are available to help reduce the frequency with which cats vomit hairballs. Most of these foods have increased amounts of dietary fiber. Insoluble fiber, specifically cellulose, increases fecal hair content as compared to other fibers when incorporated in complete foods. Kibble size is another important feature of foods designed to reduce vomiting associated with hairballs. Radiographic gastrointestinal transit studies indicate that a larger kibble size is associated with an increased tendency for hairballs to exit the stomach and be eliminated in the feces, thereby reducing the frequency of vomiting. There is little or no evidence to support the use of lubricants (e.g., petroleum jelly) or papain for the treatment of hairballs in cats. If used, laxatives and lubricants should be given intermittently because large daily doses may interfere with normal digestion and nutrient absorption.

Frequent regurgitation or vomiting of hairballs (i.e., every day) with or without diarrhea, weight loss, anorexia or abdominal pain usually indicates an underlying problem (e.g., gastric motility defect or lymphoplasmacytic enteritis). Cats with severe or frequent clinical signs should be evaluated more extensively with diagnostics including hematology, serum biochemistry profiles, radiography and upper gastrointestinal endoscopy.

Appendix N. Small and Large Bowel Diarrhea, Use of Fiber, Drugs for IBS.

Table 1. Potential causes of acute small bowel diarrhea in dogs and cats.

Dietary	Infectious agents	Miscellaneous	Toxin or drug induced
Dietary indiscretion	Bacteria	Hemorrhagic gastroenteritis	Chemotherapeutic agents
Foreign bodies	*Bacillus* spp.		Digoxin
Garbage toxicity	*Campylobacter* spp.		Heavy metals
Raw meat consumption	*Clostridium* spp.		Laxatives (magnesium oxide, lactulose)
	Escherichia coli		Nonsteroidal antiinflammatory drugs
	Salmonella spp.		
	Staphylococcus spp.		
	Yersinia spp.		
	Parasites		
	Helminths (roundworms, hookworms, *Strongyloides* spp.)		
	Protozoa (*Giardia* spp., *Isospora* spp., *Cryptosporidium* spp.)		
	Rickettsia		
	Salmon poisoning		
	Viruses		
	Canine distemper		
	Coronavirus		
	Panleukopenia		
	Parvovirus		
	Rotavirus		

Table 2. Potential causes of chronic small bowel diarrhea in dogs and cats.

Dietary	Infectious agents	Inflammatory bowel disease	Miscellaneous	Neoplasia
Adverse reactions to food	Algae	Eosinophilic gastroenteritis	Juvenile diarrhea	APUD cell tumors
Food allergy	Prototothecosis	Lymphocytic enteritis	of cats	Lymphosarcoma
(hypersensitivity)	Bacteria	Lymphoplasmacytic enteritis	Lymphangiectasia	Mast cell tumor
Lactose intolerance	*Campylobacter* spp.	Regional enteritis		
	Mycobacterium spp.	Suppurative gastroenteritis		
	Salmonellosis			
	Small intestinal bacterial overgrowth			
	Fungi			
	Histoplasmosis			
	Pythiosis			
	Zygomycosis			
	Parasites			
	Helminths (roundworms, hookworms)			
	Protozoa (*Isospora* spp., *Giardia lamblia*, *Cyrptosporidium* spp.)			
	Viruses			
	Coronavirus			
	Feline immunodeficiency virus			
	Feline infectious peritonitis			
	Feline leukemia virus			

Key: APUD = amine precursor uptake and decarboxylation.

Table 3. Characteristics of small and large bowel diarrhea.

Characteristics	Small bowel	Large bowel
Blood in feces	Melena	Hematochezia
Fecal quality	Loose, watery, "cow-pie"	Loose to semi-formed, "jelly-like"
Fecal volume	Large quantities	Small quantities
Frequency of defecation	Normal to slightly increased	Increased
Malaise	May be present	Rare
Mucus in feces	Usually absent	Usually present
Steatorrhea	May be present	Absent
Tenesmus	Absent	Usually present
Urgency	Absent	Usually present
Vomiting	May be present	Absent
Weight loss	May be present	Rare

Appendix N. Small and Large Bowel Diarrhea, Use of Fiber, Drugs for IBS, continued.

Table 4. Clinical signs associated with life-threatening acute gastroenteritis.

Abdominal pain	Fecal leukocytes
Dehydration	Fever
Depression	Melena or hematochezia

Table 5. Breed-associated small intestinal disorders.

Eosinophilic gastroenteritis	German shepherd dog
	Irish setter
Hemorrhagic gastroenteritis	Dachshund
	Miniature poodle
	Miniature schnauzer
Immunoproliferative small intestinal disease	Basenji
	Ludenhund
Intestinal adenocarcinoma	Siamese cat
Lymphoplasmacytic enteritis	German shepherd dog
	Chinese Shar-Pei
	Soft-coated wheaten terrier
	Domestic shorthair cat
Parvoviral enteritis	American pit bull terrier
	Doberman pinscher
	Rottweiler
	Labrador retriever (black)
Small intestinal bacterial overgrowth	German shepherd dog
	Beagle
Lymphangiectasia*	Yorkshire terrier
	Golden retriever
	Dachshund
	Basenji (IPSID)
	Ludenhund (IPSID)
Wheat-sensitive enteropathy	Irish setter

Key: IPSID = immunoproliferative small intestinal disease.
*Soft-coated wheaten terriers may be affected by a protein-losing enteropathy that may occur in conjunction with a protein-losing nephropathy.

Table 6. Potential causes of acute large bowel diarrhea in dogs and cats.

Dietary
Dietary indiscretion
Foreign bodies
Garbage toxicity
Drugs
Cyclophosphamide
Doxorubicin
Infectious agents
Bacteria
  Campylobacter spp.
  Clostridium spp.
  Salmonella spp.
Parasites
  Giardia lamblia
  Trichuris vulpis
  Tritrichomonas foetus
Viruses
  Panleukopenia
  Parvovirus
Miscellaneous
Hemorrhagic gastroenteritis
Colon volvulus

Table 7. Potential causes of chronic large bowel diarrhea in dogs and cats.

Infectious causes
Parasitic
  Giardia lamblia
  Trichuris vulpis
Bacteria
  Campylobacter spp.
  Salmonella spp.
Viral
  Feline immunodeficiency virus
  Feline leukemia virus
Fungal
  Histoplasmosis
  Pythiosis
Inflammatory bowel disease
Eosinophilic colitis
Lymphocytic colitis
Lymphoplasmacytic colitis
Regional enterocolitis
Suppurative colitis
Dietary (adverse reactions to food)
Food allergy (hypersensitivity)
Food intolerance
Neoplasia
Adenocarcinoma
Adenoma/polyps
Lymphosarcoma
Mast cell tumor

Table 8. Breed-associated colonic disorders.

Disorders	**Breeds**
Flatulence	Brachycephalic dogs and cats
Hemorrhagic gastroenteritis	Dachshund, miniature schnauzer, toy poodle
Irritable bowel syndrome	Working breeds, toy breeds
Ulcerative colitis	Boxer, French bulldog

Appendix N. Small and Large Bowel Diarrhea, Use of Fiber, Drugs for IBS, continued.

BOX 1. A SAFE AND PRACTICAL METHOD FOR PROVIDING SUPPLEMENTAL FIBER TO A PATIENT'S CURRENT FOOD AND LIMITATIONS OF USING CANNED PUMPKIN AS A SUPPLEMENTAL FIBER SOURCE.

Adding fiber supplements is the least desirable approach for increasing fiber intake in patients with chronic constipation. In most constipation cases, dietary fiber intake can be increased by switching to a balanced food with the desired fiber content (Tables 3 and 4, Chapter 49) or a mixture of two balanced foods can be fed using the Pearson square method to determine the amounts of constituent foods in the mixture (Chapter 1, Small Animal Clinical Nutrition, 5th edition). If fiber supplements are used, they should be added to moist foods to ensure the fiber is mixed with the food and doesn't settle out in the bowl.

For this method, a practical source of fiber is Fiber One Bran Cereal[a] breakfast cereal. Although it is a human breakfast cereal and is not nutritionally balanced for dogs and cats, it does contain carbohydrate, protein, minerals and vitamins. Thus, relative to other readily available fiber supplements such as psyllium, wheat bran or canned pumpkin, Fiber One breakfast cereal is a more balanced source of fiber. It is somewhat palatable (depending on the individual patient's preferences and amount used) and contains a good amount of insoluble fiber (almost 50% dry matter [DM] crude fiber). **Table 1** provides a dose schedule for moist food.

Use the Pearson square method for determining how much Fiber One to add to a dry pet food to achieve a specific crude fiber level. Variability in the weight density per 8-oz. measuring cup makes it difficult to create a similar reliable table for dry pet foods.

Besides not being a balanced food, canned pumpkin as a fiber source has an important volume limitation. Canned pumpkin contains 90% water and on an as fed basis has only a fraction of the crude fiber of Fiber One cereal. As noted below, to obtain a fiber level of 10 to 11%, 2 tsp of Fiber One breakfast cereal are added to an 8-oz. cup of moist food. To achieve the same amount of fiber, more than 8 oz. of canned pumpkin would have to be added to the 8 oz. of moist food, more than doubling the amount of food the patient would have to eat to ingest the same amount of crude fiber.

ENDNOTE
a. Fiber One Bran Cereal. General Mills Cereals, LLC, Minneapolis, MN, USA.

Table 1. Dose schedule for Fiber One Bran Cereal to add to a typical moist food* and resultant crude fiber level.

Added Fiber One	Total crude fiber in mixture (DM)
1 tsp	7 to 8%
2 tsp	10 to 11%
3 tsp	13 to 14%
4 tsp	16 to 17%
5 tsp	18 to 19%

Key: tsp = rounded teaspoon (~5 g).
*8 volume oz. measuring cup of a typical moist food; assumed crude fiber content of approximately 3% DM, before Fiber One cereal is added. To improve acceptance by the patient and allow the colon and colonic microflora to adapt to the increase in fiber intake, increase the amount of fiber added gradually.

Appendix N. Small and Large Bowel Diarrhea, Use of Fiber, Drugs for IBS, continued.

BOX 2. MEDICAL THERAPY TO BE CONSIDERED FOR CONCURRENT USE WITH APPROPRIATE DIETARY MANAGEMENT FOR DOGS WITH IDIOPATHIC BOWEL SYNDROME.

Most patients diagnosed with idiopathic bowel syndrome (IBS) respond favorably to increased intake of dietary fiber and can be managed successfully long term with appropriate food and intermittent pharmacotherapy. Medical treatment generally includes, either individually or in combination, antidiarrheal drugs, anticholinergics and tranquilizers.

Pharmacotherapy for diarrhea-predominant IBS includes use of motility-modifying drugs such as loperamide at 0.2 to 0.5 mg/lb, per os, or diphenoxylate at 0.1 to 0.22 mg/lb, per os, b.i.d. Loperamide is a potent antidiarrheal drug that decreases intestinal secretions, enhances absorption, stimulates rhythmic segmental contractions and increases anal sphincter tone. Stool consistency often improves significantly and pain and urgency abate after loperamide therapy. Although loperamide can be used safely on a long-term basis, several days to one to two weeks of therapy is often sufficient to normalize stools. After the first several days of therapy, it may be possible to decrease administration to once or twice daily.

Patients with signs of abdominal pain (e.g., cramping, bloating, assuming an arched-back stance, reluctance to move, loud abdominal gurgling sounds) or those with signs of general distress (e.g., pacing) can be treated with antispasmodics or combination antispasmodic-tranquilizer preparations. Antispasmodics reduce smooth muscle contractility. Abdominal pain can often be relieved by antispasmodic agents and the effects of stressors can be reduced by sedatives. Librax[a] contains the sedative chlordiazepoxide (5 mg) and an anticholinergic agent clidinium bromide (2.5 mg). The dose of Librax is 0.2 to 0.5 mg/lb of clidinium, per os, b.i.d. or t.i.d. Chlordiazepoxide is a benzodiazepine with peripheral smooth-muscle relaxant properties and central nervous system effects. This combination seems to be especially effective in relieving the discomfort that may be associated with increased colonic motor function. The drug can be given when the owner first notices that the patient has signs of abdominal pain or diarrhea or when stressful conditions are encountered and can usually be discontinued after a few days. Long-term use may be necessary (one to two doses daily) in patients affected by unpredictable flare-ups of abdominal distress.

Other anticholinergics such as propantheline (0.25 mg/kg, per os, b.i.d. or t.i.d.), hyoscyamine (0.003 to 0.006 mg/kg, per os, b.i.d. or t.i.d.) or dicyclomine (0.15 mg/kg, per os, b.i.d. or t.i.d.) have been suggested. Anticholinergics can decrease or inhibit gastrointestinal motility, which may worsen diarrhea. In people, side effects include xerostomia, urinary retention, blurred vision, headache, psychosis, nervousness and drowsiness.

Combination therapy (loperamide plus clidinium/chlordiazepoxide) may be necessary in some patients with diarrhea and abdominal pain. Sulfasalazine, especially when used in combination with loperamide or clidinium, sometimes provides symptomatic relief in patients with significant dyschezia and increased evacuation of small volumes of loose, mucoid stool. This response has been observed in patients in which multiple colon biopsy specimens and careful evaluation for pathogenic intestinal organisms have proved negative. Likewise, H_2-receptor blockers such as famotidine at dosages of 0.25 to 0.5 mg/lb, per os, every 24 hours, used in combination with clidinium or isopropamide, may provide better control of IBS-related nausea or vomiting than either drug alone.

The novel use of peppermint oil for the relief of pain in pediatric human patients with IBS has been reported. In randomized, placebo-controlled trials, enteric-coated peppermint oil capsules were found to relieve pain in 75% of affected patients. This treatment has not been evaluated in veterinary medicine.

ENDNOTE
a. Roche Laboratories, Inc., Nutley, NJ, USA.

Appendix O. Common Conversions.

Table 1. Conversions to and from metric measures.

Imperial/U.S. to metric		Metric to imperial/U.S.	
Weights		**Weights**	
1 gr (grain)	64.8 mg	1 g	15.43 gr
1 oz (avoirdupois)	28.4 g	1 g	0.0353 oz
1 lb (avoirdupois)	453.6 g	1 g	0.0022 lb
1 lb	0.454 kg	1 kg	2.2 lb

Dosages			
1 mg/lb	2.2 mg/kg	1 mg/kg	0.454 mg/lb
1 kcal/lb	2.2 kcal/kg	1 kcal/kg	0.454 kcal/lb

Volumes			
U.S.			
1 fl oz	29.57 ml	1 L	33.82 fl oz
1 cup	0.237 L	1 L	4.221 cup
1 pt	0.473 L	1 L	2.114 pt
1 qt	0.946 L	1 L	1.057 qt
1 gal	3.785 L	1 L	0.264 gal

Imperial			
1 fl oz	28.41 ml	1 L	35.20 fl oz
1 cup	0.284 L	1 L	3.520 cup
1 pt	0.568 L	1 L	1.760 pt
1 qt	1.136 L	1 L	0.88 qt
1 gal	4.546 L	1 L	0.22 gal

Table 2. Comparison between U.S. and imperial systems.

Imperial		U.S.	
1 fl oz	28.42 ml	1 fl oz	29.57 ml
1 cup	10 fl oz	1 cup	8 fl oz
1 pt	20 fl oz	1 pt	16 fl oz
1 qt	40 fl oz	1 qt	32 fl oz
1 gal*	160 fl oz	1 gal**	128 fl oz
1 gal*	4 qt	1 gal**	4 qt
1 gal*	4.55 L	1 gal**	3.78 L

*1 gal (imperial) = 4 qt = 8 pt = 160 oz = 4.55 L.
**1 gal (U.S.) = 4 qt = 8 pt = 16 cups = 128 oz = 3.78 L.

Table 3. Temperature conversions.*

°C	°F	°C	°F	°C	°F	°C	°F	°C	°F
0	32.0	10	50.0	20	68.0	30	86.0	40	104.0
1	33.8	11	51.8	21	69.8	31	87.8	41	105.8
2	35.6	12	53.6	22	71.6	32	89.6	42	107.6
3	37.4	13	55.4	23	73.4	33	91.4	43	109.4
4	39.2	14	57.2	24	75.2	34	93.2	44	111.2
5	41.0	15	59.0	25	77.0	35	95.0	45	113.0
6	42.8	16	60.8	26	78.8	36	96.8	46	114.8
7	44.6	17	62.6	27	80.6	37	98.6	47	116.6
8	46.4	18	64.4	28	82.4	38	100.4	48	118.4
9	48.2	19	66.2	29	84.2	39	102.2	49	120.2
								50	122.0

*When you know the Fahrenheit temperature, subtract 32 and multiply by 5/9 to obtain °C. When you know the Celsius temperature, multiply by 9/5 then add 32 to obtain °F.

Appendix O. Common Conversions, continued.

Table 4. Equivalent values and conversion factors.

Volumes

1 gtt*	0.05 ml	1 cup**	16 Tbs
1 tsp	5 ml	1 ml	20 gtt
1 dsp	8 ml	1 cup**	236.6 ml
1 Tbs	15 ml	1 cup***	284.2 ml

Weights

1 oz	437.5 gr	1 g	1,000 mg
1 lb	16 oz	1 kg	1,000 g

Key: tsp = teaspoon, dsp = dessertspoon, Tbs = tablespoon, gr = grains.
*Official dropper size for water at 15°C.
**U.S. cup.
***Imperial cup.

Table 5. Percent, ppm and ppb.

Percent	ppm	ppb
μg/0.1 mg	1 μg/g	1 ng/g
mg/0.1 g	1 mg/kg	1 μg/kg
g/100 g	0.4545 mg/lb	0.4545 μg/lb

Table 6. Energy conversion units.

Kilocalorie (kcal)	1,000 cal	4.184 kJ
Kilojoule (kJ)	1,000 joule	0.239 kcal
Megajoule (MJ)	1,000 kJ	239.0 kcal

Conversion from:	To:	
mg/MJ	mg/100 kcal	÷ 2.39
mg/100 kcal	mg/MJ	x 2.39
g/MJ	mg/100 kcal	÷ 0.00239
mg/100 kcal	g/MJ	x 0.00239
mg/100 kcal	g/100 kcal	÷ 1,000
g/100 kcal	mg/100 kcal	x 1,000
mg/MJ	g/MJ	÷ 1,000
g/MJ	mg/MJ	x 1,000

Table 7. Vitamins A, D and E: Conversions from international units to equivalent activity.*

Vitamins	Units	Substances	
Vitamin A	1 IU	0.300 μg of crystalline retinol (vitamin A alcohol)	0.550 μg of vitamin A palmitate
Vitamin A	1 RE*	1 μg of crystalline retinol	6 μg of β-carotene
			12 μg of other provitamin A carotenoids
Provitamin A	1 IU	0.6 μg β-carotene	1.2 μg of other provitamin A carotenoids
Vitamin D	1 IU	0.025 μg of crystalline vitamin D_3	
Vitamin E	1 IU	1 mg of synthetic racemic α-tocopherol acetate	= dl-α-tocopherol acetate
			= all racemic α-tocopherol acetate

1 mg of synthetic racemic α-tocopherol = 1 mg of synthetic racemic α-tocopherol = 1.1 IU of vitamin E
1 mg of naturally occurring α-tocopherol = d-α-tocopherol = RRR-tocopherol = 1.49 IU of vitamin E
1 mg of naturally occurring α-tocopherol acetate = d-α-tocopherol acetate = 1.36 IU of vitamin E

*On pet food labels and tables with daily nutrient allowances for pets, the vitamins A, D and E are expressed in international units (IU). These units reflect the activity of these vitamins, not their amounts. United States Pharmacopeia Units (USP) are equivalent to IU. In human foods, retinol equivalent (RE) is often used for vitamin A activity.

Appendix P. Metabolic Weight of Dogs and Cats.*

Body weights kg	lb	Metabolic weights BW$^{0.75}$	Body weights kg	lb	Metabolic weights BW$^{0.75}$
1	2.2	1.000	41	90.2	16.203
2	4.4	1.682	42	92.4	16.498
3	6.6	2.280	43	94.6	16.792
4	8.8	2.828	44	96.8	17.084
5	11.0	3.344	45	99.0	17.374
6	13.2	3.834	46	101.2	17.663
7	15.4	4.304	47	103.4	17.950
8	17.6	4.757	48	105.6	18.236
9	19.8	5.196	49	107.8	18.520
10	22.0	5.623	50	110.0	18.803
11	24.2	6.040	51	112.2	19.084
12	26.4	6.447	52	114.4	19.364
13	28.6	6.846	53	116.6	19.643
14	30.8	7.238	54	118.8	19.920
15	33.0	7.622	55	121.0	20.196
16	35.2	8.000	56	123.2	20.471
17	37.4	8.372	57	125.4	20.745
18	39.6	8.739	58	127.6	21.017
19	41.8	9.100	59	129.8	21.288
20	44.0	9.457	60	132.0	21.558
21	46.2	9.810	61	134.2	21.827
22	48.4	10.158	62	136.4	22.095
23	50.6	10.503	63	138.6	22.362
24	52.8	10.843	64	140.8	22.627
25	55.0	11.180	65	143.0	22.892
26	57.2	11.514	66	145.2	23.156
27	59.4	11.845	67	147.4	23.418
28	61.6	12.172	68	149.6	23.680
29	63.8	12.497	69	151.8	23.941
30	66.0	12.819	70	154.0	24.200
31	68.2	13.138	71	156.2	24.459
32	70.4	13.454	72	158.4	24.717
33	72.6	13.768	73	160.6	24.974
34	74.8	14.080	74	162.8	25.230
35	77.0	14.390	75	165.0	25.486
36	79.2	14.697	76	167.2	25.740
37	81.4	15.002	77	169.4	25.994
38	83.6	15.305	78	171.6	26.246
39	85.8	15.606	79	173.8	26.498
40	88.0	15.905	80	176.0	26.750

*Metabolic weight (BW$^{0.75}$) can be calculated by cubing BW$_{kg}$ and then taking its square root twice.

Appendix Q. Body Surface Area (BSA) of Dogs and Cats.

Table 1. Body surface area (BSA) of dogs.

Body weights kg	lb	BSA m²	Body weights kg	lb	BSA m²
1	2.2	0.10	36	79.2	1.10
2	4.4	0.16	37	81.4	1.12
3	6.6	0.21	38	83.6	1.14
4	8.8	0.25	39	85.8	1.16
5	11.0	0.30	40	88.0	1.18
6	13.2	0.33	41	90.2	1.20
7	15.4	0.37	42	92.4	1.22
8	17.6	0.40	43	94.6	1.24
9	19.8	0.44	44	96.8	1.26
10	22.0	0.47	45	99.0	1.28
11	24.2	0.50	46	101.2	1.30
12	26.4	0.53	47	103.4	1.32
13	28.6	0.56	48	105.6	1.33
14	30.8	0.59	49	107.8	1.35
15	33.0	0.61	50	110.0	1.37
16	35.2	0.64	51	112.2	1.39
17	37.4	0.67	52	114.4	1.41
18	39.6	0.69	53	116.6	1.43
19	41.8	0.72	54	118.8	1.44
20	44.0	0.74	55	121.0	1.46
21	46.2	0.77	56	123.2	1.48
22	48.4	0.79	57	125.4	1.50
23	50.6	0.82	58	127.6	1.51
24	52.8	0.84	59	129.8	1.53
25	55.0	0.86	60	132.0	1.55
26	57.2	0.89	61	134.2	1.57
27	59.4	0.91	62	136.4	1.58
28	61.6	0.93	63	138.6	1.60
29	63.8	0.95	64	140.8	1.62
30	66.0	0.98	65	143.0	1.63
31	68.2	1.00	66	145.2	1.65
32	70.4	1.02	67	147.4	1.67
33	72.6	1.04	68	149.6	1.68
34	74.8	1.06	69	151.8	1.70
35	77.0	1.08	70	154.0	1.72

Table 2. Body surface area (BSA) of cats.

Body weights kg	lb	BSA m²
1	2.2	0.10
2	4.4	0.17
3	6.6	0.22
4	8.8	0.26
5	11.0	0.30
6	13.2	0.34
7	15.4	0.38

Appendix R. Equations for Calculating Resting Energy Requirements of Dogs and Cats.

Table 1. Equations for calculating resting energy requirements of cats and dogs.

BW kg	$70 \times kg^{0.75}$ kcal ME	$0.293 \times kg^{0.75}$ MJ ME	$70 + 30 \times kg$ BW kcal ME	$0.29 + 0.126 \times kg$ BW MJ ME
5	234	0.98	220	0.92
10	394	1.65	370	1.55
20	662	2.77	670	2.80
30	897	3.75	970	4.06
40	1,113	4.66	1,270	5.31
60	1,509	6.31	1,870	7.82

Key: BW = body weight, ME = metabolizable energy.

Appendix S. Litter Sizes and Birth Weights of Selected Canine Breeds.*

Breeds**	Average litter sizes	Birth weights (g)
Airedale terrier	9	300
Appenzell mountain dog	10	465
Australian silky terrier	3	-
Bernese mountain dog	5	445
Borzoi	9	450
Boxer	8	440
Cavalier King Charles spaniel	4	230
Chihuahua	2-3	140
Chow chow	6	460
Dachshund	4	215
Dalmatian	5-6	-
Doberman pinscher	7	410
English bulldog	7	295
English cocker spaniel	6	230
English springer spaniel	11	375
Fox terrier	3	260
French bulldog	5	215
German shepherd dog	6	445
German shorthaired pointer	7-8	415
Great Pyrenees	≥5	705
Hovawart	11	435
Irish terrier	6	270
Labrador retriever	5	450
Maltese	3	155
Miniature dachshund	3	210
Miniature pinscher	3	-
Miniature poodle	2-3	165
Miniature schnauzer	4	155
Newfoundland	7	595
Norwich terrier	5	225
Papillon	3	120
Pekingese	2-3	-
Pomeranian	2	-
Pug	3	-
Rottweiler	7	-
Saint Bernard	7	640
Scottish terrier	5	240
Shetland sheepdog	4-5	260
Shih Tzu	2-3	-
Sloughi	3	670
Standard schnauzer	6	285
Yorkshire terrier	5	95

*Because of the very large variation in the adult body weight of dogs and number of puppies per litter, there is no direct relationship between birth weight and the body weight of the mother. Puppies from the largest breeds weigh approximately 1% of the bitch's weight, whereas a Chihuahua puppy averages 6.4% of its mother's body weight.
**Breeds listed here are those for which data were available.

Appendix T. Body Weight and Height at Withers of Selected Canine Breeds.

Breeds	Body weights (lb/kg)		Height at withers (in./cm)	
	Females	Males	Females	Males
Affenpinscher	6/3	9/4	9/23	11/28
Afghan hound	50/23	60/27	24-26/60-65	26-29/65-72
Ainu dog	na	na	16-19/41-47	19-21/49-52
Airedale terrier	42/19	55/25	22-23/55-58	23-24/58-60
Akita	75/34	101/46	24-26/60-65	26-28/65-70
Alaskan malamute	75/34	126/57	23-26/57.5-65	25-28/62-70
American cocker spaniel	24/11	28/12.5	13-15/34-36	14-16/36-39
American Eskimo dog				
Toy	na	na	9/22.5	12/30
Miniature	na	na	>12/>30	15/38
Standard	na	na	>15/>37.5	19/48
American water spaniel	25-40/11-18	30-45/13.5-20.5	15-18/37-45	15-18/37-45
Anatolian shepherd dog	90-130/41-59	110-141/50-64	28-31/70-77	29-32/72-80
Anglo-French hound				
Small	49/22	55/25	19/48	22/55
Great	66/30	71/32	24/60	27/68
Appenzell mountain dog	48/22	55/25	18-20/46-50	22-23/55-58
Ariegeois	66/30	66/30	21-23/52-58	22-24/55-60
Artois hound	40/18	53/24	20/52	23/59
Australian cattle dog	35/16	45/20	17-19/42-48	18-20/45-50
Australian kelpie	30/13.5	30/13.5	20/50	20/50
Australian shepherd	na	na	18-21/45-53	20-23/50-58
Australian terrier	14/6.5	14/6.5	10/25	11/28
Basenji	22/10	24/11	16/40	17/43
Basset hound	40/18	60/27	13/33	15/38
Beagle	26/12	31/14	13/33	15/38
Beagle harrier	44/20	44/20	17/43	19/48
Bearded collie	40/18	60/27	20-21/50-53	21-22/52-55
Beauce shepherd (Beauceron)	66/30	85/38	24-27/60-68	25-28/63-70
Bedlington terrier	17/8	23/10.5	15-17/37-41	16-18/40-44
Belgian shepherd dog				
Groenendael	62/28	62/28	22-24/56-60	24-26/60-65
Laekenois	62/28	62/28	22-24/56-60	24-26/60-65
Malinois	62/28	62/28	22-24/56-60	24-26/60-65
Tervuren	62/28	62/28	22-24/56-60	24-26/60-65
Bergamasco	57-70/26-32	70-84/32-38	22/55	24/60
Bernese mountain dog (Berner sennenhund)	88-100/40-45	110/50	23-26/57-65	25-28/62-70
Bichon frisé	na	na	9/23	11/28
Billy	55/25	66/30	23-25/57-63	24-26/60-65
Bloodhound (St. Hubertus dog)	80-100/36-46	90-110/41-50	23-25/57-63	25-27/62-68
Bolognese	5/2.5	9/4	10-11/25-28	11-12/27-30
Bordeaux dog (large)	>88/>40	>90/>45	Smaller than male	23-27/58-66
Bordeaux dog (medium)	77-88/35-40	84-99/38-45	na	na
Border collie	30/13.5	45/20.5	18-21/45-53	19-22/47-55
Border terrier	11-14/5-6	13-16/6-7	10/25	10/25
Borzoi	55-90/25-41	75-105/34-48	≥26/≥65	≥28/≥70
Boston terrier				
Lightweight class	na	≤15/≤6.8	na	na
Middleweight class	na	≤20/≤9.0	na	na
Heavyweight class	na	≤25/≤11	na	na
Bourbonnais setter	40/18	57/26	21/53	21/53
Bouvier des Ardennes	na	na	16-18/40-46	17-19/42-48
Bouvier des Flandres	60-77/27-35	77-88/35-40	21-27/53-66	24-28/61-69
Boxer	53/24	70/32	21-24/53-59	22-25/56-63
Brazilian guard dog	89/40.5	99/45	24/60	30/74
Briard	75/34	75/34	22-26/55-64	23-27/58-68
Brittany spaniel	30/13.5	40/18	17/44	21/51
Brussels griffon	5/2.2	≤12/5	7/17	8/20
Bulldog	40-50/18-23	50-55/23-25	na	na
Bullmastiff	88-120/40-55	110-130/50-59	24-26/60-65	25-27/62-68
Bull terrier	52/23.5	62/28	21/53	22/55
Cairn terrier	13/6	16/7.5	9/24	12/30
Canaan dog	40/18	55/25	19/49	24/59

Appendix T. Body Weight and Height at Withers of Selected Canine Breeds, continued.

Breeds	Body weights (lb/kg)		Height at withers (in./cm)	
	Females	Males	Females	Males
Cao de Castro Laboreiro (Portuguese watchdog)	44-66/20-30	66-88/30-40	21-23/52-57	22-24/56-60
Catalonian shepherd	44-66/20-30	66-88/30-40	17-19/43-48	18-20/45-50
Cavalier King Charles spaniel	10/5	18/8	12/30	13/33
Chesapeake Bay retriever	55-70/25-32	65-80/29.5-36	21-24/52-60	23-26/57-65
Chihuahua	≤6/≤2.7	6/≤2.7	6/16	8/20
Chinese crested dog	≤12/≤5.5	≤12/≤5.5	9-12/22-30	11-13/27-33
Chow chow	44/20	70/32	17-20/42-50	19-22/47-55
Clumber spaniel	55-70/25-32	70-85/32-38.5	17-19/42-48	19-20/47-50
Collie (rough and smooth)	44-65/20-30	55-75/25-34	22-24/55-60	24-26/60-65
Coonhound				
Black and tan coonhound	55-75/25-34	60-80/27-36	23-25/57-63	25-27/62.5-67.5
Redbone coonhound	55-75/25-34	60-80/27-36	23-25/57-63	25-27/62.5-67.5
Coton de Tulear	12/5.5	15/7	10/25	12/30
Curly-coated retriever	70/32	80/36	23-25/57-63	25-27/62-68
Czesky terrier	13/6	20/9	11/28	14/35
Dachshund				
Miniature (UK)	10/4.5	10/4.5	na	na
Miniature (USA)	≤11/≤5	≤11/≤5	na	na
Standard (UK)	20/9	26/12	na	na
Standard (USA)	16/7.5	32/14.5	na	na
Dalmatian	50/23	59/27	19/48	23/58
Dandie Dinmont terrier	18/8	24/11	8/20	11/28
Deerhound (Scottish)	66-95/30-43	85-110/38.5-50	≥28/≥70	30-32/75-80
Doberman pinscher	64/29	88/40	24-26/60-65	26-28/65-70
Dogue de Bordeaux	119/54	143/65	28/69	30/75
Dupuy setter	na	na	25-26/64-65	26-27/66-68
Dutch shepherd	66/30	>66/30	21-25/54-61	23-25/57-63
Elkhound (Norwegian)	44/20	55/25	19/49	21/51
English cocker spaniel	26-32/12-14.5	27-34/12.5-15.5	15-16/37-40	16-17/40-43
English setter	40/18	70/31.5	24/60	25/63
English springer spaniel	40/18	50/22.5	19/48	20/50
English toy spaniel	8/3.5	14/6.5	10/25	10/25
Entlebuch mountain dog	55/25	66/30	20/50	20/50
Eskimo dog	55-90/25-41	66-110/30-50	20-24/50-60	23-27/57-68
Estrela mountain dog	60-90/27-41	75-105/34-48	20-24/50-60	23-27/57-68
Eurasier	40-57/18-26	51-71/23-32	19-23/48-56	21-24/52-60
Field spaniel	35/16	55/25	17/43	18/45
Finnish spitz	25/11.3	35/16	15-18/39-45	17-20/44-50
Flat-coated retriever	55-75/25-34	55-80/25-36	22-24/55-59	23-25/57-61
Foxhound				
American foxhound	na	na	21-24/52-60	22-25/55-63
English foxhound	65/29.5	70/32	21-24/52-60	22-25/55-63
Fox terrier (smooth and wire)	15-17/6.5-8	16-18/7-8.5	≤15/≤39	≤15/≤39
French bulldog	18/8	29/13	12/30	12/30
French hound	60/27	62/28	24-27/61-68	24-29/61-71
French setter	60/27	60/27	24/60	24/60
French spaniel	44/20	55/25	21-23/52-58	22-24/55-60
German hunt terrier	16-18/7-8	19-22/9-10	16/40	16/40
German pointer (Deutscher Vorstehund)				
German shorthaired pointer	45-60/20-27	55-70/25-32	21-23/52-58	23-25/57-63
German wirehaired pointer	45-64/20-29	55-75/25-34	22-24/55-60	24-26/60-65
German shepherd dog	70/32	95/43	22-24/55-60	24-26/60-65
German spaniel	44/20	66/30	15-18/39-44	15-20/39-49
German spitz				
Small (Kleinspitz)	6/3	7/3	9/23	11/28
Standard (Mittelspitz)	25/11.5	25/11.5	11/29	13/33
Glen of Imaal terrier	35/16	35/16	14/35	14/35
Golden retriever	55-65/25-30	65-75/29-34	21-23/54-56	23-24/57-60
Gordon setter	45-70/20-32	55-80/25-36	23-26/57-65	24-27/60-68
Great Dane	121/55	176/80	≥29/≥72	≥32/≥80
Great Gascony blue	71/32	77/35	23-26/59-64	25-28/62-70
Greater Swiss mountain dog	na	na	23-27/59-68	25-29/64-71
Greenland dog	≥66/≥30	≥66/≥30	22/55	24/60
Greyhound	60-65/27-30	65-70/30-32	27-28/67-70	28-30/70-75
Griffon nivernais	50/23	55/25	Smaller than male	21-23/52-58

Appendix T. Body Weight and Height at Withers of Selected Canine Breeds, continued.

Breeds	Body weights (lb/kg)		Height at withers (in./cm)	
	Females	Males	Females	Males
Griffon Vendéen				
Petit basset	25/11.5	35/16	13/32	15/37
Basset	40/18	44/20	15/37.5	17/43
Briquet	35/16	53/24	20/50	22/55
Grand	66/30	77/35	24/60	26/65
Hamiltonstövare	50/23	60/27	18-23/45-56	19-24/49-59
Hanover hound	84/38	99/45	Smaller than male	20-24/50-60
Harlequin pinscher	na	na	12/30	14/35
Harrier	48/22	60/27	19/48	21/53
Havanese	7/3	12/5.5	10/25	11/26
Hovawart	55-77/25-35	66-88/30-40	22-26/55-65	24-28/60-70
Hungarian coarse-haired vizsla	na	na	21-24/52-59	22-26/56-64
Hungarian greyhound	50-60/22-27	60-70/27-32	na	na
Hungarian Kuvasz	≤110/≤50	≤110/≤50	26-28/65-69	28-30/70-74
Ibizan hound	45/20.5	50/23	22-26/56-65	24-28/59-69
Iceland dog	na	na	15-18/38-44	17-19/42-48
Irish red and white setter	40/18	70/32	23/59	27/68
Irish setter	60/27	70/32	23-25/57-63	27/68
Irish terrier	25/11	27/12	18/45	18/45
Irish water spaniel	45-58/20-26	55-65/25-30	21-23/52-58	22-24/55-60
Irish wolfhound	≥105/≥48	≥120/≥54	≥30/≥75	≥32/≥80
Italian greyhound	6/2.5	10/4.5	13/32	15/38
Italian segugio	39/18	62/28	19-22/47-55	21-23/52-58
Italian setter	55/25	88/40	na	na
Italian spinone	62-70/28-32	71-82/32-37	23-26/57-64	23-28/59-69
Jämthund	na	na	21-23/52-58	23-28/57-63
Japanese chin	4/1.5	7/3.5	8/20	11/28
Japanese fighting dog	100/45	200/91	≥23/≥59	≥23/≥59
Japanese spitz	13/6	13/6	Smaller than male	12-14/30-35
Japanese terrier	na	na	12/30	15/38
Jura hound	na	na	17/44	22/55
Keeshond	55/25	66/30	17/43	18/45
Kerry blue terrier	na	33-40/15-18	17-19/44-48	18-20/45-49
Komondor	80/36-50	100-150/45-68	≥26/≥64	≥28/≥69
Kooikerhondje	20/9	24/11	15/38	15/38
Kromfohrländer	26/12	26/12	15/38	18/45
Kuvasz (Hungarian shepherd)	70-90/32-41	99-110/45-52	26-28/65-70	28-30/70-75
Labrador retriever	55-70/25-32	65-80/29-36	21-24/54-59	22-25/56-61
Lakeland terrier	15/7	17/7.7	13/34	14/36
Lancashire heeler	8/3.5	12/5.4	10/25	12/30
Lapland spitz	44/20	44/20	15-18/39-44	17-20/44-49
Lapponian herder	≤66/≤30	≤66/≤30	17-19/43-48	19-22/48-55
Leonberger	80/36.3	150/68	26-30/65-75	29-32/73-80
Lhasa apso	na	na	Smaller than male	10/25
Löwchen	4/2	9/4	8/20	14/35
Maltese	4/1.8	≤7/2.7	10/25	10/25
Manchester terrier				
Toy (American-bred)	≤7/≤3.2	≤7/≤3.2	na	na
Toy (English toy terrier)	≤12/≤5.4	≤12/≤5.4	10/25	12/30
Standard (American-bred)	≤12/≤5.5	≤16/≤7.3	na	na
Standard (open classes)	≤16/≤7.3	≤22/≤10	15/38	16/40
Maremma sheepdog	66-88/30-40	77-99/35-45	24-27/60-68	26-29/65-73
Mastiff	165/75	198/90	≥27/≥69	≥30/≥75
Mexican hairless dog	na	na	16/40	20/50
Miniature bull terrier	10/4.5	40/18	10/25	14/35
Miniature pinscher	10/4.5	10/4.5	10/25	12/31
Mudi	18/8	29/13	14/35	19/48
Münsterlander				
Small	33/15	37/17	19/48	22/55
Large	55/25	55-66/25-30	23/58	24/60
Neapolitan mastiff	110/50	154/70	24-27/60-68	25-29/64-72
Newfoundland	110-120/50-55	132-152/60-69	26/65	28/70
Norfolk terrier	11/5	12/5.5	9/22	10/25
Norwegian buhund	26/12	40/18	Smaller than male	17-18/42-45
Norwich terrier	10/4.5	12/5.4	≤10/≤25	≤10/≤25
Nova Scotia duck tolling retriever	36/16.5	51/23	17/42	21/52

Appendix T. Body Weight and Height at Withers of Selected Canine Breeds, continued.

Breeds	Body weights (lb/kg)		Height at withers (in./cm)	
	Females	Males	Females	Males
Old English sheepdog (bobtail)	55/25	66/30	≥21/≥52.5	≥22/≥55
Otterhound	65-100/30-45	75-115/34-52	23-26/57-65	24-27/60-68
Papillon	3.5/1.5	11/5	8/20	11/28
Parson Jack Russell terrier	na	na	12-13/30-33	13-14/32-35
Pekingese	7-11/3-5	8-14/3.6-6.5	na	na
Pharaoh hound	na	na	21-24/52-60	23-25/57-63
Picardy shepherd	50/23	70/32	20-24/50-60	22-26/55-65
Pinscher	na	na	17/42	19/48
Pointer	46-65/20-30	55-75/25-34	23-26/57-65	25-28/62-70
Poitevin	66/30	66/30	25/62	28/70
Polish lowland sheepdog	na	na	16-19/40-46	17-20/42-50
Pomeranian	3/1.5	7/3.2	11/27	11/27
Poodle				
Toy	na	na	≤10/≤25	≤10/≤25
Miniature	11/5	11/5	>10/>25	15/37
Standard	45/20	70/32	>15/>37.5	na
Porcelaine	55/25	62/28	21-22/52-55	22-23/55-58
Portuguese setter	na	na	19-22/47-55	20-24/51-60
Portuguese water dog	35-50/16-23	42-60/19-27	17-21/42-53	20-23/50-58
Pudelpointer	55/25	70/32	≥24/≥60	≥24/≥60
Pug	14/6.5	18/8	10/25	12/30
Puli (Hungarian puli)	22-29/10-13	28-33/13-15	14-16/36-40	16-18/40-44
Pumi	17/8	28/13	13/32	17/44
Pyrenean mastiff	121/55	155/70	Smaller than male	27-32/69-79
Pyrenean mountain dog (Great Pyrenees)	85-99/38-45	100-121/45-55	25-29/62-73	27-32/67-80
Pyrenean shepherd	18/8	30/13.5	15-20/38-50	15-20/39-50
Rafeiro do alentejo	77-99/35-45	88-99/40-45	25-28/64-70	26-30/66-74
Rhodesian ridgeback	70/32	85/38.5	24-26/60-65	25-27/62-67
Romanian shepherd dog	110/50	110/50	25/63	26/65
Rottweiler	88/40	110/50	22-25/55-63	24-27/60-68
Saint Bernard	110/50	200/90.5	≥26/≥65	≥28/≥70
Saint-Germain setter	40/18	57/26	na	na
Saluki	29/13	66/30	≥22/≥54	23-28/58-70
Samoyed	37-55/17-25	44-66/20-30	19-21/47-53	21-24/53-59
Schapendoes (Dutch)	na	na	16-19/40-47	17-20/43-50
Schipperke				
Small type	7/3	11/5	10-12/25-30	11-13/27-33
Large type	11/5.4	18/8	10-12/25-30	11-13/27-33
Schnauzer				
Miniature	11/5	15/6.8	12/30	14/35
Standard	33/15	40/18	18-19/45-46	18-20/46-50
Giant (Riesenschnauzer)	66/30	77/35	24-26/60-65	26-28/65-70
Scottish terrier	18-21/8-9.5	19-22/8.5-10	10/25	na
Sealyham terrier	18-20/8-9	23-24/10-11	10/26	≤12/≤30
Shar-Pei	40/18	55/25	18/45	20/50
Shetland sheepdog (sheltie)	na	na	13/33	16/40
Shiba Inu	20/9	30/13.6	13-16/34-39	14-17/36-41
Shih Tzu	9/4	18/8	9/22	10/26
Siberian husky	35-50/16-23	44-60/20-27	20-22/50-55	21-24/53-60
Sicilian hound	22-26/10-12	26-30/12-14	17-18/42-45	18-20/45-50
Silky terrier (Australian)	8/3.6	10/4.5	9/22	10/25
Skye terrier	25/11.5	25/11.5	9/24	10/25
Sloughi	45/20	60/27	23/58	30/75
Soft-coated wheaten terrier	30-35/13-16	35-40/16-18	17-18/42-45	18-19/45-48
Spanish greyhound	60/27	66/30	Smaller than male	25-28/64-69
Spanish mastiff	110/50	132/60	Smaller than male	26-28/65-70
Stabyhoun	33/15	44/20	na	≤19/≤47.5
Staffordshire bull terrier	24-34/11-15	28-38/13-17	14/35	16/40
Staffordshire terrier (American)	na	na	17-18/42-45	18-19/45-48
Sussex spaniel	35/16	45/20	13/32	15/38
Swedish vallhund	25/11.4	35/16	12-13/30-33	13-14/32-34
Swiss scent hound (Laufhunde)	na	na	17/44	22/55

Appendix T. Body Weight and Height at Withers of Selected Canine Breeds.

Breeds	Body weights (kg)		Height at withers (cm)	
	Females	Males	Females	Males
Tahltan bear dog	15/6.8	15/6.8	12/30	16/40
Tawny brittany basset	na	na	13/32	17/43
Tibetan mastiff	≥180/≥82	≥180/≥82	≥24/≥60	≥26/≥65
Tibetan spaniel	9/4	15/6.8	10/25	10/25
Tibetan terrier	18/8	30/13.6	14/35	17/42
Vizsla (Hungarian vizsla)	44/20	66/30	21-23/52-58	22-24/56-60
Weimaraner	70/32	85/38	23-25/57-63	25-27/62-68
Welsh corgi				
Cardigan	25-34/11-15.5	30-38/13-17	10/26	12/31
Pembroke	22-28/10-13	22-30/10-14	10/25	12/30
Welsh springer spaniel	35/16	45/20	17-18/42-45	18-19/45-48
Welsh terrier	20/9	21/9.5	Smaller than male	15-16/38
West Highland white terrier	15/7	22/10	10/25	11/28
Whippet	28/13	28/13	18-21/45-52	19-22/47-55
Wirehaired pointing griffon	50/23	60/27	20-22/50-55	22-24/55-60
Yorkshire terrier	≤8/≤3.5	≤8/≤3.5	9/22	9/22

Key: na = information not available.

Index

Text in boldface denotes chapter titles. Topics are alphabetized under the main headings for each chapter. Page numbers followed by the letter b refer to boxes, those followed by the letter f refer to figures and those followed by the letter t refer to tables.